BSAVA Manual of Psittacine Birds

Second edition

Editors:

Nigel Harcourt-Brown
BVSc DipECAMS FRCVS
30 Crab Lane, Harrogate, North Yorkshire HG1 3BE

and

John Chitty
BVetMed CertZooMed MRCVS
Strathmore Veterinary Clinic, 6 London Road,
Andover, Hants SP10 2PH

Published by:

British Small Animal Veterinary Association
Woodrow House, 1 Telford Way, Waterwells
Business Park, Quedgeley, Gloucester GL2 2AB

A Company Limited by Guarantee in England.
Registered Company No. 2837793.
Registered as a Charity.

A catalogue record for this book is available from the British Library.

ISBN 0 905214 76 5

The publishers and contributors cannot take responsibility for information
provided on dosages and methods of application of drugs mentioned in
this publication. Details of this kind must be verified by individual users
from the appropriate literature.

Typeset by Fusion Design, Wareham, Dorset, UK
Printed by Replika Press Pvt. Ltd., India

Other titles in the BSAVA Manuals series:

For information on these and all BSAVA publications please visit our website: www.bsava.com

Contents

Contributors

J R Best BVSc MRCVS
Quantock View, Steart, Somerset, TA5 2PX

John Chitty BVetMed CertZooMed MRCVS
Strathmore Veterinary Clinic, 6 London Road, Andover, Hants, SP10 2PH

Brian H Coles BVSc DipECAMS Hon. FRCVS
4 Dorfold Way, Upton, Chester, Cheshire, CH2 1QS

Martine De Wit DVM
White Oak Conservation Center, 581705 White Oak Road, Yulee, FL 32097, USA

Gerry M. Dorrestein DVM PhD DipVet Pathology Hon Memb ECAMS
Department of Pathobiology, Section Pet Avian, Exotic Animals and Wildlife, Utrecht University, Yalelaan 1, 3584 CL Utrecht, Netherlands

Thomas M. Edling DVM MSpVM
PETCO Animal Supplies Inc., San Diego, CA 92121, USA

Neil A. Forbes BVetMed CBiol MIBiol DipECAMS FRCVS
RCVS Recognised Specialist in Zoo Animal and Wildlife Medicine
Great Western Referrals, Unit 10, Berkshire House, County Park Business Park, Shrivenham Road, Swindon, Wilts, SN1 2NR

Simon J Girling BVMS (Hons) DZooMed CBiol MiBiol MRCVS
RCVS Recognised Specialist in Zoo Animal and Wildlife Medicine
Cambusbarron, Stirlingshire

Nigel H. Harcourt-Brown BVSc DipECAMS FRCVS
30 Crab Lane, Harrogate, North Yorkshire, HG1 3BE

Alan Jones BVetMed MRCVS
The Cottage, Turners Hill Road, Worth, Crawley, West Sussex, RH10 4LY

Alistair M Lawrie BVMS MRCVS
The Lawrie Veterinary Group, 25 Griffiths Street, Falkirk, FK1 5QY

Michael Lierz Dr med vet MRCVS
Institute for Poultry Diseases, Freie Universität Berlin, Koenigsweg 63, 14163 Berlin, Germany

Deborah Monks BVSc (Hons) MACVSc CertZooMed MRCVS
Great Western Referrals, Unit 10, Berkshire House, County Park Business Park, Shrivenham Road, Swindon, Wilts, SN1 2NR

Aidan Raftery MVB CertZooMed CBiol MiBiol MRCVS
Avian and Exotic Animal Clinic, 221 Upper Chorlton Road, Manchester, M16 0DE

Ron Rees Davies BVSc CertZooMed MRCVS
The Exotic Centre, 12 Fitzilian Avenue, Harold Wood, Romford, Essex, RM3 0QS

April Romagnano PhD DVM DipABVP (Avian)
5500 Military Trail, Suite 40, Jupiter, FL 33458, USA

Peter W. Scott MSc BVSc FRCVS
RCVS Specialist in Zoo Animal and Wildlife Medicine
Vetark Professional, PO Box 60, Winchester, SO23 9XN

Michael D. Stanford BVSc MRCVS
Birch Heath Veterinary Clinic, Birch Heath Road, Tarporley, Cheshire, CW6 9UU

Thomas N. Tully, Jr DVM MS DipABVP (Avian) DipECAMS
School of Veterinary Medicine, Louisiana State University, Baton Rouge, LA 70803-8410, USA

Kenneth R. Welle DVM DipABVP (Avian)
All Creatures Animal Hospital, 708 Killarney, Urbana, IL 61801, USA

Foreword

Since the first edition of this Manual was published in 1996 there have been many advances in psittacine medicine and surgery and this edition fully addresses this new information. Although primarily produced for veterinary surgeons in general practice, the manual will also be very useful for those working towards a further qualification in zoological medicine or wishing to study the subject in greater depth.

Part 1 covers the identification, husbandry, anatomy and physiology of commonly kept species. Part 2 goes on to advise on the approach to the clinical case and describes the relevant diagnostic techniques. Part 3 covers hard and soft tissue surgery. Part 4 takes a systematic approach to clinical syndromes and their management. One chapter of this section focuses on problems likely to be presented in general practice in cockatiels and budgies and usefully provides advice on treatment taking into account the financial constraints often encountered in practice.

In the final section, zoonotic diseases, aspects of legislation including trading and methods of identification, and ethical issues relating to pet bird keeping, are brought to the attention of the reader.

The formatting and cross referencing throughout the Manual facilitates quick and easy accessibility of information. The photographs and line drawings are of a truly outstanding quality.

The editors and authors have to be congratulated on this comprehensive Manual. Clinical cases in psittacine birds may not be encountered every day by the general practitioner but are challenging cases when they are. The Manual certainly provides the basis for their improved care and treatment.

As usual thanks are due to the Publications Committee and the staff at Woodrow House for producing another excellent addition to the library of BSAVA Manuals.

Ian Mason BVetMed PhD CertSAD DipECVD MRCVS
BSAVA President 2004–2005

Preface

The primary aim of this Manual is to cover the medicine and surgery of psittacine birds for the general practitioner while also acting as an introductory text for those wishing to study this subject in greater depth. There have been many advances in psittacine medicine since the last edition was published in 1996 and these are reflected in the differences between the two books.

It is impossible to identify and treat the sick bird properly without understanding the healthy parrot in the wild and in captivity. The first three chapters endeavour to provide the reader with this information. In the case of nutrition, behaviour and reproduction the normal situation is discussed alongside the abnormal in each chapter.

Many psittacine patients are presented in a very sick or critical state; in the second part of the book, basic clinical information on handling and examining the patient and the taking of clinical samples are discussed, along with the initial stabilization and hospitalization of the patient. Subsequent chapters cover anaesthesia, surgery, systemic illnesses and disease by individual organ system. These are designed to be read in their entirety or to be referred to as needed.

For general practitioners the most commonly seen psittacine patients are the smaller patients. The small size and low economic value of these patients often make them the most difficult to examine and treat. We have, therefore, included a chapter devoted to the sick small psittacid, which concentrates on the common presentations and syndromes and provides a practical approach to their care.

The final chapter covers the legal and ethical aspects of owning and selling parrots as well as discussion of zoonotic disease and how this relates to the veterinarian.
For many practitioners the appearance in the surgery of a sick parrot is a sudden and unplanned event. An appendix of diagnostic algorithms is provided for various common presentations. These aim to provide a step-by-step approach for the clinician to follow and to refer them to the relevant chapter for further information. Other useful appendices include a drug formulary, a list of common and taxonomic names, and a pictorial guide to droppings.

Both editors developed their interests in avian medicine from general practice and we hope that this is reflected in a practical, easy-to-use and relevant guide to psittacine medicine.

The editors would like to thank the chapter authors not only for their excellent contributions but also for adhering to the publishing deadlines and making the editors' job as easy as possible. We would also like to thank Marion Jowett and her team at BSAVA for their encouragement throughout this project.

Lastly, but by no means least, we would like to thank our wives and families for their support and tolerance of the time spent editing this book.

John Chitty
Nigel H. Harcourt-Brown

December 2004

Species and natural history

Brian H. Coles

Introduction and general considerations

Parrots are classified into 353 species in 84 genera. They are an unmistakable group, with characteristically large heads and powerful hooked beaks, and are of ancient lineage not closely related to any other group of birds. They have short necks and zygodactyl or yoke-toed feet, so that digits II and III are directed forward whilst digits I and IV are placed backwards. This structure, together with the beak acting as a third hand, makes these birds very agile arboreal climbers, often hanging upside down while feeding.

The Psittaciformes probably evolved in the Old World – possibly Australia, where the oldest known fossil of a cockatoo has been found. Parrots probably diverged from all other birds in the Palaeocene some 60 million years ago and the order is split into two main families: the Psittacidae (the vast majority of parrots) and the Cacatuidae (the cockatoos, with 18 species in five genera). Today parrots mostly inhabit the tropical and subtropical regions of the world, though a number of species are found in the more temperate regions of Australia and New Zealand and fossils have been found in France and in North America up to the Canadian border.

Parrots range in size from the large Hyacinth Macaw, weighing up to 3 kg, to the pygmy parrots, which weigh only 10 g. Whilst sexual dimorphism occurs amongst many Australian and Asian parrots, this is not as obvious in those species found in Africa or the New World.

Distribution, habitat and sources of food

Different species of parrot occupy a range of habitats at varying altitudes, including temperate woodland, savannah, scrub, semi-desert and tropical rainforest (Figure 1.1). It is in the latter type of habitat (particularly in the Neotropics), where there is a multiplicity of fruiting trees producing a vast range of different types of fruits and flowers, that the greatest number of parrot species is found.

Taxonomy and common names	General characteristics	Habitat	Diet	Breeding		
				No. eggs	Incubation	Fledge
Family Cacatuidae 18 spp. in 6 genera **Cockatoos** (see also subfamily Nymphicinae below)	Distinctive from other parrots in having erectile crest used as threat Range in size from large **Palm Cockatoo** (1 kg) to Cockatiel (c. 90 g) Overall plumage in most species basically white, with species-specific markings Absence of green and blue in plumage Iris black in male, brown in female, pale grey in immatures **Sulphur-crested Cockatoo**: large (500–1260 g) and small species (228–315 g) **White Cockatoo** 530–610 g **Salmon-crested** or **Moluccan Cockatoo** 670–800 g	**Palm Cockatoo** mainly in forests and savannah woodland in New Guinea **Greater Sulphur-crested** N, E and S Australia in open forest, woodland and farmland **Lesser Sulphur-crested** Celebes and some other Indonesian islands, in woodland, forest edges and coastal plains **White** and **Moluccan** both in separate parts of Moluccan Islands of Indonesia	**Greater Sulphur-crested** feeds mostly in trees: seeds, nuts, fruit **Lesser Sulphur-crested** feeds in trees: fruit etc.; also forages for seeds and grain **Moluccan Cockatoo** feeds in trees: fruit, nuts, seeds **White Cockatoo** as Moluccan but also insects	3–4 (but smaller species may lay up to 7)	c. 4 weeks	c. 8–12 weeks

1.1 Types of parrot commonly kept as cage birds. (continues) ▶

Taxonomy and common names	General characteristics	Habitat	Diet	Breeding		
				No. eggs	*Incubation*	*Fledge*
Subfamily Nymphicinae **Cockatiel**	Smallest representative of the cockatoos Species type mostly brownish grey with white wing covert feathers. Male forehead, crest, cheek patches and throat yellow, with prominent orange ear coverts Female smaller crest, same basic colouring but much less yellow, also feathering barred under wings (solid black in male) Immatures resemble female until sexual maturity at 6 months	Over whole of Australia except coastal regions	Feeds mainly on ground on grass seeds, fruits, berries (even mistletoe), grain crops (considered a pest by farmers)	4–7	18–12 days	c. 4–5 weeks
Family Loriinae 11 genera, 55 spp. **Lories** and **lorikeets**	Many have long tapering tails; in some, tails only medium length and more rounded Mostly medium size (c. 20–24 cm) but smallest 13 cm and largest 42 cm Most have glossy brilliant plumage in range of red, blue, violet, olive brown, green and yellow according to species Most well known is **Rainbow Lorikeet** (blue forehead, crown and cheeks; black underside of head; yellow collar; breast red barred with black; thighs yellow barred with green; upper parts green)	Archipelago of SE Asia. Some species (e.g. **Rainbow Lorikeet**) also into N, E and S Australia	Specialized brush-tongued feeding on pollen and nectar, also fruit and flowers	1–5 Smaller species tend to lay more than larger species	23–30 days	c. 42–90 days Smaller species fledge earlier than larger species
Genus *Cyanoramphus* 6 spp. (with 8 subspp. in Red-fronted Parakeet) Commonly called **kakarikis**	Small to medium, rather chunky, with long pointed tail Overall plumage green in most, slightly darker above than beneath. All tend to have violet-blue outer flight feathers. Most have reddish patch each side of rump; many have varying red markings on head **Yellow-fronted Kakariki** typical of genus: red above cere, yellow forehead 23–26 cm, 50–113 g	New Zealand and neighbouring islands in polycarp forest and scrub	Seeds, berries, shoots, flowers Invertebrates often an important part of diet	5–9	c. 20 days	c. 6 weeks
Genus *Platycercus* 8 spp. **Rosellas**	Medium size (25–36 cm, c. 100–120 g) Long graduated tails; all show pronounced mottling or scalloped appearance of plumage on back Variety of species-specific markings in red, yellow, green and blue-violet	Different species in various parts of Australia	Predominantly seed eaters, spending much time on ground searching for food	c. 4–7	19 days	13–14 weeks
Genus *Neophema* 7 spp. **Grass parakeets**	Similar shape to Budgerigar but slightly larger (c. 20–21 cm, 44–61 g) Tendency to sexual dimorphism, particularly in **Scarlet-chested** and **Turquoisine** Except **Bourke's** (which has upper parts of body brown, abdomen pink), all have green upper plumage with yellow abdomen and species-specific markings in red, blue and yellow on remainder of body	Different species inhabit various parts of Australia; **Bourke's** and **Scarlet-chested** in large areas of central Australia	Seeds of grasses and other seeds; fruit, berries, young shoots, small insects	c. 3–5	18–20 days	c. 30–35 days

1.1 (continued) Types of parrot commonly kept as cage birds. (continues) ▶

Taxonomy and common names	General characteristics	Habitat	Diet	Breeding		
				No. eggs	*Incubation*	*Fledge*
Genus *Melopsittacus* one species: **Budgerigar**	Nominate race c. 18 cm and c. 30 g, but many captive-bred mutant strains larger (c. 26–29 cm) and heavier (c. 35–85 g) In wild, back of head, neck and body basically yellow barred black; forehead and throat yellow with row of black dots across throat; underparts greenish-yellow. Great variety of mutant colours bred in captive birds	Across greater part of Australia away from coastal areas, and Tasmania Wide variety of habitats, from forest/woodland to open grassland, grain crops, dry scrub and acacia deserts	Grass seeds (0.5–2.5 mm long), chenopod seeds Only feeds on or near the ground	4–6	c. 18 days	c. 30 days
Genus *Eclectus* **Eclectus Parrot** 1 sp., 9 subspp. (many of which breed in captivity)	Stocky (355–615 g) Male brilliant green, flanks and underwing red, maxilla orange Female black bill, dark red on head, back and tail, bright purplish body, yellow tip to tail (see Figure 18.2)	New Guinea, surrounding islands and N tip Australia Tend to live below 1000 m in woodland, parkland, even gardens	Fruit, seeds, nuts, buds, blossoms	2	26 days	12 weeks
Family Psittacula 14 spp. **Ringneck parakeets**	Heavy beak; tapering tail longer than body Sexually dimorphic. Male usually red beak, well developed ring around neck or more striking head colour **Ringneck Parakeet** (95–143 g) 1 subsp. Africa, another India: male green, with pink and black neck ring, red maxilla; female no ring, black tip to beak. Captive Ringneck Parakeets in many colour varieties **Alexandrine Parakeet** larger (200–250 g): male pink neck ring, red shoulders **Moustached Parakeet** (135–170 g): red beak, grey head, black chin, pink chest, green body; female duller	**Ringneck Parakeet** N sub-Saharan Africa, all India and Pakistan; deciduous habitats of all types **Alexandrine Parakeet** India to Thailand; lowland forest and wooded areas **Moustached Parakeet** N India and Indochina; deciduous forest	Fruits, seeds, flowers Most spp. raid orchards, cultivated fields, gardens **Ringneck Parakeet** considered most destructive pest in India	3–4	22–26 days	6–8 weeks
Genus *Loriculus* 10 spp. **Hanging parrots**	Closely related to lovebirds and look similar except beaks much finer and more pointed. So named because roost hanging upside down Size c. 11–16 cm, c. 22–35 g Overall mostly green; most spp. have red upper tail and red crown. Species-specific markings of red, blue and yellow Colour of bills black or orange, depending on species	Various parts of SE Asia and Indian subcontinent Woodland and forest	Fruits, berries, nectar, seeds	c. 2–4	c. 22 days	c. 5 weeks
Genus *Agapornis* 9 spp. **Lovebirds** Most common: **Peach-faced Lovebird** (*A. roseicollis*)	Small chunky, with relatively large bills and short rounded tails Most species not dimorphic but males tend to be slightly larger Size 15–18 cm, 43–63 g Species-specific phenotype: overall green plumage, rose-pink forehead and to just behind eyes, also cheeks and throat; rump bright blue Many captive mutant strains (e.g. Pastel Blue, Pied) Together with hanging parrots, the only two genera of parrots that collect nesting material held in plumage by female	Sub-Saharan Africa Forest edge, woodland, savannah	Cereal seeds, maize, cultivated sunflower seeds, fruit (e.g. figs, mango), buds and foliage	3–6	c. 23 days	c. 43 days

1.1 (continued) Types of parrot commonly kept as cage birds. (continues) ▶

Taxonomy and common names	General characteristics	Habitat	Diet	Breeding		
				No. eggs	*Incubation*	*Fledge*
Genus *Psittacus* **Grey Parrot** subsp.: **Timneh Parrot**	**Grey Parrot** probably most familiar of all parrots c. 402–490 g Overall colour grey, lighter around eyes and over rump. Tail red, beak black Iris yellow in adult, mJack in young bird up to 3–4 months then yellowing up to 4 years **Timneh** subsp. slightly smaller (c. 350 g) with maroon instead of red tail, upper beak horn-coloured	Nominate race across central Africa from Gulf of Guinea to W Kenya to Tanzania **Timneh** confined to Sierra Leone and Ivory Coast Feral populations in many African cities Edge of forest clearings, woodland, savannah, coastal mangroves, cultivated areas	Seeds, figs, fruits (particularly the fleshy part of oil-seed palm surrounding inner stone)	2–3	21–30 days	c. 80 days
Genus *Poicephalus* 9 spp. Most common: **Senegal Parrot** and **Meyer's Parrot**	Thickset, with short squarish tails **Senegal** (21–23 cm, 120–161 g) green upper plumage and neck, yellow chest and abdomen yellow, grey head **Meyer's** brown upper plumage, yellow patch on crown and over carpal joint, bluish-green breast and abdomen Iris of **Meyer's** orange, of **Senegal** yellow	Various species in different areas of sub-Saharan Africa **Senegal** C and W Africa **Meyer's** C and E Africa Both spp. woodland/savannah	Seeds, grain, fruit, figs, leaf buds	c. 2–4	c. 25–31 days	c. 63 days
Macaws Genus *Ara* 15 spp. Genus *Anodorhynchus* 3 spp. (including **Hyacinth Macaw**)	All are slender elegant birds with long tapering tails Range in size from relatively small (e.g. **Hahn's** c. 34 cm, 150–180 g) to **Hyacinth** (100 cm, c. 1600 g) and popular **Blue and Gold** (c. 86 cm, c. 1300 g) Most species have bare facial area devoid of most feathering (which may have been to prevent feathering becoming matted when feeding on fruit); in some species this area flushes pinkish, indicating change in mood Variety of colours in blue, red, yellow and green according to species	Large areas of Amazon Basin, many species in same locality Some spp. found in Caribbean Species separation may be by altitude Variety of habitats include flooded forest, gallery forest, deciduous pine forest, mangrove swamps	Seeds, fruit, palm nuts, figs, leaves, flowers, nectar	c.1–3	c. 24–30 days (longer for larger birds)	13–14 weeks
Conures: two main genera: *Aratinga* (19 spp.) *Pyrrhura* (18 spp.)	All small to medium size, with long graduated tails *Aratinga* larger of the two genera (28–37 cm, 155–185 g); overall plumage green with species-specific red or brown or blue markings, except for **Sun Conure** (generally yellow but forehead and sides of head and abdomen tinged orange, mostly green wings, olive green tail) and **Jandaya Conure** (only head, breast and abdomen yellow) *Pyrrhura* (24–26 cm, 72–94 g): overall plumage dusky green, with species-specific other colour markings; most have red-brown tails, some a scaly or scalloped appearance of neck and breast plumage	Mostly individual species restricted to various parts of Amazon Basin but some in Caribbean	Seeds, fruits, nuts	Usually 2–4 (can be up to 7)	c. 4 weeks	c. 8 weeks

1.1 (continued) Types of parrot commonly kept as cage birds. (continues) ▶

Taxonomy and common names	General characteristics	Habitat	Diet	Breeding		
				No. eggs	*Incubation*	*Fledge*
Genus *Forpus* 7 spp. **Parrotlets**	Small chunky, with short pointed tail Most species c. 12–13 cm, c. 20–28 g; largest is **Yellow-faced** (c. 14.5 cm, 30–38 g) Some sexual dimorphism Overall plumage green with blue to violet-blue primary covert feathers in male; some species have blue rump. In most species, head and neck paler green (in **Yellow-faced** forehead and neck yellow)	**Celestial** in drier parts along Pacific side of Andes Other species confined to various parts of Amazon Basin; **Blue-winged** inhabits very large part of this area Forest, woodland, scrub, pasture, town suburbs	Fruits, berries, buds, seeds	c.4–6	c. 17–22 days	c. 35–40 days
Genus *Pionites* **Caiques** 2 spp.: **Black-headed** and **White-bellied**	Both medium size (23 cm, 130–170 g) Bills rather narrow, upper beak markedly ridged Both species white breast and abdomen; most of wings and upper tail green, primary feathers violet-blue **Black-headed** black forehead and crown; **White-bellied** orange forehead and crown and yellow neck	**Black-headed** N part of Amazon Basin **White-bellied** S part of Amazon Basin	**Black-headed** eats seeds, fruit pulp, flowers and, occasionally, leaves	2–4	27–29 days	c. 10–11 weeks
Genus *Pionus* 8 spp. **Pionus parrots**	All medium size (c. 26–28 cm, 170–275 g) All species relatively short squarish tails with red feathers under tail Overall plumage in many species dull green/dusky brown except in **Blue-headed** and **Coral-billed** Some species have scaly appearance to feathering on neck and other species-specific markings	Individual species in various parts of Amazon Basin and Caribbean Forest/woodlands and cultivated areas	**Maximilian's** eats seeds (70%), flowers (20%), corn (8%), fruit (2%) **Blue-headed** also eats bananas	3–5	24–29 days	c. 8–12 weeks
Genus *Amazona* 27 spp. **Amazon** parrots	Stocky, with short rounded tail Overall plumage green in most, with species-specific markings in other colours **Blue-fronted** typical medium size (c. 400 g) with yellow crown, chin and throat, but blue forehead and above cere **Orange-winged** overall green, with prominent orange patch on underside of outer three secondary flight feathers c. 298–469 g	**Blue-fronted** and **Orange-winged** range over greater part of Amazon Basin, but **Blue-fronted** as far as Paraguay and N Brazil, and **Orange-winged** further N and towards coast of N and E Both found in scrub, savannah, palm groves, gallery rainforest along water courses	Fruits, flowers, leaf buds, seeds	3–4 **Blue-fronted** up to 8	23–25 days	58–60 days

1.1 (continued) Types of parrot commonly kept as cage birds.

Parrots as a whole are primarily seed eaters (Figure 1.1). Therefore, with the exception of some of the macaws, some cockatoos and Pesquet's Parrot, most of the parrots do not eat the fleshy outer part of the fruit but are concerned with getting at the highly nutritious kernel. To achieve this the fruit and then the nut is wedged by the tongue against a ridge on the underside of the upper beak, whilst the chisel-like action of the lower beak strips the husk and the flesh and then exerts considerable pressure to crack the nut (in macaws this may be a pressure of more than 200 psi). During the whole process of splitting the nut, the tongue gradually rotates the nut to apply pressure to different areas. Some of the macaws, besides eating the fruit, also eat flowers and mature leaves and take nectar. Macaws will sometimes tackle unripe fruit that contains potentially toxic tannins. To overcome these harmful effects, the birds eat clay taken from river banks and also at the same time may obtain needed minerals.

Another group of parrots includes specialist nectar and pollen eaters. These are the Loriidae, also known as lories and lorikeets and also called the brush-tongued parrots. In these birds the tongue is long and when fully extended exhibits a coating of erectile hair-like epidermal papillae, which enables the bird to brush up pollen.

Parrots mostly feed in the trees, where they are safer from predators, but they will also forage on the ground for fallen fruit and seed. Some of the smaller species, such as the Budgerigar, spend more time on the ground and never, unlike most parrots, use the foot to hold the food. Food of animal origin probably does not play a big part in the diet of most parrots, though they may take the larvae of some beetles, insects and moths, and Hyacinth Macaws will eat apple snails. However, parrots are opportunist feeders and very adaptable birds. For many years there has been a thriving population of the Ringneck Parakeet in the London suburbs and in the southern counties of England, the survival of which has been helped by bird-table feeding during the winter. Many cities worldwide also have feral populations of this parrot, which visits gardens and orchards, inhabits woodland and raids all kinds of cereal crops. It should be noted that although the parrots have a hooked beak rather like the raptors, their gape is smaller.

No species of parrot is truly migratory but some, such as the Grey Parrot, are nomadic and often fly considerable distances (up to 30 km each day) in search of food, returning to their traditional roosting sites at night.

Social life

Parrots are social animals and well recognized as being noisy. Vocalization is used in the wild to maintain flock cohesion, to reinforce pair bonds and to give warning of danger. Most parrot species live in flocks, some of which can be very large and composed of several thousand birds. Most parrots are also monogamous and form pair bonds throughout life. The pairs feed and roost and do most things together throughout the year. Within a flock there are smaller family groups which will stay together until the next breeding season. In the family group the more juvenile birds learn by observing the more experienced older birds as well as interacting with their siblings. In dry habitats the older birds will know where the nearest waterhole is in times of drought, whilst those in tropical rainforest will know the time and location of fruiting trees. Absence of early socialization with conspecifics has been shown to have adverse effects on fledglings reared with an alien species.

Breeding biology

With few exceptions, parrots are hole nesters. They may nest either in a natural cavity in a suitable tree or in the abandoned nest of another species, such as a woodpecker. The original hole may be enlarged or altered to meet the requirements of the nesting parrots.

A few species nest in holes in cliffs or banks or in termite mounds. Some of the more adaptable species will make use of holes in buildings or in old pipes. Nests can be anything from 0.5 to 2 m in depth. Darkness is believed to stimulate Budgerigars to commence egg laying and this may be important for other species as well. The nest may sometimes be lined with grass but more often has just a bed of wood chips left from remodelling of the nest hole.

Possession of a suitable nest hole is probably the most important part of the breeding cycle. The female tends to be the more aggressive of the pair in defending the nest. In most parrot species territorialism is confined to the immediate area within approximately one metre of the nest during the breeding period, though a few species nest communally, even with other species in the same tree. Courtship in most species is by food passing and allopreening (i.e. preening of the companion bird). Both male and female birds usually prepare the nest, but generally only the female incubates the eggs.

The eggs of all species of parrot are white and relatively small. They are generally laid on alternate days but in some of the larger species the intervals between egg laying may be as long as 5 days. Clutch size can be up to eleven in the smaller species but only one to three in the larger birds (Figure 1.1). Incubation starts as soon as the first egg is laid, so that chicks will be progressively older and more advanced when the whole clutch has been hatched. Some chicks may be twice the size of their siblings.

The newly hatched chicks are usually covered in down. During the first week the female will stay in the nest to hatch all the eggs and keep the hatched chicks warm. Throughout this time the male bird will feed her and she will in turn feed the chicks. In all species, feeding of the chicks is carried out by regurgitation of food from the crop, with the young bird's beak held in that of the adult and the food passing down the funnel-like groove of the lower beak into that of the youngster. From the second week, when all the eggs are hatched and the hatchlings are better able to maintain their body temperature, the female will leave the nest for short periods and the male will share in feeding the young. After this initial period, both birds will leave the nest unattended for longer periods whilst they both forage for enough food to meet the needs of their growing youngsters. Compared with other species of bird, parrots tend to grow and mature rather slowly. Although Budgerigars may be sexually mature at 6 months, some of the larger species do not reach sexual maturity for several years.

Anatomy and physiology

Nigel H. Harcourt-Brown

Integument

The outer surface of a parrot is covered with feathers. The feathers form a continuous layer that insulates, protects and enables the parrot to fly. The epidermis is thinner (approximately 13 micrometres (μm) in the feathered areas) and more fragile than that of mammals but forms and keratinizes in a similar manner. The immature nucleated cells next to the basal layer contain oil globules that are pushed out of the cell as it keratinizes. This covers the surface of the bird with a layer of oil (sebum) that has antimicrobial properties, as well as keeping the skin supple and preventing dehydration.

In the majority of psittaciforms there is a uropygial gland on the dorsal aspect of the base of the tail. It is a bilobed holocrine gland: the glandular cells break down completely to form the secretion, which is water repellent, but it has many other properties. Usually only 7% of the sebum in the plumage is from the uropygial gland. Various neotropical parrots (e.g. Amazons, *Pionus* parrots and *Brotgeris* parakeets) do not have a preen gland. Birds have no sweat glands and no true cutaneous glands. Heat loss is accomplished through the respiratory tract and the feet, especially whilst flying.

The dermis is thinner (80–200 μm) than that of mammals. It contains the feather follicles, smooth muscle and elastic tendons, which move the feathers; it also contains blood vessels and nerves.

The subcutaneous layer contains fat, often as discrete fat bodies. Amazons and some cockatoos seem to have more fat than other parrots, and exhibition Budgerigars have been bred selectively to have large fat bodies on their chest. This complicated subcutaneous layer also contains striated muscles and is responsible for feather movement.

The brood patch is a portion of skin on the caudal half of the ventral abdomen. In the female, the hormones that stimulate breeding cause this area to lose all its feathers and develop a profuse blood supply prior to laying. The brood patch is in contact with the eggs and is well supplied with nerves that sense temperature changes in the eggs, allowing the bird to control incubation by either cooling eggs that are too hot or warming eggs that are too cold. It is also able to sense nitric oxide released by the egg in response to temperature change and hypoxia.

The distal portion of the leg is covered with scaly skin. The scales (scutes) vary in size. The skin on the underside of the foot and digits is closely attached to fleshy pads that protect the phalangeal joints and flexor tendons; this allows the bird to grip firmly with its foot. The cere is a featherless portion of skin at the base of the upper beak; it is well developed in parrots, and in some species (e.g. Budgerigars) it is coloured and can indicate gender.

Feathers

The feather is a very complicated epidermal structure. It is a tough keratinized cellular derivative of the epidermis and is formed in a follicle that penetrates deep into the dermis. Once formed, it is full of airspaces as well as pigment granules and oils. The feathers are arranged in distinct areas known as feather tracts (*pterylae*). The featherless spaces (*apteria*) may be bare or covered with semiplumes and down feathers. These featherless tracts are invisible from general observation, as the contour feathers from the *pterylae* cover them.

There are several types of feather:

- *Contour feathers* form the majority of the external plumage. Each feather has a long central stalk or rachis, on either side of which are the barbs. The barbs are further divided into the proximal and distal barbules, which hold on to their adjacent barbules with hamuli or hooklets. Contour feathers cover most of the body; they are also the flight and tail feathers (Figures 2.1 and 2.2).
- *Down feathers* have a short rachis and long soft barbs. They are found under the contour feathers and form an insulating undercoat.
- *Semiplumes* are a combination of the above two types, downy at the base and with a contour feather at the tip. They are found along the margins of the contour feather tracts.
- *Powder down feathers* are continually growing white to grey down feathers. The barbs at the tip constantly break off, forming a fine white dust that coats the whole bird (including its beak) and its surroundings; this is very obvious in white cockatoos. Powder down feathers may be found in patches on the body wall under the wing (e.g. cockatoos) or may be only scattered feathers (e.g. Pionus parrots).
- *Filoplumes* consist of a long spike with a tassel of

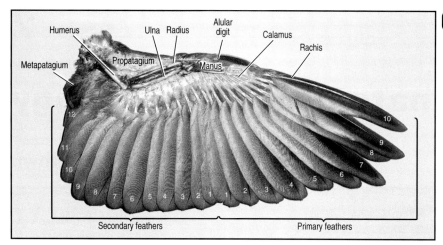

2.1 Ventral wing of a Maximilian's Pionus Parrot.

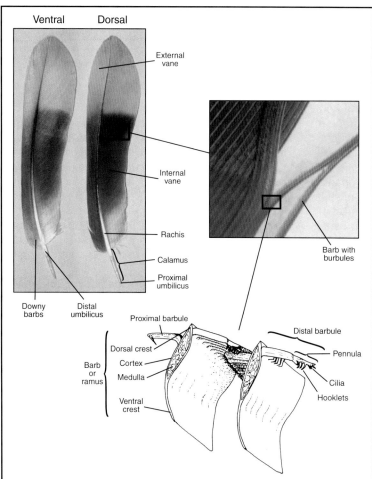

2.2 Two tail feathers (retrices), moulted on the same day by an Amazon, shown as a dorsal and a ventral view. The feathers were from each side of the tail and are a mirror-image pair. In the embedded feather, the dermis of the follicle projects into the proximal umbilicus and forms a small mound of pulp inside the calamus. This mound is stimulated (by trauma) to produce a new feather when the old calamus is lost. The umbilici mark the path of the blood vessel of the growing feather. On the inner vane of the remiges, the distal barbule has three hooklets and three ventral cilia. When the distal barbules are seen from the ventral aspect, the hooklets form a brush-like border. Each hooklet is able to hook round the C-shaped cross-section of the proximal barbule. The proximal barbule's pennulum is bent round at the end and extends towards the outer margin of the feather.

barbs at its tip. They are assumed to be sensory detectors, as they are closely associated with sensory Herbst corpuscles. They probably assess the strains and movement of the contour feathers, which is vital for flight. Each flight feather has up to 10 closely associated filoplumes.

- *Bristle feathers* are the short spiky feathers around the eye and loral region (ear). They are protective.

Plumage colour

Parrots have colourful plumage. The colour defines the parrot's species and is used to enhance behavioural signals. It also provides sexual dimorphism,

camouflage, and juvenile or adult characteristics. These traits are well developed in comparison with mammals (other than primates), and birds have excellent colour vision.

Plumage coloration is achieved in several ways. Colours may be produced by pigments: brown, yellow and black melanins are produced by melanocytes; reds and yellows are produced from carotenoids such as carotenes and xanthophils. These dietary pigments are dissolved in fat globules in the feather cells. White is due to reflection and refraction of all wavelengths of light through airspaces in unpigmented feathers. Blue pigment is rare and the bright blue in

Budgerigars is due to the Tyndall effect, a scattering of light on particles of less than 0.6 μm across (similar to the effect that produces a blue sky). Most parrots have green feathers that are a mixture of yellow carotenoids and the blue Tyndall effect. Selective breeding has made some birds lack one or other of these 'colours' so that a blue or yellow feather is the result. Ultraviolet light reflectance occurs in parrots; it is based on the structural characteristics of feathers and not on pigment.

Moult

Adult and immature plumage are usually different in both colour and shape. Feathers tend to wear out and are replaced annually. The first moult usually commences at 3–10 months of age but thereafter parrots normally moult once each year, usually starting during or just after breeding. The moult happens as a predictable sequence of feather loss. Wing and tail feathers are moulted as mirror image pairs. The wings usually take longer to moult than the tail or body feathers: complete wing moulting takes 160 days in a Galah.

Feather growth taxes the bird's resources, especially in small parrots. Moult frequently makes birds less active and they also require sufficient protein, especially sulphur-containing amino acids, to re-grow their feathers. Feathers grow from a blood-filled shaft but when they are fully formed they are isolated from their blood supply and the feather is dead. Old feathers are pushed out of the follicles by the new growing feather.

Moulting is triggered by many external factors that combine to stimulate the thyroid and gonads, whose hormones initiate moult. Once the moult has started other (unknown) local factors, secreted by the growing feather, cause the adjacent feather to moult in sequence. This is very obvious in the wing, where the first feather to fall out is usually primary 6 and the sequence moves in each direction along the wing. The developing feather has a considerable blood supply and grows out of the dermis surrounded by a cornified sheath. As the feather grows the sheath ruptures, allowing the feather to unfurl, which is helped by normal grooming using the beak and also claws. Once the feather is fully grown the blood supply disappears but the feather is held in place in its follicle by an epidermal collar of living tissue. When the feather is about to be replaced, this collar starts to proliferate and pushes the old feather out of its follicle. If the feather is pulled out prematurely the epidermal collar is torn; this damage stimulates the growth of a new feather.

Beak and claws

The beak is described in detail in Figure 2.3.

The claws at the end of each toe are similar to the beak in that they are heavily keratinized and mineralized. They are made of a thicker, harder and more rapidly growing dorsal portion and a flat softer ventral portion. As the growth is greatest in the dorsal portion the claw curves ventrally, making it ideal for grasping.

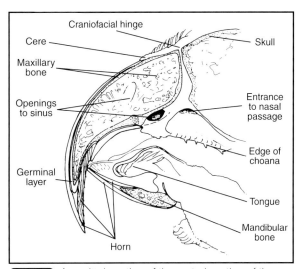

2.3 A sagittal section of the rostral portion of the head of a Grey Parrot. The horny beak or bill (rhamphotheca) is a hard, tough epidermal structure. The beak is attached to a bony base, either the mandible or maxilla, which acts as a form to produce the beak's shape. The bony base is overlain by periosteum that is bound to the dermis by a layer of collagen and elastin fibres. The typical layers of epidermis are modified and formed by keratin-filled cells, firmly held together by cell junctions that cannot break down. The stratum corneum is very thick and its keratinized cells are also mineralized with hydroxyapatite crystals.

The beak has a well developed superficial innervation in some areas but mostly is completely inert. The beak grows continually through life from both a germinal layer corresponding to the coronary band and from the germinal layer overlying the supporting bone. It becomes thicker towards its rostral end as it grows. In a large macaw it takes at least 9 months for a mark made next to the cere to reach the rostral tip. The inner and outer surfaces of the beak are formed as separate plates. The inside of the upper beak appears to have two areas of beak growth that between them form a shelf in the horn. Grey Parrots make a loud click by flicking the tip of their mandible off this shelf. The rostral part has a lamellar appearance but is smooth if the beak is wearing correctly. The shape of the beak is maintained mainly by the lower beak grinding against the inner surface of the upper beak. This happens during chewing but resting parrots will also grind their lower beak against the upper in a side-to-side rasping motion. The outer layers of the beak (cuticle) are also rubbed away by the bird wiping its beak on perches. Baby parrots hatch using their egg-tooth on the dorsal aspect of the end of the beak. It is a cone of horny cells containing hydroxyapatite that is shed as the beak grows.

Skeletomuscular system

Like the feathers, the skeleton (Figure 2.4) is light but 'engineered' to be very strong. The medullary cavity of some bones is filled with air rather than marrow.

Skull

The skull is a lightweight box with two huge orbits surrounded in many parrots by a complete bony ring. The upper jaw is formed by the premaxilla and nasal bones and can be moved relative to the rest of the skull (Figure 2.5). In large parrots there is a synovial joint at the junction of beak and skull (Figure 2.3); in smaller parrots this is combined with a flexible elastic zone. The

9

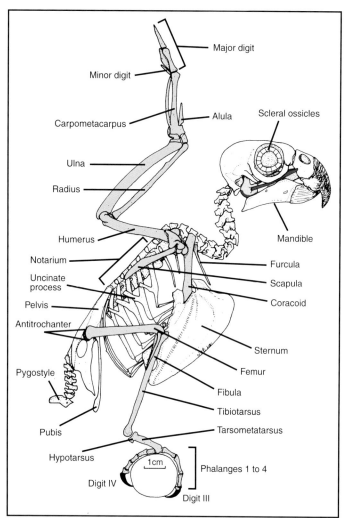

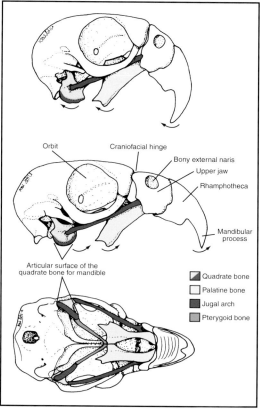

2.4 A right lateral view of the skeleton of the Blue-headed Pionus Parrot. The bird is illustrated in its normal standing position but for clarity the wing is elevated. The jaws are in normal resting occlusion. The orbit contains the scleral ossicles. Even though the skeleton is very light, the body of the bird is very strong.

The true ribs have a joint between the sternal and vertebral portions of the rib; the body wall is strengthened by uncinate processes that overlap the caudally adjacent vertebral rib. The sternum is attached by flexible joints to the sternal ribs, there is a slightly flexible joint with the coracoid and strong fibrous attachment to the most ventral portion of the furcula.

2.5 Lateral and ventral views of the skull of a Blue-headed Pionus Parrot. Parrots have very mobile jaws. The lower beak can be moved rostrally, caudally and laterally in relation to the upper jaw – it is quite possible for a parrot to place the tip of the maxilla inside the lower jaw. All these movements are interrelated by the mobility of the jaw bones and the unique jaw musculature (parrots have an extra jaw muscle compared with other birds). The muscles move the jaw bones and the skeleton of the palate. The quadrate bone (pink) is highly mobile and forms the articulation (dark red) for the mandible. The rest of the palatoquadrate bridge and the jugal arch move in concert with the upper jaw to which they are connected. When the upper jaw elevates it moves the quadrate bone, and therefore the lower jaw, rostrally as well. The jaws of parrots are not only very mobile but also immensely strong. This strength is made possible by the craniofacial hinge.

lower jaw consists of two fused mandibles. The mandibles do not articulate directly with the skull. The complex movements of the upper and lower jaws, relative to each other, allow the beak to be used in many subtle ways other than a basic scissors movement. The ligaments and muscles of the jaw are also highly specialized. The maxilla has a hollow air-filled interior that connects with the upper respiratory system.

Vertebrae, ribs and thoracic girdle

Parrots, like most other birds, have a very flexible neck. The vertebrae over the lungs are known as the notarium and, although not fused, are less flexible. The remaining thoracic, lumbar and sacral vertebrae are completely fused to form the synsacrum. The caudal vertebrae and terminal pygostyle are freely movable and support the tail feathers.

The ribs articulate with the thoracic vertebrae proximally and the well developed sternum distally. The carina (keel) forms a bony septum, on either side of which are the pectoral muscles. The sternum supports the thoracic girdle, which consists of the scapula, clavicle and coracoid bones. The coracoid acts as a strut, holding the shoulder a constant distance from the sternum. The scapulae lie adjacent to the ribs and the left and right clavicles are fused into a structure known as the furcula (it is absent in some parrots, such as lovebirds and rosellas). The furcula acts as a spring and stores energy during the down-beat as it is compressed. These three bones are joined by ligaments at their proximal ends to articulate with the head of the humerus; their jointed articular surfaces form the triosseal foramen through which the tendon of the supracoracoideus muscle passes.

Wing

The wing bones (Figures 2.1 and 2.4) are the humerus, radius and ulna, and the manus (a semi-fused three-fingered hand). There are separate radial and ulnar carpal bones and the distal carpals and metacarpals are fused into a carpometacarpus (see Figure 11.10). The alula digit (thumb) has a good range of movement; the major and minor digits form an integrated unit. The wing is very mobile when flexed but when extended it tends to move at the shoulder joint and otherwise resists dorsal and ventral forces. The shafts of the flight feathers are closely attached to the dorsal aspect of the ulna and manus; the primary feathers are more firmly attached than the secondary feathers.

The wing has its main muscle mass on the sternum (Figure 2.6). The pectoral muscle contracts to cause the down-stroke of the wing and forms 15–20% of the total body weight of the bird. Dorsal (or deep) to the pectoral muscle is the supracoracoideus muscle. Its tendon of insertion runs through the triosseal foramen and inserts on the dorsocranial edge of the humerus. During normal flapping flight, the supracoracoideus muscle rotates the humerus, causing the wing to raise its leading edge. This allows the bird to maintain its position in the air between down-strokes. During slow flight and take-off, the shoulder muscles elevate the wing. The propatagium (a triangular portion of skin) is present from the cranial aspect of the shoulder to the carpus and caudally to the elbow. The leading edge of the propatagium is supported internally by an elastic tendon that is joined by various other muscles and tendons, all of which maintain the aerofoil shape of the wing. The elbow joint has a wide range of movements when flexed, and the radius and ulna pronate and supinate.

Leg

The leg of the parrot (Figure 2.7) has a femur, a tibiotarsus (the tibia fused to the proximal row of tarsal bones) and a short fibula that does not extend below the fibular crest (Figure 2.4). The tarsometatarsus is also a short bone, formed by the distal row of tarsal bones combined with the fused second, third and fourth metatarsal bones (see Figure 11.11). The first metatarsal bone is separate. The parrot's foot is zygodactyl: digits II and III face cranially, digits I and IV caudally. The pelvis is formed by fusion of the ilium, ischium and pubis. The acetabulum is formed from a bony rim and a fibrous cup. Caudodorsal to the acetabulum is the antitrochanter, which articulates with the trochanter of the femur and prevents abduction of the limb when the bird is in a normal standing position. Because of their foot shape and short tarsometatarsus, parrots are very good at climbing and manipulating their food, but when walking on a flat surface they have a typical waddling or rolling gait, especially those (such as macaws) that walk on the caudal tarsometatarsus as well as the foot.

Like that of the wing, the main muscle mass of the leg is close to the body and so many muscles have long tendons of insertion. When the toes are flexed and gripping there is a locking mechanism between the flexor tendons and their sheath that maintains grip with a minimum of muscle activity. In parrots the long digital extensor muscle extends all four digits.

Medullary cavities and medullary bone

In growing parrots the medullary cavities of most bones contain active bone marrow. When a bird stops growing, many bones become pneumatized: diverticula from the air sacs invade and occupy the medullary cavities of many vertebrae, the pelvis, sternum and humerus.

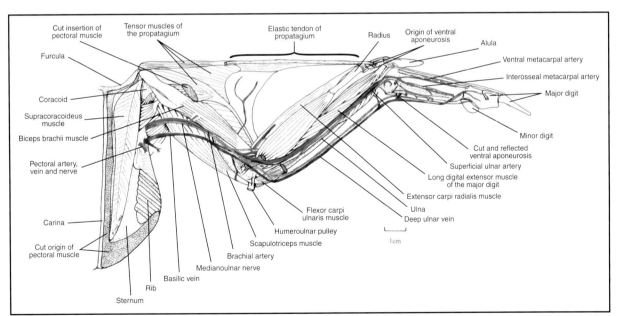

2.6 Ventral view of the wing of a Grey Parrot. Arteries are red, veins blue and nerves green. The pectoral muscle has been removed. The brachial artery gives rise to the radial and then ulnar arteries. The superficial ulnar artery gives rise to the ventral metacarpal and digital arteries. The deep ulnar vein is the major venous return from the distal wing. The supracoracoideus muscle can be seen entering the triosseal foramen in the shoulder.

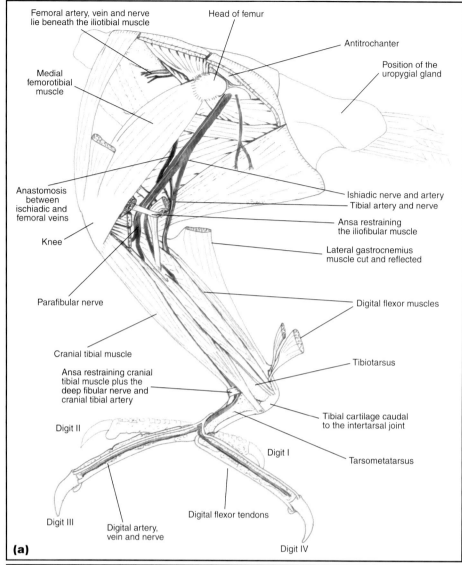

Femoral artery, vein and nerve
lie beneath the iliotibial muscle

Head of femur

Antitrochanter

Position of the
uropygial gland

Medial
femorotibial
muscle

Anastomosis
between
ischiadic and
femoral veins

Ishiadic nerve and artery

Tibial artery and nerve

Ansa restraining
the iliofibular muscle

Knee

Lateral gastrocnemius
muscle cut and reflected

Parafibular nerve

Digital flexor muscles

Cranial tibial muscle

Ansa restraining cranial
tibial muscle plus the
deep fibular nerve and
cranial tibial artery

Tibiotarsus

Digit II

Tibial cartilage caudal
to the intertarsal joint

Digit I

Tarsometatarsus

Digit III

Digital artery,
vein and nerve

Digital flexor tendons

Digit IV

(a)

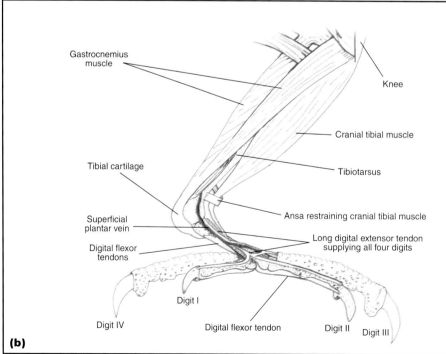

Gastrocnemius
muscle

Knee

Tibial cartilage

Cranial tibial muscle

Tibiotarsus

Superficial
plantar vein

Ansa restraining cranial tibial muscle

Digital flexor
tendons

Long digital extensor tendon
supplying all four digits

Digit I

Digit IV

Digital flexor tendon

Digit II

Digit III

(b)

2.7 (a) Lateral view of the left pelvic limb of a Grey Parrot. The limb, including the pelvis and synsacrum, has been removed from the vertebral column, and the integument removed, except for digits I and II. To illustrate the course of the main nerves, arteries and veins, iliofibular and lateral iliotibial muscles have been removed, and lateral gastrocnemius muscle and minor flexors of digits II and III have been sectioned at their origins and reflected. (b) The distal portion of the leg of a Grey Parrot has had the skin removed, except for digits III and IV. The major venous return from the distal limb is the superficial plantar vein. The distal third of the tibiotarsus is visible as it has virtually no soft tissue covering once the skin is removed.

The tendons of insertion are long and there are several adaptations where they run over joints. The iliofibular muscle (a flexor of the knee) and the cranial tibial muscle (flexor of the intertarsal joint) are both held close to their respective joints by a strap-like ansa. Alongside the tendon of insertion these ansae contain a neurovascular bundle. The gastrocnemius muscles (extensors of the intertarsal joint) insert on the hypotarsal region and their fibrous insertions cover the tibial cartilage and then the flexor tendons on the caudal tarsometatarsus. The tibial cartilage contains the minor digital flexor tendons in several tunnels; the two major digital flexor tendons run through this region in tunnels in the hypotarsus. The minor flexors provide most of the complicated toe movements, the major flexors insert on the distal phalangeal bone and produce powerful digital flexion. The digital extensor tendon is shown in Figure 11.5. There are some small intrinsic muscles in the tarsometatarsal region that also make fine movement possible.

Medullary bone (Figure 2.8; see also Figure 18.4) is labile bone that normally occurs only in female birds in the reproductive phase. Its formation is controlled by oestrogens and androgens and so it can also be formed in non-laying birds with hormonal abnormalities. It consists of interconnected spicules, resembling embryonic bone, that grow out from the endosteal surface of the long bones. Medullary bone has no Haversian system and contains less collagen than normal bone. Phases of formation and destruction alternate during the laying cycle.

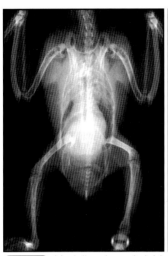 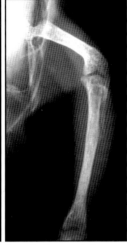

2.8 Medullary bone is laid down in the medullary cavity of bones that are not pneumatized. It is most obvious in the long bones, and in this Pionus parrot. it is absent from the humerus but present in the femur. Two weeks after these radiographs were taken the bird laid a clutch of five eggs.

Body cavities

Birds do not possess a diaphragm that can separate the body into thoracic and abdominal cavities. In birds in general there are 16 body cavities. Eight of these are connected to the respiratory system and are pneumatized (air sacs). The others, which are not pneumatized, are the left and right pleural cavities, a pericardial cavity, four separate hepatic peritoneal cavities and the intestinal peritoneal cavity. The intestinal peritoneal cavity contains the gastrointestinal tract from proventriculus to rectum, the gonads, spleen and abdominal air sacs; the kidneys and reproductive tracts are extraperitoneal.

Digestive system

Oral cavity

Parrots have a thick blunt-ended tongue that has an intrinsic musculature, which is unique amongst birds. This enables many parrots to pick up food such as seeds and manipulate the food against the jaws. The tongue also contains fat and cavernous vascular tissue. In lories and lorikeets the tongue is curled into a groove and carries several hundred bristles that help to collect pollen and nectar.

Salivary glands are numerous and widely distributed within the palate, tongue, floor and corner of the mouth, cheeks and pharynx. The glands are compound tubular structures with multiple lobules. Each lobule is composed of many secretory tubules that open into a common cavity that then drains via a single duct. These ducts are numerous and can be seen with the naked eye as small openings all over the mouth. They are stimulated by the parasympathetic nerves and secrete mainly mucus.

Oesophagus

The oesophagus lies on the right side of the neck and is modified at the thoracic inlet to form the crop (Figure 2.9). Peristaltic waves move the food down the oesophagus and mix the contents of the crop.

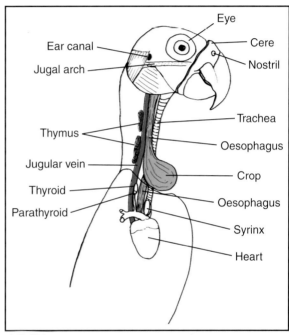

2.9 A lateral view of the right side of the neck of the Grey Parrot. The thymus is well developed in the young bird and is present on each side of the neck. It regresses as the bird gets older. The right jugular vein is usually the larger of the two. The oesophagus, heart and syrinx are all very close to each other. All the structures illustrated in the neck are subcutaneous.

Stomach

The stomach is divided into a proventriculus and ventriculus (gizzard) (Figures 2.10 and 2.11). Cranially the proventriculus is glandular and contains oxynticopeptic cells that secrete hydrochloric acid and pepsin; caudally it is muscular. The intermediate zone opens into the gizzard. In parrots the gizzard is extremely muscular and has internal and external adaptations for grinding food with grit (Figure 2.11). The internal surface is covered with the cuticle (koilin layer), which is a carbohydrate–protein complex and not keratin. The pyloric part of the stomach is between the muscular part of the gizzard and the duodenum. It contains endocrine cells. Radiographic studies have shown that the food is propelled in alternate directions between the proventriculus and the gizzard in a series of cycles.

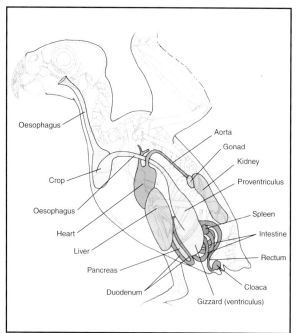

2.10 Left lateral view of the viscera of a Blue-headed Pionus Parrot.

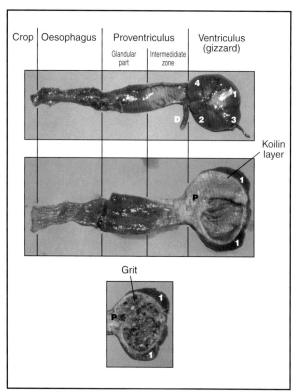

2.11 External and internal views of the alimentary tract from oesophagus (distal to the crop) to duodenum of a typical parrot (*Pionus senilis*). The glandular part of the proventriculus can be identified by its darker colour and a honeycomb pattern on its surface; the intermediate part is paler. The body of the gizzard has two thick muscles (1, 2) and two thinner areas (3, 4) that correspond to blind-ending sacs within the gizzard. The entrance to the pyloric part of the stomach (P) and duodenum (D) is in the cranial part of the gizzard. The koilin layer is well developed in parrots. If parrots have access to grit, the healthy gizzard will always contain it.

Intestines

The duodenum is a U-shaped loop of bowel. The jejunum and the ileum are arranged in a series of U-shaped loops, or coils. At the junction between the ileum and the jejunum is the vitelline diverticulum (the remnant of the yolk sac and the yolk duct) (Figure 7.7). The intestinal wall has three types of epithelial cells: chief cells, which have a brush border and are absorptive; goblet cells, which are mucus secreting; and endocrine cells, which in combination with those in the stomach and pancreas form a diffuse endocrine organ. Chemical digestion and absorption of food take place in the small intestine. The large bowel is short; the paired vestigial caeca arise at the junction between the jejunum and the rectum. The intestine empties into the cloaca (Figure 2.12). The length of the intestines of the Eclectus Parrot is nearly twice that of the other large parrots.

Pancreas

The pancreas has three lobes. The dorsal lobe lies above the ventral lobe in the duodenal loop (Figure 15.16a) and a small splenic lobe runs from the cranial part of the pancreas towards the spleen. The pancreas secretes the same exocrine digestive enzymes as mammals: amylase, lipase and proteases, including trypsin. It also produces insulin and glucagons but insulin has little effect on glucose metabolism, which is mainly controlled by steroid hormones.

Liver

The liver has right and left lobes (the right lobe is larger). Each lobe is drained by a bile duct and these unite. In most parrots (not cockatoos) the gall bladder is absent and the right lobe's bile duct becomes the main drainage to the duodenum.

Urinary system

Parrot kidneys lie in the left and right renal fossae of the synsacrum. Each kidney is divided into cranial, middle and caudal divisions (Figure 2.13). Each division consists of many lobules, which may be seen as small lumps on the renal surface; the lobule is the fundamental unit of the kidney. The blood supply to the kidney is very complex.

Uric acid rather than urea is the end point of avian nitrogen metabolism. It is formed in the liver. Although some is excreted through glomerular filtration, 90% is actively secreted by the renal tubule. Uric acid mixed with salts forms spheres a few micrometres across that mix with mucus to become a colloidal solution, which prevents the insoluble urates from precipitating in the ureter.

Uric acid excretion is vital for an embryo developing in a shelled egg. It is moved to, and stored in, the allantois as a crystalline anhydrous deposit, allowing water from excretion to be recycled. As it is insoluble, uric acid will not poison the closed system of the egg (as would happen with urea). After hatching, uric acid excretion requires more water loss from the kidney in the bird than urea excretion does in mammals.

There are two types of nephron. The 'mammalian' type is found in the medulla of the lobule and has a well developed glomerulus plus a nephronal loop. The

14

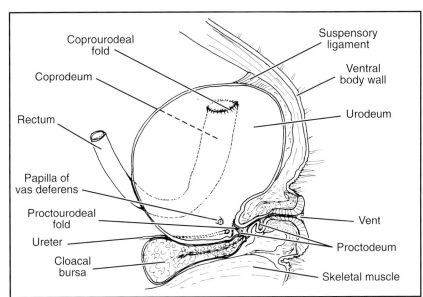

Coprourodeal fold

Coprodeum

Rectum

Papilla of vas deferens

Proctourodeal fold

Ureter

Cloacal bursa

Suspensory ligament

Ventral body wall

Urodeum

Vent

Proctodeum

Skeletal muscle

2.12 An internal left lateral view of the cloaca of a 9-month-old male Grey Parrot. The bird is in ventral recumbency. The urodeum is dilated to almost its maximum capacity to mimic the endoscopic view. The cloaca is the terminal portion of the urinary, reproductive and alimentary systems. In parrots the three chambers of the cloaca are not arranged in a tube-like line and the urodeum is the largest chamber. The rectum opens into the coprodeum with no obvious junction. The coprodeum is larger than the rectum; it is closely attached to the outside of the left side of the urodeum and opens into it on the ventrolateral aspect. The junction between coprodeum and urodeum has the ability to open and close. The urodeum is the middle compartment. The ureter and reproductive ducts open into the urodeum. The ureters open relatively dorsally through a small mound. Each vas deferens opens through a small papilla on the lateral aspect close to the exit to the urodeum. The left oviduct opens at the same site and develops with a membrane over the opening that usually disappears when the bird is mature. The right oviduct is permanently sealed. The proctodeum is the final compartment and is short. It is separated from the urodeum by a well developed semicircular uroproctodeal fold. The cloacal bursa (bursa of Fabricius) is a pouch-like diverticulum with a central duct that opens into the proctodeum in young birds. The bursa is larger than the cloaca in 6-week-old parrots but slowly regresses and is a tiny remnant by the time the bird is sexually mature. The termination of the cloaca is the vent, which is kept closed by well developed muscles. In poultry the coprodeum can empty directly through the vent by eversion of the urocoproctodeal fold; eggs are also laid directly from the oviduct through the proctodeum. Sometimes parrots make a straining noise when they defecate, which is not usually a sign of abnormality. In the parrot's cadaver the exit to the coprodeum can be positioned against the entrance to the proctodeum and this may happen due to increased coelomic pressure which with no diaphragm would make the bird vocalize. The coprourodeal fold is said to close whilst eggs are laid; in parrots, new-laid eggs are never stained with faeces and this fold contains muscle.

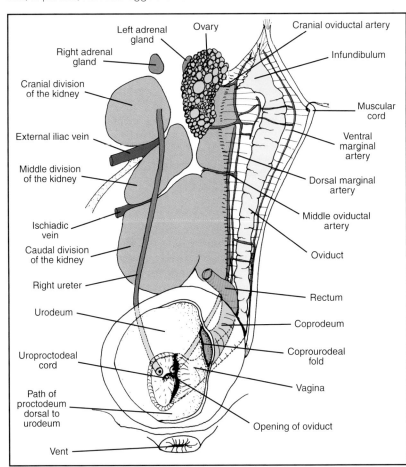

Left adrenal gland

Right adrenal gland

Cranial division of the kidney

External iliac vein

Middle division of the kidney

Ischiadic vein

Caudal division of the kidney

Right ureter

Urodeum

Uroproctodeal cord

Path of proctodeum dorsal to urodeum

Vent

Ovary

Cranial oviductal artery

Infundibulum

Muscular cord

Ventral marginal artery

Dorsal marginal artery

Middle oviductal artery

Oviduct

Rectum

Coprodeum

Coprourodeal fold

Vagina

Opening of oviduct

2.13 A view of the urogenital tract of a sexually mature female Grey Parrot. The bird is in dorsal recumbency and the overlying alimentary tract has been removed. The oviduct is pulled to the left by the muscular cord to show the oviduct and its arterial supply. The ventral marginal artery is in the ventral ligament, the dorsal arteries run in the dorsal ligament. The oviductal veins are omitted. Some of the uterine artery complex has been omitted for clarity and the caudal arterial supply of the oviduct is hidden by the cloaca. A fully developed oviduct is twice the length of the bird's body and lies in a sinuous folded manner rather than as illustrated. It can be difficult to see any external differences that demarcate the regions of the oviduct, although they are very different internally. It is also difficult to find any remnants of the right oviduct and ovary. Full-sized mature oocytes would be almost as large as the ovary on this drawing. Oocytes enlarge and mature sequentially, so during laying there is only one fully grown egg but usually a number of medium-sized oocytes waiting to mature.

15

'reptilian' type is found in the cortex of the lobule and has a less developed glomerulus and no nephronal loop. In experiments it has been shown that some birds, when subjected to salt-loading, direct blood away from the reptilian nephrons, which cannot concentrate salt in their tubular filtrate because they have no nephronal loop. Other species have alternative mechanisms (Goldstein and Skadhauge, 2000).

The renal portal veins and efferent venous flow from the glomerulus form the peritubular capillary plexus. This plexus surrounds the proximal tubules; urates are removed from the venous blood and are secreted into the proximal tubule. Two-thirds of the blood entering the kidney is from the venous system. Because there is a pair of valves in the portal circulation and there are muscular sphincters in the afferent veins, the blood flow through the kidneys can be controlled. All, part or none of the venous blood can enter the kidney tissue. This may be useful during increased exercise, as it can increase the venous return to the heart and also enable greater blood flow through the limbs to allow heat loss.

The urine (colloids in mucus and water) flows slowly and viscously down the ureter and enters the urodeum (Figures 2.12 and 2.13) and can then be transferred by retroperistalsis into the coprodeum and even the rectum, where it is stored until defecation. During this time, water and salts are reabsorbed in the coprodeum and the bowel. In most birds, 10–20% of the water and up to 70% of Na^+ is reabsorbed with additional secretion of 20% of K^+. Wild Budgerigars that are adapted to living in dry conditions are able to retain an even greater percentage of water: at room temperature on a dry seed diet they do not need to drink.

Reproductive system

Male
The male reproductive organs are a pair of equally active testes next to each adrenal gland at the cranial division of the kidneys. In many parrots the right testis is smaller than the left, because germ cells migrate from the right gonad (ovary or testis) to the left during development. Inactive testes are small with no obvious blood supply. When sexually active they are much larger with well developed blood vessels. Sperm is collected in the epididymis and passes into the convoluted ductus deferens, which enlarges distally into a sperm receptacle, the seminal glomus. In this structure the temperature can be 6°C below that of the surrounding tissues. There are no accessory genital glands.

Female
In the female parrot, only the left side of the reproductive tract is fully and functionally developed (Figure 2.13). The blood supply to the ovary is large and the vessels are quite short. The ovary is closely attached to the body wall, next to the adrenal gland and cranial division of the kidney. The ovary has many obvious follicles; these are small in immature birds and are enlarged by the presence of yolk in adult birds when breeding. The follicle develops suspended on a stalk of smooth muscle, blood vessels and nerves. It contains a large primary oocyte surrounded by a multi-layered

wall that is potentially divided by the stigma. At ovulation the stigma is split; the (secondary) oocyte is 'grabbed' by the infundibulum, a task made easier by the discrete size of the left abdominal air sac which encloses the ovary. If the oocyte is shed but not enveloped by the infundibulum it is usually reabsorbed.

The oviduct is supported by the dorsal ligament and the ventral ligament and has five parts.

- The first part, the infundibulum, picks up the oocyte after it has been shed by the ovary and surrounds it with a first layer of albumen (egg white). Fertilization of the oocyte by the sperm is limited to a period of about 15 minutes, being the period between release of the oocyte from the ovary and it being covered with albumen. This is possible because sperm are contained in folds in the mucosa of the oviduct.
- The egg passes through the magnum, where the rest of the albumen is added.
- In the isthmus the shell membranes are produced, which cover the egg and also determine its final shape.
- The egg then enters the shell gland, where it spends 80% of its time in the oviduct. Firstly the egg absorbs water and enlarges to a plumped egg shape. Then the calcium carbonate and protein shell is produced and is finally covered with a cuticle giving the egg its shiny appearance (Figure 2.14). The shell contains thousands of tiny pores that run from the shell membranes to the surface, allowing the embryo to respire. In parrots the shell is white.
- The final part of the oviduct is the muscular vagina that in many species has spermatic fossulae, which are capable of sperm storage. In many species (e.g. Budgerigar) viable sperm can be stored and released for several days. After mating, some of the sperm is stored; some is able to reach the infundibulum within a few minutes.

It is traditional to describe the egg moving down the oviduct. In reality, because of the length of the oviduct and size of the egg, the egg is relatively static in the coelomic cavity whilst the oviduct moves over it by peristalsis.

Cardiovascular system
Parrots, like most birds, have to be able to sustain sudden and prolonged high levels of muscular activity. The heart of birds is much larger and beats faster than that of mammals of comparable size and the rate can vary very quickly. Birds have a high cardiac output, seven times greater in a Budgerigar than a human or dog at maximum exercise. This high cardiac output is combined with a higher arterial pressure (180/140 mm Hg). Avian cardiac muscle cells are much smaller in diameter than mammalian cells.

The four-chambered heart lies ventral to the lungs in a relatively midline position in the body. It is surrounded by pericardium that is attached to the sternum and the liver's peritoneal sacs. The right atrioventricular valve is a muscular flap on the free wall of the ventricle; the other valves are similar to those of mammals.

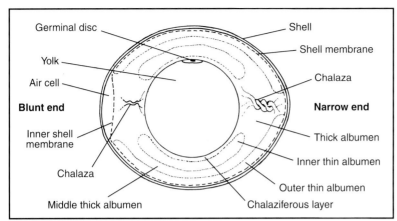

2.14 Parrot eggs are white and relatively small and have little difference between the blunt and narrow ends. Most parrots lay their eggs on alternate days. The eggs are incubated (usually by the female) from the time that they are laid. Parrots brood their eggs continually and turn them regularly.

The hard outer shell is shaped to resist external forces but is easily broken by force from within. The outer layer of the shell is the cuticle: a thin, hard, continuous outer covering of lipid and protein that gives the egg its smooth sheen. It is responsible for repelling water and bacteria. The testa is the calcified portion (98% $CaCO_3$ and 2% protein matrix) and has a complicated structure. This part of the shell provides most of the calcium required by the embryo. The surface of the testa has pores that open on to the surface (under the cuticle) and also connect with canaliculi that run right through the shell to the membrane. They allow gaseous exchange. The pores are most numerous at the blunt end of the egg. There are two shell membranes: the inner membrane rests on the albumen; the outer membrane is thicker and is attached to the shell. As soon as the egg is laid, cooling allows separation of the membranes at the blunt end to form the air cell.

The clear proteinaceous albumen forms about 75% of the egg in parrots. It is divided into compartments. The yolk is surrounded by a thick viscous albumen layer which, as the female parrot regularly turns hers eggs, becomes twisted and condensed and forms chalazae. The chalazae resist the tendency of the yolk to float to the most dorsal aspect of the egg. The thick albumen tends to be a shock-absorber too. There are two compartments of more liquid albumen that contain more water and less ovomucin; they prevent the embryo from drying out and allow more rapid mixing and diffusion of nutrients and gases to supply the early embryo. The albumen is a source of water and mineral ions for the growing embryo and additional nourishment. It is completely used during incubation. Lysozymes and similar proteins in the albumen prevent bacterial infection of the egg.

The yolk is orange and on its surface is a visible germinal disc; radiating from this area is the more watery white yolk, which is less dense. During turning, the yolk's structure makes the part containing the germinal disc stay most dorsal (closest to the incubating bird). The yolk is covered by two membranes. It is 50% solids, 99% of which are protein, and is the main nutrient source for the embryo. In the latter stages of growth the yolk is connected directly to the embryo's intestine.

Calcium for the egg's shell is obtained from the duodenum and upper jejunum or from reabsorption of bone. If there is sufficient calcium in the diet the intestine is the main source. In cases where the diet does not contain sufficient calcium, further calcium is obtained from the medullary bone and, failing this, from cortical bone. Medullary bone is a labile buffer for calcium demand and even in diets with adequate calcium it is used while demands for calcium are at their highest. It is quickly replaced by calcium absorbed from the gut. Whilst laying, poultry will preferentially consume a diet supplemented with oyster shell grit. Preference for calcium-rich food during this time has been shown in other species of bird as well. During the last third of incubation the chorioallantoic membrane, which lies over the inner shell membrane, secretes a weak acid that dissolves the inner lining of the shell and provides the embryo with calcium to form its skeleton.

The arteries and veins are similar in distribution to those of mammals. There are species differences; for instance, in cockatoos the left carotid artery is much smaller than the right. Two venous anastomoses are notable. A jugular anastomosis, just caudal to the head, allows the blood in the left jugular vein to be shunted to the much larger right jugular vein. An anastomosis between the femoral and ischiadic veins allows the femoral vein to be the main venous return of the leg.

The high-pressure blood supply for glomerular filtration comes from the three renal arteries. There is also a lower pressure supply from the external iliac vein (mostly derived from the femoral vein) and renal portal vein that finally surrounds the renal tubules, allowing the secretion of urates. The portal veins enter into a ring-like renal portal system. The renal portal valve is able to cause blood to be shunted through the whole kidney or parts of the kidney. At times of maximum energy demand, the blood can even bypass the kidney altogether.

Lymphatic system

Lymphatic vessels are less numerous in birds than in mammals. Within the trunk these vessels are closely associated with arteries, whereas outside the trunk they accompany veins. The lymphatic ducts drain into the venae cavae. Parrots have no lymph nodes but there are nodules of lymphoid tissue in the lymph vessels as well as lymphoid tissue in the spleen and bone marrow. Primary lymphoid tissue is formed in the thymus and cloacal bursa.

The thymus (Figure 2.9) consists of several paired lobes at the base of the neck. It produces mainly thymus-dependent (T) lymphocytes, which originally migrated there from the yolk sac, and some bursa-dependent (B) lymphocytes.

The cloacal bursa (Figure 2.12) is unique to birds. It is a dorsomedial diverticulum in the proctodeum and is also best developed while the bird is growing. In parrots it is a thin-walled sac and is the source of the majority of the B lymphocytes. The bursa involutes slowly and is usually just a remnant of tissue by the time the bird is fully grown. After this, B cells come from the bone marrow.

True lymph nodes are rare in birds and when they do occur they are in a pair near the thyroid and a pair near the kidneys. There are mural lymphoid nodules in the walls of the lymphatics, and there are aggregates of lymphoid tissue in the alimentary tract and occulonasal region and variable amounts in all the other organs.

The spleen is situated on the right side of the bird, at the junction of the proventriculus and gizzard. It phagocytoses erythrocytes and produces lymphocytes and antibodies but is not erythropoietic.

Respiratory system

The body of the bird contains the viscera within their peritoneal cavities and a number of air-filled sacs (Figure 2.15). The two lungs are a mass of interconnected airways that commence at the primary bronchus and finally enter the air sacs via holes (ostia). There are eight air sacs: one cervical, one clavicular, two cranial thoracic, two caudal thoracic and two abdominal. The

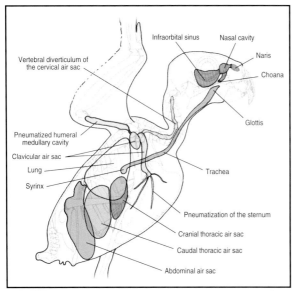

2.15 Right lateral view of the respiratory organs of the Blue-headed Pionus Parrot.

cervical and clavicular sacs enter the vertebrae, humerus and other soft tissue structures mainly outside the main body cavity. Caudoventral to the lungs are the thoracic and abdominal sacs. The exact structure of the sacs and the pneumatization of the body differs between genera and even species; for instance, the femur is pneumatized in birds of prey but not in parrots. The air sacs have two principal functions: reduction of the bird's weight; and ventilation by acting as bellows to pull air through the lungs, but not gaseous exchange. The respiratory movements elevate and depress the sternum and also expand and contract the rib cage. This expands and contracts the air-filled sacs but does not change the volume of the lungs.

The upper respiratory tract provides a filter system (nostril and conchae) to warm, moisten and filter the air. The nasal passages also connect to an extensive air-filled infraorbital sinus (Figure 2.16). The air passes through a slit in the roof of the mouth (choana) to the larynx. The larynx can open and shut but has no ability to make noises, though it modifies them. The trachea has complete tracheal rings that are calcified. It ends in the syrinx, which is a complicated movable structure. Internally the parrot's syrinx arises as a valve, beyond which are the lateral tympaniform membranes and then two primary bronchi, one supplying each lung. Externally the syrinx has several muscles that are attached to the modified tracheal and bronchial cartilages and this system produces the voice. The primary bronchi give rise to smaller and smaller airways, all of which are variously interconnected but finally pass through the lung to empty into the air sacs. This complex system of airways, plus an aerodynamic valve, allows a unidirectional path through the majority of the lung tissue for the majority of the air (Figure 2.17).

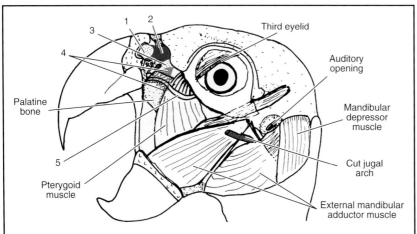

2.16 Lateral view of the head of a Grey Parrot. The jugal arch and lateral wall of the infraorbital sinus have been removed. The medial wall of the sinus overlies the pterygoid muscle and palatine bone. The nasal passages have been opened by removal of the overlying bone.
1: The vestibular region contains the rostral nasal concha and is lined by non-ciliated stratified squamous epithelium. It receives secretion from the nasal gland. It filters, warms and humidifies inspired air.
2: The respiratory region contains the middle concha and is lined with mucociliary epithelium. This is the primary defence against infection of the lower respiratory tract. In Grey Parrots there is no caudal concha and the olfactory nerves are probably in the caudodorsal nasal passage wall. The cilia propel mucus caudally and then ventrally (in chickens at 10 mm/min). Beneath the epithelium is a richly vascular bed that warms the air. Because this area also retains fluid from the nasal gland, it plays a major role in water and heat economy as well as air filtration and olfaction.
3: This area is a common chamber between the above (1 and 2), the respiratory passages to the choana (4), and the aperture of the infraorbital sinus. The infraorbital sinus is moist with a rich supply of mucus glands at the aperture; the mucociliary current at this opening is very rapid.
4: This ventral part of the respiratory passage leads into the choana and is medial to the palatine bone and pterygoid muscle. The nasolacrimal duct opens into this area.
5: The nasopalatine branch of cranial nerve V runs across the medial aspect of the infraorbital sinus. The infraorbital sinus has a number of potential air-filled extensions around the skull, including into the maxillary bone, and also an extension around the vertebrae as far as the crop and shoulders.

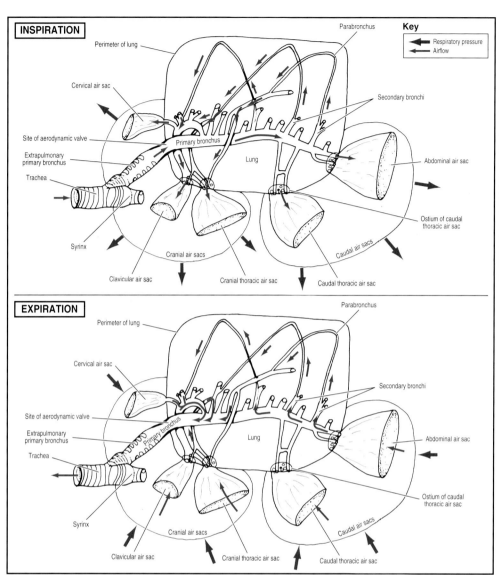

INSPIRATION

Perimeter of lung

Cervical air sac

Site of aerodynamic valve

Extrapulmonary primary bronchus

Trachea

Syrinx

Clavicular air sac

Cranial air sacs

Cranial thoracic air sac

Primary bronchus

Lung

Parabronchus

Key
Respiratory pressure
Airflow

Secondary bronchi

Abdominal air sac

Ostium of caudal thoracic air sac

Caudal air sacs

Caudal thoracic air sac

EXPIRATION

Perimeter of lung

Cervical air sac

Site of aerodynamic valve

Extrapulmonary primary bronchus

Trachea

Syrinx

Clavicular air sac

Cranial air sacs

Cranial thoracic air sac

Primary bronchus

Lung

Parabronchus

Secondary bronchi

Abdominal air sac

Ostium of caudal thoracic air sac

Caudal air sacs

Caudal thoracic air sac

2.17 Movement of air through the lung of a bird. Inspiratory movements increase air sac volumes and expiratory movements decrease them. The volume and shape of the lung remains the same. Because of the arrangement of the parabronchi and the possible presence of an aerodynamic valve, the air is moved unidirectionally through the parabronchi and therefore the area of gaseous exchange.

The final unit of gaseous exchange is the smallest section of the airway: the air capillary. The air capillaries form an anastomosing three-dimensional network of airways through which the air flows. The air capillaries completely fill the spaces between the blood capillary network. Airway size is controlled and helped by smooth muscle in the larger airway walls and a surfactant that covers the air capillaries and is secreted by cells in the walls of the airways.

There are other major features of the avian respiratory system that make gaseous exchange in birds far superior to that in mammals (Box 2.1). Birds are able to fly vigorously under conditions that would cause extreme hypoxia in mammals.

Inspiration and expiration are active processes. The ribs move craniolaterally and push the sternum cranioventrally. Although there is no diaphragm, this still increases the internal volume of the bird and draws air into the air sacs. Expiration is caused by active contraction of muscles that forces air out of the system. During anaesthesia, birds in sternal recumbency have to raise their whole body to inspire; birds in ventral recumbency have a decreased ability to inflate some air sacs and so also have compromised ventilation.

The avian lung does not change shape during the respiratory cycle and, so, neither do the airways. The terminal units of gaseous exchange (air capillaries) are smaller (3–10 μm) than the alveolus of mammals (35 μm or larger). The airways are covered by a trilaminar substance, unique to birds, which acts as a surfactant that keeps the fluid content of the airways low: it prevents the airways collapsing under the effect of surface tension, keeps the protective fluid layer sufficiently thin that it does not diminish the airway diameter significantly, and decreases the risk of pulmonary oedema. The small sized airways encourage a greater oxygen diffusion gradient.

In mammals the air in each alveolus is only changed as a proportion during each respiratory cycle. In birds there is a one-way passage of air through the lung. As there are no blind-ending alveoli, there is no dead space during the respiratory cycle and all the air is involved in gaseous exchange.

The blood–gas barrier (capillary endothelial cell/basal lamina/respiratory epithelial cell) is one third thinner in birds than in mammals.

Within the air capillary bed the blood flow tends to be counter to the direction of the air flow, forming greater diffusion gradients. This is known as cross-current gas exchange.

Avian lung has a 20% greater volume of capillary blood per gram weight than mammalian lung. The blood content of the lungs is also constant during the respiratory cycle, unlike that of mammals.

Box 2.1 Comparison between the avian and mammalian lung.

Central nervous system

The central nervous system of birds is similar to that of mammals. The brain is not as large as the mammalian brain in animals of a similar size, but larger than the reptilian brain. There is a very poorly developed cerebral cortex. The rostral colliculus (optic lobe) is huge and the total cross-sectional area of the optic nerves is greater than that of the cervical spinal cord. The olfactory region is poorly developed (see Chapter 19).

The spinal cord is morphologically similar to that of all other vertebrates. It consists of central grey matter surrounded by three columns of white matter (dorsal, ventral and lateral). Birds have marginal nuclei that surround the grey matter and these are likely to be ventral commissural neurons that project information across the cord and may be multi-synaptic neurons that transmit non-localizing pain fibres along the column. The spinal cord is the same length as the vertebral column and has no cauda equina. It is surrounded by the meninges. The epidural space is filled with a gelatinous rather than liquid substance. A large venous sinus runs along the dorsal aspect of the vertebral canal and is voluminous in the area of the medulla oblongata; it anastomoses with the renal circulation. The glycogen body is found at the separation of the dorsal columns of the lumbosacral cord; the two types of nerve fibres that make up the glycogen body are thought to regulate vascular reflexes and have a neurosecretory role.

The wing is supplied from a brachial plexus (see Figure 19.2). The brachial plexus gives rise to both a ventral and dorsal fascicle, so that the wing is surrounded with nerves, whereas the majority of the leg has a caudolateral supply. The pelvic limb is supplied from a lumbosacral plexus that runs between the kidneys and the pelvis before it reaches the leg.

Senses

Vision is the bird's most important sense and in most species the eye is huge. The ear is not as well developed as the eye but has some role, as auditory cues are important to parrots.

The eye and vision

Predated species, such as parrots, tend to have narrow heads with the eyes set laterally. In parrots the visual field is 300 degrees plus, but they have the narrowest field of binocular vision known in birds: between 6 and 10 degrees.

The eye (Figure 2.18) has a small anterior chamber and the cornea is thinner than in mammals. The posterior chamber is much larger but in parrots the eye is flat, rather than globular or tubular. The shape of the eye allows the retina to have all-round visual acuity (unlike mammals, which have a single region of acute vision). The ciliary body suspends the lens and contains two striated muscles: the anterior and posterior sclerocorneal muscles. The eyeball and its internal muscles are supported by bony scleral ossicles adjacent to the cornea.

The lens is soft and has a central body surrounded by an annular pad, from which it is separated by a fluid-filled space. Accommodation is effected by the posterior sclerocorneal muscle, which forces the ciliary body against the lens, thereby increasing the curvature of the lens. Not only is the lens soft but also it will allow ultraviolet light to pass through.

As the muscles of the eye are striated muscle, including that controlling the iris, birds have conscious control over their iris. Many parrots use their iris as a behavioural signal, especially Amazons; the iris can give a flash of colour.

The retina consists of a large number of cones and some rods. Each cone has its own ganglion and the brain receives a one-to-one signal, giving excellent visual acuity. In contrast, several rods are synapsed to a single ganglion, which allows a small amount of light to trigger an impulse. This gives good night vision. As in mammals, there is a central area in most birds that is devoid of rods. The cones contain an oil droplet, which appears to function as a cut-off filter to absorb short-wavelength light and allow the transmission of longer-wavelength light. Budgerigars have only orange, yellow and pallid greenish droplets. Experiments using coloured seeds show that they see blue but are not red-sensitive. This may be due to their lack of red

2.18 A view of the ventral portion of the left eye of a Grey Parrot. The suspensory ligaments have been omitted on the temporal (right) side of the eye to show the underlying ora serrata. The cartilaginous layer of the sclera abuts to the inner aspect of the scleral ossicles. The scleral ossicles are surrounded by fibrous tissue that becomes the cornea. The inner surface of the iris contains lots of melanin granules; this pigmented layer continues around the ciliary body and finally forms the layer of pigment in the choroid. The optic nerve is overlain by the pecten so it cannot be seen with an ophthalmoscope. The nerve is flattened as it goes through the sclera. The lens forms as a vesicle; the body of the lens arises from the posterior pole and grows until it almost fills the vesicle. In the latter stages of development the annular pad forms as a peripheral ring. The gap between the annular pad and the body of the lens is the remnant of the original lens vesicle. This eye was 16 mm in diameter.

Labels: Body of lens; Cornea; Anterior chamber; Iris anterior layer; Iris pigmented layer; Sclerocorneal junction; Sclerovenous sinus; Scleral ossicle; Ora serrata; Lens vesicle; Retina; Choroid; Cartilage layer of sclera; Fibrous layer of sclera; Optic nerve; Ciliary body; Annular pad of lens; Sclerocorneal muscles; Zonnular fibres; Vitreous membrane; Vitreous body; Pecten

oil droplets. Birds can see colours produced by ultra-violet (UV) light. This is useful in tropical vegetarian birds: forest fruits become UV light-reflective when ripe. Many parrots have UV-reflecting plumage that indicates age and gender.

Most non-predatory birds look closely at an object by turning their head and using a single eye. However, birds do have extrinsic muscles that move their eyes. Parrots are able to move their eyes to look more downwards, upwards or forwards (for example, they can see the end of their beak and look at their food as they select it and pick it up). This can change their visual field by several degrees. The pattern of retinal cells varies with the species and is related to the flying and hunting behaviour of the bird. Whilst flying, many birds are able to view the ground and the horizon at the same time, with both in focus even though they are different distances away from the bird. Not only does

this use different parts of the retina, but the visual impulses also go to different parts of the brain.

The pecten is a thin black pleated structure (7–14 folds in parrots) found in the posterior chamber, whose base is always in contact with the optic disc and overlies the optic nerve. It is a highly vascular structure that is considered to supply nutrients and oxygen to the relatively avascular posterior segment. Tissue fluid has been shown to move out of the pecten into the posterior chamber.

A semi-transparent nictitating membrane protects and cleans the eye (see Figures 2.16 and 19.7). It is moved voluntarily by two muscles under the control of cranial nerve VI. There is a gland associated with the membrane and as the membrane sweeps across the eye it distributes secretions from this gland; as it returns it funnels the secretions towards the tear duct.

3

Husbandry

Alan K. Jones

Introduction

Parrots seen in veterinary practice may be divided broadly into two groups: species that are not very far removed from wild-living birds (most larger parrots); and those that have been bred in captivity for many generations and are very different from the wild original (Budgerigars, Cockatiels and many small parakeets). The various husbandry techniques available for these birds will be discussed, together with their relevance to the general practitioner. The housing method can have a significant impact on possible diseases encountered.

Housing

Husbandry methods may be divided into: collections of birds in aviaries; and pet birds in small numbers in indoor cages.

Aviaries

Layout

Aviaries may be indoor or outdoor, or commonly a combination of both. The latter comprises a building containing compartments with sleeping quarters and/or nest box, plus food and water bowls. Extending from this building and accessed through a closeable pop-hole is an outside flight of wire-mesh construction. Species such as Cockatiels and Budgerigars may be kept in communal groups and are generally sociable birds. It is important in such communal aviaries to provide plentiful perching, feeding, drinking and nesting spaces, to prevent fighting and possible destruction of nests, eggs and chicks (Figure 3.1).

Advantages	Disadvantages
Presence of several birds of one species may *positively* influence breeding activity by: • Allowing wider choice of mate selection • Mimicking natural flock behaviour • Mutual stimulation of breeding condition	• High potential for aggression during breeding season (may lead to loss of extremities, or death) • Suppression of breeding activity if the flight is overcrowded • Dominant birds will pair off and breed but will prevent others from so doing

3.1 Advantages and disadvantages of communal aviaries in the breeding season.

Most larger parrots and parakeets are kept in pairs, in a bank of aviaries with adjacent flights. This allows the keeper control over specific pairings of birds and will avoid any competition for food and nest sites. Neighbouring birds should be compatible, since many will be naturally aggressive to each other, or may be prevented from breeding by the sight of other species. It is important that flights are 'double-wired', i.e. the metal mesh is fixed in two layers with a minimum 3 cm gap. This will prevent birds attacking their neighbours' toes, and will also prevent predators such as cats, rats and birds of prey from reaching parrots through the wire.

Construction

Suitable wire mesh is available by the roll, or in ready-made panels. The thickness or 'gauge' of the wire will vary according to the species kept. Large macaws, for example, require thicker (13 gauge) wire than grass parakeets (16 or 19 gauge). The mesh should be of good quality: cheaper varieties are a source of zinc poisoning (Chapter 20).

The mesh is attached to a framework of metal or wood. Wood should be treated with a bird-safe preservative (e.g. tannalized, or water-based fence paints). Birds' beaks (especially of species like large macaws, or Alexandrine and Derbyan parakeets) are highly destructive, so exposed wooden frames should be protected by sheet metal, or metal may be used to make the frame.

Ideally the mesh frames will be mounted on solid low walls of brick or blockwork (Figure 3.2), to reduce the risk of invasion by rodents. The floor covering may

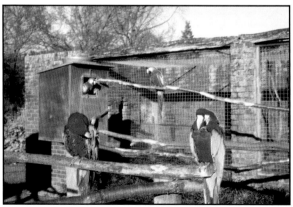

3.2 Scarlet Macaws housed in an outside aviary; note the nest box. Some free-flying Green-winged Macaws are seen in front of the aviary.

be earth or turf, shingle or bark chips, concrete or paving. Earth will predispose to infestation with intestinal parasites, as worm eggs will persist in the soil. Wood products may harbour spores of *Aspergillus* spp. Stones, concrete or paving will reduce these disease risks, provided that they are regularly hosed down and droppings are not allowed to accumulate. Alternatively, birds may be kept in 'suspended aviaries' (Figure 3.3), with a mesh floor fitted above ground level so that droppings and waste food pass through and cannot be reached by the birds. Ample perching should be provided in the flight to ensure that birds do not spend too much time on the wire, since this can damage their feet. It is also necessary to ensure that vermin cannot climb up the supporting legs of the flight. This method is not best suited to birds that naturally forage on the ground, such as Roseate Cockatoos, though these species are obviously most vulnerable to infestation.

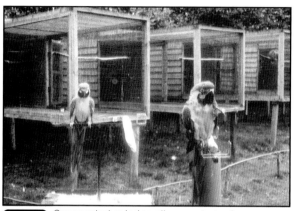

3.3 Suspended aviaries allow waste to drop through the wire floor. Some free-flying Blue and Gold Macaws are seen in front of the aviary.

The roof of the flight may be of mesh entirely open to the elements, provided there is an internal house in which the birds can roost and shelter. Alternatively, part or all of the roof may be covered. Access to fresh air, sunshine and rain will greatly improve feather and skin condition, though birds will require shade from strong direct sun. Against this are potential health risks of raptor or vermin attack; or contamination of the flight with pathogens from wild birds' droppings. On balance the health benefits to be gained from an 'outdoor life' outweigh these possible health risks.

Siting

Siting of the aviary complex is important. Local environmental factors, such as the direction of the sun or the prevailing wind, must be considered. What may offer a cold and miserable environment in one area may provide welcome shade and shelter in hotter climates.

Adjacent vegetation may be significant: leaf fall will make a mess of the flight and overhanging foliage will create a gloomy environment, with continual water drip and consequent algal growth. It will also offer a route for squirrels and rats to reach the aviary roof, while branches breaking off in storms could damage the construction. In general, plants inside the flight are not compatible with parrots, since they will rapidly be destroyed.

The proximity of airports, busy roads or local industries could have a deleterious effect on the health of the birds. Human neighbours are also important:

- Parrots are noisy, and complaints from neighbours can lead to unpleasantness and even the cessation of birdkeeping.
- Nearby cats, noisy dogs or children may disturb the birds, especially while they are breeding, leading to loss of eggs or chicks.
- Neighbours who have frequent barbecues or bonfires pose a real threat with the toxic smoke that could blow into the flights and kill birds.

Aviaries that are totally indoors incur the problems of any intensive rearing system, i.e. inadequate ventilation will predispose to the rapid spread of infectious agents, especially respiratory diseases (Figure 3.4). Against this is the advantage of being able to control temperature, humidity and lighting (which should include ultraviolet light) (Box 3.1).

Advantages	Disadvantages
• Space and the ability to fly • Sunshine and fresh air (if with an outside flight) • Generally fitter birds • May exhibit more 'natural' behaviour	• Need to be acclimatized to outdoor life • Possible attack by or disease transmission from predators or wild species • Vulnerability to theft • Violent weather and other environmental hazards • Possible difficulty in monitoring health and behaviour without disturbing birds

3.4 Advantages and disadvantages of keeping birds in outdoor aviaries.

- All parrots kept indoors should be provided with artificial full-spectrum light (producing both UV-A and UV-B) for normal vitamin D metabolism and breeding behaviour.
- UV-A (315–400 nm) is important for normal vision in birds, allowing them to visualize UV-reflective plumage. This allows for normal breeding behaviour.
- Exposure to UV-B (285–315 nm) is important for endogenous synthesis of vitamin D in birds. This is particularly important for Grey Parrots, which are known to suffer regularly from disorders of calcium metabolism in captivity.
- The bulb should be kept within 30 cm of the bird.
- Light should be provided for at least 60 minutes daily. It is perhaps advisable to mimic the photoperiod for the bird's country of origin.
- Bulbs providing radiation of 295 nm wavelength are the most efficient for vitamin D synthesis. Commercially available bulbs include Arcadia bird full-spectrum (36W FB36) and Philips Flutone tubes (TLD/96S).
- Excessive exposure to UV-B will not lead to vitamin D toxicity.
- Avoid placing physical materials between the bulb and the bird that might block UV-B radiation. Most glasses and plastics do not transmit UV-B radiation.
- Replace bulbs every 6 months, as the ability to produce UV-B is lost long before the capacity to produce visible light.

Box 3.1 Provision of ultraviolet radiation for captive parrots. Courtesy of M. Stanford.

Cages

These, in one form or another, provide housing for the majority of pet parrot species. There is a plethora of designs and sizes available, with a range of prices and finishes, and good examples are often more expensive than the birds.

There is ongoing discussion as to whether or not creatures that are designed to fly should be confined at all in cages, but if they are to be kept in a domestic environment there is no doubt that an appropriate cage is the safest way to house them. The cage should be considered a sanctuary and resting place for the bird and, as far as is possible, the pet should be allowed freedom outside that home, on a stand or with the owner. There are legal requirements linked to the Wildlife and Countryside Act 1981 as to minimum cage size (Chapter 22), which state that a bird should be able fully to open its wings in all three dimensions. Thus a macaw with a 90 cm wingspan must have a cage no smaller than 90 × 90 × 90 cm. This is the absolute minimum, and then used only for limited periods, perhaps as a temporary holding cage.

It is useful to have a small cage or box for transporting the bird (Chapter 4). This container may also be used to put the bird somewhere quiet to rest and sleep, which is useful if the house is noisy or busy, and beneficial in giving seclusion to birds that pluck when stressed (Chapters 16 and 17). Large cages are difficult to transport and so they should be robust enough to withstand repeated dismantling and reassembly, for cleaning or moving.

Cage design

In terms of wire strength, the same criteria of construction appropriate to their occupants apply to cages as to aviaries. An important aspect is that the sides should be flat rather than curved: round or oval cages are not comfortable for parrots. The majority of cross-wires should be horizontal rather than vertical – most parrots spend time climbing, and this will be easier with the former.

The cage material should be easy to clean, with few crevices to harbour dirt and germs. Lightweight plastic trays may be hygienic but they crack easily and are not robust enough for long-term use. Many cages are made of plastic-coated wire, which looks attractive when new but will not withstand for long the attention of a parrot's beak. The underlying metal then becomes exposed and usually rusts: the flakes of plastic, exposed metal and dirt-traps are all health risks.

Large cages may be designed to stand directly on the floor, or smaller ones to be placed on a table or shelf. Others will have legs to raise the cage to a suitable height. This undercarriage may incorporate useful shelving, which will also improve stability by bracing the legs. Castors on the legs will facilitate moving these cumbersome objects. The design may feature trays underneath, or 'skirts' of metal to catch scattered food (Figure 3.5).

Cage equipment

Comfort and safety of the bird are paramount and there are several risk factors to consider. Poorly designed fastenings or fancy embellishments may trap digits (of owners or birds) or may allow the bird to escape. Dirt-harbouring crevices have already been mentioned. However, by far the most important safety aspect, as already mentioned for aviaries above, is the possibility of zinc poisoning from the cage material. Cages that have a powder-coated finish are safe; owners need to ensure that so-called 'zinc-free' cages are in fact so.

Most cages come supplied with perches cut to fit inside, usually made of smooth wood or plastic. These may be easy to clean but should be replaced with

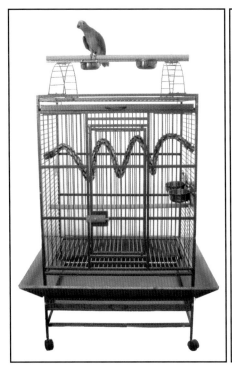
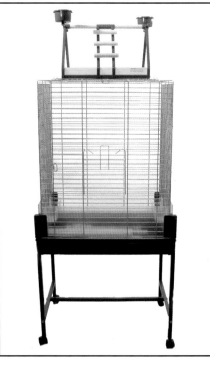

3.5 Good quality commercially available cages. Note the large size, integrated 'playstand' and 'skirt' for catching waste. There is room for many toys, perches and feeders.

natural wood branches (from non-toxic species and a safe source) as quickly as possible. Suitable woods are ash, hazel, birch, willow, eucalyptus, chestnut, sycamore, elder and *untreated* fruit trees. The diameter should be appropriate to the species, such that the toes may curl comfortably around the perch without being either over-stretched or too tightly flexed. Variation in diameter within this comfortable range, as well as the irregular shapes of natural wood compared with metal or plastic, will improve condition of the feet as well as giving the birds physical occupation as they chew the wood. This may mean that the perches require regular replacement, but the birds will be happier and fitter.

A 'play stand' for the bird gives additional stimulation and freedom (Figure 3.6). This may be a commercial product (generally a circular pan with perch and feeding bowls attached) or a home-made construction using natural branches. Trays or skirts to collect debris may be fitted, and the perches may be hung with various toys.

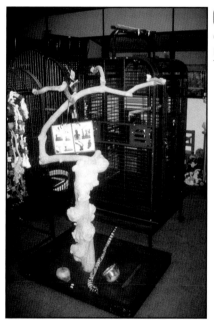

3.6 Commercial playstands with toys.

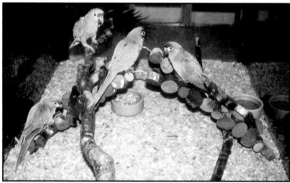

Food and water containers are generally supplied with the cage. These may be plastic, ceramic or stainless steel and may be attached in various ways. Parrots enjoy tipping over and emptying out their bowls and so simple D-cups (Figure 3.8) hooked over the wire are unsuitable for long-term use. Dishes may be inserted through an opening in the side of the cage and held in place with an external clip. Better are swivel feeders,

where a holder is rotated through 180 degrees from inside to outside the cage, enabling the attached bowls to be removed, cleaned and replaced without entering the cage itself (Figure 3.7). The swivel mechanism is secured from outside. These same criteria apply to food and water supplies for aviary birds: swivel feeders make the care and maintenance of outdoor birds quick and easy, without having to enter each aviary in turn.

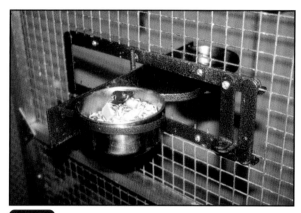

3.7 Swivel feeders are recommended.

Problems for indoor birds

Birds kept indoors are prone to problems shared by their aviary-housed relatives, including dietary or toxic conditions and exposure to noisy pets or children – the latter perhaps even more so. They also experience a range of conditions unique to their domestic environment.

Paramount is the lack of sunlight and fresh air, coupled with a warm dry indoor atmosphere (especially in winter, when heating is on), predisposing to poor feather quality, resulting in dull colours, brittleness and irritation and culminating in feather plucking (Chapter 16). This will be exacerbated by poor diet and boredom. Practitioners see far more feather conditions in indoor birds than in those kept outside, and while this may partly be explained by the former being solitary hand-reared birds with emotional 'hang-ups', the indoor environment and atmosphere have a considerable effect.

The companionship of humans or other birds – or rather its lack or inappropriate nature – will lead to stress-related illness. Parrots are kept often in minimal space (Figure 3.8) and not allowed out for fear

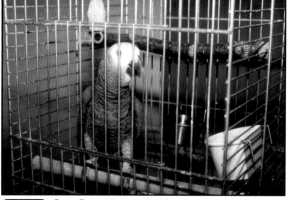

3.8 Grey Parrot in a typical inadequate small cage. Note the D-cup food holders on the bars.

of biting or damage to the home, thus leading to a vicious circle of further confinement. If birds *are* allowed freedom in the household, they may encounter hazards such as other pets, fires and chimneys, saucepans, mirrors and windows, or escape through open doors. Other domestic hazards include salt, chocolate, alcohol, cigarette smoke (marijuana toxicity has also been seen in a pet parrot), poisonous plants (Speer and Spadafori, 1999) and the deadly fumes from overheated non-stick cooking utensils or burning cooking oils.

Choice of bird and source

Wild or captive-bred

Parrots are still imported from their native countries, but regulations for quarantine and importation are changing slowly (Chapter 22). It is probable that there will be an increase in the licensing and registration requirements to keep psittacine species, similar to that required for raptors, with closed rings and recorded numbers.

Wild-caught birds commonly carry infectious diseases such as salmonellosis, Pacheco's disease, chlamydophilosis and intestinal parasites, and will be of uncertain age and temperament. They will not be tame but potentially can be tamed.

Captive-bred birds appear to offer an ideal choice for the pet market; they are acclimatized, used to humans, and do not further endanger natural populations. In practice, this ideal has not been fulfilled for a number of reasons. Firstly, many of these birds are not as robust as their wild-bred counterparts, especially those that are incubator-hatched and hand reared (Figure 3.9). This branch of aviculture is still comparatively new, and not all the answers for raising strong, healthy parrot babies are yet known (see Chapter 18). Secondly, there has been a rapid spread of other infectious diseases through bulk rearing of baby birds and disseminating the offspring through pet shops. Naturally occurring viruses with a long incubation period, such as psittacine beak and feather disease (PBFD), polyomavirus and proventricular dilatation disease (PDD), are now widespread in aviculture because of increased availability of captive-bred parrots (Chapter 13).

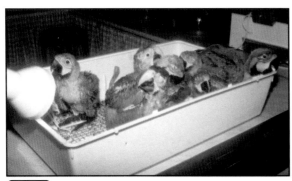

3.9 Hand rearing young macaws.

Many home-bred birds will develop severe psychological problems with sexual maturity, since they are still innately wild species. Hand rearing parrots does not make them domesticated: this requires generations of selective genetic alteration to render them suitable to accept confinement. As these birds mature, they become confused as to their identity, having difficulties relating to both humans and other birds. This can lead to inappropriate sexual behaviour, aggression, screaming, destructiveness, or feather plucking. Such birds often will be passed on repeatedly as being unmanageable, and may be put to sleep or abandoned in a 'sanctuary' (Chapter 17).

Type of bird

As well as the above comments, it is essential to realize the commitment to the longevity of a parrot and its potential for noise, mess and destruction. Generally these are not cheap pets, but if owners buy from the cheaper end of the market they may repent their purchase expensively, since their pet may be unfit, of poor background, and potentially carrying infectious disease (Speer and Spadafori, 1999).

Sexing

Sex and age should be identified. The former is important if the owner requires a specific bird to breed, and (in general) many larger parrots when sexually mature relate better to human owners of the opposite sex rather than the same sex. Young birds that have been hand reared often respond to people of the same gender as the rearer, though quite how birds recognize their owner's sex is uncertain.

Some parrot species are visually dimorphic: Budgerigars have different cere colour, grey Cockatiels have plumage differences, Ringneck Parakeets have a cervical ring of coloured feathers in the adult male, and white cockatoos have iris colour differences. However, all these are visible only in the adult bird; juveniles of both sexes have similar appearances. Some of the newer colour mutations of Cockatiels and Budgerigars do not have the obvious sexual colour variations. An exception is the Eclectus Parrot (see Figure 18.2), in which the marked plumage differences are evident as soon as the chick fledges.

Monomorphic species (the majority of parrots) may be sexed either by DNA analysis of a blood or feather sample, or by endoscopy ('surgical sexing') (Chapter 18). Such birds may be sold with certification of the test, linked to an identity ring worn on the leg.

Ageing

Baby birds of all species, but especially white cockatoos, are appealing and may provoke an impulse buy. Such birds are immediately tame and tractable, but will not necessarily remain that way. The Grey Parrot and large macaws have grey irises as juveniles; these start to turn gradually to yellow from 6 months old, and are usually fully yellow at 1 year old (Figure 3.10). The scales on the feet are softer; the lower mandible is proportionately larger than the upper maxillary beak; and the beak generally is smooth and shiny in juvenile parrots as compared to adults (Figure 3.11).

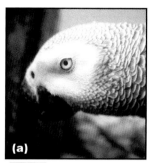 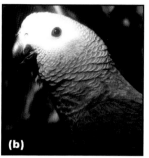

3.10 (a) Adult Grey Parrot with yellow iris; (b) juvenile with grey iris.

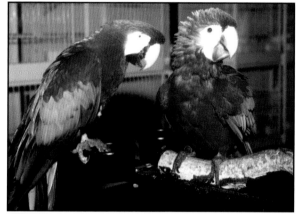

3.11 Scarlet Macaw: note the differences in head shape and beak proportions between the adult (left) and the juvenile (right).

Choice of species

Of the common species available, Figure 3.12 is a brief summary of their characteristics and suitability for captivity. For biological details, see Chapter 1. The comments in Figure 3.12 are generalizations; inevitably there will be exceptions in all cases with individual owners and their birds.

General care and welfare

- *Diet* is very important: poor nutrition and related nutritional diseases are at the root of most problems seen in avian practice. This subject and the use or otherwise of *grit* are discussed fully in Chapter 15.
- The importance of *water* to a bird's plumage has been mentioned: regular *bathing or spraying* is essential to prevent drying and deterioration of feather quality, with consequent feather plucking.
- *Parasite control* is covered in detail in Chapters 13, 15 and 16; external parasites are commonly suggested as a cause in feather-plucking parrots, but in practice this is unusual. Treatment for internal and external parasites might be required in recently imported birds, aviary collections or ground-feeding species, but rarely are they a problem in established indoor pet parrots.
- *Environmental enrichment* is important and necessary. These are highly intelligent creatures, requiring continual mental and physical stimulation for their wellbeing. Regular contact with other birds and/or humans is desirable; if the owner is absent, the radio or television may be left playing (but it is also important to allow the bird adequate rest: over-stimulation can be as stressful as inactivity). Toys and puzzles should be provided. Favourite food items may be hidden inside tubes, woodblocks or empty nut shells. There are many acrylic, wood, leather and rope toys available from pet stores (Figure 3.6) but cheap and easily replaced items such as cardboard boxes, cardboard rolls or pine cones will provide endless occupational therapy.

Large macaws	Require substantial space and can be noisy Most are surprisingly gentle birds, with exception of Scarlet Macaw Long-lived (40–50 years); destructive Have a distinctive smell to the plumage
Dwarf macaws (e.g. Red-shouldered, Yellow-collared)	Generally good small parrot species, but can also be noisy and destructive Commonly feather-pluckers
Cockatoos	Black species rarer, specialist birds, kept only by dedicated enthusiasts White species very common and readily available but not ideal as house pets Many turn from cuddly babies to neurotic, demanding, feather-plucking, screaming, aggressive and destructive misfits and end up being passed from home to home in downward spiral of misery – not fault of bird but primarily due to lack of understanding by human carer(s) as to physical and mental needs of species Produce a lot of powder down
Pionus parrots	Small, attractive, generally quiet and trouble-free birds Distinctive hyperventilation when alarmed that may be mistaken for upper respiratory disease
Poicephalus parrots and caiques	Grouped together because of size and suitability, although the former from African continent (Meyer's, Senegal, Jardine's) and latter from South America Both make good family pets, being not too demanding, with great character and playfulness Caiques can be noisy

3.12 Common species kept in captivity. (continues) ▶

Amazons	Archetypal 'green parrot' Live 35–40 years Wide variety of species, of generally interesting character and reasonable temperament May occasionally be aggressive, but usually good family pets, with no particular fixation on one person Can be noisy (but it is at least a 'musical' noise!) Tend to obesity in cages Very susceptible to hypovitaminosis A with associated sinus problems Distinctive plumage smell
Grey Parrots	'African Grey' the commonest pet parrot, silver-grey plumage, red tail, black beak Slightly smaller Timneh Grey, darker grey body, maroon tail, horn-coloured beak Highly intelligent, good talkers and mimics, but demanding and often become 'one-person' birds Live 35–40 years Should not be owned if owners out at work all day Need continual mental and physical stimulation if not to become frustrated feather-pluckers Often fussy feeders Susceptible to hypovitaminosis A and hypocalcaemia Produce a lot of powder down
Eclectus Parrot	Interesting birds, with marked sexual dimorphism Generally quiet, appear to be studiously observing world around them, with occasional sudden vocal contribution Prone to feather problems and hypocalcaemia Eat more fruit than other common species, therefore have messier droppings Deserve to be more popular
Lories and lorikeets	Fruit and nectar-eating birds, colourful, playful and lively, but *messy* owing to their diet More suited to outside aviaries
Conures	Two groups, generally kept in aviary situations *Aratinga* species are *very* noisy and do not make good indoor pets *Pyrrhura* species smaller and generally quieter, and may make pet birds if taken on young. Playful
Budgerigar	Familiar caged pet in variety of colours, but also large numbers kept by enthusiasts for showing and breeding. Latter birds tend to be larger, yet less fit than 'domestic' variety Prone to adiposity, and tumours of all types, plus viral and genetic feather problems
Cockatiel	Very common, both as house pets and aviary birds, with numerous colour mutations Quite noisy, but sociable Prodigious egg-layers – can become problem in household environment (Chapter 18) Yellow and white varieties prone to skin and feather conditions Produce dust
Other parakeets	Includes ringneck group, small Australian species (Bourke's, Splendids, and other *Neophema* species) and larger Australian species (rosellas) Rosellas and ringneck parakeets may be found for sale as pets in shops, but this should be discouraged. None of these should be considered as indoor caged birds, but are well suited to aviary collections *Neophema* and related species particularly very popular, attractive, easy to keep, and mostly quiet Quaker parakeets are colony birds, but do as individuals make entertaining and easy family pets

3.12 (continued) Common species kept in captivity.

Identification methods

The identification of an individual bird may be important for a number of reasons, including the following:

- To enable breeders to pair specific birds, or to recognize offspring from particular parents
- To trace the origin or supplier
- To provide confirmation of ownership.

Since parrots fly, and thereby escape easily, it is common for 'stray' birds to require identification. Regrettably, there is also a large potential for parrot theft, owing to the high monetary value of these birds. When a stolen bird is located, positive proof of its identity is required to secure a conviction for theft and to reunite the bird with the correct owner. (Addresses for the National Theft Register and the Independent Bird Register are given at the end of this chapter.)

Various techniques are available for marking a bird:

- *Tattooing* has been used (as with greyhounds and farm animals) but tattoo ink appears not to persist in avian skin as well as it does in mammals. Rubber stamping the owner's telephone number across the flight feathers, as practised in racing pigeons, would work as a temporary measure until the bird moults.
- *Photographing* specific features of the bird is useful where there is a recognizable characteristic, such as a deformed beak or missing toes. Facial feather lines in the large macaws appear to be as unique as human fingerprints and may be photographed (Figure 3.13).

- Birds that have been sexed by the DNA method may have their *DNA profile* stored, since this is unique to the bird, and may assist in future identification or relationship disputes. This requires a specific request to the laboratory concerned.
- *Microchip* implantation is used increasingly in avian species, and is a simple, reliable and virtually foolproof method of identification. Full details of the technique and discussion of sites for implantation are given in Chapter 6. The chips are well tolerated by birds, and current types appear to have no complications. Early varieties from different manufacturers caused some confusion with different scanners, but modern types conforming to ISO standards are both universally readable and non-migrating.

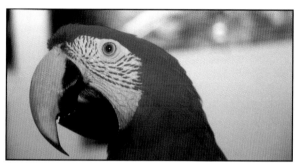

3.13 Facial feather lines on this Green-winged Macaw can be used to identify the individual bird.

Ringing

The current most common method of identifying birds is with a leg ring (leg band). Rings are worn between the foot and the hock, on the non-feathered tarsometatarsus. Rings may be *closed* or *open*. Closed rings consist of a continuous circle of metal, which may only be attached when the bird is a small chick. At this age the toes are small and soft enough to allow passage of the ring over the foot on to the tarsometatarsus.

Open (or 'split') rings are manufactured as an incomplete circle and may be fitted to the lower leg in an older bird, using a plier-like closing tool (Figure 3.14). These rings would be used for simple identification of individuals; as a legal requirement for import or export; or to confirm sexual differentiation following scientific sexing techniques. The advantage over the microchip is that the ring is externally visible.

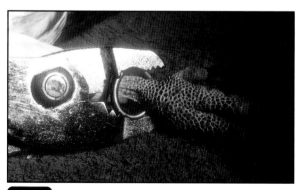

3.14 Ring-closing pliers used to apply a leg ring.

Rings may be plastic but these are only really suited to passerine species or waterfowl, since they are easily removed by a parrot's beak. Aluminium bands, with a flat cross-section, are suitable for smaller parrots but may be bitten through and removed by larger birds. Worse, strong beaks may compress these rings, tightening them on to the leg and creating serious injury, with potential loss of a foot (Chapter 6). This metal may be coloured, and registered colours are used to indicate the year of hatch in Budgerigar societies. There is also a number/letter code, which may include breeder's initials or telephone number, plus the year of hatch and a letter indicating ring size. Later alphabetical symbols (e.g. U, V, W) are larger sizes than preceding letters (R, S, T) (Figure 3.15). There is, however, no universally accepted coding method, nor is there in the UK a central register of all numbers issued. Thus identifying the source of a ring on a stray bird may prove difficult.

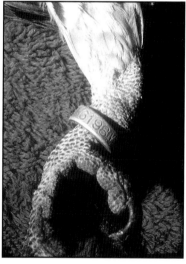

3.15 Aluminium breeder's ring.

Many of the larger parrots are ringed with stainless steel bands, which are tougher and cannot be crushed (Figure 3.16). These may be made in flat cross-section, or more usually they are circular in profile. Closed rings are used on babies, usually bearing the breeder's initials. Split types are placed on older birds and, stamped with a number/letter code, are the most common type used to identify birds for import/export, or to record the results of surgical sexing.

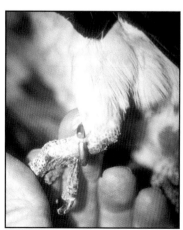

3.16 Stainless steel sexing ring.

These rings are not easily coloured and so, by accepted convention, cock birds are ringed on their *right* legs and hen birds on their *left* legs, allowing for easy visual distinction. However, since similar rings are used by breeders or importers without regard to the sex of the bird, simple distance inspection should not be relied upon as an indicator of a sexed bird. The ring code should be read, to confirm the initials of the veterinary surgeon who performed the procedure (Figure 3.17).

AEUK	Avic Euro (Importers and dealers)
BII	Bird International (Breeders/exporters from Philippines)
PSUK	Parrot Society UK (Issued to PS members to identify their birds)
SEXED/SEXD	Sexed at Pegasus Birds, dealers in Essex
EBHR	English Bred/Hand Reared
Veterinary surgeons' sexing rings:	
ADM	Dermod Malley
ABVET	Andreas Brieger
AEAC	Avian & Exotic Animal Clinic, Manchester
AL	Alistair Lawrie
AKJS	Alan K Jones
BCS	Brian Stockdale
BHVC	Birch Heath Veterinary Centre
CJH	Chris Hall
DNA	DNA sexed via Avi-Gen
JRB	Richard Best
MGB	Matt Brash
NF	Neil Forbes
NHB	Nigel Harcourt-Brown
PWS	Peter Scott
WHWW	William Wildgoose

3.17 Commonly encountered ring prefixes. (Any other combinations are likely to be breeders' initials or importation rings.)

One final type of ring commonly encountered is the Swiss-made open ring that is fitted to adult birds and then held closed with a rivet. These are also used for post endoscopy-sexing identification, and come in two different colours. Black is used for males, and gold for females (Figure 3.18).

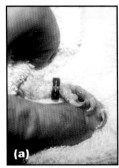 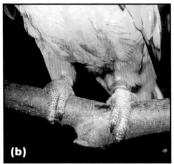

3.18 'Swiss-style' riveted sexing rings as used by Andrew Greenwood: (a) male (black); (b) female (gold).

Useful addresses

Registers

National Theft Register
(coordinated by John and Anita Hayward)
PO Box 243
Bicester
OX26 1ZN
tel. 01869 325699

Independent Bird Register
The White House Business Centre
Hatton Green
Hatton
Warwick
CV35 7LA
tel. 0870 6088500
www.ibr.org.uk

Ring manufacturers

AC Hughes Ltd
1 High Street
Hampton Hill
Middlesex
TW12 1NA
tel. 020 8979 1366
www.achughes.com

Lambournes
Marche Way
Battlefield Enterprise Park
Harlescott
Shrewsbury
SY1 3JE
tel. 01743 443883
email: sales@lambournes.net

JE Bandings Ltd
Unit 4, Bessborough Works
Molesey Road
West Molesey
Surrey
KT8 2HF
tel. 020 8941 5444

Societies

The Parrot Society UK
92a High Street
Berkhamsted
Herts
HP4 2BL
tel. 01442 872245
www.theparrotsocietyuk.org

Publications

Cage & Aviary Birds (weekly)
IPC Media
King's Reach Tower
Stamford Street
London SE1 9LS
tel. 020 7261 6116
email: Birds@ipcmedia.com

Birdkeeper (monthly)
IPC Media
King's Reach Tower
Stamford Street
London SE1 9LS
tel. 020 7261 6116
www.birdkeeper.com

Parrots (monthly)
Imax Publishing Ltd
Unit B2, Dolphin Way
Shoreham-by-Sea
West Sussex
BN43 6NZ
tel. 01273 464777
www.parrotmag.com

4

Handling

J.R. Best

Basic principles of handling

The principles governing the handling of psittacine birds for a clinical examination or veterinary procedure are similar to those governing the handling and restraint of any animal, namely to restrain the animal with the minimum risk of injury or distress to both the animal and the handler. Psittacine birds, especially the smaller species, are delicate animals and it is important to bear in mind that the bird might be injured or debilitated and therefore susceptible to further injury or distress by unsympathetic handling. Successful handling of difficult patients requires a confident and firm, but not rough, approach and this can only be gained through experience.

Whereas smaller psittacine birds are capable of inflicting painful bites, larger birds are powerful individuals with beaks that are capable of inflicting serious wounds. Few psittacine birds are actively aggressive, though most will vigorously resist attempts at capture and respond defensively by biting. It is essential, therefore, in capturing and during subsequent handling to ensure rapid and complete control of the head of the bird, whilst also restraining the wings and feet.

Whenever possible, birds should be handled within rooms with closed doors and windows. Reduction of the light level within a room might assist in the capture of an active bird from a cage and also the retrieval of a bird that has escaped during handling. Similarly, red light, such as in a dark room, might calm the bird. The approach to handling psittacine birds should take account of their nature and husbandry; hence a tame hand-reared pet bird that is used to regular and gentle handling would require a different approach to that for an aviary or caged bird that is only very rarely handled (Chapter 17). However, whether tame or not, *all* larger parrots are capable of inflicting serious injury.

Handling birds (especially pet birds) in a room away from their owners is often a wise precaution. Many owners find it very distressing to see their birds handled and their presence could possibly cause the bird to associate the unpleasant experience with its owner, thus damaging a fragile bird–human bond. Some experienced bird keepers can prove to be valuable assistants in handling their own birds. During an examination the responsibility for the safety of both the patient and assistants is that of the veterinary surgeon and this must be borne in mind when forming a policy for the handling of birds within the practice.

Most medium-sized to large psittacine birds are restrained in towels or cloths by methods described below, but caution must be exercised to prevent the following potential problems:

- Respiration being compromised by excessive pressure placed on the thoracic wall through being held too tightly
- Respiration being compromised by being held in dorsal recumbency for long periods, especially in birds with abdominal masses or coelomic fluids
- Collapse due to congestive heart failure, especially in older birds, obese birds and dyspnoeic birds
- Hyperthermia developing either through prolonged handling (especially if the head is covered) or following a strenuous attempt to evade capture. It has been shown that hyperthermia can occur in Amazons after only 4 minutes of handling (Greenacre and Lusby, 2004).

These dangers should be carefully explained to owners before a high-risk patient is handled. Oxygen should be readily available in the event of an emergency.

Reducing disease transmission

Health and safety implications in handling psittacine birds are primarily the risks of physical injury but also include the real risks of zoonotic infection to handlers and assistants. The use of disposable examination gloves reduces the risk of infection to personnel handling birds and their accommodation but also reduces the risk of cross-infection between patients. To prevent cross-infection, separate freshly laundered towels and cloths should be used for individual birds and kept with, and used only on, that bird whilst it resides in the surgery. Towels are available that do not reflect ultraviolet light and, as birds are sensitive to such light, these towels may cause less stress. It should be noted that most washing powders contain UV enhancers.

Additional precautions, notably the use of surgical facemasks, goggles or eye-shields, should be taken in the presence of birds likely to be carrying air-transmitted infections, especially potential cases of chlamydophilosis (Chapter 22).

Capture

The initial stage in handling a psittacine bird usually involves removal from the cage or box used for transportation. This is the stage at which there is the greatest risk of escape and it is essential to ensure that all windows and doors to the room are closed and that disturbance from outside the room is unlikely.

Whenever possible, it is a distinct advantage to encourage clients to present a bird at the surgery within its own uncleaned cage. This provides a secure container from which to capture the patient and also gives the clinician an opportunity to assess the bird from a distance, gain an impression of its standard of husbandry and an indication of clinical signs, including posture, respiration and the nature of its droppings (Chapter 5). Although patients requiring hospitalization will benefit from being managed in a specialized avian unit, the bird's own cage will provide familiar accommodation in which it could be kept for short-term hospitalization for observation or administration of medication.

Most cages have a door through which the bird can be captured with minimal risk of escape. Removal of toys and perches from the cage will greatly ease capture. It is often impossible to capture and remove birds through a small side door to a cage; however, many cages can be turned on their side with the base removed, through which the bird can be caught once all perches have been removed and a cloth draped over the opening to prevent an escape.

In all but the smallest of psittacine birds (e.g. Budgerigars, grass parakeets), it is preferable to use a towel or cloth to capture the bird from a cage. The thickness and size of the towel or cloth vary with the size of bird. The use of thick leather gloves to capture and handle psittacine birds, although favoured by some aviculturists, is not generally recommended for veterinary attention, as gloves greatly restrict dexterity and the protection afforded against bites by larger parrots is poor.

The approach to the bird should be quiet and confident, with the handler using a reassuring tone of voice and avoiding any sudden movements. Whilst inside a cage the bird is coaxed to climb the bars and is then grasped from behind around the neck using a towel or cloth (Figure 4.1). Small and medium-sized birds can be caught with one hand but larger parrots will require a two-handed approach and possibly the use of two towels. Once the bird has been restrained and when its feet are free of the bars, it can be removed from the cage. The towel or cloth used should be large enough to cover the head and to encircle the bird completely, thus restraining its wings and legs. Most birds will stop struggling once their head is covered and the body is enclosed.

The capture of birds that are presented in purpose-built wooden transport boxes, with sliding doors on the top or rear, should be straightforward. Many birds are presented in front-loading plastic cat-transport boxes and these can cause difficulties, especially with smaller psittacine birds, which can easily escape past the handler's arm through the relatively large opening of the door. This risk can be diminished by draping a towel

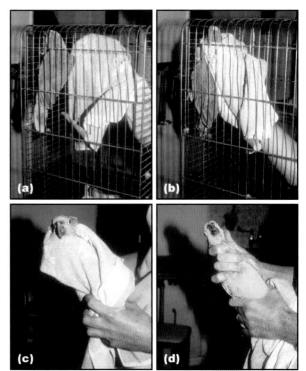

4.1 (a) The bird (in this case a Yellow-headed Amazon) is coerced into a corner of the cage. A towel is draped over the handler's (open) hand. (b) As the bird turns away from the hand it is grasped firmly behind its head. The palm of the hand is against the bird's back. (c) Using the other hand the towel is wrapped around the bird's body, thus restraining its legs and wings. Its feet and beak are extricated from the bars and the bird is removed from the cage. (d) The 'hold' (without the towel in place): the bird is held firmly but not tightly; the thumb and forefinger prevent it turning its head, with the thumb against its cheek and the index finger encircling the neck below the head. The rest of the hand holds the wings so that the bird cannot flap.

over the entrance of the cage, with the door slightly ajar, before attempting to capture the bird.

Cardboard boxes and top-opening cardboard or plastic pet carriers also present a potential for escape during capture. It is preferable to drape a towel or cloth over the top of the container and to open the flaps one by one beneath the covering towel or cloth. The bird can then be captured by gently lowering the towel or cloth and grasping it firmly behind the neck.

The capture of birds from an aviary is, in the majority of cases, most easily and safely performed using a hand-held net (see below). Most aviaries incorporate a built-in shelter connected to the flight into which birds can be encouraged so that they can be captured. Breeding birds in aviaries are provided with nest boxes in which birds will often hide or roost and which, depending on the design, can be used for capturing by blocking the entrance once the bird is inside.

Birds that escape during handling and that are freely flying within a room may be caught using a hand-held catching net for small and medium-sized birds (suitable nets with padded rims are available from pet stores dealing with products for the aviculture trade) or an angler's landing net for larger birds.

With a hand-held net the bird can be caught whilst perched or in flight; once within the net the bird should be trapped by turning the handle through 180 degrees to close the entrance. Larger parrots tend eventually to land on the floor and can then be coaxed into a corner and caught with a net or by covering with a thick blanket or two large towels. If practicable, darkening the room and locating the escaped bird using a torch will greatly reduce the stress to the bird and its captors. It is important to allow the recaptured bird to 'rest' before using anaesthesia; otherwise, the 'adrenaline rush' may predispose to arrhythmia.

Handling for examination and treatment

The basic principles of handling psittacine birds are as follows:

- Ensure that a secure area within the surgery is selected for the capture of a bird from a cage and subsequent handling.
- Check that windows and doors are closed and that unannounced entry into the room is avoided.
- Ensure that all necessary equipment for examination is at hand and, if assistance is necessary, employ trained practice personnel, not the owner.
- Use a darkened room to capture a very active or distressed bird.
- Use a clean fresh cloth, towel or blanket of sufficient size to cover the bird's head and enclose its wings, body and feet.
- Grasp the bird behind its head and neck, holding the cloth so that its head is covered and sufficient material is free to wrap around the wings and body.
- Do not handle a bird for prolonged periods (possibly for periods of no longer than 4 minutes). Replace the bird in a cage immediately if at any time it shows signs of respiratory distress.
- Exercise great care when handling old birds, obese birds and dyspnoeic birds.

Once captured and restrained, most psittacine birds can be handled for examination or for the performance of a procedure. Many procedures require the help of an assistant in the restraint of the patient and it is essential for the safety of the bird and the operators that any person assisting is well aware of the techniques of handling psittacine species and especially the dangers of handling larger parrots. Owners very rarely make safe confident assistants and, with the real risks of injury and the threat of subsequent litigation, such practice should be strongly discouraged, other than in exceptional circumstances.

An adequately sized towel, with a generous thickness, allows the bird to be held safely behind the neck, so controlling the head and beak and, at the same time, covering the head to restrict vision and enclosing the wings, body and legs to control struggling (Figure 4.1). During handling many birds, especially tame pets, can be calmed by gently and repeatedly stroking the crown of the head. Once effectively restrained in this manner most birds will allow restricted examination of the head, body and limbs. Such restraint is adequate for many routine procedures, such as trimming of beaks and nails, placement of gavage tubes, intramuscular and subcutaneous injections, venepuncture and induction of inhalation anaesthesia.

Following handling, care must be taken to prevent any damage or further injury when returning a bird to its cage. If it is able to perch, the bird should be gently released from the towel or cloth so that it can climb directly on to a perch or the bars of the cage.

Sedation or general anaesthesia is indicated for many procedures, especially those that are potentially painful or prolonged or require a passive patient, including radiography. Sedation and general anaesthesia are discussed in Chapter 8.

Small psittacine birds

Handling the smaller species of psittacine birds (Budgerigars, lovebirds and grass parakeets) present few special problems other than those of capturing small birds in large cages and of minor yet painful bites. Most are pet birds presented within a cage that is usually full of toys and perches, and capture is made easier by the removal of these impediments. Frequently the cage will contain several birds and care must be taken to prevent their escape during and after capture of the target bird. Whenever possible, darkness (as described above) is especially useful to assist the capture of small birds in cages.

The use of a small, soft cloth, as described previously, will prevent the handler being bitten. With experience and confidence it will be found that many Budgerigars, especially tame pets and trained exhibition birds, and most grass parakeets are easy to capture with bare hands. Once captured, birds can be handled for examination or for the performance of simple procedures using the 'ringer's grip' (Figure 4.2). The bird's neck is held, within the cloth, between the first two fingers and its wings and body are gently restrained with the closed hand.

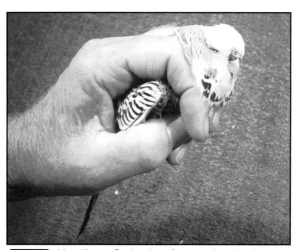

4.2 Handling a Budgerigar for examination: the 'ringer's hold'.

Parakeets and medium-sized parrots

Although many of the parakeets and medium-sized (Cockatiels, Grey Parrots and Amazons) to large parrots that are presented for veterinary attention are hand-reared pets and able to be handled to a certain extent by their owners, it is generally unwise to attempt to handle them for examination without them being securely restrained. As discussed earlier, if assistance is required, then, for safety and legal reasons, it must be given by a competent person, preferably not the owner.

Whenever possible, the bird should be captured from within a confined container (cage or travelling box) and restrained as described previously (Figure 4.1). The presentation of a pet bird at a veterinary surgery on its owner's arm, or, more often, shoulder, should be discouraged. Birds presented in this way can often be restrained in a towel whilst being held by the owner; however, this method lacks the degree of control needed to minimize the risk of the bird being injured and the handler being bitten.

Examination and many simple procedures can be effectively performed with the birds restrained within a towel of suitable size, but with difficult patients or for prolonged or painful procedures sedation or general anaesthesia of suitable subjects is indicated.

Large parrots

The techniques discussed for medium-sized parrots apply equally to large parrots (large cockatoos and macaws) with the caveat that bites from large parrots can cause serious injuries. Great care and caution must be exercised when handling such birds, no matter how tame they appear with their owners.

Capture of some difficult larger parrots, especially those that roll on to their backs and defend themselves with their beak and feet, is safer using the thickness of two towels or blankets and using a two-handed approach to restrain firstly the head and neck and then the wings, body and feet. Once the patient has been restrained, one towel or blanket can be removed to allow easier handling for examination.

Capture of an escaped parrot

Advice is frequently sought on possible action to be taken when a parrot escapes – usually a pet bird that has escaped from a house whilst flying freely within a room or whilst being carried outdoors by an over-trusting owner. It should be emphasized at this point that the majority of parrots that have had their wings clipped by normal methods are still capable of a degree of flight, especially when frightened and when flying outdoors into a head wind. This should be made clear to owners requesting wing clipping for their birds.

Most escaped pet parrots may fly only short distances and usually stay where they land, keeping still and quiet, whereas smaller parakeets may be more mobile and vocal. Early morning is often the best time to locate a lost bird, as there are fewer disturbances and more chance of hearing the bird calling. Tame birds may respond to their owner's voice or return to their cage when it is placed in a prominent position. If located, lost birds may be approached more closely after dark with the aid of torches and then captured with hand-held nets. A bird that has escaped from an aviary may be encouraged to enter an open safety-porch that has been baited with food or by the use of its mate as a decoy. Hosing an escaped bird with water may facilitate recapture by reducing the bird's flying ability.

Advertising, especially using the local media, is frequently successful in locating a lost bird and the use of implanted transponders ensures identification of ownership.

5

The initial presentation: triage and critical care

Aidan Raftery

Introduction

Triage is derived from the French word *trier*, meaning 'to sort out'. It has evolved in emergency medicine to mean the process of identifying quickly those patients who have life-threatening conditions and require immediate attention, as opposed to those who can wait (Figure 5.1).

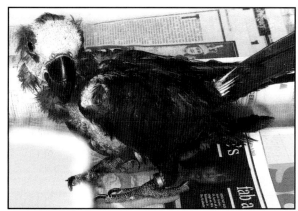

5.1 Eclectus Parrot with generalized feather loss and skin reddening but no signs requiring immediate evaluation. (Compare Figure 18.2)

Information for receptionists

The receptionist is the first point of contact between client and veterinary practice. In veterinary practices accepting avian cases, receptionists require:

- Guidelines for recognizing avian medical emergencies. These must be simple and divide cases into safest interval for treatment (Figure 5.2)
- Information on which species the practice is equipped to treat, and which veterinary surgeons within the practice are accepting avian patients
- A list of avian veterinary surgeons to whom cases may be redirected when avian veterinary knowledge within the receptionist's practice is unavailable.

To allow a full evaluation of the bird at the surgery, the receptionist should request the owners to bring:

- The bird in its own cage if possible or, if not, a picture or video of its cage. The cage should not be cleaned and ideally there should be paper on the floor to allow best visualization of droppings

See as soon as possible:
- Acute change in number and appearance of droppings
- Acute decrease in food intake
- Change in attitude, personality or behaviour
- Fluffed posture
- Decreased vocalization
- Change in breathing or abnormal respiratory sounds
- Acute enlargement or swelling of any body part
- Bleeding or injury
- Vomiting or regurgitation
- Discharge from eyes or mouth

See within 24 hours (if the above-mentioned signs are not present):
- Decrease or increase in water consumption
- Change in weight or general body condition
- Discharge from nostrils
- Change in number and appearance of droppings
- Decrease in food intake

If there is any doubt, consult the veterinary surgeon or a veterinary nurse with avian medicine qualifications/experience. The receptionist should not give medical advice over the phone.

5.2 Receptionist telephone triage to assist the veterinary receptionist or nurse untrained in avian nursing to determine how urgently the patient should be seen. It is based on the major complaint that the owner communicates.

- A fresh dropping sample, on paper in a pot
- Sample of the food fed
- Any treatments already administered
- Vitamin, mineral and any other supplements being given.

If the bird has had veterinary treatment at another veterinary practice, arrangements should be made for the medical history to be available at the time of consultation.

The following points should be borne in mind in the design and management of the waiting room and consulting room:

- All birds to stay inside their secure carriers until within the consulting room
- No open windows or unscreened fans
- Separate areas so that psittacine patients can avoid noisy dogs and staring cats
- Low ceilings and properly fitting lockable doors
- Red lighting available, to help when capturing nervous patients.

History taking

A structured avian clinical examination should be developed and every patient should be examined assiduously. While taking the detailed history, there is time to observe the bird for any abnormalities. Behaviour, movement, body shape, respiratory depth and rate and the bird's reaction to its environment should be noted.

The history-taking list given in Figure 5.3 is a guideline. As the clinical investigation progresses the clinician may need a more detailed history of the relevant system (see individual system chapters).

---

1. Signalment

- Age (if known)
- Sex; how sex established (sexually dimorphic species, DNA testing of blood or feather pulp sample, surgical sexing or unreliably by interpretation of the bird's behaviour)
- Reproductive history if female (laid any eggs, how many and how often)
- Species; captive bred or wild caught; parent reared or hand reared
- Source: direct from breeder, pet shop or other source
- Length of ownership, previous history, when purchased.

2. Environment

- Cage: set-up, position, size and metal used in its construction
- Perches: size, appropriateness of their position and composition
- Photoperiod, and type of lighting to which bird is exposed
- Hygiene: frequency and method of cleaning
- Owner–animal interaction
- In-contact birds (including visits to pet shops, aviaries or boarding facilities)
- Toxin exposure: does it spend time out of its cage when potentially it could have access to toxins, or does it live in the kitchen where airborne toxins generated by cooking could be significant?

3. Diet

- What is fed; consider what is actually eaten
- Purchased loose or in sealed bag
- Food preparation and storage methods
- Water source, any supplements added, and whether water can be contaminated by droppings or bird's bathing
- Hygiene: frequency of cleaning and replenishing food and water containers.

4. Presenting signs

- Record the reason the bird is being presented for veterinary examination
- If signs present, establish when first noticed
- Have signs progressed, remained unchanged, or improved?
- Has owner noticed any other changes (e.g. in droppings, vocalization, food/water intake, behaviour)?

5. Medical history

- Previous medical history of patient must be reviwed (including treatments carried out by owner and any previous veterinary treatment).

5.3 Guidelines for history taking.

Clinical examination

Birds often hide signs of illness and may be very ill by the time that the owner notices that there is a problem. Conversely, owners of strongly bonded birds may notice signs early on that the bird may hide from strangers (Figure 5.4).

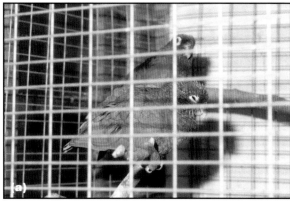
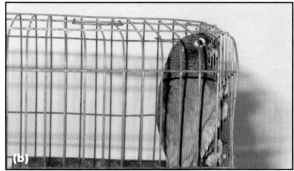

5.4 (a) The female of this pair of Maximilian's Pionus Parrots, with her eyes half-shut and unresponsive, was too weak to stay on her perch. She was caught and put into a cage, then transported to the surgery. (b) On the consulting room table 20 minutes later, the same bird was able to climb around the cage and look alert. She died within a short period of time from yersiniosis.

The bird should be observed before it is handled. Assessing the bird's attitude, conformation, stance, movement and respiratory rate and effort is best done from a distance, to reduce the effect on the bird's behaviour.

Capture and restraint

After remote observation, the patient must be caught and restrained (Chapter 4) in order to carry out a complete physical examination. In the critically ill bird, handling time must be minimized and only a brief clinical examination may be possible (see 'Stabilization of the critical case' later in this chapter). It is important to decide what will be needed for handling, for the examination and for collecting diagnostic samples and have everything set up in advance.

It is essential to have the assistance of a veterinary nurse competent in handling parrots. The increased struggling associated with inexperienced handlers during capture and restraint can have significant consequences. Some psittacids, especially the larger macaws, are very strong and the assistant needs to be physically able to restrain the patient; otherwise there is a very high risk of injury to the assistant, the veterinary surgeon and the patient. Owners should not be allowed to restrain their birds, for the safety of all concerned and in some cases to preserve their relationship with the bird.

Weight

All avian patients should be weighed each time they are examined. Hospitalized birds should be weighed daily, first thing in the morning. Trained birds will stand on a perch attached to the scales; others will have to be placed in a weighing box (Figure 5.5).

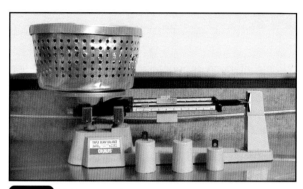

5.5 Balance scales with animal box.

Weight alone should never be used as a measure of body condition. Other factors such as pectoral muscle mass and palpation of the coelomic space have to be considered.

Physical examination

The clinician must be familiar with what is normal for the species (Chapters 1 and 2). It is advised that the aspiring avian clinician make arrangements to examine many healthy individuals of the species that they are going to treat. It is only by being familiar with the normal that the clinician will be in a position to recognize the abnormal.

Sex

The sex of those species that are sexually dimorphic should be recorded (Chapter 3). Monomorphic species can be sexed by DNA analysis or alternatively during coeloscopy examination (Chapter 9), which is often used in the investigation of a sick bird.

Beak

The beak should be symmetrical and smooth. Shape and appearance are species dependent, as is the growth rate. There are differences in the normal length even among similar species; for example, the Green-winged Macaw has a larger beak than the Scarlet Macaw, which has a similar body weight. Both of these species have a mainly ivory coloured upper beak with black tips at the wearing edge and these can be compared with the massive black beak of the Hyacinth Macaw (see Figures 11.20 and 11.21).

In some species (e.g. Grey Parrot) the relatively large amount of powder down produced give their black beaks a greyish appearance. In these species a shiny black beak may indicate a disease process affecting the powder down feathers (Chapter 16), whereas in other species a shiny black beak is normal (Figure 5.6; see also Figure 13.4).

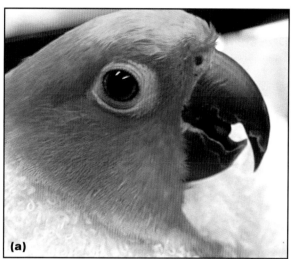

(a)

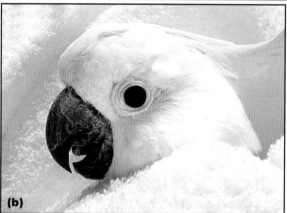

(b)

5.6 (a) The normal shiny beak of a Jenday Conure. (b) The normal dusty grey beak of a Triton Cockatoo.

Beak deformities may have many aetiologies. Neonates are most commonly seen with deviations of the beak. In adult birds deformities can be seen caused by trauma (Figure 5.7), such as fractures, growth plate damage resulting in grooves or deviations (Chapter 11) and iatrogenically by incorrect beak trims (Chapter 6). Nutritional deficiencies can

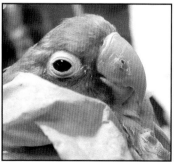

5.7 Lovebird with bite wound on the beak.

cause a rough flaky beak that crumbles when a metal speculum is used to open the oral cavity (Chapter 12). Cnemidocoptic mites (especially common in Budgerigars) and chronic hepatopathies are also common causes of poor beak quality (Chapters 16 and 20). There are several viral diseases that can affect the beak (Chapter 13). Neoplastic lesions, especially squamous cell carcinomas and melanomas, can cause distortion of the beak.

Oral cavity

The oral cavity can be most easily opened for inspection by holding the bird with one hand while the other hand holds an oral speculum in place (Figure 5.8).

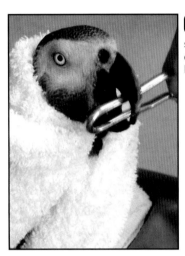

5.8 Using a metal speculum for oral examination of a Grey Parrot.

An alternative method is to use two gauze loops (Figure 5.9). An extra pair of hands is necessary for this method, but it is less likely to cause damage when the beak is of poor horn quality. Alternatively, general anaesthesia may be necessary to examine the oral cavity properly. A light source will be needed to examine this area.

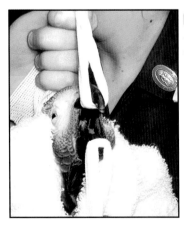

5.9 Gauze loops used to examine the oral cavity.

The mucosa of the oral cavity should be smooth and moist, and pink if not naturally pigmented (Figure 5.10). The choana, which is the opening into the nasal cavity through the hard palate, should be symmetrical. Any asymmetry of the opening might be associated with

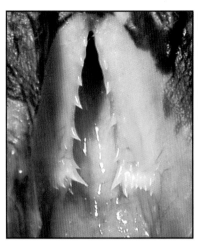

5.10 A normal (non-pigmented) choana in a Galah. There are species differences in shape and number of papillae.

chronic infection or neoplasia. Symmetrical distortion and non-patency of the slit, i.e. choanal atresia, are occasionally seen in Grey Parrots (Chapter 2).

The choanal papillae can be seen projecting caudomedially from the edge of the slit. Blunting of these papillae should be noted; it can (among other conditions) be associated with hypovitaminosis A (Chapter 12). Any discharge from the choanal slit is abnormal and is usually associated with a rhinitis or sinusitis. Samples for cytology and microbiology can be taken from the rostral part of the slit to help to establish the aetiology.

The slit just caudal to the choanal opening is the infundibular cleft, into which the right and left pharyngotympanic (eustachian) tubes open. This is very difficult to examine in the conscious bird.

The tongue of most parrots is thick and fleshy. Swellings and thickenings especially along the sides are often associated with the squamous metaplasia of hypovitaminosis A (Figure 5.11).

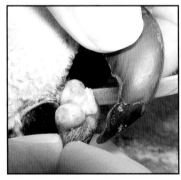

5.11 Multiple abscesses on the tongue of a Grey Parrot.

If possible, the laryngeal opening should be examined. It should be symmetrical and covered in smooth moist mucous membranes. There should not be any discharge from the trachea. Lower respiratory tract disease should be suspected if the larynx is seen to be constantly open, especially when combined with a voice change or loss.

Gross changes in oral cavity disease are rarely specific and bacterial infections are often secondary (Figures 5.12 and 5.13).

Nutritional	Hypovitaminosis A
Non-infectious	Trauma Foreign bodies Local irritants
Viruses	Herpesvirus Polyomavirus Poxvirus
Bacterial	Opportunistic secondary invaders
Fungal	*Candida albicans* *Aspergillus* spp.
Neoplasia	Mainly epithelial or mesenchymal

5.12 Oral cavity disease.

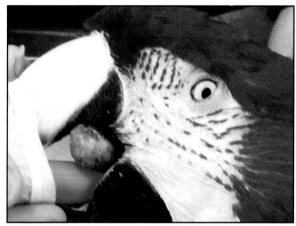

5.13 Green-winged Macaw with oral tumour. Note the cere in this species and compare with the Amazon in Figure 5.15.

Eyes

An ocular examination is an important part of the general clinical examination and is obligatory in birds with traumatic injuries. Ocular lesions make it more likely that the bird will have a traumatic incident; conversely, traumatic incidents (especially head trauma) commonly result in ocular damage

Initial assessment of vision should take place before the bird is restrained. Can it find its food and water? Can it avoid novel obstacles? Often a bird that has gradually lost its sight will have become familiar with its normal surroundings, but it will bump into new items in its cage. Blind or partially sighted birds will behave differently outside their cages and will be reluctant to fly. If loss of vision is suspected, the bird should be tested to see whether it will follow a moving object. The menace response and the pupillary light reflex are not reliable in psittacids.

In many species the periocular area is devoid of feathers and can be vividly pigmented. For example, in the Sulphur-crested Cockatoo this area is pale blue. Blue and Gold Macaws have lines of small black feathers in a white periocular area (this species will 'blush' when excited: the white periocular area turns pink). Any periocular swellings should be noted. Differentials would include infraorbital sinusitis, neoplasia, trauma, lacrimal gland inflammation, *Cnemidocoptes* infestation and avian pox.

- The eyelids should be symmetrical and free from any swellings, discolorations and discharges.
- The transparent nictitating membrane should be seen moving briskly across the eye and is responsible for blinking and spreading the tear film.
- The conjunctival tissues should be pale pink and free from discharges.
- The cornea is similar to the mammalian cornea and should be clear and bilaterally symmetrical.
- The posterior chamber must not be neglected. This is the most common area injured by head trauma.

Iris colour depends on the species, and in some species it depends on age and sex. Immature birds of many species have a different coloured iris from adults; for example, in Grey Parrots it starts out grey and changes to yellow with maturity (Figure 3.10). In many cockatoo species, iris colour can help to differentiate between the sexes of mature birds. For example, in Greater Sulphur-crested and Umbrella Cockatoos the iris is dark brown in males and dark red in females, whereas in Moluccan Cockatoos the iris is black in males and dark brown in females.

Chapter 2 gives details of ocular anatomy and Chapter 19 has a more detailed description of the ophthalmic examination.

Ears

Both external ear canal openings should be examined; they are located on the side of the head just under the eyes. The opening is hidden by feathers (the ear coverts).

The head should be rotated relative to the body to find the optimum position to visualize the external ear canal. If abnormalities are found, endoscopic examination of the external ear canal may be needed. Generally a 1.2 mm zero degree semi-rigid endoscope is the best choice.

Generally ear infections are rare but if an infection is diagnosed the patient should be checked for any predisposing immunosuppressive disease processes. Infraorbital sinusitis, especially when involving the postorbital diverticulum, can sometimes cause swelling in the ear (Chapter 14). Trauma may cause bleeding. Neoplasms are seen occasionally. Cnemidocoptic mites can occasionally cause proliferation of the skin in and around the external ear canal (Figure 5.14). Microscopic examination of a skin scraping is usually diagnostic.

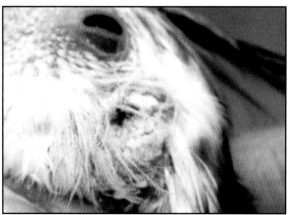

5.14 Cnemidocoptic mite-induced changes to a Cockatiel's ear.

Cere

The cere is the thickened area at the base of the maxillary beak. The external nares are contained within the cere in psittacids. In some species, such as Cockatiels, the cere is a well developed structure; in others, e.g. lovebirds, it is smaller and hidden by feathers. It is important to be familiar with the normal for the species being examined (Figures 5.13 and 5.15). In male Budgerigars the cere turns blue with maturity (cere colour varies with some colour mutations). In older Budgerigar hens it often hypertrophies; if this is occluding the nares, removing excess horn will be necessary. High levels of oestrogens in males from, for example, oestrogen-secreting tumours can cause the blue cere to turn brown and hypertrophy.

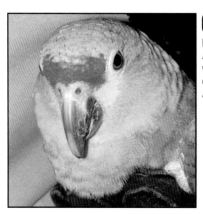

5.15

Red-lored Amazon. Note the well developed cere typical of Amazons.

Nares

The openings should be bilaterally symmetrical. Each naris should be examined for the presence of discharges, which can be seen as staining on the feathers or as plugs blocking or restricting the opening. Chronic sinusitis (bacterial or fungal) can cause soft tissue erosion, resulting in a much enlarged opening that may be filled with a rhinolith that has to be removed (Chapter 14).

Head and neck

The skin and feathers of the head and neck should be observed for any abnormalities. Abnormal swellings should be investigated. Infraorbital sinusitis will often result in a soft tissue swelling, most commonly anterior to the eye but the site depends on which diverticulum of the sinus is swollen (see Figure 11.24). Cnemidocoptic mites can cause scaly skin around the beak and ears (Figure 5.14).

Cervicocephalic air sac distension may cause distension of the neck, whereas a tear in the air sac or fracture of one of the pneumatic bones may lead to subcutaneous emphysema. There are normal featherless areas of skin called apteria, which owners sometimes 'find' and are concerned that they are abnormal. The apterium overlying the jugular vein is very useful when jugular blood samples are required. This area can also be usefully transilluminated to examine the soft tissue structures in this area (e.g. for visualizing crop contents: birds are sometimes presented because the owner has suddenly noticed the lumps caused by seeds in a normal crop).

Crop

The crop should be carefully palpated for the presence and consistency of its contents (forceful palpation may cause regurgitation, with a significant risk of aspiration). It is unusual for the crop to be empty, unless food has been withheld. The clinician should be familiar with the normal variation in crop consistency between birds on different diets.

- If the consistency of the crop contents are doughy, there may be a crop stasis (Chapter 15).
- Foreign bodies present within the crop are often palpable.
- Crop burns are most commonly seen in nestlings being hand reared (Figure 5.16). These are usually presented as fistulas through the crop wall, but sometimes they are presented earlier when only the discoloration of the dead skin is noticeable.

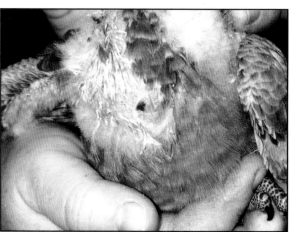

5.16 Skin necrosis in a Grey Parrot caused by hot liquid, given by crop tube; this later developed into a crop fistula when the dead skin sloughed.

- Bite wounds are another common cause of crop fistulas. Small fistulas may heal with medical management, but often surgical repair is necessary (Chapter 10).
- Thickening of the crop wall may be caused by fungal and/or bacterial infections, trichomoniasis (most commonly in Budgerigars) and neoplasia. Samples can be obtained by aspirating crop contents through a sterile crop feeding tube.
- Perforation of the crop or cervical oesophagus can occur in birds that are being tube fed. The instrument perforates the crop or oesophagus and the bolus of food is deposited subcutaneously.
- In Budgerigars it is common to find both lipomas and xanthomas in the skin overlying the area of the crop. Moistening the area with alcohol will temporarily dampen down the feathers and make it easier to visualize and help to determine whether the crop is involved. Cytology is usually necessary to confirm the diagnosis.

Pectoral musculature and keel

The pectoral musculature is palpated to help evaluate the bird's body condition. In the absence of a historical weight for the individual, pectoral muscle mass gives the best indication of body condition. Damping the feathers in the area with an alcohol-soaked cotton wool ball will improve visualization.

Species prone to obesity will often lay down fat in this area, which is readily visualized under the thin skin. When fat is found in this region the bird can be judged, as obese, as fat is more readily laid down internally. Asymmetry between the sides may indicate atrophy due to disuse of one wing, neurological disease or a condition of the pectoral musculature itself, including trauma, neoplasia or infection (bacterial, fungal or parasitic; e.g. with the muscle cysts of the protozoan parasite *Sarcocystis*).

Haemorrhage in the pectoral muscles may be traumatic in origin. Conditions that affect blood clotting (e.g. chronic hepatitis) will predispose to haemorrhages. Polyomavirus infection, especially in the larger parrots can also cause haemorrhages in the pectoral musculature (see Figure 7.18).

The prominence of the keel depends on the species being examined and to a lesser degree on individual variation. It should be straight, with no indents or deviations. Changes in shape usually result from flying injuries. Many have been caused at the fledgling age: when the bird was learning to fly, a diet marginal in calcium resulted in softer bones, making deforming injuries to the keel more likely.

The pectoral musculature and keel is an area where cockatoos often mutilate themselves. The investigation of self-mutilation should include biochemistry and haematology and whole body radiography. A pectoral muscle biopsy may be needed for microbiology and histology. This behaviour, if not caused by organic disease, can also be caused by a psychological disorder (Chapters 16 and 17). Placing a collar to prevent the mutilation without attending to the underlying condition or providing an alternative releasing behaviour will only aggravate the bird's mental condition.

Coelomic area

This area should usually have a concave profile, except in the chick, where it has a convex profile. Coelomic cavity fluid or a mass such as organomegaly, neoplasia or an egg may result in a distended profile. Gentle palpation may identify the bulging as fluid or as a solid mass. When fluid is present, rupture of the air sac membrane could result in flooding the lungs. If there are follicles present on the ovary, overzealous palpation can easily rupture a follicle and lead to egg yolk peritonitis. When a solid mass is palpable this may be neoplasia, organomegaly or an egg, or it may be an organ displaced by a pathological process behind it.

When fluid is present, diagnostic samples should be taken for analysis. Ultrasonography, radiography and a biochemistry/haematology profile are often essential parts of the investigation of distension of the coelomic cavity. Endoscopy is sometimes needed to reach a definitive diagnosis but is contraindicated when there is fluid present.

Vent

The vent is the external opening of the cloaca. The rectum, ureters and the male and female reproductive tracts open into the chambers of the cloaca (see Figure 2.12). The dorsal and ventral lips form the vent, a transverse opening which in the normal bird is held closed by the tone of the sphincter muscles. No tissue should be seen to be protruding and there should be no discharges present. Soiling or feather loss around the vent is abnormal and its cause should be investigated.

Examination of the cloaca is limited to the vent and the posterior compartment of the cloaca, the proctodeum. A moistened cotton bud can be used to evert the mucosa of the proctodeum. Endoscopy is needed to examine the cloaca more effectively (Chapter 9).

Tissue seen prolapsing through the vent may be cloacal tissues, oviduct, ureter, rectum, an intussusception or tissue masses (Figure 5.17). A correct diagnosis is essential before treatment can be initiated (Figure 5.18).

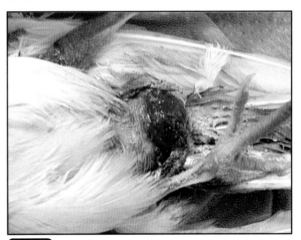

5.17 Cockatiel with a cloacal prolapse.

Prolapse of cloacal tissues	Caused by chronic straining, poor muscle tone or sexual frustration
Prolapse of oviduct	Usually a complication of egg laying (Differentiating oviductal from rectal prolapse can be difficult; endoscopy might be needed)
Prolapse of rectum	Seen with any condition causing prolonged tenesmus Intussusception on rare occasions may prolapse and be difficult to differentiate from rectal prolapse Both presentations are surgical emergencies and require immediate attention (Chapter 10)
Prolapse of tissue masses	Papillomatous lesions most common masses seen protruding through vent; occur most often in Amazons and macaws Diagnosis can be confirmed by applying acetic acid, which causes tissue to blanche if a papillomatous lesion Other tissues may require cytology or biopsy to achieve definitive diagnosis
Bacterial or yeast cloacitis	Sometimes diagnosed but usually secondary to another condition, either in cloaca or elsewhere

5.18 Prolapses through the vent.

Cloacoliths are urate stones or mixed faecal/urate stones that occupy the cloaca. They form when there is a disease process causing delayed or incomplete emptying of the cloaca, or where it is completely obstructed. Efforts must be made to identify the underlying cause or it will recur.

Pelvic limb

Initial assessment of the pelvic limb should start before the bird is restrained. Is the bird bearing weight equally on both feet? Is it walking normally?

With the bird in restraint, both legs should be palpated to compare the muscle mass for symmetry. Any area of swelling or atrophy should be noted. Atrophy can be caused by chronic disuse or by a neurological problem. Swollen areas may be due to abscessation, neoplasia, haematoma or muscle cysts caused by *Sarcocystis*.

The skin overlying any muscle abnormalities should be examined for colour change that may indicate bruising. Bruised areas turn a vibrant green colour after approximately 2 days. This may indicate trauma and there may be a bone fracture at the site. All the bones of the limb should be carefully palpated, and joints tested to evaluate whether their range and direction of movement are normal (Chapter 2).

Swollen joints need to be investigated by radiography and cytology. If sepsis is suspected, a culture and sensitivity of the joint aspirate is indicated. Where deposits of uric acid crystals are the cause (i.e. gout) these can often be seen through the skin. The cause of gout should always be investigated to allow an appropriate treatment plan and prognosis to be formulated.

Careful palpation of the bones may identify bony deformities. In the adult bird angular deformities are often a result of juvenile osteodystrophy and are due to a diet marginal in calcium and vitamin D_3 during their growing phase, or premature exercise on the immature skeleton (Harcourt-Brown, 2004). Radiography often reveals angular deformities of the skeleton that are not appreciated on palpation. The most commonly affected bone is the tibiotarsus (Harcourt-Brown, 2003). In the adult bird many of these angular deformities are subtle and non-progressive and do not need attention. However, extreme deformities need correction to establish normal limb function (Chapter 11). When angular deformities of a bone are diagnosed in a growing bird, they should be attended to immediately. Waiting for the skeleton to mature before treatment may lead to greater deformity, and growing bones have a greater ability to remodel and heal (Chapter 18). Any nutritional and management shortcomings should also be corrected.

Where a fracture is suspected the clinician should exercise great care on examination of the limb. In general, avian bones are surrounded by little tissue, resulting in the sharp ends of the fracture more easily penetrating the skin, reduced support for bone fragments and the blood supply being more easily disrupted, with haematoma formation being common. Radiography is essential when a fracture is suspected and should be performed as soon as the patient is stable (Chapters 9 and 11).

Feet

The psittacine foot is zygodactyl and each digit terminates at a nail (Chapter 2). The nails should be smooth and of an appropriate length and shape. They may have to be clipped regularly, but there should be an attempt to provide an environment where normal wear makes clipping unnecessary.

The skin of the foot (and of non-feathered leg) should have a regular scale pattern on both the dorsal and plantar surfaces. There are pads on the plantar surface at the metatarsophalangeal articulation and on the digits. These are specialized thickenings to bear the weight and withstand compression. There is a prominent pattern on their weight-bearing surfaces which should be visible even in the older bird (Figure 5.19). If the pattern has disappeared and the skin on the pads is smooth and shiny (Figure 5.20), the causes need to be investigated and corrected at this stage before it progresses further. Inadequate perches, reduced exercise (Chapter 3), obesity (Chapter 12) or any disease that will reduce blood circulation to and from the foot or cause the bird to sit still for extended periods will cause these changes, which may progress to 'bumblefoot' (Chapter 11).

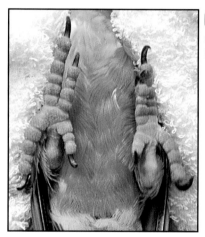

5.19 Normal plantar surface of the psittacid foot.

Each toe should be palpated and movement of the joints assessed. Swellings at joint level can be caused by the accumulation of uric acid crystals (gout; Chapters 7 and 20), bacterial sinusitis or bony and soft tissue changes secondary to trauma, neoplasia or inflammation. Radiography, cytology, bacteriology, biochemistry and haematology may be necessary to achieve a diagnosis.

Swellings of toes may occur with constricting bands of fibrous tissue (Figure 5.20). This is most frequently seen in immature birds being hand reared (Chapter 18). When seen in adults the management remains the same as in the paediatric patient. Leg rings sometimes cause a constriction leading to swelling of the entire foot. This is most commonly seen in the Budgerigar. Sometimes the incorrect size of ring has been applied, but often proliferative skin changes, caused for example by cnemidocoptic mites, have resulted in accumulations of dead skin under the ring, eventually leading to a constriction that initially blocks venous drainage (Figure 5.21).

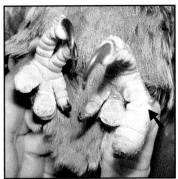

5.20 Adult Severe Macaw with a constricting band of fibrous tissue (arrowed) causing swelling of the distal digit. Note reddening and flattening of papillae on the surface of the feet.

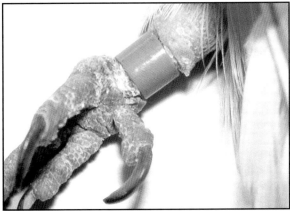

5.21 Budgerigar ring with built-up keratinous material causing restriction of venous drainage.

Trauma is common from bite wounds or through a flighted bird landing on top of a closing door. Self-trauma can be secondary to another lesion or to a neuritis. Granulomatous lesions in the coelomic cavity or renomegaly may cause a neuritis of the nerves supplying the foot, causing pain that often leads to self-trauma. Renal adenocarcinoma in the Budgerigar is a common example where the resultant neuritis, from pressure of tumour invasion, causes lameness that is usually unilateral.

Wings

Is there a history of the bird's flying ability deteriorating, or it becoming reluctant to fly? Other disease processes will often affect flying ability through general weakness and will predispose the bird to flying injuries. A complete clinical examination, including an ocular examination, is essential to rule out other disease processes.

How the wings are held while the bird is perching should be observed. A drooping wing may indicate a problem in the wing, the thoracic girdle (i.e. scapula, clavicle or coracoid bones) or the pectoral muscle, or a neurological deficit. Pain may also cause wing dysfunction, mimicking that of neurological deficits.

As in the leg, the muscles should be carefully palpated for any areas of swelling or atrophy. The joints should be palpated for swelling, heat and pain and to evaluate their range and direction of movement. The bones of the thoracic girdle and of the wing should be palpated for any deformities. Fractures of the humerus may result in subcutaneous emphysema, as a diverticulum of the clavicular air sac extends into its medullary cavity.

The primary and secondary flight feathers should be palpated at their insertions on the ulna, carpometacarpus and the digits. Any deviation from normal can be more easily visualized by damping the feathers with spirit (sparingly, to avoid chilling).

The propatagium should also be palpated. This is the triangular area of feathered skin between the shoulder and carpal joints. Its anterior leading edge contains the elastic propatagial ligament, which is very important for normal flight. Any swellings should be investigated. The elasticity of the propatagium and its ligaments is easily appreciated during the examination. Ventrally the propatageal area is a common site of self-mutilation, leading to a localized chronic ulcerative dermatitis. These lesions are commonly seen in lovebirds, Cockatiels and Grey Parrots (Chapter 16).

Feathers

The history should record answers to the following questions:

- When was the last moult?
- Was it a complete moult, or were there feathers that were not replaced?
- What is the frequency of moulting in this individual?
- How long does the moulting process take?

In the normal psittacid there should be a moult every 12 months. The length of the moulting process varies between species and according to whether or not they are reproductively active. The sequence of feather replacement in a moult is also predetermined, allowing an assessment of how far the moult has progressed. Birds with subclinical conditions, on poor nutrition and in an inappropriate environment will moult less frequently and each moult will take longer or may not be completed. Further questions include:

- For how long have the feather abnormalities noted by the owner been present?
- Are the feather changes progressive?
- Where on the bird did they start and which feather types are involved?
- Is there a seasonal pattern and at which time of the year were the changes first seen?

Colour change

Sometimes feathers will change colour, or after a moult the new feathers may be a different colour. The most commonly seen example is in the Grey Parrot, when some red feathers appear that should be grey. Often there is no obvious cause, but it can sometimes be caused by circovirus infection (see Figures 13.7 and 16.19). Testing for circovirus infection should be part of the investigation in these cases.

Green feathers can sometimes be replaced by yellow after a moult. This can be due to viral, nutritional or internal disease. When the problem is resolved these feathers will return as green at subsequent moults. Green feathers will sometimes turn black due to a fungal growth on the feathers: organic debris accumulates on the feathers and is colonized by airborne fungal spores.

Decreased frequencies of moulting and abnormal preening are among the predisposing causes, which should be investigated.

Normal changes from juvenile to adult plumage must not be confused with the abnormal (del Hoyo *et al.*, 1997; Juniper and Parr, 1998).

Feather loss

Birds are often presented because owners have found an apterium (an area of skin that normally does not have any feathers). The scapular apterium is the commonest one that is confused with feather loss.

Generalized feather loss is diagnosed when lost feathers are not replaced. A careful examination of the skin will be needed to differentiate between cases where the bird is plucking out the newly emerging feather or where there is a failure of the epidermal collar in the follicle to grow a replacement feather. Where failure of feather growth is suspected, the possibility of systemic disease should be investigated.

Cases involving self-inflicted feather loss and damage are very common. It is essential in these cases that the bird is given a full clinical examination and that its nutritional status is evaluated. They are often seen after many months of home treatments where owners have been attempting to treat 'boredom'. Unfortunately most of the hobbyist's books incorrectly state the main cause of feather plucking as boredom. These cases can be particularly challenging to bring under control. The abnormal behaviour has to be managed in parallel with investigating the underlying cause. It is important to see these cases early before the behaviour becomes habitual.

If an organic disease has been ruled out, a psychological disorder may be the trigger of the behavioural problem. It is important to attempt to make a diagnosis (Chapters 3, 16 and 17).

Feather abnormalities

Abnormal feathers are seen for a variety of reasons. Genetic disorders are rare, though colour mutations are highly prized by aviculturists and many species are available in a range of colours (Chapter 3). In the Budgerigar, feather duster disease is a genetic disorder where there are excessively large feathers.

- *Feather cysts* in psittacids are most commonly seen in Blue and Gold Macaws (Chapters 10 and 16).
- *Stress lines* in the vanes of feathers are the result of an insult to the feather follicle while the new feather is developing (Chapter 16). Traumatic or inflammatory damage to the blood feather resulting in localized haemorrhage will often give rise to horizontal black lines that usually extend across both the vane and the shaft.
- *External parasites* (i.e. lice and mites) are rarely seen in pet psittacids in the UK.
- *Folliculitis* of multiple follicles can result in a range of abnormal feather developments. Feathers develop with constrictions of the shaft

which result in its fracture, retained feather sheaths, pulp cavity haemorrhage and shortened clubbed and curled feathers. These signs are generally manifestations of systemic disease (Chapter 13). Localized disease processes will result in feather pathology being confined to a small area.

- *Haemorrhage from a feather* can occur when it is damaged at the development stage commonly known as a blood feather. This should not be confused with pulp cavity haemorrhage as mentioned above, which will usually be seen in multiple feathers.

Poor plumage condition can be seen in birds for a variety of reasons. Some may have abnormal plumage that needs investigation; others are not preening effectively. Some of these birds live in unsuitable conditions and their plumage smells of contaminants such as cooking grease and cigarette smoke. In some birds the poor plumage condition is due to prolonged moulting intervals, which need to be investigated.

Skin

Psittacids are infrequently presented to the veterinary surgeon for abnormalities of the skin. The commonest skin pathology seen is due to self-trauma, which can be due to either physiological or psychological disease. For example, chronic ulcerative dermatitis of the wing web area from self-mutilation is commonly seen in lovebirds, Cockatiels and Grey Parrots. The work-up for this condition should include biochemistry and haematology, whole-body radiographs and a faecal analysis, as giardiasis is not an uncommon cause (especially in lovebirds and Cockatiels). Cockatoo species are often seen with large ulcers in their pectoral musculature caused by self-mutilation.

Bruising of the featherless skin around the eye, seen most conspicuously in the Grey Parrot, can be caused in the struggle while being captured or by the restraining grip. It can also be caused by a clumsy or ataxic bird falling over. Trauma to the leading edge of the carpus is another injury commonly caused during attempted restraint, where the bird knocks the carpus against a hard surface, sometimes breaking the skin. These injuries should be recognized before handling the bird, as the injury most commonly happens when the owner is struggling to get the bird into the travel cage prior to its visit.

Masses in or under the skin can be neoplastic lesions or abscesses. In some species (e.g. Budgerigars and Cockatiels), xanthomas, which are a non-neoplastic lesion, are common. Abscesses are usually caseous in birds, and may have either a bacterial, a mycobacterial or a fungal cause. Fine-needle aspiration of the mass with cytology and culture of the aspirate may be needed to arrive at a diagnosis.

Swellings around the eye are often related to disease processes in the sinuses (Figure 5.22). Air under the skin may be due to a fracture of a pneumatic bone or rupture of an air sac. This is most common in the neck area, where rupture or distension of the cervicocephalic air sac is the usual cause.

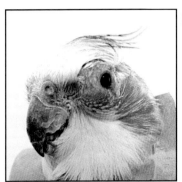

5.22 Swelling and redness of the nares and periocular area due to a localized lesion in the preorbital diverticulum of a Cockatiel.

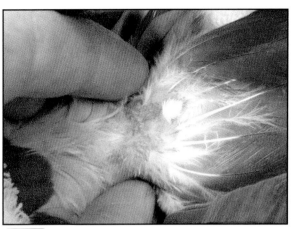

5.23 Normal uropygial gland in a Grey Parrot.

Hyperkeratosis of the featherless skin of the legs, cere and around the beak is most commonly caused by cnemidocoptic mites in Budgerigars. In severe cases it can involve the ears, and occasionally the skin around the uropygial gland and the vent. The diagnosis is easily confirmed as the mites are readily identified microscopically from a skin scraping. In extreme cases there may be a primary predisposing cause. Herpesvirus can cause pale thickened patches of skin on the legs and feet; this can be seen in cockatoos, macaws and Grey Parrots (Schmidt *et al.*, 2003). A biopsy is necessary to confirm the diagnosis.

Thermal insults – both heat and cold – will cause darkening of the skin. Frostbite usually affects the extremities, typically the toes. They will become black and be cold to the touch, and sometimes a serosanguineous fluid will leak from the area. Burns do not cause blistering as seen in mammalian skin, due to the lack of a large capillary plexus beneath the epidermal border (Spearman and Hardy, 1985). Skin damaged by high temperature will be darker in colour, leathery in appearance and feel hardened and less flexible to the touch (Figure 5.16).

Occasionally birds are seen with generalized inflamed skin, which is often extremely pruritic. Most of these cases appear to be skin reactions to internal infections and clear up when the underlying disease is treated.

Uropygial gland

The uropygial gland is not as well developed in psittacids as in some other orders. Indeed it is absent in some commonly seen species (e.g. Amazons). When present, the gland should be examined as part of the physical examination. It is a lobed structure protruding dorsally at the base of the tail feathers (Figure 5.23). Neoplasms are the most common problem seen. Both carcinomas and adenomas are common and are most frequently seen in the Budgerigar. Occasionally an impacted uropygial gland may be seen (see Figure 16.26).

Cardiovascular system

Evaluation of the cardiovascular system is an important part of the physical examination. Mucous membrane colour can be assessed in the oral cavity, skin of the face and the vent area, where these areas are not pigmented. Yellow coloration of mucous membranes is usually due to pigments in the food; birds do not develop jaundice externally.

Capillary refill time (which should be < 1 second in the normal bird) can be evaluated on the skin of the feet if non-pigmented. Perfusion status can easily be evaluated by observing the refill time of the basilic or the ulnar veins where they run over the medial aspect of the elbow. With normal perfusion, refill time will also be < 1 second following digital pressure.

Auscultation is achieved over the pectoral muscles. Heart rates vary from 110 to 300 beats per minute, depending on the species, though this will be much lower in the larger species when they are relaxed or when they are under general anaesthesia. Excitement will result in a dramatic increase in heart rate, often making it very difficult to count heart rates. Muffled heart sounds are easily appreciated, indicating either pericardial fluid or soft tissue insulating the sound. Murmurs are more easily detected in tame large species or in any species under general anaesthesia, when the heart rate should be much slower. Arrhythmias are also sometimes detected. A sinus arrhythmia is normal but all other arrhythmias should be investigated (Chapter 20).

Signs that may indicate cardiac disease (though disease may be asymptomatic) include:

* Cough (but may be mimicking)
* Dyspnoea
* Lethargy
* Syncope
* Bulging coelomic space
* Exercise intolerance
* Sudden death.

Respiratory system

Evaluation of the respiratory tract (Chapter 14) includes the upper airways (as covered above under oral cavity, nares, and head and neck). The respiratory rate and effort should be observed before handling. Patency of the upper airways can be evaluated by occluding each naris in turn while keeping the bird's beak shut. Obstructions to the flow of air will cause increased respiratory sounds or, if there is a complete obstruction, lack of air movement. Gentle pressure should be applied on the different pockets of the infraorbital sinus while watching for fluids being forced out of the nares or lacrimal duct. The choana should be rechecked for discharges after this exercise.

With tracheal lesions, increased respiratory noise can sometimes be heard, even at rest. Increased respiratory effort may cause the bird's tail feathers to move up and down with each breath, sometimes referred to as 'tail bobbing'. Disease processes that reduce the size of the air sacs will also cause an increased respiratory effort (e.g. organomegaly). Coughing can be a symptom of tracheal or syringeal pathology, or the bird may be mimicking a mammalian cough. Voice change is commonly associated with disease processes involving the syrinx.

Auscultation is not as useful as in mammals, due to the anatomy of the avian lung and to the fact that there is only limited movement during the respiratory cycle. However, the lungs, air sacs and trachea should always be auscultated for any abnormal sounds. Wheezes, clicks, crackles and squeaks may be heard with lower respiratory tract disease. A paediatric stethoscope will enhance auscultation and should be placed dorsally and laterally over the ribs on both sides. The air sacs are best auscultated on the ventral and lateral surfaces.

If recovery of normal respiratory rate after restraint for examination takes longer than 3 minutes, there is a reduced respiratory capacity. Acute respiratory distress is an emergency, the initial management of which is detailed below. Rarely can a diagnosis of respiratory disease be reached by a clinical examination alone (Chapter 14).

Stabilization of the critical case

Often it is safest to deal with a critical case in stages, allowing the bird to rest in between. The bird has to be transferred to a critical care cage, which usually allows a brief initial one-minute examination. Proficiency in handling is essential at this stage to minimize struggling.

- Check for oculonasal discharges and swellings.
- Examine the oral cavity briefly; palpate the crop, pectoral muscles and coelomic space.
- Assess vascular perfusion by observing basilica or ulnar vein refill time.
- Auscultate the heart, lungs and air sacs.
- Observe the vent and use the grasping reflex of the feet to estimate the degree of debility.
- If the bird is relaxed, weigh it and expand to a full clinical examination.

It may be essential to attempt to stabilize the bird before performing a full clinical examination and collecting diagnostic samples. It is important to be prepared for critical cases:

- Decide what will be needed for handling the bird and have everything set up in advance to minimize handling time.
- Prepare for resuscitation with drug doses calculated and drawn up.
- Work as a team (veterinary surgeon and nurses). The team needs to be familiar with the procedure to be carried out and with avian resuscitation techniques (Chapter 8).

Essential equipment for avian emergency medicine (not normally found in a small animal clinic) includes the following:

- Gram scales: digital or balance, sensitive to 1 g, minimum range 10–2000 g (depending on species accepted as patients)
- Avian hospital cages (capable of maintaining high temperature and humidity)
- Avian oral specula (assortment of sizes)
- Crop-feeding tubes (assortment of sizes)
- Nebulizer (capable of producing particles < 3 μm)
- Selection of avian foods
- Commercial avian critical care enteral feeding formulations
- Parenteral fluid warmer (Figure 5.24)
- Support staff trained in avian nursing.

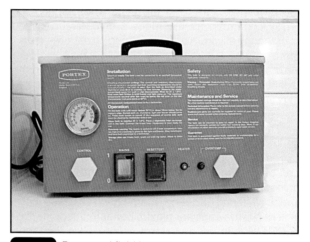

5.24 Parenteral fluid heater.

Stabilization

Hypovolaemia/shock
Correcting the hypovolaemia is an immediate priority. Birds in hypovolaemic shock typically have pale mucous membranes, prolonged venous refill time and a rapid heart rate. Vascular access may be difficult and placement of an intraosseous catheter may be necessary.

Give immediately, via the catheter as a slow bolus over 5 minutes:

- Lactated Ringer's (10 ml/kg) combined with 5 ml/kg haemoglobin-based oxygen carrier (5 ml/kg)
- OR Lactated Ringer's (10 ml/kg) combined with hetastarch (5 ml/kg).

Dehydration
Fluids for dehydration can be given intravenously, intraosseously or orally. Maintenance is 50 ml/kg daily. The deficit is estimated and replaced over 24 hours.

Hypothermia
Anorexic birds rapidly become hypothermic. Birds normally have a higher body core temperature than mammals. All avian emergencies should be placed in a warm (30°C) critical care cage.

Hypoxia

Oxygen enriching the air in the critical care cage will benefit most avian emergencies. Dyspnoeic birds will stabilize rapidly. A facemask or a clear plastic bag can be used but this may be stressful. Where there is severe respiratory distress caused by an obstruction in the trachea or syrinx, an air sac breathing tube must be placed if there is no response to oxygenation within 30 minutes or if the bird is continuing to deteriorate (Chapter 8).

Inanition

Birds rapidly become exhausted when not eating. Nutritional support starts with an initial bolus of glucose or dextrose. When hypovolaemia has been corrected, enteral nutrition can be given initially by crop-feeding tube, using one of the commercial products formulated for psittacids that has been made up according to the manufacturer's recommendation (Figure 5.25). The ideal product should be easily absorbed and require minimal or ideally no digestion by the patient.

Product	Manufacturer
Critical Care Formula	Vetark Professional, UK
Emeraid Critical Care	Lafeber Company, USA
Emeraid Nutri-Support	Lafeber Company, USA
Emeraid Carbo-Boost	Lafeber Company, USA
Poly-Aid	The Birdcare Company, UK
Guardian Angel	The Birdcare Company, UK

5.25 Commercially available critical care enteric products for psittacids.

Fluid therapy

Crystalloid solutions

Glucose–saline (i.e. 5% glucose + 0.9% saline) is an ideal solution to include in the initial bolus, as the glucose is an immediate carbohydrate source and the physiological saline solution will rapidly replace lost fluid in the extracellular and intracellular fluid spaces and temporarily expand the circulation fluid volume.

Lactated Ringer's solution, as well as providing electrolytes and fluid, provides lactate that is metabolized in the liver to bicarbonate. Bicarbonate helps to correct the acidosis seen in most avian emergencies (Jenkins, 1997). If possible the acid–base balance should be measured prior to its use. It can be used as a maintenance fluid.

Colloids

Colloids (haemoglobin-based oxygen carriers, whole blood or synthetic colloids) are used to expand plasma volume. They contain large molecules that do not readily pass out of the vasculature. Both natural and synthetic colloids are available. Their use is essential in the treatment of hypovolaemic shock. The combination of colloids and crystalloids in the treatment of hypovolaemic shock therapy reduces the crystalloid requirement by 40–60% (Raffe and Wingfield, 2002). When the PCV falls below 20% in acute conditions or below 12% with chronic disease processes, a colloid with oxygen-carrying ability should be chosen.

Synthetic colloids: These (e.g. Haemaccel, Intervet UK) are more economic to use than the alternatives. Their major disadvantage is that they do not transport oxygen to the tissues. Availability, cost and low risk are major advantages when compared with whole blood or plasma (Wingfield, 2002).

Oxygen-carrying colloids: Haemoglobin-based oxygen carriers (e.g. Oxyglobin, Biopure Netherlands BU) have the advantage of being readily available for use in emergencies, having a colloid effect in addition to being a potent carrier of oxygen. Their main disadvantage is cost (Raffe and Wingfield, 2002). There have been no clinical trials to establish safe dose rates but Oxyglobin has been used in psittacids in hypovolaemic shock at doses of up to 30 ml/kg divided over 24 hours.

Blood is a complete and physiological volume expander with the disadvantage of poor availability, high cost, the possibility of spreading disease and carrying a risk of transfusion reactions (Raffe and Wingfield, 2002). Ideally, donors should be from the same species and have a disease-free status. If these are unavailable, a donor from the same genus could be used. Pigeons have been used as donors for a single transfusion. A volume 1% of body weight can be safely collected from the donor. Acid citrate dextrose at a dose of 0.15 ml/ml of blood can be used as an anticoagulant (Jenkins, 1997). Check for agglutination or haemolysis before repeat transfusions by mixing donor and recipient red cells and serum on a microscope slide.

Routes for fluid therapy

- *Enteral fluid therapy* is preferred if the patient is not critically ill or hypovolaemic, has a functioning gastrointestinal tract, is not in severe dyspnoea and has a level of consciousness to prevent reflux from the crop. It has the advantage of being the most physiological route and will also help to maintain normal gut structure and function. Enteral fluids are given by a crop-feeding tube. The major disadvantage is the risk of aspiration (Proulx, 2002).
- *Intravenous fluid therapy* is the preferred route for critically ill patients. It has the advantage of easy placement of the catheter (with practice). Large volumes can be given slowly as a bolus. The major disadvantage is that the catheter must be protectively bandaged to prevent it being removed by the bird.
- *Intraosseous catheters* are easier to place in small patients and when peripheral circulation has collapsed. Both colloids and crystalloids can be given by this route, with equivalent responses to the intravenous route. The major disadvantage is that placement is painful, but in emergency situations the catheter may have to be placed without an anaesthetic. Osteomyelitis is also a risk. Intraosseous catheters must also be protectively bandaged to prevent them being removed by the bird.

In situations where equipment or experience is deficient, it must be stressed that when fluids are needed it is preferable that they are given by the route available rather than not be given. However, intra-coelomic fluids are always contraindicated in birds, due to the presence of air sacs. Chapter 6 gives details of the crop tubing technique and injection and catheter placement methodologies.

Hospitalization

Hospitalization facilities are essential for practices accepting avian cases. A high percentage of avian patients require hospitalization and critical care management.

- The ideal avian hospitalization cage should have temperature and humidity control.
- It must be easy to capture the bird from the cage.
- The cage should be able to withstand thorough cleaning and disinfection.
- The perch must be removable for housing very ill birds and for disinfection.

The hospitalized parrot should be positioned out of sight and sound of predators (i.e. dogs, cats, ferrets and birds of prey). Purpose-built avian hospital cages are available; alternatively, cage requirements can be improvised from an aquarium or incubator (Figure 5.26).

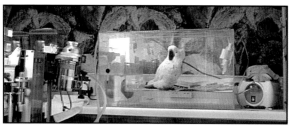

5.26 Critical care incubator with oxygen-enriched air and nebulizer set-up.

Emergency situations and their initial management

Collapsed bird

1. Perform a brief examination when transferring from transport cage to critical care cage, as detailed in the 'Stabilization' section above.
2. Place in a warm (30°C) humid oxygen-enriched critical care cage with perches removed and familiar food and water within reach.
3. Collect brief history and signalment.
4. Place intravenous or intraosseous catheter.
5. Collect blood for diagnostics.
6. Give 5% glucose saline (5 ml/kg) and lactated Ringer's (5 ml/kg) as a slow bolus via the catheter.
7. Establish a full history for the bird.
8. When stable, do a full clinical examination.

Acute respiratory distress

1. Perform a brief examination when transferring from transport cage to critical care cage, as detailed for 'Stabilization' above.
2. Place in a warm (30°C) humid oxygen-enriched critical care cage with perches removed and familiar food and water within reach.
3. If tracheal or syringeal blockage, prepare team and equipment to place an air sac tube (Chapter 8).
4. When stable under isoflurane anaesthesia (following placement of an air sac tube):
   - Place intravenous or intraosseous catheter.
   - Endoscopically examine the trachea and the syrinx if appropriate.
   - Take radiographs.
   - Collect blood for diagnostics.
   - Give glucose saline (5 ml/kg) and lactated Ringer's (5 ml/kg) via the catheter as a slow bolus.

Refer to Chapter 14 for further guidance.

Seizures

There are many possible causes for a bird having seizures. Syncope is often confused with seizure activity in parrots. Diagnostic samples should be collected before treatment if possible, as treatment may compromise their diagnostic value (Chapter 19).

1. Obtain a brief history, checking exposure to lead and other toxins. Record pattern and history of the seizure activity along with any other symptoms over the last 3 months. If acute onset, check possibility of exposure to high environmental temperatures.
2. Perform full clinical examination if possible. If triggering seizures, do a brief examination.
3. Place intravenous or intraosseous catheter.
4. Collect blood for biochemistry and haematology profile.
5. Give 5% glucose saline (5 ml/kg) and lactated Ringer's (5 ml/kg) as a slow bolus via the catheter. For Grey Parrots, also give calcium gluconate (50–100 mg/kg) slowly via the catheter.
6. Give diazepam (0.1 mg/kg) as a bolus via the catheter to arrest the seizure activity.
7. Place in a 30°C critical care cage enriched with oxygen if no history suggestive of heat stroke.
8. Remove perches, place soft bedding on the floor, and also place food and water at floor level.
9. Obtain a complete history and, when the bird is stable, perform a full clinical examination.

Egg binding

1. Diagnosis may not always be confirmed by palpation. Radiography may be necessary.
2. Perform a full or brief clinical examination, depending on the condition of the bird.
3. Provide analgesia.
4. Place in a warm (30°C) humid oxygen-enriched critical care cage with perches removed and familiar food and water within reach.

5. Lubricate by using blunt cannula to place warmed water-soluble gel into the cloaca.
6. Give glucose saline (10 ml/kg) by crop-feeding tube.

Refer to Chapter 18 for further guidance on dealing with egg binding and its complications.

Bone fracture

1. Give analgesic.
2. If compound fracture, start antimicrobial cover.
3. Perform a full clinical examination.
4. Place in a warm (30°C) humid oxygen-enriched critical care cage with perches removed and familiar food and water within reach.
5. A figure-of-eight wrap can be used for temporary stabilization of a wing fracture distal to the elbow joint. A body wrap is needed for proximal fractures.
6. Give glucose saline (10 ml/kg) by crop-feeding tube.

Refer to Chapter 11 for fracture management.

Acute blood loss – hypovolaemic shock

Birds in hypovolaemic shock typically have pale mucous membranes, prolonged capillary refill time, increased heart rate, a falling haematocrit and often a history of blood loss (Lichtenberger et al., 2003).

1. Perform a brief examination when transferring from transport cage to critical care cage, as detailed for 'Stabilization' above.
2. Place in a warm (30°C) humid oxygen-enriched critical care cage with perches removed.
3. Place intravenous or intraosseous catheter.
4. Collect brief history and signalment.
5. Give immediately, via the catheter as a slow bolus over 5 minutes:
   - lactated Ringer's (10 ml/kg) combined with 5 ml/kg haemoglobin-based oxygen carrier (5 ml/kg)
   - OR lactated Ringer's (10 ml/kg) combined with hetastarch (5 ml/kg)
   - OR whole blood (10–15 ml/kg), ideally from a healthy donor of the same species.
6. Establish a full history for the bird.
7. When stable, do a full clinical examination.

6

Basic techniques

John Chitty

Introduction

This chapter will discuss various basic techniques that are often required in avian medicine. Some may form part of an examination or diagnostic investigation, while others may be the primary reason for the bird being presented (e.g. clipping wing or beak). It is important not only to learn correct techniques but also to understand the issues surrounding these and the reasons for presentation.

Injection techniques

Intramuscular injection
This is the most common route by which injectable drugs are given to pet birds. In general, injections are given into the pectoral muscle mass rather than the leg, because the muscle mass is larger and because of concerns over the presence of a renal portal venous system resulting in effects on the drug pharmacokinetics.

In preparation for injection, the feathers should be parted and the skin cleansed. The needle is inserted into the mid to caudal portion of the muscle and the substance is injected into the *middle* of the mass, i.e. passing caudal-to-cranial parallel with the sternum (Figures 6.1 and 6.2). Prior to injection the operator should draw back the plunger to ensure that the substance is not being inadvertently injected into a blood vessel.

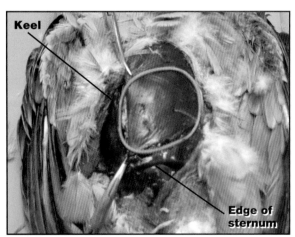

6.1 In this dissection of an Amazon, the correct site for intramuscular injection or for microchip insertion is shown in the mid to caudal region of the pectoral muscle mass.

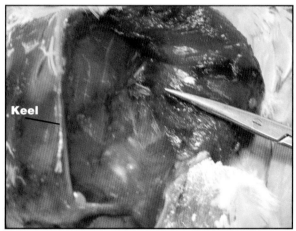

6.2 The superficial pectoral muscle is reflected, showing the large plexus of nerves and blood vessels that should be avoided when injecting in this region.

The smallest suitable needle should be used with respect to the viscosity of the drug and size of bird. In general, needles of 23 gauge (G) or smaller are used, but 21 G needles may be used in larger birds when injecting viscous drugs.

Care should be taken with the following:

- *Irritant substances* (Figure 6.3). In the experience of the author, certain drugs (e.g. enrofloxacin (Baytril; Bayer, Newbury, UK), doxycycline (Vibravenos; Pfizer, Sandwich, UK) and some long-acting oxytetracycline preparations may be extremely irritant. Post-mortem examination of birds

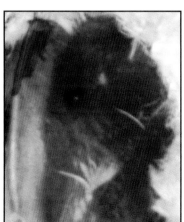

6.3 In this cadaver specimen, a muscle reaction can be seen following a single injection with Baytril 2.5% (Bayer).

that have received multiple intramuscular injections of these compounds may show extensive areas of bruising. In the live bird, high levels of plasma creatinine kinase may be seen following even a single injection of 2.5% enrofloxacin.

- *Volume.* Injection of 0.1 ml into a 500 g bird is equivalent (on a weight:weight basis) to a single injection of 14 ml into a 70 kg human being. Although this argument is extremely simplistic and the pectoral muscle mass is comparatively much larger than any in humans, care should be taken when injecting large volumes as this may be a source of pain in an already sick bird.

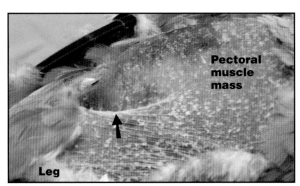

6.4 The precrural fold is arrowed (head to the right). Note the available 'space' under this fold for large volumes of fluid.

Therefore, repeated injections of irritant drugs should preferably be avoided, using the oral route as soon as practicable. If this is not possible, or if it is felt that oral absorption would not be reliable, the intramuscular route should be used but injection sites should be varied. In these cases, and where injection volumes are small, use of leg muscles is acceptable. The cranial tibial muscle should be used (see Figure 2.7).

Large-volume drugs (> 1 ml/500 g body weight) should be split between sites or placed subcutaneously. Irritant drugs, especially Vibravenos, should not be injected via this route as skin slough is likely.

Subcutaneous injection

This is a very useful route for fluid therapy and large-volume drugs. Absorption from subcutaneous sites is rapid and large volumes of fluid (up to 20 ml/kg) may be absorbed within 15 minutes. The absorption rate may be increased by adding hyaluronidase at 150 units/litre.

The injection site is prepared as described above. The ideal site is the large precrural fold (Figure 6.4). Care should be taken not to enter the body cavity inadvertently while injecting.

Intravenous injection and blood collection

Intravenous injections may be given into, or blood may be collected from, the sites described in Figures 6.5 and 6.6 (for exact anatomical location, see Figures 2.6, 2.7 and 2.9). These veins are all superficial and are found easily.

Site	Restraint	Pros	Cons	Tips
Right jugular vein (Figures 6.6a,b and 2.9)	Bird restrained or anaesthetized, neck extended. Parting of feathers reveals vein running under large apterium. Placement of digit at base of neck raises the vein	Easy. Large volumes can be taken. Haemostasis relatively simple. Only recommended technique in small birds (< 150 g).	Very difficult for left-handed operators. Struggling birds may cause laceration of vein and fatal subcutaneous haemorrhage; general anaesthesia may be appropriate. Restraint may be stressful to sensitive or dyspnoeic birds	Anaesthesia may be recommended for this technique. Gentle digital pressure applied afterwards to avoid haematoma formation.
Superficial ulnar/ basilic vein (Figures 6.6c and 2.6)	Bird restrained or anaesthetized and placed on its back. One wing extended and vein visualized. Operator raises vein with free hand.	Easier for left-handed operators. Restraint relatively simpler.	Fragile vein and may be hard to draw large volumes, especially in smaller birds. Haemostasis can be hard to achieve and bird should be replaced in cage to allow it to calm down and blood pressure to drop (preferable to prolonged handling). Unlike jugular venipuncture, this haemorrhage unlikely to be fatal and is readily visible; but small losses may cause lot of mess and distress to owners. In conscious older cage-bound bird care must be taken when extending wing as it is easy to break humerus	Drop of tissue glue may be helpful to facilitate haemostasis.
Superficial plantar metatarsal/ caudal tibial vein (Figures 6.6d and 2.7)	Bird restrained and leg extended. Operator can raise vein with free hand.	Superficial, simple to find and raise but vein harder to visualize as skin not transparent in this region. Restraint easy.	Very fragile and only possible to draw small volumes. Haemostasis difficult.	Only of use where other veins damaged or where very small volumes of bloods required. Tissue glue may facilitate haemostasis or light temporary dressing may be applied.
Toe clip	Bird restrained and nail cut short enough that nail bed is penetrated. Nail should be cut in opposite manner to that described for a nail trim (see later) to increase bleeding.	Easy.	Unsuitable for collection for biochemistry/ haematology due to contamination from tissue fluid or from urates/faeces on claw. Impossible to collect large volumes. Technique may cause pain and haemostasis important, as is risk of introducing infection.	May be of use when collecting very small volumes (e.g for sexing, circovirus testing, or collection for 'Immunocomb' *Chlamydophila psittaci* testing). Vein should be cauterized afterwards; silver nitrate or potassium permanganate appropriate. Attention should be paid to welfare aspects of this technique

6.5 Venipuncture sites.

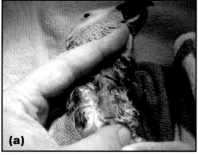
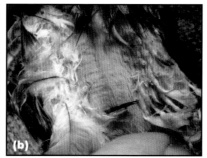
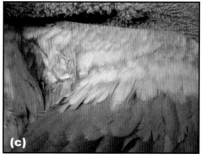
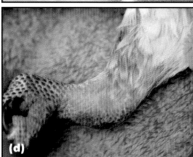

6.6 (a) Restraint of a Grey Parrot for jugular venipuncture. An assistant holds the towel-wrapped body while the operator extends the neck with their left hand. The thumb of the left hand is used to raise the vein. (b) Right jugular vein. Note the large superficial vein lying in an apterium. (c) Superficial ulnar vein. (d) Superficial plantar metatarsal vein. See also Figures 2.6, 2.7 and 2.9.

The right jugular lies beneath an apterium on the lateral neck, while the superficial veins in the distal leg are located beneath the scaly skin. The ulnar vein lies in a relatively featherless area over the medial elbow, though one or two feathers may need to be removed to facilitate exposure. Wetting the skin with a spirit-soaked swab improves visualization and wetting the feathers will keep them out of the way. Care must be taken not to overdo this, as hypothermia may result.

Two operators are required for injecting or bleeding conscious medium to large birds. For very small birds a simple one-handed holding technique greatly facilitates the procedure (Figure 6.7).

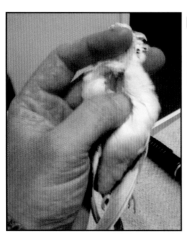

6.7 Single-handed technique for accessing the right jugular vein in a Budgerigar.

All these veins may be suitable for intravenous injection of drugs or fluids. As a simple rule the basilic vein is used for intravenous injection and the right jugular for blood collection. When bleeding very fat birds (especially Amazons), where intradermal fat may obscure the vein, use of the ulnar vein is indicated. Great care should be taken with haemostasis in these cases, and in any other bird where liver disease is suspected, as many have coagulopathies.

Blood is generally collected using a 2.5 or 1 ml syringe. A 23–25 G, $^5/_8$ inch needle is used; the size depends on the size of bird but a larger needle should be used where possible for haematology collection, to avoid damage to blood cells.

As with mammals, up to approximately 1% body weight may be safely removed (e.g. up to 4 ml from a 400 g Grey Parrot). It is important to note that this figure is based on healthy birds; the figure should be slightly reduced for sick or dehydrated birds.

Injected drugs should be given slowly to avoid embolic effects.

Intravenous catheter placement

In some cases, placement of an intravenous catheter may be considered, either for continuous or bolus fluid therapy, or where repeated use of intravenous drugs is required. Either the right jugular or basilic vein (Figure 6.8) may be used. The former may be more difficult to maintain without extensive dressings and the latter is preferred in birds larger than 300 g.

Catheters may be taped or sutured into position. Surprisingly, most birds leave these in place (NA Forbes, personal communication).

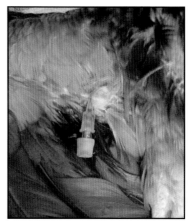

6.8 Catheter inserted in the basilic vein (courtesy NA Forbes).

Intraosseous injection

This is an alternative route for continuous or bolus fluid therapy by which fluids are injected into the medullary cavity of either the ulna (Figure 6.9) or the tibiotarsus (the pneumatized humerus must *not* be used). Uptake into the main circulation is virtually instantaneous, due to the central venous sinus. Intravenous drugs may also be given by this route, but not if they are cytotoxic or irritant.

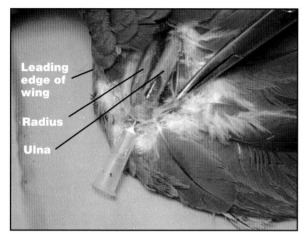

6.9 Dissection showing position of an intraosseous needle. It has been inserted into the ulna via the dorsal condyle just proximal to the carpus on the dorsal surface of the wing.

These sites are easier to access and maintain than the intravenous route. However, as the fluid needs to be given under pressure, some specialized equipment is required: either a syringe pump or 'Flowline' (Arnolds, UK) apparatus.

The bird should be anaesthetized (unless extreme urgency is required) and the site prepared aseptically. A needle is introduced into the bone. This can be either a specialized bone needle or a standard injection needle (18 G, 1.5 inch for birds > 700 g; 21 G, 1 inch for birds between 200 and 700 g; 23 G, 1 inch for birds < 200 g; this technique is not recommended for birds < 100 g).

- *Ulna*: The dorsal condyle just proximal to the carpus should be identified. With the carpus flexed, the needle is driven through this proximally into the medullary cavity, where it can be 'felt' *in situ*. To confirm correct positioning, a small volume of fluid may be injected while watching the basilic vein, where the fluid bolus may be seen.
- *Tibiotarsus*: The cranial cnemial crest is identified just distal to the stifle and the needle is inserted through this distally into the medullary cavity. As the 'tibial plateau' on the lateral side is wider than the medullary cavity, the needle should be inserted from the craniomedial aspect of the proximal tibiotarsus. This route may appear to be simpler than the other but it is more difficult to confirm that the needle is in place other than 'feeling' it within the bony cavity.

In either case the needle is taped or bandaged in place.

Care should be taken when using this route in osteoporotic birds, as iatrogenic fractures may result. Care should also be taken in needle maintenance, as osteomyelitis may result from introduced infection. It is advised that the equipment should not be left in place for more than 3 days.

Crop tubing

This is a simple and effective means of providing oral drugs or fluids or for feeding sick birds. It should be noted that anaesthetized birds should be allowed to recover fully before they are subjected to crop tubing.

Metal crop tubes are recommended, as plastic tubes may easily be damaged or broken and swallowed by the bird. However, they should be used with care, as oesophageal perforation is possible with rigid tubes. The largest possible tube size should be selected, to help to avoid glottal insertion.

The bird should be restrained in a towel and its beak should be opened by using the thumb and index finger placed in the commissures. In very large birds a mouth gag may be used (Chapter 5). The neck is extended and the tube is passed lateral and dorsal to the glottis (Figure 6.10). Should resistance be encountered or the bird become distressed, the tube should be withdrawn and the process tried again. The tube should be felt within the crop before the fluid bolus is administered.

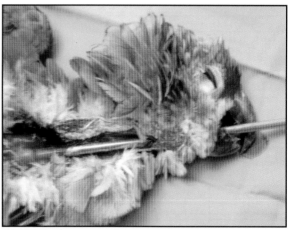

6.10 Placement of a crop tube, shown in a cadaver. Using a straight tube the angle to which the neck must be extended can be seen. Ideally the tube should be placed along the right-hand side of the neck, as this facilitates passage along the oesophagus into the crop.

Fluids should be pre-warmed and given slowly to avoid regurgitation. The volume should not exceed 20 ml/kg body weight in each dose but the process may be repeated as soon as the crop empties.

This technique may also be used to obtain a diagnostic crop washing. The tube should be inserted and warmed saline passed into the crop. A small volume is aspirated and submitted for diagnosis.

Microchip placement

Microchipping is an effective means of identifying the individual bird that is difficult for the bird or a person to modify or damage.

Prior to insertion, the bird should be scanned in case it is already microchipped. Many guidelines have been issued by different authorities in different countries on implantation sites. As a result, microchips may have been implanted in the right pectoral muscle, base of the neck or either thigh; therefore, the whole bird should be scanned before concluding that it is not already microchipped. If in doubt, radiography of the whole bird is the only way to prove conclusively that there is no microchip present.

The British Veterinary Zoological Society recommends that the microchip should be inserted into the left pectoral muscle mass. This may be done with the bird conscious or anaesthetized; the author recommends that all birds weighing < 200 g should be anaesthetized for this procedure.

The feathers are parted and the skin is prepared aseptically. The needle is inserted in the caudal third of the muscle mass and directed cranially so that the microchip is placed in the approximate middle of the mass between superficial and deep pectoral muscles (Figure 6.1). To avoid the large plexus of nerves and blood vessels in this region (Figure 6.2), it is extremely important not to place the microchip too far cranially (Monks, 2002).

Occasionally, haemorrhage may be a problem. This may be avoided by stretching the skin to one side so that the holes in skin and muscle are not aligned. The skin hole may be closed with a suture or with tissue glue.

Digital pressure on tissue overlying the needle as it is withdrawn reduces the chance of the microchip being withdrawn with the needle.

Wing clipping

This frequently requested procedure is a very easy one to perform but the implications and ethics of doing so are complex. There is a wide variety of views both on whether wing clipping should be performed (Figure 6.11) and, if done, how it should be done (Figure 6.12). In summary, wing clipping should not be regarded as a long-term management tool for the convenience of the owner unless it enables the owner to give the parrot a more extensive, fulfilling life (Hooijmeier, 2003). The technique also has uses for short-term training and behavioural modification.

Advantages
Safety. Bird cannot hurt itself while flying
Damage. Bird less able to damage home, making it more desirable pet
Security. Bird cannot escape
Freedom. Increased safety and security enables owner to take the bird out of cage or house more often
Training. Bird is more dependent on owner, thus more amenable to training or behaviour modification

Disadvantages
If pet has to be 'modified' to fit into home, is it the right pet (or right home) anyway?
No clip totally removes ability to fly; clipping often increases chances of injury during attempted flight
Birds moult out clipped feathers and grow new ones
Interim period of reduced flight often induces complacency in owner, resulting in doors and windows being left open when bird can fly again
Clipping reduces freedom as it creates an 'invisible cage' (many believe birds need to fly to fulfil certain behavioural needs); birds can be trained to come back or be trained to harness (see Figure 22.6), both of which enable bird to be taken out
Wing trims not totally reliable and clipped birds much more vulnerable if they do escape
Clipped bird may be less fit and more prone to obesity than one who is fit and flying
Many start feather chewing after bad clip

6.11 Advantages and disadvantages of wing clipping.

Technique	Advantages	Disadvantages
One-winged (unilateral)	Much more effective at deflighting bird	Bird very unbalanced and increased chance of injury (e.g. split keel) from spiralling fall
Two-winged (bilateral)	Better balanced so better able to fly Less chance of injury following fall	
Removing outer primary flight feathers (6–10)	Fewer feathers need to be removed and by breaking up leading edge of wing flight is disrupted. Result is reduction in 'lift' with less effect on 'thrust', enabling safer descending glide	Result less attractive as outer feathers removed and obvious that bird is clipped. Some argue this method does not take account of natural moulting sequence of feathers, meaning new feathers tend to come through 'unguarded' and be more prone to damage and bird may be more likely to start feather chewing. Note that moulting sequences vary from species to species
Removing inner primaries (1–5)	More cosmetic appearance May be more considerate of moulting sequences; certainly outer feathers will guard the new growing feathers	Affects 'thrust' not 'lift', so may not enable gliding descent

6.12 Wing clipping methods.

It is important that a wing trim is not simply booked in as a 'quick procedure' but taken as an opportunity to introduce training and management procedures to the owner. In the author's practice two appointments are made: a half-hour one to discuss management and training; and a short one to perform the trim. Charges, naturally, should reflect the time spent. Most owners are not hostile to this; in fact, most seem pleased that the veterinary surgeon is interested and that they and the bird will benefit from procedures learnt.

The aim of the veterinary surgeon is that this should be the only wing clipping that the bird ever receives. The following points should be discussed with the owner:

- No wing clip is 100% effective. In fact, a good clip enables a gliding descent, so the bird will still be able to fly. Security in the house should therefore not be relaxed and the bird should be carefully supervised outside. In general, the stronger and more accomplished a flyer the bird is, the less successful the clip will be
- Microchipping is highly recommended
- The house is still not safe. Many birds are very comfortable walking on the floor and all are capable of climbing
- Basic training should include step-up/step-down and returning on command (see Chapter 17).

Selection of the method used should be based on the following criteria:

- *Species of bird.* Those with high ratios of wing surface area to body weight require more feathers to be removed. The classic example is the Cockatiel: even where every feather has been clipped on both wings, the bird's flight might be relatively unaffected. In this species a one-winged clip is more appropriate
- *Purpose of clip.* How 'deflighted' does the bird need to be?
- *Experience.* For every argument there is a counter-argument and many very experienced avian veterinary surgeons favour clipping methods that others regard as dangerous. Therefore each should find their own preferred method(s), which should be modified or changed as experience shows problems. If the owner (especially an experienced aviculturist) has strong feelings about the style of clip they favour, this should be taken into account and discussed prior to performing the procedure; owners are not always right but may have a valid point of view.

This author favours the bilateral technique adopted by the Association of Avian Veterinarians (if there are potential problems, there is a large worldwide organization to offer support). Exact details are available on a laminated wall chart from the AAV but are summarized as follows:

- Long-tailed, slim-bodied birds (e.g. macaws, parakeets): clip primaries 5–10 (see Figure 2.1)
- Heavy-bodied, short-tailed birds (e.g. Amazons, Grey Parrot): clip primaries 6–10 (Figure 6.13)

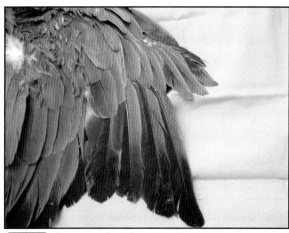

6.13 Amazon wing trim: primaries 6–10 are removed from each wing. Note that no cut ends protrude beyond the covert feathers. Compare normal wing in Figure 2.1.

The bird should be flight tested after clipping. If it can still fly further than 7.5 m, another primary should be taken from each wing. The bird is then tested again and the feathers are trimmed until the flight distance is < 7.5 m. In either of the two groups it should not be necessary to trim beyond the first primary; in the second group it is rarely necessary to go beyond the fourth primary.

Whichever method is chosen, the following are essential:

- Feathers should be cut singly, using a small pair of sharp scissors or nail clippers (Figure 6.14). This reduces the chance of damage (or even accidental amputation) of the wing tip. It also reduces the chances of damaging other feathers.
- Feather ends should be 'sharp' and not left splintered.
- Blood feathers should never be cut:
  - Should one or more be found in the region to be clipped, an alternative technique should be used
  - Should many be found, the clip may be deferred until the feathers have grown through

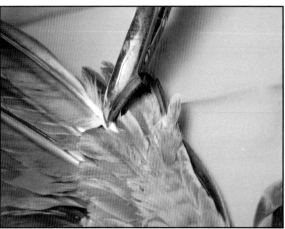

6.14 Correct method of cutting feathers. A sharp pair of nail trimmers is used to cut each feather individually and below the level of the covert feathers.

- If just one is coming through, a neighbouring feather may be left alongside it as a 'guard'; it can then be clipped at a later date.
- Feathers should not be cut flush with the skin but a small length of calamus should be left to provide some protection for adjacent growing feathers. However, it should not be left protruding beyond the intact covert feathers. Failure to 'hide' these cut ends appears to be a factor in stimulating feather chewing.

Imping

In some cases where wing clipping has occurred there may be a failure of the clipped feathers to moult (possibly due to reduced mass of the feather) or the bird may be chewing the cut ends. Imping is used to replace remiges (flight feathers) damaged by wing clipping or chewing. It restores the full length of feather and this may remove the stimulus to chew, stimulate moulting of these feathers, and restore flight. The latter may provide further mental stimulation for the bird, which may be another aid in stopping chewing.

The best source of new feathers is from the same bird, and owners should always be advised to keep moulted remiges, as they may come in useful later. Failing this, feathers from the same species should be used. However, there is a disease risk in imping feathers from one bird to another. Therefore feathers should only be stored from birds that are negative for psittacine beak and feather disease (PBFD), polyomavirus, proventricular dilatation disease (PDD) and paramyxovirus (PMV). Feathers can be sterilized using ethylene oxide or they can be frozen prior to use in order to reduce contamination. As a last resort, feathers from a different species may be used, though they may look odd.

Imping is simple but fiddly and is best performed under anaesthesia, as it may be time consuming and it is easiest with a stationary patient. The basic technique (Figures 6.15 and 6.16) is as follows:

1. The stump of the damaged feather is trimmed so that the exposed end is smooth.
2. The replacement feather is trimmed so that it 'fits' on to the end of the old calamus, creating a new feather of the same length as the original. For this reason the equivalent feather should be used if possible (e.g. primary 1 to primary 1, primary 2 to primary 2).
3. The replacement is 'grafted' on to the old. A plastic or dowelling rod (or small-diameter knitting needle or kebab skewer) is trimmed and whittled so that it fits snugly into the base feather at one end. The other end is similarly trimmed so that it fits into the calamus of the new feather. Cyanoacrylate (tissue) glue is applied to each end and the rod is inserted into the calami. This stage must be done quickly before the glue dries. It is extremely important that the apposition of the old and new feathers is exact and that the replacement feather is oriented correctly.

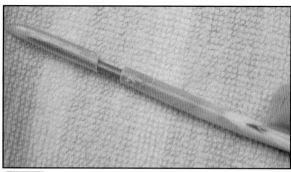

6.15 The imping technique. A rod (in this case a plastic knitting needle) is glued into the remnant of the calamus. A replacement feather is measured and cut to size, then secured to the rod.

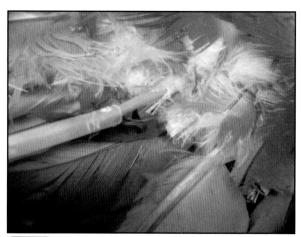

6.16 Imping. A replacement feather is being attached to the chewed calamus of a primary feather in this Scarlet Macaw.

These grafted feathers can be surprisingly strong and are quite capable of allowing flight. Even more surprising is the frequency with which birds tolerate the new feathers.

Bleeding blood feathers

This is a common problem and should be the primary differential diagnosis for any bird presented with profuse bleeding.

It is important that the bleeding is controlled in the correct manner. While ligation or application of haemostatic compounds to the affected feather may be effective in the short term, these feathers frequently bleed again and often become infected. This may trigger feather chewing and in some cases dystrophy or cyst formation. The feather should therefore be removed as soon as possible. It is generally done with the bird conscious.

The damaged blood feather is grasped and pulled out slowly while being slightly twisted. This technique stops haemorrhage by twisting and stretching the artery that enters via the base of the feather. It also stimulates the development of a new feather. Any residual bleeding from the follicle is controlled by gently squeezing the follicle for a few seconds.

Claw clipping

In general, specialist bird nail clippers or very small cat nail clippers may be used (Figure 6.17). For the larger parrots a grinding tool (on high speed) is preferred, in which case the nail can be shaped using the grinder but care must be taken not to damage the skin of the foot. Haemorrhage is less likely, as the heat from the grinder will aid in cauterizing the nail.

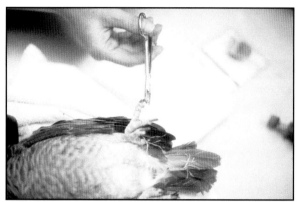

6.17 Small nail trimmers being used to trim the nails of a Grey Parrot. Note that the nail is being cut side-to-side and that only the tip is being removed. Alternatively a grinding tool may be used.

Where clippers are used, the nail should be cut from side to side (Figure 6.18). This results in a squeezing of the nail over the artery and reduces haemorrhage. The artery is often found near the end of the nail; it is easy to see and avoid in white nails (e.g. certain Amazon species) but less so in black nails. Therefore small amounts should be taken off each nail until either a desired length is reached or bleeding starts.

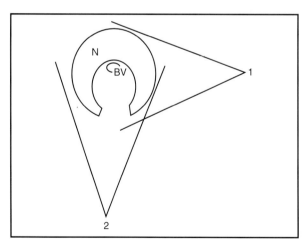

6.18 Cross-section of a nail. For clarity, the soft ventral plate is not shown. N, nail (hard dorsal plate); BV, blood vessel; 1, direction of clip for obtaining a small blood sample; 2, direction of clip when trimming the nail (note how the blood vessel is constricted by surrounding nail by the action of the clippers).

There is no 'set length' to achieve when clipping nails and each case should be judged individually. In general there is no need to perform clipping under general anaesthesia unless the nails are grossly overgrown and haemorrhage will be unavoidable in bringing the claws back to a normal length. In these cases anaesthesia avoids the need for prolonged restraint.

Haemorrhage may be stopped by using silver nitrate powder or sticks, or potassium permanganate powder or crystals. Where bleeding does occur it may be useful to remove all perches so that the bird hangs on the bars of the cage, thereby reducing its chances of knocking off the clot from the end of the toe. The bird should be closely monitored until bleeding has stopped.

It should be borne in mind that there may be important underlying causes for overgrown nails:

- *Perch width.* This should be appropriate to the bird's size and individual preference. If perches are inappropriate, overgrown nails may be seen in conjunction with pressure lesions on the feet
- *Failure to perch properly,* e.g. due to arthritis
- *Malnutriton or liver disease.* Abnormal keratin metabolism may result in an adult bird suddenly developing overgrown nails. Amazons appear particularly prone, in conjunction with hepatic lipidosis.

Clipping should be done again if and when required; there is no set interval and many birds will never need a clip. Avoidance of the need for clipping is based on provision of suitable perching and a good diet. A concrete perch may be useful for wearing down nails but in some cases, where the bird is not perching properly, these perches may damage the skin.

Beak clipping

This is more correctly referred to as 'beak shaping'. The beak is a precisely shaped tool capable of both power and great sensitivity. It is kept in shape by:

- Its own action (wear of upper against lower beak)
- Grinding of the beak against itself by the bird
- Grinding of the beak against the perch by the bird.

There should be no need to reshape beaks routinely. The need will arise only if the beak has overgrown or become deformed (e.g. scissor beak) from the following:

- Malformation in young birds (rare)
- Damage to beak and/or cere such that beak growth is affected or permanent deficits in beak tissues result. This may be from trauma or disease (e.g. scaly face in Budgerigars)
- Iatrogenic causes: unnecessary or badly done beak clipping may damage sensitive tissues, resulting in worsening of the problem; for example, bruising of the rictal phalanges (found on the upper beak at the commissures) is a common cause of scissor beak (Speer, 2003b) as the pain from this causes the bird to use its beak differently

- Abnormal keratin metabolism (e.g. malnutrition or liver disease). It is important to assess thoroughly any adult bird presenting with an overgrown beak.

Repair methods (Chapter 11) may be considered where problems stem from deformity or damage but in some cases regular shaping may be better tolerated than a prosthesis.

As stated above, the procedure is better termed 'beak shaping' as the aim is to return the beak to the normal shape *for that species* rather than simply making the beak shorter. It therefore follows that normal anatomy (see Figures 2.3 and 2.5) should be known before starting the procedure; although the basic design is the same for all psittacine species, there is variation.

It is highly recommended that the beaks of all but the smallest birds are shaped using a low-torque, low-speed grinding tool and a range of shaped grinding pieces (Figure 6.19). For small birds a pair of bird nail trimmers and nail files may be used.

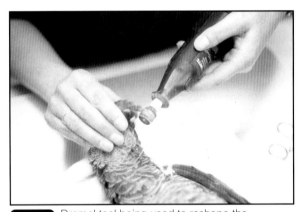

6.19 Dremel tool being used to reshape the overgrown beak of a Grey Parrot.

Beak layers should be taken back carefully and slowly, to avoid entering the sensitive underlying tissues. Where haemorrhage is encountered, the area should be cauterized with potassium permanganate or silver nitrate and no further tissue should be removed in this region.

Being more aggressive when clipping, and removing more tissue, does not mean that clipping needs to be performed less frequently (Figure 6.20). It will often result in further damage, thus increasing the number of clipping or shaping procedures required. A more sympathetic approach, where the beak is 'reshaped', may lead to more frequent treatments in the short term, but in the long term it may be possible to restore the beak to a normal or near-normal shape, and this will ultimately reduce the frequency of clipping.

It is also recommended that the procedure is carried out under anaesthesia, as careful shaping is nearly impossible in the conscious bird (especially larger species) without damaging the beak, tongue or handler. Anaesthesia also minimizes stress to the bird. A single injection of carprofen should be given to any bird that bleeds during or following beak reshaping.

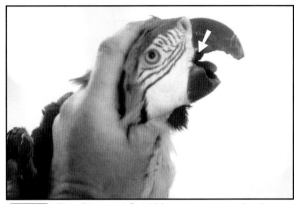

6.20 This Blue and Gold Macaw was seen by the author for a second opinion following an aggressive beak clip the previous day. The bird was unable to prehend food due to the pain from the damage to the end of the beak and the left rictal phalanx. It is obvious that this is not the correct shape for a normal macaw and the haemorrhage from the damaged areas has not been controlled, meaning an infection of these regions is a possibility. The rictal phalanges (arrowed) are very sensitive and a bird will shift loading to the other side of the mouth, resulting in uneven wear and a scissor beak such as formed within 6 weeks of this clip. The bird then required reshaping of the beak every 4 to 6 weeks to control this situation, showing that an aggressive clip does not necessarily result in fewer procedures being necessary.

Ring removal

A variety of identification rings may be attached to birds' legs (Chapter 3). Damage to these rings by the bird's beak or other external causes, swelling or crusting of the underlying skin, or movement of the ring to an inappropriate place (e.g. over the intertarsal joint) may result in constriction of and damage to underlying tissues. Further swelling results in increased constriction, and so on. Unless the ring is removed, severe damage to underlying structures can cause loss of the foot.

Where a ring of inappropriate size has been placed, and also in macaws (which walk on the entire ventral surface of the tarsometatarsus), an underlying pressure necrosis of the skin may result. This can progress to a deep infection or abscess.

In some cases owners may request the rings to be removed in order to prevent problems occurring. It is important that the legal consequences of removing an identification ring are considered and that appropriate action (e.g. placement of a microchip) is taken where this is necessary (Chapter 22). Any removed ring should be retained and returned to the owner. Where possible, cutting should take place away from the engraved area so that the identification remains clear.

Removal of leg rings is not always simple, especially where there is a lot of swelling (removal of the tough stainless steel rings used on larger species is difficult enough anyway). Routine equipment found in clinics may not be appropriate, as many clippers, cutters and saws will damage underlying tissues directly or through twisting of the ring when cutting. The latter may be the most common cause of iatrogenic fractures during this procedure.

Practices seeing birds should invest in specialist ring cutters (Figure 6.21) and a dremel tool with cutting burs for removing tougher rings. Where this equipment cannot be obtained, a small hacksaw blade may be used to cut steel rings but it should be noted that it is easy to damage underlying tissues using this method. Small pliers, narrow-jawed bulldog clamps or old artery forceps may be used to grip and bend the cut ring away from the leg.

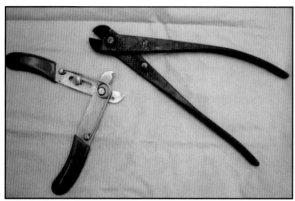

6.21 Ring cutters. The lower pair has a notch to prevent ring twisting and can be used for all but stainless steel rings. The upper pair is much heavier, with a sharp cutting edge; the grips are shaped to allow easier use. This pair can be used to cut some stainless steel rings.

It is recommended that this procedure is always carried out under general anaesthesia to stop the patient struggling.

When using a cutting bur, it is vital to avoid heat damage to the underlying tissues. The ring should be surrounded with wet swabs and regularly checked for overheating. If it feels hot, cutting should be stopped and the ring cooled with water before recommencing.

Euthanasia

As in other areas of veterinary medicine, euthanasia of the sick bird is an option for the clinician where therapy is not possible, practicable or affordable and the bird is suffering. Similarly it may be felt that euthanasia of birds suffering from behavioural diseases may be a kinder option than being rehomed to a rescue shelter.

Whatever the indication, euthanasia must be carried out in a humane manner. It should also be carried out in a manner that takes into account the feelings of the owner. There is often a very strong emotional bond between owner and bird and this may be a very difficult time for all parties (Harris, 1997).

Cervical dislocation and decapitation of smaller birds are not humane methods in such cognisant birds. Instead, an overdose of anaesthetic should be given. Ideally this should be done by intravenous injection of pentobarbital but the restraint required may be distressing to the owners, should they be present. It is therefore useful to induce anaesthesia prior to this injection. If owners are present, it may be prudent to consider additional health and safety aspects of waste anaesthetic gases. Sedation using intramuscular ketamine may also be used.

Intracoelomic injection of pentobarbital may result in rapid death but it often does not and these injections may be associated with considerable pain to the bird. This method cannot, therefore, be recommended. Intracardiac injection of pentobarbital may be achieved in smaller psittacine birds but inadvertent intrapulmonary injection will result in considerable distress to bird and owner.

Where the body is required for post-mortem examination, euthanasia may be achieved by overdosage of a volatile anaesthetic agent. Both intracoelomic and intracardiac injection will result in tissue disruption, which may not be desirable should such an examination be required.

7

Clinical pathology and necropsy

Gerry M. Dorrestein and Martine de Wit

Introduction

A complete patient evaluation consists of a thorough history, physical examination and necessary diagnostic tests. These diagnostic tests are highly variable and are best collected according to the needs of the patient and clinical suspicions. Not all patients presented will survive; many avian practitioners carry out a post-mortem examination (PME) in their practice, during which careless observation and sampling can result in useless or misleading information. Changes in anatomical pathology are the substrate of the disease and understanding these changes gives clinicians an extra dimension in selecting the right diagnostic tool and therapeutic approach for future patients.

This chapter is intended to connect clinical and laboratory findings to pathological changes and *vice versa*. It guides the practitioner towards an understanding of the clinical changes, using pathological findings as examples, and suggests additional tests, where appropriate, to come to a diagnosis. It also helps the practitioner to perform a PME and to collect the correct samples to come to an understanding of the clinical symptoms. Much of the systematics and approaches are based on the authors' daily dealings with veterinary students in their clinic and necropsy room in the final year of the students' education.

The tools in this chapter are haematology, cytology, clinical chemistry, urinalysis, additional laboratory tests and morphological techniques such as PME, cytology and parasitology. The chapter does not go into detailed laboratory techniques and backgrounds, but refers to in-house possibilities in a well equipped veterinary practice.

Choice of tests and samples

The clinical value of a given diagnostic sample and test is determined by collection and processing as well as accurate interpretation of the results (Figure 7.1). In addition to the more common samples such as blood and faeces, many other techniques can give valuable information that can lead to a diagnosis. These include, but are not limited to, abdominocentesis, tissue and bone marrow biopsy, crop wash, nasal flush, sinus aspiration, tracheal wash, air sac wash and urine collection. Similar tissues can be collected at a PME. Although there are many different recommendations for parasite handling, storage and fixation, in the authors' laboratory all parasites are collected in glycerine alcohol (9 parts 70% ethanol and 1 part glycerine).

Basic tests performed on most of these materials are: macroscopic evaluation (opacity, colour, smell); microscopic examination of wet mounts (0.9% saline) and stained smears (before and after spinning); microbiology (after evaluation of the stained smear for making the right choice of a culture medium); and, in some cases (biopsy), a histopathological examination. The most common materials sampled are blood and faeces (faecal examination is discussed in Chapter 15).

Blood

Blood examination can be essential in establishing a diagnosis. A general psittacine blood examination includes a complete blood count (CBC), plasma uric acid, bile acid, calcium and enzyme (aspartate aminotransferase, gamma glutamyl transferase, glutamate dehydrogenase, creatine kinase), assays and protein electrophoresis (Figures 7.2–7.5).

	Advantages	Disadvantages
In-house	Rapid results, especially electrolytes, acid–base, blood gases, cytology	Unqualified/inexperienced staff? Lack of reliability/repeatability of some tests on some machines Maintenance of wet chemistry machines Poor quality control Difficulties in performing haematology due to nucleated red blood cells
External	Experienced/qualified staff, especially cytologists Good quality control Reliable/repeatable test protocols	Not all laboratories experienced in handling avian samples *or* interested in doing so Prolonged transport to the laboratory resulting in death of microorganisms, degradation of blood samples, etc. Delay in receiving results

7.1 In-house *versus* external laboratory.

Haematology[a]	Amazon	Grey Parrot	Macaw	Cockatiel
White blood cell count ($\times 10^9$/l)	5–17	6–13	10–20	5–11
Haematocrit (l/l)	42–53	41–54	42–54	41–59
Heterophils (%)	31–71	45–73	50–75	46–72
Lymphocytes (%)	20–67	19–50	23–53	26–60
Monocytes (%)	0–2	0–2	0–1	0–1
Eosinophils (%)	0	0–1	0	0–2
Basophils (%)	0–2	0–1	0–1	0–1
Biochemistry	**Amazon [b]**	**Grey Parrot [b]**	**Macaw [b]**	**Cockatiel [a]**
Uric acid (mmol/l)	72–312	93–414	109–231	202–648
Urea (mmol/l)	0.9–4.6	0.7–2.4	0.3–3.3	
Bile acid (mmol/l)	19–144	18–71	25–71	44–108
Aspartate aminotransferase (AST) (IU/l)	57–194	54–155	58–206	128–396
Creatine kinase (CK) (IU/l)	45–265	123–875	61–531	160–420
Gamma glutamyl transferase (GGT) (IU/l)	1–10	1–4	1–5	
Glutamate dehydrogenase (GDH) (IU/l)	< 8	< 8	< 8	
Calcium (mmol/l)	2.0–2.8	2.1–2.6	2.2–2.8	2.05–2.71
Glucose (mmol/l)	12.6–16.9	11.4–16.1	12.0–17.9	12.66–24.42
Total protein (g/l)	33–50	32–44	33–53	21–48
Albumin:globulin ratio	2.6–7.0	1.4–4.7	1.4–3.9	

7.2 Laboratory reference ranges ([a] Fudge, 2000a; [b] Lumeij and Overduin, 1990).

Parameter	Derivation	Comments
Bile acids	Extracted from portal circulation by the liver	Sensitive indicator of liver function; elevates and decreases rapidly
Bilirubin	Major bile pigment. Birds are not jaundiced	Elevation indicates obstruction
Calcium	Ionized and protein-bound[a]	Ionized calcium normally maintained at consistent level
Creatinine	Derived from creatine metabolism. Levels usually very constant	Severe renal disease: infection, decreased filtration, toxic drugs, renal neoplasia
Glucose		Elevated in diabetes
Urea	Protein catabolism. Excreted through glomerular filtration	Excreted in urinary water and therefore reabsorbed. Unreliable for renal function but elevation may signify dehydration
Uric acid	Major product of protein catabolism. Excreted by renal tubules	High uric acid = renal disease. Normal values lower in vegetarians than in carnivorous species

7.3 Blood biochemistry. [a] As most calcium is protein-bound, low albumin will automatically mean low total calcium; it is therefore most useful to measure ionized calcium.

Enzyme	Location	Causes of release
Alanine aminotransferase (ALT)	Present in many tissues	Non-specific cell damage
Aspartate aminotransferase (AST)	Liver, heart, skeletal muscle, brain, kidney	Liver or muscle disease, vitamin E/selenium deficiency
Alkaline phosphatase (ALP)	Duodenum, kidney. Low hepatic activity. Tissue-specific isoenzymes	Increased cellular activity (not damage), liver and bone disease
Creatine kinase (CK)	Skeletal and cardiac muscle, brain	Muscle damage, convulsions, vitamin E/selenium deficiency, lead toxicity, intramuscular injections
Gamma glutamyl transferase (GGT)	Biliary and renal tubular epithelium	Hepatocellular damage and some renal diseases
Glutamate dehydrogenase (GDH)	Skeletal and cardiac muscle, liver, bone and kidney	Hepatic necrosis, haemolysis, muscle damage

7.4 Enzyme interpretations.

Change in fraction	Associated with
Decreased albumin	Decreased production (such as liver insufficiency), increased (gastrointestinal) loss (such as proventricular dilatation disease), or increased use (such as chronic inflammation)
Elevated α-globulins	Acute inflammation or infection, reproductively active female
Elevated β-globulins	Acute inflammation or infection
Elevated γ-globulins	More chronic inflammation or infection

7.5   Common abnormalities on plasma protein electrophoresis.

A complete blood count includes packed cell volume (PCV), total protein (total solids), albumin, white blood cell count (WBC) and the percentages of heterophils, lymphocytes and monocytes. Additional tests are selected based on the clinical findings and the results of the general screening and other laboratory tests. Where there is uncertainty about sample type and handling, the laboratory performing the analysis should be contacted. This is especially true for the analysis of toxic agents, where the choice of containers is important for some (zinc) and the choice of anti-coagulant is critical for others (lead).

Haemocytology, including cell morphology (Figure 7.6) and blood parasites, can add important information to clinical and blood examinations and may be mandatory in establishing the therapeutic plan. Laboratory testing for infectious diseases is essential in suspected ill birds, in post-purchase examinations and in the management of aviaries. Evaluating clinical laboratory findings to come to a clinical diagnosis or prepare a differential list of expected pathological changes *before* starting a PME is important to gain a better understanding of the physiology of avian diseases.

Cytology

Haemocytology and cytology are both based on the study of individual cells. In disease situations they can give information about pathophysiological changes caused by the disease. Both techniques provide a simple, rapid, inexpensive method of diagnosis that can be performed in the veterinary practice. Frequently, the aetiological agent causing the lesion can be identified. However, the veterinary surgeon should be aware of the limitations of diagnostic cytology:

- It does not always provide a definitive diagnosis
- It does not give information concerning the architecture of the tissue (cells in the same smear may have originated from different areas of the organ or lesion), the size of the lesion, or the invasiveness of a malignant lesion
- The cells observed may not necessarily represent the true nature of the lesion. An example of this is the imprinting of the ulcerated surface of a neoplastic mass that reveals the cytological features of inflammation and infection only.

Cytopathology should not compete with histopathology; the two should complement each other in achieving the final diagnosis. Occasionally one is unable to characterize the cells in a specimen; a repeat smear or biopsy may be required to define the lesion.

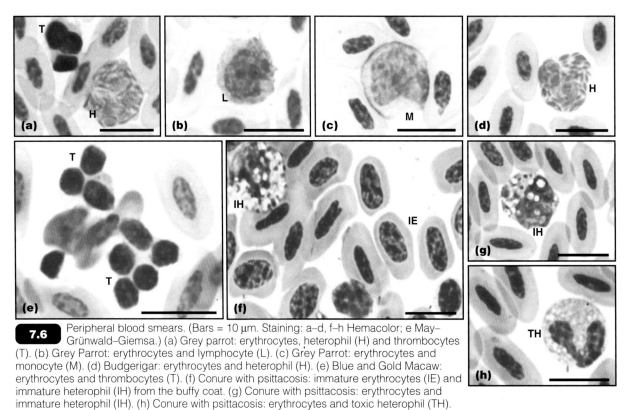

7.6   Peripheral blood smears. (Bars = 10 μm. Staining: a–d, f–h Hemacolor; e May–Grünwald–Giemsa.) (a) Grey parrot: erythrocytes, heterophil (H) and thrombocytes (T). (b) Grey Parrot: erythrocytes and lymphocyte (L). (c) Grey Parrot: erythrocytes and monocyte (M). (d) Budgerigar: erythrocytes and heterophil (H). (e) Blue and Gold Macaw: erythrocytes and thrombocytes (T). (f) Conure with psittacosis: immature erythrocytes (IE) and immature heterophil (IH) from the buffy coat. (g) Conure with psittacosis: erythrocytes and immature heterophil (IH). (h) Conure with psittacosis: erythrocytes and toxic heterophil (TH).

At PME, cytology is an invaluable tool for defining the presumptive diagnosis and for starting treatment in the flock situation. It is indispensable for a rapid investigation of possible bacterial, mycotic or yeast infections. The diagnosis of many protozoal infections (e.g. *Giardia* (Figure 7.7), *Atoxoplasma*, *Microsporidium* and *Plasmodium* spp.) depends on demonstrating these organisms in impression smears of a selection of organs. This technique is also an invaluable aid for a quick differentiation between tumour and inflammation.

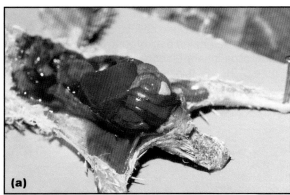

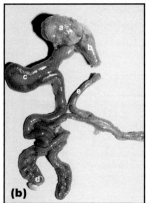 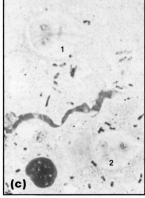

7.7 (a) Budgerigar fledgling with *Giardia* enteritis; (b) a = ventriculus (gizzard); b = proventriculus; c = duodenum plus pancreas; d = small intestine with Meckel's (vitelline) diverticulum; e = ileum; (c) 1, 2 = *Giardia*. (Original magnification 1000x oil immersion)

In the clinic a cytological examination of swellings, discharges from eyes, nostrils and wounds, fluids, mouth, crop and cloacal swabs, and faecal smears can give much additional information about the nature and the aetiology of a process or symptom. Cytological samples of the alimentary tract of live birds can be obtained using a cotton swab or by aspiration (cloaca, proventriculus, crop). At PME, samples of the alimentary tract are obtained by scraping any lesions with a cotton swab or spatula blade. The material can also be used for microbiological culture and microscopic examination. It is important that cytological specimens are taken from fresh sources, since cells degenerate rapidly following the death of the patient or removal of the tissue.

Cytological evaluation is always an adjunct to other diagnostic procedures. A definitive diagnosis often requires information from the clinical history, physical examination, evaluation of samples obtained from the bird, radiographs, surgical investigations, PME and histopathology.

Sampling techniques and sample preparation

Blood smears

Blood for haematological evaluation can be obtained by several methods (Chapter 6). Blood smears should be made with fresh, non-heparinized blood (heparin interferes with the proper staining of the blood cells), which can be obtained either from the needle used to obtain the sample or from blood collected directly into a non-heparinized microhaematocrit tube. EDTA-treated blood can also be used (Figure 7.8). The smear can be made using the standard two-slide wedge technique or by using the slide and cover glass method. After spreading the blood, the smear is air dried.

Heparinized blood	EDTA and clotted blood
Smaller sample required as it gives more plasma	Large sample required Less serum available
Total protein higher	Fibrinogen absent
Separate immediately, as cells break down releasing enzymes and electrolytes	Allow clot to retract (usually 1 hour at room temperature) and centrifuge in a gel tube
Can post; plasma should be separated	Can post; serum should be separated
Potentially poor cytology, so prepare air-dried smears	Better cytology but air-dried smears still useful

7.8 Comparison of heparinized and EDTA-treated blood for avian histology and biochemistry.

Cytology samples

A successful cytological examination is only possible if the following four conditions are achieved:

- Representative sample
- Good quality smear
- Good staining technique
- Correct evaluation of the cytological findings.

Fine-needle aspiration

Fine-needle aspiration often provides a good cytological sample for a rapid presumptive diagnosis without radical tissue removal, and this can be performed in the examination room.

Contact smears

Contact smears are made by imprinting the removed mass or the tissue obtained from the scraping of an exposed lesion *in situ* or at PME. At a standard PME, impression smears are made from the cut surfaces of liver, spleen and lungs, and also from an endgut scraping. All this material can be collected on one slide. Extra impressions are made from macroscopically altered organs. Impressions of organs should be made from a freshly cut surface, which should be fairly dry and free of blood. This can be achieved by gently blotting the surface with a clean paper towel. Imprint slides can then be made by gently touching the glass with the mass or by touching the microscope slide on to the surface of the

63

mass. It is important not to use too much pressure and to air dry the slide quickly. Several imprints of the same organ should be made on each slide.

If the imprints show poor cellularity, more cells may be obtained by scraping the mass with a scalpel blade to improve exfoliation of the cells. The imprinting procedure can be repeated, or imprints can be made from the material remaining on the scalpel blade.

Direct smears

Direct smears can be made from aspirated fluids (e.g. ascites or cyst contents). They can be made using the wedge method or the coverslip method commonly used for making blood smears. A 'squash-prep' procedure should be used to make smears from thick tenacious fluid or from fluid that contains solid tissue fragments. Fluids that have low cellularity require concentration methods to increase the smear cellularity. Sediment smears made after slow-speed centrifugation (500 rpm for 5 minutes) of the fluid or smear made with cytocentrifuge equipment will usually provide adequate cytological specimens.

Fixation and staining

Once a sample has been collected and a smear has been made, the specimen must be properly fixed to the slide. If smears are to be sent to a diagnostic laboratory, they must be air dried, properly packed (broken slides are fairly common) and accompanied by a distinct identification and case history.

The method of fixation depends upon which staining procedure is to be used. Fresh air-dried blood smears and cytology slides are adequate for Romanowsky stains, e.g. Giemsa stain and many quick stains. At least two slides should always be made and at least one of them left unstained in case special staining is needed.

Cytologists use a variety of stains and staining methods, including acid-fast (*Mycobacterium* spp.), Giemsa (cells), Gram (microorganisms), modified Giminez (*Chlamydophila* spp.), Stamp (*Chlamydophila* spp.) and Sudan III (fat globules) (Campbell, 1995). Proper fixation must be applied if specific stains are used. To obtain this information the diagnostic service should be contacted.

The cytological descriptions in this chapter are based primarily on slides stained with a modified quick Wright's stain (Hemacolor, Merck). The great advantage of the rapid stains is the short staining time (usually 20 seconds), which allows rapid examination of the specimen and provides satisfactory staining quality. These stains are suitable for use in practice where a simple staining procedure is desirable. Many rapid stains also provide permanent reference smears for comparison with other cytological specimens.

Examination

Once the smears have been stained and dried, they are ready for microscopic examination. For a reliable evaluation of the haematological or cytological changes in the sample it will often be necessary to consult a haematologist or cytopathologist, but recognition of many aetiological agents is often easy and can give a presumptive diagnosis.

Scanning and low magnifications (100× or 250×) are used initially to obtain a general impression of the smear quality. At these magnifications, the examiner is able to estimate the smear cellularity, identify tissue structures or large infectious agents (i.e. microfilariae or fungal elements), and determine the best locations for cellular examination. Oil immersion (1000×) magnification is used to examine cell structure, bacteria and other small objects.

In addition to viewing cellular structure, the cytologist should determine background characteristics, the amount of peripheral blood or stain precipitation present (Figure 7.9), the thickness of different areas in the

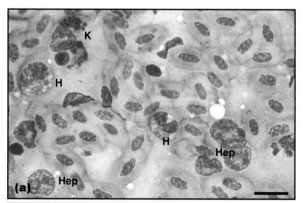

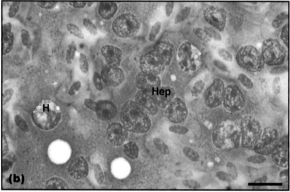

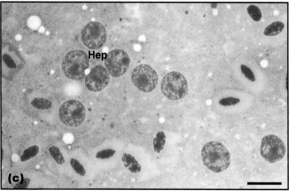

7.9 Macaw liver cytology. (a) Too much blood; too many erythrocytes. (b) Smear too thick – difficult to distinguish individual liver cells. (c) Excellent smear: liver cell nuclei are totally free and the eccentric location of the nucleolus should be noted. (Hep = hepatocytes; K = Kupffer cell with haemosiderin; H = heterophils). Bars = 10 μm.

smear, and the distribution of the cells. The background characteristics may be useful in defining the nature of the material being examined. Protein aggregates create a granular background with the quick stains. Bacteria, crystals, nuclear material from ruptured cells and exogenous material (e.g. plant fibres, pollen, and talcum or starch crystals from examination gloves) may be seen in the non-cellular background of the smear. Excessive peripheral blood contamination of a specimen will dilute and mask diagnostic cells, making interpretation difficult.

Stain precipitate on the smear should not be confused with bacteria or cellular inclusions (Figure 7.10). Stain precipitate varies in size and shape and will be more refractive than bacteria or most cellular inclusions. The thickness of the smear will affect the appearance of the cells and the quality of the smear. Thick areas do not allow the cells to expand on the slide and so they appear smaller and denser when compared with the same cell type on thinner areas of the smear. Therefore, examination of the cells in thick smears should be avoided. The cellular distribution should also be noted.

Microbiological cultures

Frequently, avian veterinarians are requested to collect from multiple-organ systems for microbiological culture.

Choanal cleft and cloacal aerobic cultures are often included in routine laboratory screening with psittacine birds, but any tissue or fluid can potentially be sampled. It is most important that the sample is taken only from the intended site, as cleanly as possible, and not the surrounding structures, to help to prevent contamination. A sterile swab of appropriate size should be used, moistened with sterile water or non-bacteriostatic saline. Biopsy or necropsy tissue and fluids may require different sampling and handling, depending on the material. A routine rapid stain of tissue from the sample area will give an indication of which microorganism can be expected and will help to select the proper culture media. In an in-house laboratory (but also after receiving back the results from a reference laboratory) the stained smear can be used for interpretation of the findings. Cultures must be carefully interpreted, and the significance of a given organism's growth should be based on clinical history, physical examination and other supporting diagnostic tests.

The collection and culture medium should be appropriate for the suspected microorganism. For routine aerobic and anaerobic bacterial cultures, commercially available sterile swabs and appropriate transport media should be used. Blood and MacConkey agar plates are standard media for most in-house aerobic bacterial cultures. The blood agar plate should be inoculated first, as MacConkey agar inhibits most

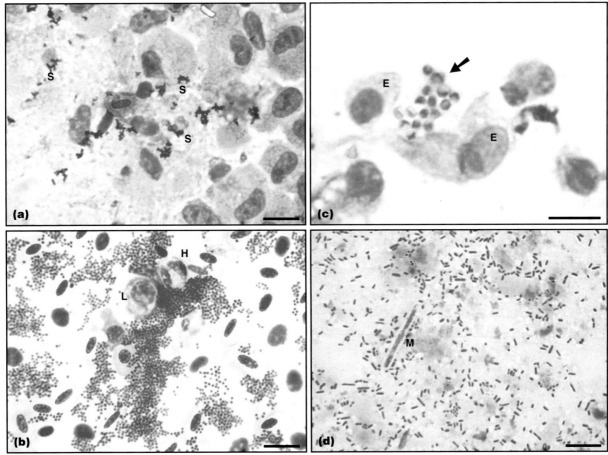

7.10 (a) Intestine: enterocytes and crystals of stain (S). (b) Endocarditis, *Streptococcus* sp. (L = lymphocyte; H = heterophil). (c) Lung *Aspergillus* spores (arrowed) and bronchial epithelial cells (E). (d) Intestine: rod-shaped bacteria and the 'megabacterium' *Macrorhabdus ornithogaster* (M). Bars = 10 μm.

non-enteric Gram-negative rods (except *Pseudomonas*) and all Gram-positive microorganisms. Most Gram-negative enteric bacteria (*Escherichia coli*, *Klebsiella* and so forth) grow well on MacConkey agar.

Viruses, certain bacterial organisms (e.g. *Chlamydophila*, *Mycobacterium*), many fungi and protozoal organisms require special culture media; the reference laboratory should be contacted for specific collection, handling and transport instructions. In general, if there is uncertainty about the need for special culturing techniques, fluid and tissue samples can be frozen. For longer storage an ultrafreezer at −70°C can be found at many diagnostic laboratories. With the exception of most dermatophytes and *Malassezia* sp. (a yeast organism recently found to cause thickening and flaking of the skin with variable feather loss in psittacine and passerine (canary) species), all medically important fungi (including *Aspergillus* as moulds and *Candida* as most common yeast) will grow on blood agar incubated aerobically at 37°C. Sabouraud and dextrose agar is used specifically to inhibit most bacterial proliferation and to promote fungal growth.

Clinical pathology of psittacids

Polyuria/polydipsia (PU/PD)

Primary polyuria is directly related to renal disease. Systemic disorders such as diabetes mellitus, stress, liver disease, hypercalcaemia or psychogenic polydipsia can cause secondary polyuria. Targeting laboratory examination of these patients includes urine analysis, CBC and plasma biochemistry (Figure 7.11).

Plasma proteins

Albumin (synthesized in the liver)
    Decreased in chronic disease, liver failure and starvation
    Increased in dehydration and during egg formation
Globulins
    Increased in chronic hepatitis, acute and chronic infections
The use of heparin raises the protein by approximately 5 g/l due to the presence of fibrinogen

---

Urea

Excreted through the glomerulus
Reabsorbed from the rectum
Unreliable for renal function and a guide to dehydration

Creatinine

Derived from creatine metabolism
Levels are usually very constant
Increases in severe renal disease

Uric acid

Major nitrogenous waste product in birds
Approximately 90% is secreted into the proximal tubules
A small portion is filtered by the glomeruli
Elevated plasma levels can be related to:
• Damage of more than 50% of the proximal tubules
• Severe dehydration
Increased plasma uric acid with normal plasma urea is likely indicative of renal disease. Elevation of both plasma uric acid and urea indicates dehydration

---

7.11   Biochemistry related to kidney disease.

The urine of a bird with polyuria can be collected easily from a fresh dropping on a non-absorbent surface. Standard urine stick tests can be used for the detection of glucose, haemoglobin and protein (Figure 7.12).

Specific gravity	1,005–1,020
pH	6.0–8.0
Protein	Trace amounts
Glucose	Negative or trace
Ketones	Absent
Bilirubin	Absent
Urobilinogen	0.0–0.1
Blood	Negative or trace
Urinary sediment	Abnormal: white or red blood cells, epithelial cells, casts, bacteria

7.12   Normal urine parameters (Hochleithner, 1994).

The avian glomerulus is impermeable to most proteins, including albumin; therefore, no protein, or only a trace, should be present in avian urine. Glomerulonephritis can result in marked protein loss. Tubular damage can induce a mild proteinuria. In the normal avian kidney, all glucose is reabsorbed in the proximal tubule; therefore, tubular diseases can cause distinct glycosuria. Glycosuria can also occur when hyperglycaemia is present and the absorption capacity of the tubules is exceeded. Haematuria may be present with inflammatory or neoplastic diseases of the kidney, ureter or cloaca. Further differentiation between primary and secondary causes of polyuria requires blood examination. For an accurate diagnosis of the cause of PU/PD, additional diagnostic procedures such as radiography, endoscopy and biopsy are often necessary.

Uric acid and urea

Uric acid, the major nitrogenous waste product in birds, can be measured to evaluate renal function. Blood creatinine concentrations are not reliable in the evaluation of avian renal function. Approximately 90% of uric acid is secreted through the proximal tubules; only a small portion is filtered by the glomeruli. It is believed that, as in mammals, the avian kidney has substantial excess capacity. Elevated plasma uric acid levels in the parrot can be related to either damage of > 50% of the proximal tubules or severe dehydration.

Determination of plasma urea may be beneficial in differentiating between kidney disease and dehydration. Urea, synthesized by the liver, is excreted by glomerular filtration, so reabsorption increases with dehydration. Increased plasma uric acid with normal plasma urea is likely to be indicative of renal disease. Elevation of both plasma uric acid and urea indicates dehydration, but renal disease may still be present.

Glucose

Plasma glucose can be measured to investigate other possible causes of PU/PD. Storage of whole avian blood has little effect on glucose measurement. However, if the sample should be stored more than several hours, it is advisable to separate plasma and blood cells to prevent lowering of glucose levels. Occasionally, parrots demonstrate transient hyperglycaemia; therefore birds with hyperglycaemia should be tested again in 2 days. Often, stress hyperglycaemia cannot be distinguished from diabetes mellitus, but repeated measurements of glucose levels > 55 mmol/l may be associated with diabetes mellitus. Determination of blood glucagons and insulin levels is important for diagnosing diabetes mellitus, but tests for these hormones are not available routinely. Histology of the pancreas with atrophy or inflammation of the pancreatic islets confirms diabetes mellitus.

Calcium

PU/PD due to hypercalcaemia can be caused by egg laying, excess of dietary calcium or vitamin D_3, or malignancies. When performing a PME on a parrot with hypercalcaemia, attention should be paid to the status of the ovary and oviduct. Over-supplementation with calcium and vitamin D_3 can lead to dystrophic calcification of the renal tubules (Figure 7.13). A PME of these patients should also focus on hyperplasia or neoplasia of the parathyroid glands (Figure 7.14).

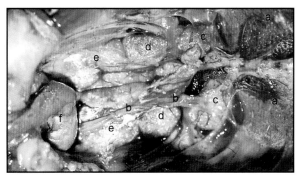

7.13 Juvenile nephritis in a Blue and Gold Macaw due to vitamin D intoxication. Note the urate tophi visible on the surface of the kidney (a = lungs; b = oviduct; c = cranial renal lobes; d = medial renal lobes; e = caudal renal lobes; f = cloaca).

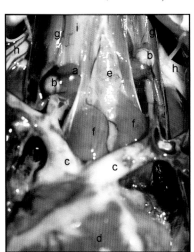

7.14

Hyperparathyroidism in a Grey Parrot (a = thyroid gland; b = parathyroid gland; c = aortas; d = heart base; e = trachea; f = syrinx; g = jugular vein; h = plexus brachialis; i = oesophagus or crop).

Total plasma protein influences plasma calcium concentrations. Total plasma calcium measured in most laboratories consists of an ionized fraction and a protein-bound fraction. About one-third of total plasma calcium is protein bound and biologically inactive; therefore, elevated protein concentrations can falsely increase the total calcium concentration, while the biologically active calcium concentration remains normal.

Green–yellow droppings

Green to yellow droppings (Appendix 2) can indicate anorexia or liver disease. Biliverdin is the most important bile pigment in birds. Anorexia leads to a higher concentration of faecal biliverdin and thus to a greenish discoloration of the faeces. Diffusion of biliverdin pigments from the faeces may result in green discoloration of the urine. Over 90% of the bile is reabsorbed in the jejunum and ileum and enters the enterohepatic cycle. In parrots with impaired clearing capacity of the liver, increased excretion of biliverdin results in a green staining of urates and urine (biliverdinuria). Hepatitis, hepatic neoplasia, fibrosis, lipidosis or haemochromatosis can cause impaired liver function (Chapter 20).

Determination of avian plasma enzymes can give information on current liver damage (Figure 7.15). Elevations in plasma enzyme activities are related to leakage of enzymes from damaged liver cells, but do not necessarily indicate impaired liver function. Damage of liver cells is usually related to hepatitis or liver neoplasia. On the other hand, chronic liver fibrosis or lipidosis produces little acute hepatocellular leakage and damage. Plasma enzymes useful in the detection of liver cell damage include aspartate aminotransferase (AST), gamma glutamyl transferase (GGT) and glutamate dehydrogenase (GDH).

Plasma AST is a very sensitive indicator of liver cell damage but specificity of this enzyme is low, because it is also present in muscle tissue. Trauma, injections or rough handling can also lead to elevation of plasma AST. To differentiate between liver and muscle damage, plasma creatine kinase (CK) can be measured. CK has a high sensitivity and specificity for muscle damage. If both AST and CK are elevated, muscle damage is present and liver disease is not proven.

Although GGT is a specific indicator of liver damage, avian GGT activity is low. The most liver-specific enzyme is GDH, but its sensitivity is low. GDH is located within the mitochondria of the liver cells. Elevated plasma GDH activity indicates severe liver cell damage and necrosis, which can occur with viral, bacterial or mycotic hepatitis. However, in circovirus infection of young Grey Parrots, liver enzyme activity is not elevated; the acute liver necrosis is caused by an extensive coagulation necrosis that prevents enzymes from reaching the circulation.

Determination of plasma bile acid concentration provides information on the clearing capacity for bile acids by the liver. Impaired liver function with elevated plasma bile acids can be caused by pathological changes such as liver fibrosis or lipidosis. It should be noted that plasma liver enzyme activities can be normal in fibrosis and similar severe liver disease, as no acutely damaged liver cells are present.

Plasma proteins

Albumin (synthesized in the liver)
  Decreased in chronic disease, liver failure and starvation
  Increased in dehydration and during egg formation
Globulins
  Increased in chronic hepatitis, acute and chronic infections
  The use of heparin raises the protein by approximately 5 g/l, due to the presence of fibrinogen

---

Alanine aminotransferase

Not diagnostic, too widespread and easily elevated

Alkaline phosphatase

Duodenum and kidney, low hepatic activity
Tissue-specific isoenzymes
Released by increased cellular activity
Juvenile or egg-laying birds show normal elevation

Gamma glutamyl transferase

Biliary and renal tubular epithelium
Most species: < 5 IU/l is normal
                5–10 IU/l is inconclusive
                > 10 IU/l is abnormal
The levels must be interpreted with the other enzymes

Aspartate aminotransferase

Liver, skeletal muscle, heart, brain, and kidney
Combine interpretation with other tests
Elevated with haemolysis
Last to elevate and last to recover in liver disease
Takes 72 hours to elevate
Always combined with CK

Lactate dehydrogenase

Skeletal and cardiac muscle, liver, kidney, bone, RBCs
Five tissue specific isoenzymes
Non specific but elevated in parrots with hepatic disease
Elevated with muscle damage
In liver disease, levels rise and fall more quickly than AST
Half-life of 24 to 36 hours
Parrots normal values 350 IU/l

Bile acids

Liver specific
Rapid and sensitive increase and decrease
Fasting may be a problem
<75 µmol/l is normal
75–100 µmol/l is inconclusive
>100 µmol/l is definitely elevated
Postprandial elevations occur in psittaciforms without a gall bladder. Assay considerations do not appear to differ based on the presence or absence of the gallbladder (Fudge, 2000b)

Bilirubin

Many avian species cannot convert biliverdin to bilirubin
But parrots have bilirubin present
Normal range < 10 µmol/l
< 5 µmol/l serum colourless
Carotenoids in serum or plasma can mimic jaundice

7.15 Biochemistry related to liver disease.

Radiography and ultrasonography can be helpful in the diagnosis of liver disease, but liver biopsies for histology are essential to establish a definitive diagnosis (Chapter 10).

The dyspnoeic parrot

CBC and biochemistry alone cannot reveal specific respiratory diseases but can add information to other tests such as radiography, tracheoscopy and endoscopy. Acute and chronic inflammation of the respiratory system can lead to leucocytosis and changes in plasma protein electrophoresis.

Heterophilia is the first haematological change seen in inflammatory disease, followed by lymphocytosis and/or monocytosis in more chronic stages of disease. Stress responses can also induce heterophilia. Therefore, the avian leucocyte count should be reviewed carefully with the recent history. Increase of the heterophil:lymphocyte ratio may be a measure of physiological stress. Avian patients with aspergillosis often demonstrate elevation of the globulin fractions on plasma protein electrophoresis, which causes a decrease in the albumin:globulin ratio (Chapter 14). It must be emphasized that elevation of globulins represents non-specific inflammation or infection with viral, bacterial, parasitic or fungal aetiology. In some cases with dyspnoea, especially in older Amazons, no abnormalities are found with the routine diagnostic procedures including blood panels, except for an elevated PCV. If other causes for high PCV are ruled out, it is possible that the bird suffers from lung atrophy. In cases with lung atrophy, PCV measurements of 60% and higher are found repeatedly. The diagnosis can only be confirmed with lung biopsy or on PME.

Gastrointestinal problems

Blood panels do not specifically identify gastrointestinal (GI) diseases. Inflammations may be detected with CBC and plasma protein electrophoresis. Biochemistry may reveal underlying diseases of other organs. Faecal assessment should be part of every avian clinical examination and is mandatory for birds with GI disease. Parasites can be detected in fresh faeces with direct saline smears and flotation. Cytology may indicate abnormal bacterial flora and yeast infection. Bacterial and/or fungal culture can identify the causative pathogen.

In the regurgitating avian patient, a crop swab should be taken. A direct smear, cytology and culture can be performed to detect flagellates, bacteria or yeasts. A crop biopsy is indicated if proventricular dilatation disease (PDD) is suspected. Histopathological changes of PDD include lymphocytic infiltrations in the neural plexuses. The crop biopsy sample should be taken from an area with blood supply, which increases the chance of including enough neural plexuses for histological evaluation. Determination of plasma amylase and lipase may be helpful in the assessment of pancreatitis, and pancreatic necrosis or carcinoma; however, pancreatic biopsy is necessary to diagnose pancreatic disorders.

The weak Grey Parrot

In parrots with a history of weakness, which can range from falling off the perch to tetany, the plasma calcium should be measured. The classical history of hypocalcaemic tetany involves a Grey Parrot on a deficient seed diet without supplementation of vitamins and minerals (Chapters 12 and 19). Plasma calcium levels < 2 mmol/l can induce clinical symptoms of weakness. In these parrots, hyperplasia of the parathyroid glands (Figure 7.14) is present, without demineralization of the skeleton. The plasma calcium should be assessed with the measurement of plasma protein levels. A protein-bound inactive fraction is incorporated in the total plasma calcium; thus, low protein concentrations falsely decrease the total calcium concentration, while the active calcium concentration remains normal. The measurement of ionized calcium levels is a more accurate reflection of the bird's calcium status. In Grey Parrots, the normal range for blood ionized calcium was found to be 0.96–1.22 mmol/l (Stanford, 2003b).

Blood samples for ionized calcium measurement should be stored in heparin and analysed as soon as possible after venipuncture, because changes in the pH of the blood sample can affect the accuracy of the ionized calcium levels. However, samples can be sent out to external laboratories if blood collection tubes are filled to minimize contact with air, or centrifuged to separate plasma from cells.

Diagnostics of infectious diseases

Tests for specific infectious diseases include chlamydial and viral diagnostics.

Chlamydophila psittaci

Psittacids with clinical signs of *Chlamydophila psittaci* infection have an acute hepatitis (Chapter 13). Plasma protein electrophoresis can demonstrate elevated liver enzymes and a decreased albumin:globulin ratio due to hyperglobulinaemia. CBC shows leucocytosis.

In-house test procedures for diagnosing *C. psittaci* involve cytological staining or specific antigen detection. These tests determine the shedding of *C. psittaci* in swabs of conjunctiva, choana and cloaca. In an impression smear of the swab, *Chlamydophila* stains red with Stamp or Machiavello stain (modified Ziehl–Neelsen) (Figure 7.16). Commercially available ELISAs can detect *Chlamydophila* antigen in the swab. Most of these ELISAs were originally developed for the detection of human *Chlamydia trachomatis* and *C. pneumoniae*, but are also suitable for the detection of *Chlamydophila psittaci*. Immunofluorescence (IF) tests are also available.

The disadvantage of the cytological staining and antigen detection tests is the fact that only shed organisms can be detected. False-negative results can occur due to intermittent shedding, or inhibition of shedding by antibiotic treatment. Specialized laboratories provide polymerase chain reaction (PCR) tests to detect *C. psittaci* DNA. Serological tests measuring antibodies against *C. psittaci* are also available but, for an immediate diagnosis in the individual bird, serology is not useful, although high antibody titres are an indication that *Chlamydophila* is present. When using serology, paired sera are mandatory and this delays the diagnosis.

Making and staining impression smears from the spleen and air sacs allows a rapid preliminary method for diagnosis of chlamydophilosis from post-mortem material. False positive and false negative results are both possible and so confirmation of this test must be performed using PCR or isolation of pathogen. However, the described method is very useful for a quick first diagnosis within veterinary practice, especially if the bird died from psittacosis.

A small sample of spleen and a piece of air sac (both handled separately) is placed between two slides and squeezed. This squash technique produces an impression smear on each of the two slides. Both are stained according to Stamp:

1. The impression smear is air dried followed by heat fixation (the smear is heated three times through a flame).
2. Stain for 10 minutes using 1:4 filtered carbol–fuchsin solution.
3. Rinse with water.
4. Cover the smear with 3% acetic acid for 2 minutes.
5. Rinse with water.
6. Stain with a filtered 3% malachite green solution for 20–30 seconds.
7. Rinse with water.

After drying the smear it can be examined with a light microscope. *Chlamydophila* structures are detectable as little red spots within the tissue cells (other bacteria and the cells appear green). It is important to evaluate both smears of each organ, as the structures might only occur on one. Negative results are always questionable and must be confirmed by other methods.

7.16 Staining technique for the rapid preliminary diagnosis of *Chlamydophila psittaci* infection.

Chlamydophilosis represents a significant zoonotic risk and at PME it is recommended that, after opening the coelomic cavity, an examination is made for the presence of this infection before proceeding further. In many cases of *Chlamydophila* infection there are visible lesions, such as pericarditis, air sacculitis and hepatitis (hepatomegaly, often with serofibrinous deposits over the surface). In some cases, however, no such lesions are apparent. The spleen is the organ of choice when testing for chlamydophilosis. An impression should be made, air dried and stained by modified Ziehl–Neelsen and examined under a high power (1000×) oil immersion objective (Figure 7.17). *Chlamydophila* organisms appear as clusters of tiny magenta-pink bodies within the blue–green staining cytoplasm of the host cells.

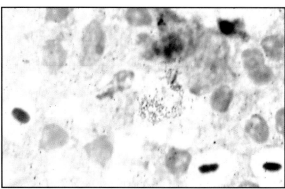

7.17 *Chlamydophila* elementary bodies stained red (Stamp) in an impression smear from the liver of a *Neophema* with psittacosis.

The traditional confirmatory test has been cultural examination but this has been largely replaced by the PCR test, which detects chlamydial DNA.

Circovirus infection (psittacine beak and feather disease)

A PCR is available for the detection of DNA from psittacine circovirus infection, the causative virus of psittacine beak and feather disease (PBFD). The assay is performed with heparinized blood. A positive PCR in a bird with clinical signs confirms that the symptoms are caused by the circovirus infection. If an adult bird without clinical symptoms tests positive on PCR, it is possible that this is due to a transient infection. It is advisable to retest these birds after 90 days. If the PCR is negative after 90 days, the bird has removed the virus. If the PCR is still positive after 90 days, the bird should be considered permanently infected with the virus. PBFD, the chronic form of the circovirus infection, can also be diagnosed by biopsy of follicles from dysplastic feathers: basophilic inclusion bodies indicate the PBFD virus. The virus can be seen with an electron microscope but cannot be cultured.

In juvenile Grey Parrots (and other African parrots) with acute signs of a circovirus infection, immediate diagnostic testing may be necessary. It is a very common finding in baby Greys purchased from pet shops. Within minutes, CBC can give an indication of circovirus infection. Severe anaemia and a white blood cell count of 0 or 1×10^9/l strongly suggest an acute circovirus infection in these juveniles with acute lethargy. In cases where the bird has no heterophils and is also anaemic, a negative PBFD PCR test on blood should be investigated further. In many of those cases the PCR on bone marrow will be positive. At PME, these juveniles demonstrate hepatic necrosis (Figure 7.32) and often secondary infections such as bacteraemia or an acute aspergillosis. Bursa, bone marrow and liver samples should always be taken at PME: some of each tissue should be frozen, some of each should be fixed in buffered formalin, and some sent for PCR. If there is a financial constraint, bone marrow should be PCR tested first. If basophilic inclusion bodies are seen in the bursa on histology, circovirus infection should be suspected.

Polyomavirus infection

Polyomavirus infection can be detected with a PCR. Viraemia can be detected in blood samples and the virus can also be found in cloacal swabs. After the virus is no longer present in the blood, it can still be shed in the cloaca for up to 4 weeks. However, cloacal polyomavirus DNA can be shed intermittently and thus can be missed. If a bird dies from a polyomavirus infection, PME demonstrates haemorrhages and hepatic necrosis. Intranuclear inclusion bodies are found in different organs, but mostly in spleen and the glomerulus epithelial cells of the kidneys (Figure 7.18). These two organs should always be collected at PME, especially when a polyomavirus infection is suspected or needs to be confirmed histologically or by using the PCR test.

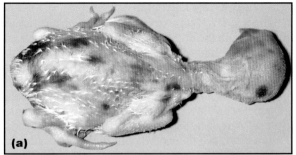
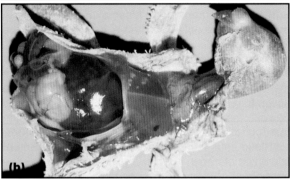
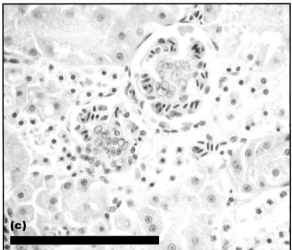
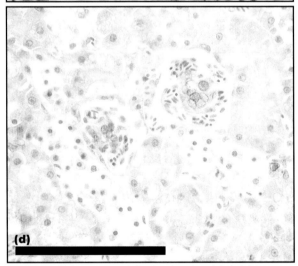

7.18 Polyomavirus infection in a lovebird chick: (a) subcutaneous haemorrhages; (b) hydrops ascites; (c) histology of kidney intranuclear inclusion bodies, HE, 1000× (oil immersion); (d) histology of kidney intranuclear inclusion bodies, ABC polyomavirus, 1000× (oil immersion). Bars = 100 µm.

Diagnostic PME and pathology

A complete PME is often the best method for truly evaluating and understanding a disease process. The ultimate goal is to take that information and experience and apply it to living patients (Echols, 2003). This section guides the reader through the PME step by step and discusses the different possibilities in each step, combining clinical findings and pathological changes. It also suggests the samples to be taken and how to proceed to reach the final diagnosis. **If the clinician suspects that a bird has died from paramyxovirus (Newcastle disease) or avian influenza, the carcass must remain unopened and DEFRA must be notified (Chapter 22).**

In addition to the obvious goal of determining a cause of death, a PME can provide valuable information concerning case management and therapy. In some cases a PME is essential due to potential legal actions. To obtain the maximum value from a PME, consultation with a pathologist and histopathology is necessary. In an ideal situation, with no economical restraints, clinicians would be able to submit whole birds to the pathologist for PME and histopathology. In many cases the clinician will have to carry out the PME and select tissues for submission. Since the maximum amount of information is desired, certain guidelines should be followed (Schmidt et al., 2003).

To make a diagnosis, the pathologist uses the clinical history (including haematology, blood chemistry, morphological techniques, therapeutic measurements), the gross description of the lesions, culture results and other data as well as the cytological and histological appearance of the lesions. Absence of any of these or incorrect submission of tissues will hamper this process. The quality of information received from examination of the samples is directly proportional to the quality and choice of the specimens submitted and the information that accompanies them.

When euthanasia of a bird is proposed, haematological samples should be collected prior to euthanasia. Larger samples may be obtained from the jugular vein or, under anaesthesia, from direct heart puncture through the thoracic inlet. The blood serum or plasma should be separated and submitted or saved and frozen pending PME results. This may be helpful in diagnosis of endocrine disorders or viral infections. Routine haematological tests may also be performed on these samples.

The method of euthanasia should be indicated to the pathologist. Since intracoelic injections of barbiturate solutions can create extensive lesions, the best euthanasia method is an overdose of an inhalant anaesthetic gas, as this leaves the least amount of artificial changes to the body.

- The PME should be performed as soon as possible after death.
- To promote rapid cooling of the carcass, thoroughly soak the plumage in cold water to which a small amount of soap or detergent has been added to aid complete wetting of the plumage and skin (it also prevents spreading of infectious material by feather dust).
- When the carcass is ready to be sent to a pathology laboratory, place it in a plastic bag, squeeze out all excess air, seal or tie the bag, refrigerate, and contact the laboratory for further instructions.
- If the carcass has been cooled immediately upon death and can be submitted to the laboratory within 72–96 hours of the time of death, it should be refrigerated (*not* frozen) and packed with sufficient ice or cool packs to keep it cold until arrival at the laboratory.
- If delivery to the laboratory is expected to be delayed beyond 96 hours, the carcass should be frozen immediately rather than simply refrigerated. Frozen tissue specimens or carcasses must be packed with ice packs (or other frozen coolants) to keep them frozen until arrival at the laboratory.
- If the carcass is extremely small (e.g. embryos, nestlings or very small adult birds), the entire carcass may be submitted for histological examination. This is best accomplished by opening the body cavity, gently separating the viscera and fixing the entire carcass in formol saline solution.

Whether the practitioner is performing the PME or simply collecting diagnostic material, preparation must be systematic. The correct selection of material for further examination and correct method of sampling, storage and shipping of material will increase the quality of results tremendously. When adequate time to do a proper PME or adequate facilities to carry out the procedure correctly and safely are not available, it is likely that mistakes will be made, systems missed or hygiene and safety compromised. In that case it may be preferable to submit the carcass to a specialist pathology laboratory.

A written report of the PME findings helps the clinician to keep track of the disease status of a bird collection.

It is important to note that even a negative finding is significant, since it means that all the signs that are being sought are not present.

Preparation

To perform a PME, it is advisable to use a well lit and well ventilated area (preferably under a fume hood) in a separate room and to wear adequate protective clothing and gloves.

Aerosols from feathers, faeces and exudates can be infectious. If there is any possibility of a zoonotic disease (e.g. chlamydophilosis and mycobacteriosis), a mask and possibly more extensive protection should be worn. It is also important to contain the feather dander and faeces in cases of avian polyomavirus and psittacine circovirus infections, so as not to contaminate the premises, clothing or adjacent birds.

Disinfectant solutions should be readily available for clean-up after the PME, but neither these solutions nor their fumes should come in contact with tissues being collected, as they may lyse cells and destroy microorganisms needed for culture. Formalin fumes should not be allowed contact with tissues that are to be cultured or with blood or tissue cytological smears, as this can severely distort staining and interpretation.

Instruments

It is helpful to have two sets of instruments that are designated for PMEs and not used around living birds. One set is used for opening the bird and the other to collect internal organ samples for culture and virus diagnostics. Both sets should be thoroughly cleaned and sterilized after use.

The instrument packs should include two scalpel blades and handles (one for cutting, one for burning organ surfaces before taking a microbiology sample), thumb-forceps, scissors and, in one set, a rongeur-type instrument for cutting bone and removing the brain (Figure 7.19). A set of ophthalmic instruments and a head loupe are invaluable in the PME of small birds, neonates and dead-in-shell embryos. Other useful equipment includes a gram scale, a hand-lens or dissecting microscope, and absorbent paper tissues.

In addition to instruments, the following should be on hand:

- 10% neutral buffered formalin (= 4% formaldehyde)
- 70% ethyl alcohol for wetting and disinfecting the feathers and skin
- 70% ethyl alcohol mixed with 10% glycerin is used for collecting parasitological specimens

- A bottle with saline (0.9% NaCl) with a pipette (for parasitological examination)
- Appropriate containers.

Other equipment for ancillary diagnostic procedures includes:

- Syringes and needles to obtain samples for serology, haematology, or cytology
- Clean glass slides for impression smears
- A stain set for cytology (e.g. rapid stains plus Stamp or Macchiavello)
- Clean glass slides and coverslips for wet mounts (parasitology)
- Burner for heating and sterilizing one scalpel blade before taking a sample for microbiology
- Sterile swabs or culture tubes with appropriate transport media for bacterial or fungal culture
- Transport media or material for PCR of chlamydophila, mycobacteria, polyomavirus and circovirus
- Petri dishes or freezer-proof tubes for submission of tissues for viral isolation.

A digital camera for documentation of gross lesions or where litigation is possible might be useful. In the latter case:

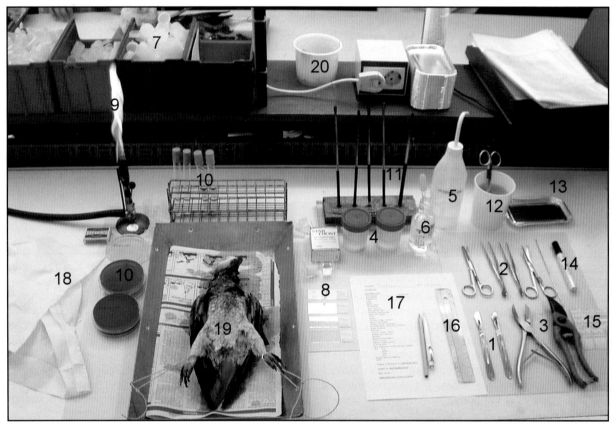

7.19 Necropsy layout: (1) two scalpel blades and handles; (2) one pair anatomical and one pair surgical forceps and two pairs scissors; (3) bone-cutting forceps; (4) containers with 10% buffered formalin; (5) 70% ethyl alcohol for wetting and disinfecting feathers and skin; (6) saline with pipette for wet mounts; (7) additional containers; (8) clean marked glass slides for cytology and wet mounts (parasitology); (9) burner for heating and sterilizing a scalpel blade and wire loop for culturing; (10) culture media for bacteriology and mycology; (11) wire loops for microbiological sampling; (12) container with disinfectant for the instruments; (13) aluminium foil plates for holding small organs or tissues; (14) waterproof marker; (15) preprinted labels; (16) ruler; (17) copy of PME work-form and checklist; (18) paper towels for cleaning in between; (19) prepared bird before starting necropsy; (20) container with disinfectants for discarding used glass slides.

- Always use a label showing the bird's laboratory reference number and the date.
- Use blue or green paper as a background for the carcass or organs.
- To provide a scale, use a plastic ruler or disposable paper measuring tape.

In general it is better to take photographs during the PME, preferably with an assistant to help so that the clinician does not have to remove the gloves before using the camera. On the other hand, in many cases it is possible to do most of the PME using forceps and scissors without touching the carcass.

To save time and prevent interruptions in the flow of the procedure, glass slides, sealable bags and formalin jars should be labelled with the owner's name and a note of the tissues enclosed before the PME is commenced. To record the findings during the PME, scribbling paper can be used and discarded with the carcass after finishing the PME and writing the final report.

PME protocol

The particular routine used for gross PME of birds can vary, but in each case all organs should be examined (Rae, 2003). The use of a checklist will ensure that all organs and systems are examined. All findings should be documented and this checklist should become part of the medical record.

Impression smears are a useful adjunct to a complete PME (see cytology section above). In the authors' protocol, two sets of impression smears are made from liver, spleen, lung and rectum; organs with pathological changes are automatically added; and for all columbiforms and psittaciforms an immunofluorescence staining test (IFT) of impression smears for *Chlamydophila* spp. of the same organs is done.

The choice of tissues for histopathological examination can be determined by several philosophies:

- Economic reasons. This is a poor rationale; it is better to collect samples of everything (all organs, the grossly normal and abnormal) and, after consulting the pathologist, send in the selected tissues and keep the others 'just in case'. Then, at the very least, the diagnosis does not get cremated with the carcass.
- Completeness. This is especially valid for scientific research. Collect all the tissues listed in Figure 7.20.
- A standard selection completed with a choice based on the PME findings. This list is practical and will in most cases lead to sufficient diagnostic support.

Tissues from organ systems that appear to be involved in the problem, based on clinical signs and/or gross lesions, are a priority. If tissues from an organ system that was obviously involved are not submitted, there may be frustration when a meaningful diagnosis is not obtained. When lesions are present, the sample should include some normal tissue as well.

Tissues collected routinely

Heart
Liver
Lungs
Spleen
Kidneys
Proventriculus
Ventriculus (gizzard)
Duodenum
Pancreas
Cloacal bursa (in juveniles)

Additional tissues (depending on gross lesions observed)

Skin, including feather follicles
Pectoral muscle
Thyroid glands
Parathyroid glands
Thymus
Trachea
Air sac
Adrenal glands
Testes
Ovary and oviduct
Oesophagus
Crop
Small intestine
Rectum
Cloaca
Leg muscle
Ischiadic (sciatic) nerve
Bone marrow
Brain

7.20 Tissues collected on PME for histopathology.

Normally selected tissues are fixed in an adequate amount of 10% neutral-buffered formalin (1:10 by volume) for histopathological examination. The best way is to fix the tissues/organs in large pots so that they can be fixed in a large quantity of formalin. Before the viscera are posted (after fixation for 12–24 hours), the pots should be drained off and the fixed tissues placed in a bag. This method gives good fixation in a large volume, but is cheaper on postage. Any specimen must be < 5 mm thick for good fixation. Formalin will not penetrate well into the brain through the unopened calvarium or into the marrow of bone unless the bone has been cracked. Wet formalin-fixed tissue may be conveniently stored and shipped in plastic heat-sealed bags.

Tissues for histopathology should *not* be frozen. Freezing and thawing changes the gross nature of the tissues as well as making histopathology much less useful.

Tissues for toxicological analysis *should* be frozen:

- Collect liver, pancreas, kidney, brain and fat and freeze individual samples separately
- Also collect crop or proventriculus or ventriculus samples and freeze
- If needed, tissue from other GI areas should be collected in separate, non-metal containers. They may be frozen at −20°C after being wrapped in aluminium foil

- Freezing for virus isolation is best done at −70°C. If this cannot be accomplished, the tissues for viral isolation should be sent (by rapid mail) in sterile containers on wet ice. Pending the diagnostic investigation, most commercial laboratories can hold tissues frozen at −70°C if asked.

History

Before starting the PME itself, the clinician should draw up a differential list of clinical diagnoses or be aware of the affected organ systems. Based on the clinical signs and the laboratory findings, a list of possible pathophysiological processes that can cause the clinical pathological changes will suggest what samples are needed for supporting or confirming a particular diagnosis.

When the owner comes with a dead bird, all information and history about the case should be taken in the same way as when a live patient is brought into the practice. This includes identification (species, age and/or purchase date, leg ring or microchip), information about housing, feeding and any environmental changes, observed clinical symptoms, medical history and pertinent laboratory data when available. The cage or packing material should be inspected for the presence of parasite or other relevant information.

The most relevant data should be summarized on the work sheet. The differential list should be made and the most important organ systems involved should be identified. In many cases a dead bird is presented with a history of sudden death. This history should be evaluated in light of the gross changes seen, so that tissues can be selected properly (Schmidt *et al.*, 2003):

- If there are changes suggestive of chronicity, the GI tract and liver may be the primary problems
- If the bird appears to be in good condition and there are no gross changes, organs such as the heart, respiratory system, brain and endocrine glands need to be examined, as disease of these organs is often the cause of sudden death
- In the absence of any clinical or gross indication of which organs to select and where there are limitations due to economical considerations, liver and spleen are recommended, as these organs are involved in many systemic disease problems
- In birds under the age of 1 year, it is essential that the bursa of Fabricius (see Figure 2.12) be examined, as it is an indicator of the condition of the bird's immune system and often contains

specific viral inclusion bodies of circovirus not seen in other organs.

In cases where litigation is possible and the PME is done in the clinic:

- Document everything seen thoroughly
- Save leg band(s) and microchips
- Take photographic evidence of all stages of the PME, even if no changes are seen
- Collect many different samples
- Store the carcass afterwards in the freezer until the case is closed
- Send a complete set of tissues to the laboratory and save an alternate set
- Save material for possible toxicological analysis, and do any other ancillary tests indicated, such as microbial studies and PCRs.

External examination of the carcass

- Wash the carcass in warm water and liquid detergent. This reduces significantly the risk of inhaling dust particles containing microorganisms, in particular *Chlamydophila psittaci*. It also facilitates detailed examination of the body surface and, when the carcass is opened, prevents dry feather contamination of the viscera.
- After recording the band number etc. palpate for obvious swellings or fractures, and confirm that all joints are fully mobile. Check for proper bone mineralization by attempting to bend a long bone. In females, radiography is a good way of assessing medullary bone.
- Record information about general bodily condition, weight, muscle mass, joints, integument (including beak and claws), plumage, body orifices (eyes, ears, nostrils and vent), uropygial gland (in some species), trauma and abnormalities (Figure 7.21).
- Be aware that abnormal plumage results in an extreme energy loss because of the lack of insulation.
- Judge the feeding status based on the muscles on the keel and the filling of the crop and intestines.
- Take survey radiographs if heavy metals (e.g. rifle bullets or ingested lead) are suspected.

Finding	Diagnosis	Tests
Broken feathers	Feather plucking	Normal feathers on the head
Altered feathers with concentric pinching	Psittacine circovirus infection (PBFD). Polyomavirus infection is a differential in lovebirds and parakeets	Histology of skin with feather follicles PCR of a pulled feather
Pink contour feathers in Grey Parrots	Possible psittacine circovirus infection. Differential = damage to pigment-forming cells. In Vasa Parrots the brown feathers turn white for the same reasons	Histology of skin with feather follicles and bursa (in juvenile birds) Circovirus PCR test on bursa or bone marrow, liver or feather Histopathology of liver

7.21 Examples of alterations found during external examination. (continues) ▶

Finding	Diagnosis	Tests
Stress bars in the wing and tail primaries	Nutritional defect, illness, or parasitism	
Blood feathers, plucked and in the follicle, along with any skin lesions		Bacteriology (Chapter 16) and collect and place in formalin for histology
Changes of the skin and nares	*Cnemidocoptes* infestation, yeast infection	Wet mount, cytology, culture, biopsy
Signs of trauma or bruising		
Skin haemorrhages (Figure 7.18)	In juveniles, related to polyomavirus infection	
Unfeathered portion of the legs and the feet	Avipox lesions (very rare in psittacines), bumblefoot, herpesvirus pododermatitis, and self-mutilation.	
Examine the site of the uropygial gland at the base of the tail in some species	Often a site of chronic inflammation and neoplasia	Bacteriology and histology
Salivary gland enlargement at the base of the tongue	Vitamin A deficiency	Histological examination with metaplastic changes
Chronic necrotic lesions at the tongue and in the beak commissure (Figure 7.22)	Mycobacterial infection (often *M. bovis*)	Smear of deep scraping stained with acid-fast staining, histology, PCR
Swelling above eye or dilated nostrils with plug	Vitamin A deficiency	Histological examination with metaplastic changes in salivary glands
Conjunctivitis and sinusitis	Chlamydophilosis, bacterial (*Mycoplasma?*) or fungal infection. (For *Chlamydophila* infection, see liver lesions)	Stamp stain, cytology, bacterial or fungal culture
In Cockatiels: sinusitis, temporomandibulitis and myositis of the mandibular muscles	*Bordetella avium* or other bacteria	Cytology, culture, histology
Conjunctivitis (very rare in psittacine birds)	Avipox lesions	Cytology, histology and culture
Abdominal or other swellings	Tumours, egg-related peritonitis	Post-mortem
Cloacal mucosal prolapse	Papilloma	Histology

7.21 (continued) Examples of alterations found during external examination.

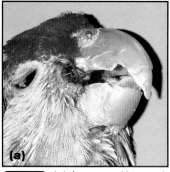 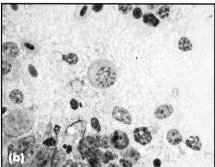 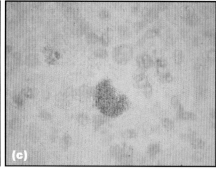

7.22 (a) Amazon with mycobacterial tongue infection. Impression smears with (b) ghost cells (Hemacolor, original magnification 1000×) and (c) acid-fast bacteria (Ziehl–Neelsen, original magnification 1000×).

Preparation of the bird

Small birds are wetted and plucked; all other birds should be wetted with alcohol (70%) before the PME. This is done to allow for better visualization of the skin, to part the feathers to permit incision of the skin, and to prevent loose feathers from irritating or harming the prosector (from zoonosis) and contaminating the viscera.

The bird is positioned on its back. In small birds the wings and legs are pinned to a dissecting board with nails or needles; large birds are fixed on a metal tray with pieces of rope. A useful tip is to pin or bind the legs over the wing tip; this keeps the feathers out of the way. A safety cabinet should be used if one is available.

The necropsy

General considerations (Schmidt *et al.*, 2003) are as follows:

- Post-mortem tissue changes must be distinguished from true ante-mortem lesions. The amount of time between death and PME, the ambient temperature and freezing of the carcass are factors that must be considered. Post-mortem changes can affect subsequent histological examination of tissues
- A relative lack or excess of blood contributes to the size, colour and consistency of any organ.

Colour changes may occur before or after death. The differences will be noted with experience

- The consistency of any organ may be affected by both ante-mortem conditions (including cell infiltration and connective tissue proliferation) and the amount of time that lapsed between death and PME
- Tissue loss may lead to symmetrical or asymmetrical changes in organ size and weight. Loss can indicate necrosis or atrophy and excess tissue may be due to hypertrophy, hyperplasia or neoplasia
- Ornithologists and biologists weigh the bird and organs and take standard ornithology measurements: beak to tail (if plumage is good), chordal or tibial length. Weighing should be done before the carcass is wetted. Condition would also be scored. For pet birds, the condition is based simply on the amount of pectoral muscle present: cachectic (absence of muscle) to fully trained muscle (and some stages in between) and the amount of body fat
- It is useful to weigh the carcass and also to take at least one and preferably two measurements so that the bird's size can be estimated. For instance, normal Grey Parrots weigh 350–600 g and vary commensurately in size; without a measurement of length it may be difficult to know whether a 400 g bird is thin or normal. Condition scores can be affected by storage.

General procedures for conducting a thorough PME include the following:

- Use a gram scale for measuring the size of organs
- Open all tube-like structures
- Cut all parenchymatous organs in slices of 1.5–2 mm to find small focal lesions
- Keep tissue for formalin fixation at < 3–5 mm thick (maximum 10 mm)
- Keep ratio of tissue to formalin at 1:10
- Collect tissue samples during the PME to prevent desiccation. Do not wait until the gross examination is finished
- Remember to collect and submit specimens from a broad spectrum of organs and systems
- Routinely collect heart, lung, liver, spleen, kidney, gonad and adrenal, proventriculus and gizzard, and a piece of intestine (duodenum and pancreas) for histopathology
- When suspecting a viral problem, freeze the tissue as soon as possible to −70°C (or temporarily to −20°C) or collect tissue on wet ice until shipment.

The 13 steps of the necropsy are set out below, with examples of pathology for each step.

Step 1: Subcutis

- Make a midline incision in the skin along the sternum from the mandible to the cloaca. Take care to avoid the oesophagus and crop.
- The skin is reflected using toothed dissecting forceps and a scalpel to expose the subcutis and fat, crop, pectoral muscles, keel, abdominal wall, and medial aspect of the legs.
- Note the colour of the muscles, fat deposits, abdominal volume and size of liver, subcutaneous haemorrhages, oedema, abscesses, bruising or evidence of injections in the pectoral muscle, and parasites in subcutis or pectoral muscle. Especially when the bird is being force-fed, look for signs of regurgitation (air sac) or feeding via the trachea, crop perforation or crop burnings. Judge the amount of food in the crop.

Examples of breast muscle pathology are given in Figure 7.23.

Finding	Diagnosis	Tests
Pale parallel stripes in leg or breast muscle	*Leucocytozoon* spp. or sarcosporidiosis	Cytology reveals bradyzoites
Large dark spot distal to keel at right side in abdomen	Swollen liver	Diagnosis: see later

7.23 Breast muscle: examples of pathology.

Step 2: Coelomic cavity (in situ)

- Starting at the level of the coracoid bone, make a longitudinal incision through the pectoral muscle down either side of the thorax.
- Grasp the sternum with thumb forceps and slightly elevate, maintaining tension on the abdominal skin.
- Using a scalpel blade, make a transverse incision just caudal to the edge of the sternum, being careful not to lacerate the liver.
- Remove the keel and pectoral muscle in one piece by cutting with heavy rongeur, scissors or poultry shears through the ribs, coracoid bones and clavicle, and note the air sacs that are now being exposed. Be careful not to cut the brachiocephalic arteries, particularly in freshly dead birds, or blood will enter the lungs via the thoracic air sacs.
- The exposed organs should now be examined visually *in situ* before they are any further disturbed.

For examples of liver pathology, see Figures 7.31 and 7.32.

Because chlamydophilosis represents a significant zoonotic risk, it is recommended that at this point an examination is made for the presence of this infection, before proceeding further:

- If the bird has a history or lesions suggestive of chlamydophilosis, microscopic examination (impressions of spleen, stained with a modified Ziehl–Neelsen) should be performed before continuing with the PME

- If the spleen smear proves positive for *Chlamydophila* it is questionable whether one can justify completing the PME in a clinical setting. The carcass should be wrapped in disinfectant-soaked paper towels and transferred to a polythene bag for safe disposal or storage in the freezer for confirmation by a referral laboratory.

At this point, compare the *in situ* view with the radiographs when they are available and confirm or reconsider the conclusions and abnormalities seen on the radiograph. Special attention should be paid to the situation of the air sacs when clinically the diagnosis of (mycotic) air sacculitis has been made. Normal air sacs appear as glistening transparent membranes.

This is also the moment to verify the clinical diagnosis relating to heart conditions, calcium endocrinological diseases (parathyroid), thyroid gland, liver problems and to note the pancreas in the duodenal loop, hydropic changes and severe GI problems. Be aware of artefact lesions caused by injection of barbiturates or other euthanates as brownish discoloration, often with crystalline deposits.

- Take smears from any abnormal material or exudate, and also from the air sacs when alterations are seen.
- If coelomic fluid is present, collect it with a sterile syringe for analysis.

Examples of air sac and pericardium pathology are given in Figure 7.24.

Finding	Diagnosis	Tests
Opaque and wet air sac	*Chlamydophila* infection	Cytology of collected material stained with modified Ziehl–Neelsen, IFT, PCR See also clinical findings and liver pathology
Opaque air sacs often with purulent deposits	Bacterial infection	Rods or cocci in cytology smear; culture and sensitivity test
Air sacs covered with several white/yellow plaques	Fungal infection (Figure 7.25)	Wet mount showing hyphae, scraping of material as stained smear, culture (Sabouraud's medium)
Air sacs solid with white/yellow material	Chronic fungal infection, mostly aspergillosis	Wet mount showing hyphae, scraping of material as stained smear, culture (Sabouraud's medium)
Air sacs, especially cervical and prescapular, with small black dots occasionally seen in lovebirds	*Sternostoma tracheocolum* infestation	Magnifying-glass and wet mount
Air sacs filled with food	Forced feeding	Wet mount and histology
Suppurative pericarditis	Bacterial infection (including *Chlamydophila*)	Cytology of collected material stained with modified Ziehl–Neelsen, IFT, PCR See also clinical findings and liver pathology
Pericardial sac filled with fluid (hydropericardium)	Inanition, cachexia, polyomavirus (in juveniles) (see Figure 7.18)	Muscle wasting, oedema and gelatinous fat-tissue, spleen and kidney histology
Pericardium and other serosae with white mucoid chalky deposits	Visceral gout, pericarditis, uricaemia	Macroscopy, wet mount with crystals (polarized light); often in combination with nephritis See also clinical blood values PU/PD

7.24 Air sac and pericardium: examples of pathology.

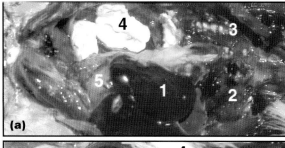

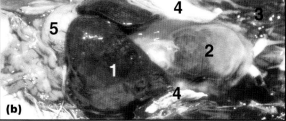

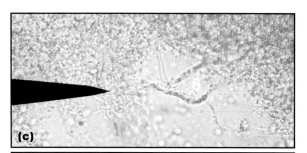

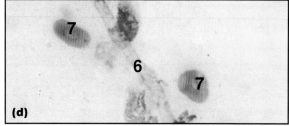

7.25 Aspergillosis. (a) Chronic air sac aspergillosis in Amazon lungs and air sacs. (b) Chronic air sac aspergillosis and hydropericardium in a cockatoo. (1 = liver; 2 = heart; 3 = lungs; 4 = air sacs filled with fungal material; 5 = gizzard). (c,d) Scrapings of fungal material showing hyphae in a wet mount (c; original magnification 10×) and (d) stained with Hemacolor (original magnification 1000×) (6 = fungal hyphae; 7 = erythrocytes).

Step 3: Thyroid, parathyroid glands and thymus

- Identify the thyroid and parathyroid glands located cranial to the heart and lateral to the syrinx adjacent to the carotid arteries bilaterally (see Figure 7.14) and collect for histology. Normal parathyroids are barely visible.
- Look for the thymus in juvenile birds laterally and at both sides of the neck, cranial of the thyroid gland as multiple grey lobes, and collect for histology.

Examples of pathology of the thyroid, parathyroid and thymus are given in Figure 7.26.

Step 4: Spleen

- The spleen can be found by grasping the gizzard with forceps, elevating and incising through the attached membrane/air sac and then rotating it towards the right side. This exposes the spleen in the angle between the proventriculus, gizzard and liver.
- Evaluate the size, colour and shape; note any pale foci. The normal spleen in the psittacine bird is round, small and pale (no blood reservoir in birds).
- Remove and measure the spleen and divide it into three samples: one each for virology,

Chlamydophila diagnostics and histopathology.
- Make impression smears from a fresh cut surface after blotting to remove excess of blood.

Examples of pathology of the spleen are given in Figure 7.27.

Step 5: Heart and large vessels

Special attention should be paid to the heart when clinical symptoms such as respiratory distress were obvious, or the radiograph shows cardiomegaly, or when hydrops ascites were present.

- After noticing the pericardial lesions, heart blood can be collected using a sterile syringe and needle for bacteriology.
- Remove the heart and large vessels and cut across the apex to check for an 'open' lumen and to assess the thickness of the ventricular walls.
- Open the heart and large vessels in the direction of the blood flow.
- Look for thrombi, valvular endocarditis lesions and pale areas in the myocardium. Remember: the right atrioventricular valve in birds is a muscular structure.
- Open the large vessels to look for atherosclerosis (mainly aorta, pulmonary artery or carotids and especially in Grey Parrots and Amazons).

Finding	Diagnosis	Tests
In Budgerigars and juvenile macaws	Goiterous thyroid glands	Histology
Parrots (especially Grey Parrots)	Hyperparathyroidism (see Figure 7.14)	Histology
Other species, especially juvenile parathyroid hypertrophy	Metabolic bone disease	Histology
'Abscesses' next to trachea	*Salmonella*, *Escherichia coli* or other bacterial infections in thymic remnants	Rod-shaped bacteria in cytology, culture, histology

7.26 Thyroid, parathyroid glands and thymus: examples of pathology.

Finding	Diagnosis	Tests
Spleen-swelling together with air sac opacity	*Chlamydophila* infection	Cytology of collected material stained with modified Ziehl–Neelsen, IFT, PCR
Very large swollen and cherry red spleen in parrots	Herpesvirus infection (= Pacheco's disease) or *Sarcocystis*	Liver necrosis with intranuclear inclusion bodies or protozoa, cytology, histology, IFT, virus isolation
Normal size, totally necrotic spleen	Reovirus infection	Histology
Swollen and pale spleen	(Bacterial) septicaemia	Cytology with bacteria, culture
Multiple irregular yellow foci in the spleen	Mycobacteriosis	Similar foci in other organs, in cytology non-staining rods, acid-fast staining positive. Differentiate avian/bovine strains by culture or PCR
Large firm spleen	Neoplasia	Cytology, histology
Enlarged friable spleen with multiple, miliary necrotic foci	Salmonellosis, yersiniosis	Similar foci in liver; cytology with rod-shaped bacteria; culture
Small, grey spleen	Lymphoid depletion, stress, viral infection	Cytology, histology, virus identification

7.27 Spleen: examples of pathology.

Finding	Diagnosis	Tests
Heart		
Epi- or endocardial haemorrhages	Septicaemia or agonal event (polyomavirus, circovirus)	Continue PME
Gelatinous, serous pericardial fat	Starvation, chronical illness	Continue PME
Pale foci or streaks in myocardium	Degenerative myopathy Related to vitamin E/selenium deficiency	Histology
Changes (inflammation, necrosis) in the myocardium	Myocarditis Caused by septicaemia or viral disease (e.g. West Nile virus, PDD)	Cytology, histology, microbiological isolation, continue PME
Cardiomyopathy with muscle cysts Enlarged lumen of left ventricle and only little difference in thickness of ventricle walls	*Sarcocystis* or *Leucocytozoon* Heart failure (Figure 7.29)	Cytology, histology Congestion of lungs and/or liver
Vessels		
Yellowish raised intimal plaques on wall inside large vessels; vessels stiff	Atherosclerosis (Figure 7.30)	Macroscopy, histology
Mineralization of large vessels	Renal disease or hypervitaminosis D	Clinical renal panel, kidney pathology

7.28 Heart and large vessels: examples of pathology.

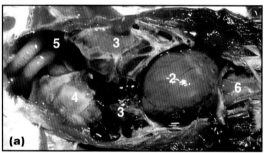
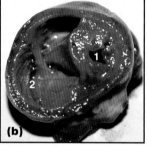
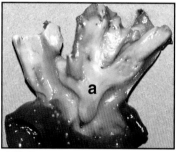

7.29 Grey Parrot with heart decompensation (1 = right ventricle; 2 = left ventricle; 3 = liver; 4 = gizzard; 5 = ascites; 6 = syrinx).

7.30 Atherosclerosis in a grey parrot (a = sclerotic plaque).

Examples of pathology of the heart and large vessels are given in Figure 7.28.

Step 6: Liver

- Evaluate the clinical pathological results for liver disease.
- Separate liver from the viscera by holding the hepatic peritoneum in the forceps and cutting them with scissors.
- In a freshly euthanased bird, blood spreading into the carcass after cutting the portal vein can hide many changes. In such a case it may be better to wait some hours before doing the PME or remove the blood from the vein using a syringe.
- Examine the liver for evidence of swelling, discoloration, inflammation, congestion and diffuse or focal lesions.
- At this point also aseptically collect liver samples: one sample each for bacteriology, virus isolation or DNA probe (PCR) testing, *Chlamydophila* testing, and histopathology. Sear a small area of one lobe of the liver and take a sample using a wire loop (see Figure 7.19) or sterile Pasteur pipette. If there are discrete lesions try to take a sample through the edge of a lesion.
- If there are no on-site cultural facilities, remove one lobe of the liver, using a sterile scalpel blade and forceps, and transfer it directly into a sterile sample pot.
- Hold the sample in a refrigerator at 4°C until it can be posted, preferably with an ice pack in an insulated container together with the other samples (each in its own sample pot).
- To make cytological preparations: take a small piece from one half of the liver, hold it in forceps, blot off any excess blood using filter paper and make impression slides from the cut surface on to three microscope slides. Stain by Hemacolor and modified Ziehl–Neelsen (for *Chlamydophila* diagnostics). The third slide can be use for an extra staining or sent to a laboratory for confirmation by immunostaining for *Chlamydophila*.
- Use any remaining tissue for cytology and toxicology, if indicated.

Examples of pathology of the liver are given in Figure 7.31. Gross liver pathology is illustrated in Figure 7.32.

Finding	Diagnosis	Tests	Comments
Enlarged red variegated liver with pale areas	Hepatitis	Cytology with many inflammatory cells; microbiology, material in freezer, histology	Elevated activity of liver enzymes
Orange liver in Grey Parrot with leucopenia	Acute circovirus infection	Histology, cloacal bursa for inclusion bodies, PCR	No increased liver enzyme activity
Enlarged liver with necrotic foci	Hepatitis caused by *Chlamydophila* infection, herpesvirus or adenovirus infection	Cytology, culture, histology activity and yellow urates	Often highly increased liver enzyme levels
Very extensive acute liver necrosis	Peracute or acute hepatitis by bacterial septicaemia, polyoma-, herpes- or reovirus	Macroscopy, cytology, histology, virology, culture	Often highly increased enzyme activity and yellow urates
Focal yellow proliferation with often central necrosis	Mycobacteriosis	Similar foci in other organs, in cytology non-staining rods, acid-fast staining positive	No increased enzyme activity or yellow urates
Small round necrotic foci	Salmonellosis or yersiniosis	Cytology with rod-shaped bacteria; culture, histology	
Evenly enlarged, often variegated, pale liver	Leucosis	Macroscopy (other organs often affected); cytology and histology	
Evenly enlarged, often variegated, pale soft liver	Degeneration	Cytology hepatocytes with vacuoles; histology.	
Enlarged orange-yellow liver	Fatty liver, lipidosis	Macroscopy, cytology, histology with Sudan III stain	Little increased enzyme activity
Small, pale and firm liver	Chronic liver fibrosis	Histology	No increased enzyme activity, but yellow urates

7.31 Liver: examples of pathology.

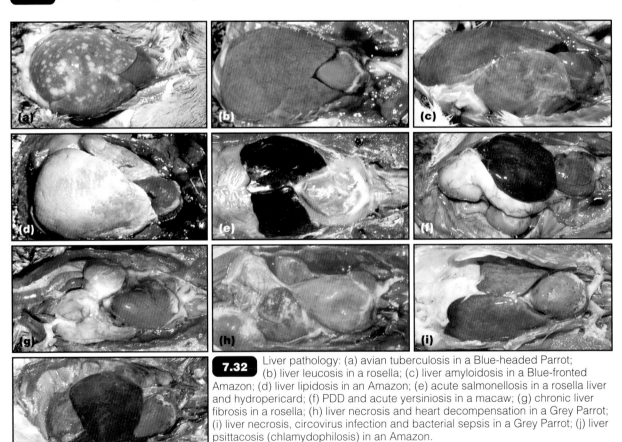

7.32 Liver pathology: (a) avian tuberculosis in a Blue-headed Parrot; (b) liver leucosis in a rosella; (c) liver amyloidosis in a Blue-fronted Amazon; (d) liver lipidosis in an Amazon; (e) acute salmonellosis in a rosella liver and hydropericard; (f) PDD and acute yersiniosis in a macaw; (g) chronic liver fibrosis in a rosella; (h) liver necrosis and heart decompensation in a Grey Parrot; (i) liver necrosis, circovirus infection and bacterial sepsis in a Grey Parrot; (j) liver psittacosis (chlamydophilosis) in an Amazon.

Step 7: Gastrointestinal tract

With the heart and liver removed, the GI tract is more accessible. The size and appearance of the crop, proventriculus, gizzard, duodenum and pancreas should be noted, but it is best to leave detailed examination of these organs until later. Therefore:

- Sever both the bronchi, reflect the trachea and reflect the GI tract to the right side of the bird to view the adrenals, gonads, kidneys and the lungs. Do not cut the rectum.
- If the intestines cannot be reflected because of peritoneal adhesions, check for a possible point of entry of infection, such as perforation of the gizzard or accidental damage to the intestine following laparoscopy.
- In a case of egg peritonitis, there will be masses of yellow inspissated yolk interspersed between adhering loops of intestine.

Step 8: Urogenital system

The adrenals (orange to yellow) are often obscured by active gonadal tissue, so it is easier to collect the cranial division of the kidney with the adrenal and gonad(s) attached for histopathology.

- Sex the bird visually. In most species, only the left ovary and oviduct develop (see Figure 2.13) but both testes develop in male birds. The gonads may be pigmented (brown or black) in some species (e.g. some cockatoos).
- Record the general size of the follicles and note discoloured, inflamed or shrunken follicles. In that case, sample for bacteriology, including selective media for *Salmonella*.
- Is the oviduct hypertrophied? Open the oviduct to look for exudate and tumours, and collect samples for cytology, bacteriology and histopathology as needed.

Examples of pathology of the genital tract are given in Figure 7.33.

Finding	Diagnosis	Tests
Swelling inside oviduct	Egg binding, egg concretments	Open the oviduct
Irregular swellings related to kidney or gonads	Tumour Common in Budgerigars, often related to paralysis of one leg	Macroscopy and histology

7.33 Common genital tract: examples of pathology.

The kidneys are nestled in the renal fossae of the synsacrum (see Figure 2.13), with the lumbosacral nerve plexus lying deep to the caudal division of the kidney. The ureters run down the ventral surface of the kidney bilaterally.

- Especially when clinically the uric acid concentration in the blood was elevated, or where visceral gout was diagnosed on observation *in situ*, pay extra attention to the kidneys. Differentiate between renal pathology and dehydration.
- In addition to the kidney/adrenal/gonad tissue collected for histopathology, aseptically collect additional renal samples for virology (polyomavirus–paramyxovirus infection), toxicology (lead, zinc) and bacteriology (if exudate is present).
- After removal of the kidneys evaluate the lumbosacral plexus, especially in cases of pelvic limb weakness or malfunction. Sample these nerves in formalin for histopathological evaluation.

Examples of pathology of the kidney are given in Figure 7.34.

Finding	Diagnosis	Tests
Pale normal-sized kidneys with fine reticular pattern of white urates over surface and in tubules (use magnifier)	Urate congestion, dehydration	Histology (fixation 100% alcohol)
Irregular pale swollen kidney with white foci often combined with visceral gout	'Renal gout; nephritis (see Figure 7.13)	Histology (fixation 100% alcohol)
Irregular swollen kidney with multifocal abscessation	Bacterial infection	Cytology, culture, histology
Enlarged hyperaemic kidneys	Acute nephritis	Histology
Pale swollen friable kidney	Kidney degeneration	Histology
White, firm small kidneys	Chronic kidney fibrosis	Macroscopy; histology
Granulomas	*Aspergillus* spp.	Scraping of cut surface of granuloma Hemacolor, culture (Sabouraud's agar), histology
Irregular swelling and growth	Tumour Causing clinically leg paralysis by pressure on the sciatic nerves	Cytology and histology

7.34 Kidney: examples of pathology.

Step 9. Respiratory tract

Examine the lungs *in situ* before removing them. Pay especially careful attention to this organ system when clinically there was an obvious dyspnoea.

- If the lungs appear congested or show discrete lesions they should be cultured for bacteria and fungi. Samples are best taken with the lung *in situ*, using a hot scalpel to sear the surface.

- If a viral condition is suspected (e.g. paramyxovirus), place lung tissue plus a portion of the trachea in a sterile container and store at 4°C until posted to a reference laboratory with other sampled organ tissues (brain and duodenum with pancreas).

The lungs are fixed in place within the avian thoracic cavity and are not freely movable. Removal requires gentle teasing of the lung tissue away from the ribs. In many cases lungs have changes in the dorsal part only and these can be missed if the lung is not removed. The avian lung is one tissue in which gross lesions may appear quite significant, but on histopathological evaluation turn out to be just passive congestion. Conversely, grossly normal lungs may contain significant histological lesions. Therefore, always include lung for histopathology, and because lesions can be focal or multifocal, it is best to include a large portion of at least one lung.

- Cut through the lungs at intervals and make an impression smear of the lung (along with impressions from liver, spleen and a smear from the intestines). This impression of the lung is also used to evaluate the blood cells for pathological changes and blood parasites (*Plasmodium*, *Haemoproteus* and *Toxoplasma* pseudocysts).
- At this point open the bird's beak, insert a pair of large scissors into the oropharynx and cut through one side of the mouth.
- Reflect the mandible and examine the oropharynx, including the choanae, the tongue and the glottis.
- Insert a pair of sharp scissors into the glottis and cut down the trachea both dorsally and ventrally, dividing it into two longitudinal halves. It is important to do this carefully and cleanly, checking in particular for haemorrhage, exudate, foreign bodies (seeds in Cockatiels), granulomas and parasites, items of inhaled food and also for white caseous–fibrinous material adherent to the mucosa, in the syrinx or bronchi. Such material is usually mycotic and, if present, should be examined microscopically (stain crushed preparations) and culture on to Sabouraud's medium.

Examples of pathology of the lung, trachea and oral cavity are given in Figure 7.35.

Finding	Diagnosis	Tests
Lung (Figure 7.36)		
Dark-coloured grey lungs	Lung oedema Often result of chronic cardiac failure	On cut surface transparent sero-haemorrhagic fluid, affected tissue sinks in water, cytology, histology
Dark-coloured wet red lungs	Lung congestion Watch for congestion in other organs and acute alterations of heart DDX polytetrafluoroethylene toxicosis, acute mycotic infection and *Sarcocystis* infection	From cut surface only blood; affected lung floats in water, lungs are supple and evenly bright red; cytology, histology
Dark firm lungs often variegated and focal changes	Pneumonic foci	Affected areas firm and sink in water, cut surface cytology (inflammation cells); histology, culture.
Diffuse pneumonia (in common with tracheitis and bronchitis) in Cockatiels	*Bordetella avium*	Culture (fastidious grower), histology
Dark, supple, collapsed, dry lung	Atelectasis	On cut surface only a dark colour of surface of lung and dried up
Scattered through the lungs white-yellow foci	Aspergillosis, mycobacteriosis	Wet mount with hyphae, acid-fast rods (in routine quick staining, non-stained rods); culture, histology, PCR
Irregular scattered necropurulent pneumonic foci with a hyperaemic zone	Bacterial pneumonia e.g. *Salmonella* or *Yersinia*	Cytology and culture
Trachea		
In syrinx of parrots white caseous–fibrinous material	Syringal mycosis After trauma or based on metaplasia due to vitamin A deficiency	Wet mount with hyphae, culture (Sabouraud's agar), histology
In trachea: red worms	*Syngamus* spp. All very rare in psittacine birds	Microscopic examination of material, histology
In trachea: black dots	*Sternostoma* mites	
In trachea: mucus and fibrin	Avipox	
Mouth		
Tongue with yellow 'abscesses' at location of salivary glands	Metaplasia, due to vitamin A deficiency	Wet mount, diet history, histology

7.35 Respiratory system: examples of pathology.

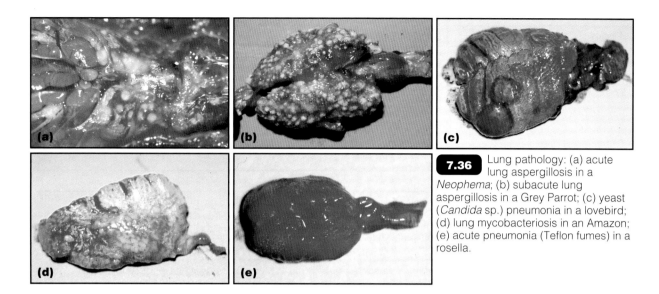

7.36 Lung pathology: (a) acute lung aspergillosis in a *Neophema*; (b) subacute lung aspergillosis in a Grey Parrot; (c) yeast (*Candida* sp.) pneumonia in a lovebird; (d) lung mycobacteriosis in an Amazon; (e) acute pneumonia (Teflon fumes) in a rosella.

Step 10. Gastrointestinal tract

- Going back to the pharynx, extend the cut downwards for the length of the oesophagus and into the crop, looking for lacerations and punctures, perioesophageal abscesses and other abnormalities.
- The crop contents can be collected in a plastic bag and frozen, if there is any suggestion of a toxic ingestion. A large section of crop, to include a big vessel and adjacent nerve, should be collected for histopathology, since PDD lesions are often confined to the nerve.
- At this point the oesophagus distal to the crop can be transected.
- Caudal traction of the distal oesophagus and sharp dissection of the mesenteric attachments can be used to remove the entire GI tract.
- Continue the dissection to make a circular incision around the vent, leaving a margin of intact vent skin and the bursa of Fabricius attached to the tract. The bursa is present in young birds, usually less than 6–12 months of age, and is located dorsal to the cloaca (see Figure 2.12). The bursa should always be collected when it is present and divided in half for histology and freezer (PCR of circovirus or polyomavirus).
- Open the distal oesophagus with scissors, continuing into the proventriculus and gizzard (with koilin layer) (see Figure 2.11). Examine the contents for amount, foreign bodies and heavy metals. Collect and freeze the contents for possible toxicological analysis. Rinse the mucosa with water and make wet mount and dried smears of mucus and/or mucosal scrapings.
- Do not separate the proventriculus and gizzard. The isthmus (see Figure 2.11) is a common place for avian gastric yeast (formerly known as megabacteria) and gastric carcinoma. Collect a large specimen of proventriculus, isthmus and

gizzard (all in one piece), containing at least one large serosal nerve and blood vessel, for histopathology (for differentiation between PDD and other reasons for a dilated proventriculus).
- Open the pylorus and proceed into the duodenal loop. The largest limb of the pancreas lies in the duodenal loop mesentery, while the small splenic pancreatic lobe is located adjacent to the spleen.
- Collect a transverse section through the duodenal loop, with pancreas attached, in formalin and one piece for toxicology.
- Continue opening the intestine through the jejunum and ileum to the rectum. In neonates, the yolk sac and stalk should be evaluated for the degree of absorption. Collect a sterile sample of the yolk material for culture, make a stained smear and place the rest of the yolk sac into formalin.
- Collect opened untouched sections of intestine for histopathology.
- Make wet mounts of intestinal contents (usually two different sides) and stained smear of mucosal scrapings for microscopic evaluation (parasites and ova, oocysts (very rare in psittacine birds), cryptosporidia, flagellates (*Giardia*), yeast and motile bacteria) and bacterial culture.
- Open the cloaca to look for papillomatous lesions, cloacoliths, trauma and inflammatory lesions.

Intestinal samples should include: wet mounts (diluted with saline) from at least two different sites; smears for rapid staining and possibly for acid-fast stain; and contents for aerobic and possible anaerobic (spores in cytology) or *Campylobacter* culture. Also collect tissue and ingesta for virology (EM negative contrast, virus isolation, or PCR).

Examples of pathology of the GI tract are given in Figure 7.37.

Finding	Diagnosis	Tests
Crop		
Thickened wall with white material (Turkish towel)	Yeast infection, candidiasis	Wet mount smear, cytology, culture.
Thickened wall with grey/yellow material	Trichomoniasis (Figure 7.38) Especially in Budgerigars and small parakeets, sometimes with trapped air bubbles	Wet mount, cytology, histology
Local red mucosal thickening	Papillomas	Histology
Stomach (proventriculus and gizzard)		
Dilated proventriculus and gizzard, often stuffed with seeds (sunflower)	Proventricular dilatation disease (PDD)	Histology
Empty proventriculus with excess of mucus, especially at isthmus region	Avian gastric yeasts ('megabacteria')	Wet mount and cytology
Irregular koilin layer that is difficult to remove from wall	Endoventricular mycosis	Deep scraping wet mount, cytology, culture
Intestine		
Haemorrhagic, black contents in entire small intestine	Haemorrhagic diathesis (massive leakage of blood into the intestine)	History (fasting for longer period), macroscopy
Thickened wall with or without blood in lumen	Enteritis	Wet mount and cytology; parasitology; microbiology
Thin wall with haemorrhagic contents or stuffed with worms	Ascaridiasis (Figure 7.39) Beware: in psittacines very rarely coccidia, often *Ascaridia*	Demonstration of worms in wet mount
Thickened areas of bowel or multifocal granulomas	Mycobacteriosis	In cytology non-staining rods, acid-fast staining positive, histology, culture or PCR
Haemorrhagic content	Lead intoxication, *Clostridium* infection, *Pseudomonas* infection, *Giardia* spp.	Lead in gizzard; lead analysis liver and kidneys; cytology, culture
Cloaca		
Congested, swollen red mucosa	Papilloma	Histology
Pancreas		
Irregular pancreas with haemorrhages	Paramyxovirus pancreatitis Especially in *Neophema* spp. with torticollis	Histology

7.37 Gastrointestinal tract: examples of pathology.

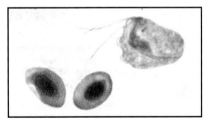

7.38 *Trichomonas* from the crop of a budgerigar; the flagella are clearly visible. Two erythrocytes are also present. (Hemacolor, original magnification 100×)

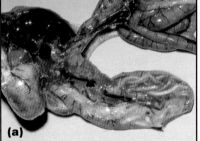

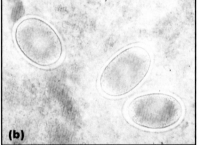

7.39 Intestinal parasites (*Ascaridia*) in a rosella: (a) infestation of intestines; (b) eggs, wet mount, original magnification 40×.

Step 11: Nasal and infraorbital sinuses

- Check the nasal and infraorbital sinuses by cutting through the upper beak caudal to the nostrils and inspect the conchae for symmetry and presence of mucus or purulent material.
- Collect material for culturing and compare the result with the findings in a stained smear from that material. It is impossible to collect uncontaminated samples from the sinuses, and therefore cultural examination is always of doubtful value.
- Collect material for histological examination when there are pathological changes.

An example of pathology of the sinus is given in Figure 7.40.

Finding	Diagnosis	Tests
Presence of turbid mucus	Bacterial or mycotic sinusitis	Wet mount, cytology, culture

7.40 Sinus: example of pathology.

Step 12: Neurological examination
The brain and spinal cord can be very important in the diagnosis of some diseases, especially PDD. When clinically neurological symptoms have been found or from the history the bird could have flown into a window before being found dead, it is always essential to open the skull.

- After removing the skin, examine for evidence of traumatic injuries. Be aware of areas of haemorrhage within the calvarium, which are common agonal changes and do not imply head trauma.
- The dorsal calvarium should be carefully removed with rongeurs.
- Visualize the brain *in situ* for any obvious abnormalities, such as abscesses, which should be cultured, and intracranial or submeningeal haemorrhages.
- Remove the brain by inverting the skull and transecting the ventral and cranial attachments. When this is difficult, especially in young or small birds, open the cranium and place the skull in fixative and send the brain *in situ* to the pathologist. When indicated, collect a portion of the forebrain for virology and toxicology, before fixing the rest in formalin.
- To inspect and collect spinal cord, cut the vertebral column with cord *in situ* into several pieces and fix in formalin. This process will allow easier removal using rongeurs, with minimal damage to the less fragile, fixed spinal cord.
- In birds with a head tilt or neurological disease, fix a large portion of the petrous temporal bone containing the middle ear and send it to the pathologist.

Step 13: Musculoskeletal system
Bone marrow is most easily collected from the tibiotarsus for both cytology and histology:

- Clean the bone and use rongeurs to break the bone.
- After collecting a bit of bone marrow for a smear, fix the bone marrow *in situ* in formalin.
- Once fixed, the previously fragile bone marrow can be dissected out and examined histologically. In bone marrow, leukaemic or aplastic processes and occasionally circovirus inclusions or TB lesions can be found. Bone marrow is also an excellent place to look for circovirus, especially in birds whose bursa has involuted.

- Samples of skeletal muscle should be collected when changes are seen or suspected based on clinical biochemical indications (CK) for histopathology. Muscular lesions may include trauma, haemorrhage, degeneration, mineralization and injection or vaccine site reactions. Myositis, degenerative myopathy, and *Sarcocystis* infection can be diagnosed histologically.
- The muscles of the legs and sciatic nerve running on the posterior surface of the femur should be examined, especially when paralysis of the hindlegs is seen clinically.
- Finally, check all the major limb joints. Any bone or joint lesion demonstrated radiographically should be opened and sampled for culture and histopathology. Be aware of the medullary bone changes in breeding females. The flexibility of bones (e.g. tibiotarsus, ribs) can be used to assess poor mineralization when calcium deficiency is very advanced. The rachitic 'rosary' at the costochondral or costovertebral junction and deformation of the keel or other long bones are obvious lesions of metabolic bone disease.
- Other findings in the joints are nematodes (*Pelecitus* sp.), bacterial arthritis (stained smear and culture), and articular gout (large deposits of urate crystals).

Final activities
This completes the gross PME, and the remaining parts of the carcass can be placed in a plastic bag and frozen until diagnostic testing has been completed.

- Examine wet mounts as quickly as possible. Warming (maximal body temperature) before examination will help in detecting moving flagellates, as it increases their motility.
- Stain any exudates and/or impression smears collected.
- When suspecting psittacosis, send a collection of liver, spleen and lung for *Chlamydophila* diagnostic tests (modified Ziehl–Neelsen, PCR and fluorescent antibody test).
- Send tissues, exudates or swabs for bacterial or fungal culture as indicated. With the exception of samples for *Campylobacter*, which does not survive freezing well, these samples can often be frozen if not sent for culture immediately.
- A pool of parenchymal tissues (liver, spleen, lung, kidney and brain) and a separate pool of intestinal contents should be refrigerated or frozen for possible virus isolation of DNA probe testing.
- Select a group of formalin-fixed tissues with lesions or a group of tissues that commonly contain histological lesions that could lead to diagnosis and submit them for histopathology. This often includes tissues such as heart, liver, kidney, spleen, lung, bursa (always when available), brain, duodenum/pancreas and proventriculus/ventriculus. Save the remaining formalin-fixed tissues, just in case the diagnosis is not made with the first set.

85

- Samples collected for ancillary diagnostics should be packed, labelled and stored properly, until shipment. See that each sample is provided with the essential documentation.
- Make a detailed PME report (Figure 7.41)

including establishing connections to the clinical findings and use this to document the samples.

Try to establish a relationship between the clinical history and the post-mortem findings.

PME Report Form and Checklist

1. Bird species, weight, age/leg band number, sex, and summarized history

2. Date of PME, your name

3. Macroscopy:

    External examination

        General body condition: muscle mass: robust, well muscled, moderately muscled, thin, emaciated, depot fat

        Feathers/integument/ectoparasites

        Palpation of skeleton

        Body openings/oral cavity

    Internal examination

        In situ description (take pictures)

        Fat/subcutis/body wall

        Coelomic cavity (air sacs/pleura/peritoneum)

        (Para)thyroids, thymus

        Spleen (size, colour)

        Heart, aorta, other vessels

        Liver

        Reproductive system (gonads, reproductive tract)

        Respiratory tract (nasal/sinus, choanal, larynx, trachea, syrinx, air sacs, lungs)

        Urinary tract (kidneys, ureters) and adrenal glands

        Digestive tract (beak, tongue, oropharynx, oesophagus, crop, proventriculus, gizzard, duodenum and pancreas, small intestine, yolk sac, caeca, rectum (colorectum), cloaca, bursa of Fabricius, vent)

        Special senses (eyes, ears, nares)

        Musculoskeletal system: muscles, skeleton (sternum, ribs, vertebrae, long bones), bone marrow, joints

        Brain, pituitary, spinal cord, meninges, peripheral nerves

4. Wet mounts (crop, rectum etc.)

5. Cytology (liver, spleen, lung, rectum)

6. Chlamydophila examination

7. Tentative (differential) diagnosis

8. Ancillary diagnostics: bacteriology, mycology, virology, parasitology, toxicology, others

9. Tissue saved:

10. Tissues submitted for histopathology:

7.41 PME report form and checklist.

8

Anaesthesia and analgesia

Thomas M. Edling

Introduction

Not too many years ago, avian clinicians strived to ensure that procedures requiring anaesthesia lasted no longer than 30 minutes. This was because there was a significant probability of grave complications in maintaining a bird under anaesthesia for a longer period of time. Thankfully, times have changed and it is now commonplace (or feasible) for birds to be anaesthetized for periods exceeding 2 hours. This change is due to advances in avian anaesthesia, which include the use of safer new inhalation agents, improved ventilation methods and better monitoring techniques, all of which help the clinician effectively to prevent apnoea and hypoventilation, the most commonly experienced difficulties during anaesthesia.

Because birds inherently have a small functional residual capacity (FRC), periods of apnoea are life threatening. Without airflow through the lungs, gas exchange does not occur, and the physiological balance of the patient cannot be maintained by the respiratory system. To help to alleviate this concern, the clinician can use intermittent positive pressure ventilation (IPPV) to help to maintain the patient appropriately during anaesthesia.

An additional essential aspect of avian anaesthesia is accurately monitoring the patient. Birds must be appropriately monitored so that proper responses to changes in the animal's physiological state can be addressed in a timely fashion. Accurate monitoring techniques are essential, as there is no formula involving respiratory rate and tidal volume that can be used to determine the ventilatory status of the patient correctly. Currently, the only method to assess the ventilatory status of any animal precisely is the measurement of arterial carbon dioxide. It has been shown that capnography could be used to measure arterial carbon dioxide effectively in the avian patient (Edling *et al.*, 2001).

Another aspect of anaesthesia that requires monitoring is arterial oxygenation. Without question, maintaining adequate arterial oxygen levels is critical, but it is very important to understand that satisfactory oxygenation is not equivalent to adequate ventilation. Birds can be well oxygenated while critically hypercapnic.

Fortunately, recent advances in avian anaesthesia such as capnography, IPPV, electrocardiography, pulse oximetry and Doppler flow monitoring have given the clinician the tools to perform avian anaesthesia safely and effectively, with a much greater probability of a successful outcome.

Preanaesthetic planning

History and physical examination

A complete and thorough history is perhaps the most important information one can acquire prior to anaesthesia. This should be followed by a physical examination.

- While obtaining the history, quietly observe the patient as it perches in its cage. Watch for signs of awareness, attention to its surrounding environment, body position, feather condition and respiratory rate and depth.
- After the initial observations, perform a thorough physical examination. Special attention should be given to the nares, oral cavity, choanal slit, glottis, abdomen, cloaca, and muscle mass covering the keel. The heart, lungs and air sacs should be auscultated for signs of disease.
- If the physical examination, history or other parameters warrant, a more in-depth evaluation should be performed (e.g. complete blood count, biochemical analysis, faecal Gram stain).

Acclimation

Placing a patient into a new or different environment can be stressful. Many patients will not become acclimatized to the new environment during the period of time available. In these cases, the bird's stress level will elevate and its disease state may worsen. The bird may refuse to eat and drink and will need to be given supportive care. When managing the high-stress bird, it is best to bring it into the clinic as close as possible to the time of anaesthesia while still allowing time for a complete physical evaluation. Preliminary testing, such as blood work, can be done prior to the day that anaesthesia will be performed.

Fasting

Ensuring that the crop is empty prior to anaesthesia is very important, due to the possibility of regurgitation. There is controversy as to the length of time a bird should be fasted prior to induction of anaesthesia. Because of a bird's high metabolic rate and poor hepatic glycogen storage, it has been recommended that fasting be limited to no more than 2–3 hours. However, when working with Cockatiels and larger birds in good physical condition, removing their food the night before and their water 2–3 hours prior to the anaesthetic procedure does not appear to have any harmful effects (Franchetti and Kilde, 1978).

Restraint

Many owners judge the veterinary surgeon's clinical abilities on the physical appearance of their bird after the visit. Improper capture or restraint techniques can result in physical trauma. The most common method of restraint is with a soft, tightly woven towel (Chapter 4).

Air sacs and positioning

Air sacs do not contribute significantly to gas exchange and therefore do not play a major role in the uptake of inhalation anaesthetics, nor do they accumulate or concentrate anaesthetic gases as once surmised. While a bird is in dorsal recumbency, normal ventilatory patterns are altered due to the reduction of effective volume. This is primarily from the weight of the abdominal viscera compressing the abdominal and caudal thoracic air sacs. Similar but more extreme ventilatory problems occur when the patient is placed in ventral recumbency. This is due to the majority of the weight of the bird's body pressing on the sternum and severely restricting its movement. Patients in both dorsal and ventral recumbency can be adequately ventilated through the use of IPPV.

It is possible to provide inhalation anaesthetics from either the trachea or a cannulated air sac, due to the cross-current gas exchange in the avian respiratory system. Cannulation also offers an effective means to ventilate an apnoeic bird with an obstructed upper airway.

Intermittent positive pressure ventilation

IPPV is an effective method for maintaining a normal physiological state during inhalation anaesthesia. It can be accomplished either manually or through the use of mechanical ventilators. Although expensive, mechanical devices are more consistent and free the clinician or nurse to do other critical duties during anaesthesia.

There are two basic types of assisted ventilation machines: the volume-limited, which delivers a set tidal volume, irrespective of airway pressure; and the pressure-limited, which delivers a constant tidal volume until a predetermined airway pressure is reached. With a pressure-limited ventilator, as the airway becomes occluded the machine will deliver a lower tidal volume for the same airway pressure. Similarly, changes in lower respiratory compliance over time may alter tidal volume at a given pressure. Thus, gradual hypoventilation may result without the operator becoming aware. In contrast, if the endotracheal tube becomes occluded during volume-limited ventilation, the resulting high airway pressure will trigger an alarm that can alert the operator. If the system leaks, gradual hypoventilation will develop due to a loss of a portion of each tidal volume.

With a volume-limited ventilator, caution is required during surgical procedures in the coelomic cavity where there is a significant opening in an air sac. Because these ventilators only deliver a preset volume of anaesthetic gas, it is almost impossible to control ventilation and thus anaesthesia, because most of the anaesthetic gas leaks from the opening in the air sac. Although difficult, it is possible to control ventilation under the same circumstances with a pressure-limited ventilator, because this type of system will continue to supply anaesthetic gas until a preset pressure is achieved.

It has been hypothesized that during IPPV the direction of gas flow within the avian lung can become reversed. Because the cross-current gas exchange system is not dependent on the direction of flow, a reversal of gas flow will not adversely affect gas exchange (Ludders et al., 1989a).

Inhalant anaesthetics

Inhalation agents

Inhalation anaesthetic agents are used to produce general anaesthesia and their safe use requires knowledge of their pharmacological effects and physical and chemical properties. Anaesthetic doses required for surgery produce unconsciousness (hypnosis), hyporeflexia and analgesia while providing optimal control of anaesthesia, rapid induction and recovery, and relatively few adverse side effects (Muir and Hubbell, 2000a).

There are currently two agents predominantly used by avian practitioners for inhalation anaesthesia: isoflurane and sevoflurane. A third agent, desflurane, has recently become available, but due to its specialized vaporizer and pungent odour it is doubtful whether it will be commonly used in avian practice. All three of these inhalation anaesthetic agents produce dose-dependent central nervous system, respiratory and cardiovascular effects.

Isoflurane

Isoflurane is the agent of choice for avian practitioners, due to its low relative cost, comparatively rapid induction and recovery, low blood solubility and minimal metabolism. In addition, it does not sensitize the heart to catecholamine-induced arrhythmias (Muir and Hubbell, 2000b). It is an excellent choice in a practice with only one type of inhalation anaesthetic agent. It is very safe and effective for the vast majority of avian anaesthetic procedures, it is almost entirely excreted by the respiratory system and it has minimal effects on organ systems. Induction occurs very rapidly (1–2 minutes) at a concentration of 3–5%. Maintenance at 1.5–2% is adequate for most birds. Recovery is also very rapid, though there seems to be a direct relationship between total anaesthetic time and recovery time.

Sevoflurane

Sevoflurane has also been shown to be an excellent anaesthetic agent, as it has a lower blood gas partition coefficient (0.69) than isoflurane (1.41) and is therefore less soluble in blood, although it is less potent (MAC 2–3%). This accounts for the shorter recovery time and time to standing compared with isoflurane (Greenacre and Quandt, 1997). In critical or prolonged surgical procedures, the use of sevoflurane can help to increase the chance of a successful outcome due to the faster recovery time when compared with other inhalation anaesthetics. In addition, sevoflurane does not cause respiratory tract irritation (as do isoflurane and desflurane) and therefore reduces the stress involved with mask induction.

However, it is significantly more expensive for what are relatively minor advantages. It has also been shown to depress plasma ionized calcium levels significantly (M. Stanford, personal communication).

Desflurane
Desflurane is a less potent (MAC 6–8%) anaesthetic agent that requires a specialized temperature-controlled and pressurized vaporizer to deliver the anaesthetic agent to the patient accurately. It has the lowest blood gas partition coefficient (0.42) of the three agents and tissue solubility (desflurane and sevoflurane blood–brain tissue coefficient = 1.3 and 1.7, respectively) (Eger EI, 1993). These physical attributes provide for a faster recovery time than isoflurane and sevoflurane, especially after prolonged anaesthetic procedures. In humans the pungency of desflurane causes respiratory tract irritation, coughing, breath holding and laryngospasms and thus it is not used for mask inductions (Eger EI, 1993).

Halothane
Halothane is no longer considered to be a safe and reliable anaesthetic agent in avian species as it sensitizes the heart to catecholamine-induced cardiac dysrhythmias. Fatalities due to pre-existing high levels of circulating catecholamines in stressed birds have been associated with the use of halothane. The cardiac dysrhythmias can and do cause cardiac depressions which are very difficult to overcome in an anaesthetized patient and commonly lead to cardiac arrest.

Nitrous oxide
Nitrous oxide used alone is incapable of producing anaesthesia in birds. It has been used in combination with halothane to speed induction and decrease the concentration of other anaesthetic agents necessary for induction and maintenance.

Even when using these reliable agents, anaesthesia remains risky because it depresses ventilation at concentrations required for surgery (Ludders et al., 1989a). Specifically, as the concentration of the inhalation anaesthetic increases, the P_aCO_2 also increases, which manifests clinically as a respiratory acidosis (Scheid and Piiper, 1989).

Anaesthetic potency
The most common measure of the potency of an inhalation anaesthetic is the agent's minimum alveolar concentration (MAC). The MAC is generally defined as the minimum alveolar concentration that produces no response in 50% of patients exposed to a painful stimulus. MAC values are measured as the end-tidal concentration of anaesthetics and are not vaporizer settings. In birds, the term minimum alveolar concentration is not appropriate because birds do not have an alveolar lung. It has been suggested that, in avian species, MAC be defined as the minimum *anaesthetic* concentration required to keep a bird from purposeful movement during a painful stimulus (Scheid and Piiper, 1989). The MAC for isoflurane in cockatoos is 1.44% (Curro et al., 1994).

Another method of comparing the potency of anaesthetic agents is by the measurement of their ability to cause respiratory depression and apnoea in an animal. The anaesthetic index (AI) can predict this effect: the lower the AI, the greater the chance of apnoea. The AI for isoflurane in dogs is 2.51 and in cats 2.40 (Steffey and Howland,1978), in horses 2.33 (Steffey et al., 1977) and in ducks 1.65 (Ludders et al., 1990). These values signify that isoflurane is more of a respiratory depressant in birds than in mammals.

This illustrates one of the great advantages of isoflurane over halothane in birds. Using halothane, respiratory and cardiac arrest will occur at approximately the same time; i.e. if the breathing stops the heart has normally stopped. With isoflurane, respiratory arrest will usually occur first, giving the anaesthetist a short time in which to intervene before the bird dies.

Breathing circuits and gas flow
Non-rebreathing circuits such as Norman elbow, modified Rees, Ayre's T-piece and Bain circuits are typically used during avian anaesthesia. These systems rely on high oxygen flow rates to remove carbon dioxide. They offer advantages over a rebreathing circuit, such as an immediate response to vaporizer setting changes and a lower resistance to breathing. Oxygen flow rates in a non-rebreathing circuit should be two to three times the minute ventilation or 150–200 ml/kg/minute (Muir and Hubbell, 2000c).

Induction methods
Mask induction is the most common technique used to induce inhalation anaesthesia in companion birds. The extremely efficient respiratory system makes mask induction the ideal method for avian patients. It is very quick, easy and effective. The masks can range from commercially available masks for small animals to plastic bottles and syringe cases (Figure 8.1a). The size and shape of the mask depends on the size and shape of the bird's head and beak. During induction, the entire head of the bird should be placed inside the mask, being careful not to cause damage to eyes and beak (Figure 8.1b). A disposable latex glove can be placed over the opening of the mask with a hole cut into the centre of the glove for insertion of the bird's head (Figure 8.1c). The hole should be roughly the same diameter as the bird's neck. When fashioned properly, the glove will provide a seal around the patient's neck tight enough to allow for IPPV. The tight seal also helps to reduce the amount of waste gas released into the environment. Waste gas should be properly scavenged using appropriate equipment.

For patients that are difficult to control, other methods of induction include induction chambers and the use of clear plastic bags to enclose a cage completely and induce anaesthesia. Both these techniques can be effective but they have their disadvantages: the anaesthetist cannot physically experience how the bird is responding to induction or have the ability to auscultate the animal; also the patient is not physically restrained and can injure itself during the excitement phase of anaesthesia.

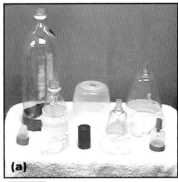
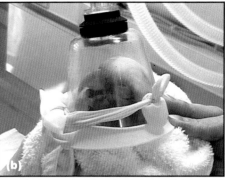
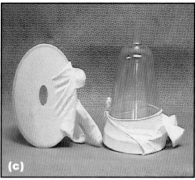

8.1 (a) Induction masks can be made from a variety of existing articles, such as plastic bottles, syringe cases, pill containers and plastic containers. The variety is limited only by the shape of the bird's head and by imagination. (b) Mask induction of a Galah. Note that the head is completely enclosed in the mask, and that the opening of the mask is covered with a latex glove. (c) Standard small mammal face mask with a latex glove fitted across the opening to create a tight-fitting induction mask. The hole cut in the glove should be slightly smaller than the neck size of the bird, and the bird's head should fit completely inside the mask. When fitted correctly, it is possible to provide IPPV in some circumstances.

Several induction techniques have been described in the literature including the use of preoxygenation techniques and slowly increasing the concentration of the gas anaesthetic agent until the desired effect has been attained. This method has the disadvantage of taking longer to achieve a loss a consciousness, which increases the excitement level of the patient and epinephrine-induced concerns.

The most common induction method (and the one the author prefers) is simply to place the induction mask over the head of the bird with a high oxygen flow rate (1–2 l/min), adjust the anaesthetic vaporizer concentration to a high concentration depending on the anaesthetic agent (4–5% for isoflurane, 7–8% for sevoflurane) and securely restrain the bird in a towel for the few seconds it takes to achieve the loss of consciousness. The vaporizer setting is then reduced to a setting lower than the MAC while the patient is being prepared for the procedure. When performed correctly, this method reduces the induction time and the stress level on the bird.

Intubation

Intubation of avian species is a relatively simple process that is easily mastered. Once anaesthesia has been induced by the mask induction technique described above:

1. Remove the mask and turn off the anaesthetic gas.
2. Have an assistant hold the bird's beak open.
3. Reaching into the bird's mouth, gently grasp the bird's tongue and pull it forwards.
4. At the base of the tongue is the glottis. When the bird breathes, the glottis will open: insert the tip of the endotracheal tube into the glottis, passing it into the trachea.

There are several reliable methods for securing the endotracheal tube to the bird. A good technique is as follows:

1. Pass a small (5 mm width) piece of one-sided plastic tape, sticky side toward the tube, centring it between the tube and the tongue as close to the point where the tube and the tongue meet as possible.
2. Pass each end of the tape around the top of the tube from each side, by simultaneously wrapping and crossing over the top of the tube, but under the upper beak.
3. Finish by wrapping the ends of the tape around the outside of the lower beak.

The sticky side of the tape will wrap around the tube and the lower beak, providing a secure but easily removable anchor. This will help to prevent the endotracheal tube from becoming dislodged and will also reduce the likelihood of tracheal damage (see also Figure 15.7).

Another important aspect to address at this juncture is the care of the patient's eyes. Most avian patients have eyes that protrude from their head, making them prone to physical injury. To help to reduce eye damage, the eye that is closest to the table should be encircled by a 'doughnut' of soft material. An ophthalmic lubricant is useful.

The diameter of the selected endotracheal tube should be such that the tube will almost completely fill the glottis/trachea. This will help to provide a tight seal and ensure that the anaesthetic gas goes into the patient and not into the operating theatre. A tube that is too large will damage the delicate tracheal tissues and can lead to strictures shortly after anaesthesia.

Another important item to consider is 'dead space', i.e. the space in the endotracheal tube, anaesthetic machine tubes and the trachea of the bird that does not contribute to gas exchange. It is very important to use the shortest endotracheal tube possible to reduce this dead space to a minimum, as too much dead space can lead to a more difficult anaesthetic procedure.

When short (10 minutes or less) non-invasive procedures such as radiography, blood collection and physical examinations are to be performed, intubation is usually not necessary. In these circumstances it is even more critical that there is a good seal between the anaesthetic mask and the patient's neck. This seal will allow the performance of limited IPPV without an endotracheal tube. When the procedure is longer than 10 minutes or invasive, intubation is essential.

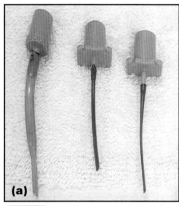
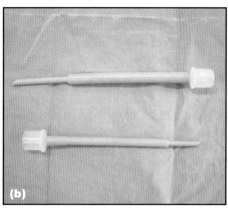
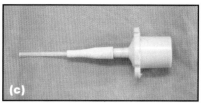
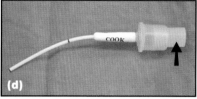

8.2 (a) Examples of endotracheal tubes. Cole (left) and red rubber catheter endotracheal tubes can be fashioned for smaller patients. (b) Stepped tubes, which have the advantage of the step closing the glottis and are therefore suitable for use with mechanical ventilators. These tubes are uncuffed and so the airway space is maximized. (c) Suitable tube for a small psittacid (down to Cockatiel size) made from a urinary catheter. (d) Commercially produced endotracheal tubes can be as small as 1.5 mm in diameter. This tube is 2 mm in diameter and is suitable for large Budgerigars. Note the stiffening stylet (arrowed).

Most birds with body weights of 100 g and higher can be intubated with minimal difficulty using readily available manufactured endotracheal tubes specifically for avian species or for human paediatric patients. Although challenging, it is possible to intubate birds weighing as little as 30 g. The smaller birds can have an endotracheal tube fashioned from a red rubber catheter or intravenous catheters of the appropriate diameter. Some manufacturers also make small endotracheal tubes that are appropriate for small birds (Figure 8.2).

Care must be taken to ensure that the trachea is not damaged during intubation. The endotracheal tube should provide a good seal with the glottis but should not fit too tightly. If the tube is cuffed, the cuff should either not be inflated or be inflated with tremendous care. Because of the limited flexibility of the complete cartilaginous rings, an over-inflated cuff will cause damage to the tracheal mucosa. Tracheal damage may not become apparent for several days following intubation, when the bird will present with dyspnoea due to a stricture in the tracheal lumen.

The most common problem associated with intubation of companion birds during inhalation anaesthesia is airway occlusion. Small endotracheal tube diameters and cold dry gases increase the probability of a complete or partial airway obstruction by mucus. This is not prevented by atropine premedication. As the airway becomes occluded, the expiratory phase of ventilation becomes prolonged (Ludders and Matthews, 1996). The obstruction can be corrected by extubating the patient and cleaning the endotracheal tube. The use of IPPV generally reduces the likelihood of endotracheal tube occlusion due to the constant forced movement of air into and out of the patient.

Air sac cannulation

Where surgical access is required to the head, neck and, especially, the trachea it is possible to cannulate the abdominal air sacs and provide anaesthesia via this route. The access site is identical to that used for left

lateral laparoscopy (see Figures 9.10–9.13). After induction the bird is maintained on an open mask while the site is prepared for surgery. A small incision is made in the skin. The underlying muscle layers and the air sac wall are penetrated bluntly using a pair of haemostats. The tube is introduced and sutured in place (Figure 8.3).

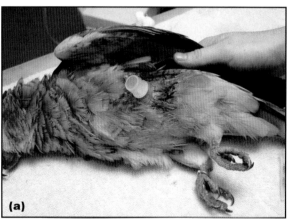
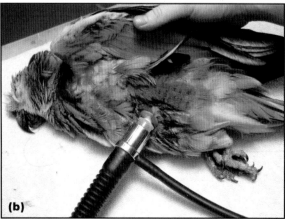

8.3 (a) Air sac tube into the left caudal air sacs of a Blue-fronted Amazon. (b) A T-piece circuit can be attached, enabling maintenance of anaesthesia and thus allowing easy access for the surgeon to remove a syringeal aspergilloma from this bird. The tube has been sutured in place so that it can be left *in situ* after surgery. (Photographs courtesy of John Chitty.)

A variety of tubes may be used. While tubes suitable for medium to large parrots are available commercially, 'home-made' tubes may also be used with some success. A suitable tube for Budgerigars and Cockatiels may be made from a cut-down dog or cat urinary catheter or a large-bore venous catheter. For larger birds, conventional endotracheal tubes may be sterilized and cut down to size. Side holes should also be made in the tube.

After the tube is implanted, anaesthesia is provided by attaching a conventional Ayre's T-piece to the air sac cannula. It is generally necessary to reduce gas flow to approximately one-third the rate used when performing tracheal intubation. IPPV may be provided using mechanical ventilators when using air sac tubes. It may also be harder to monitor anaesthesia using this technique, as respiratory movements will normally stop. It is therefore essential to monitor heart rate and peripheral blood flow. If desired (e.g. if there is tracheal obstruction or inflammation) the air sac tube may be left in place at the end of the procedure. (Bizarrely, parrots usually leave the tube in place unless the trachea is patent.) When reinducing anaesthesia in a cannulated bird, conventional mask induction is normally used but the air sac tube should be blocked until the bird is anaesthetized.

This technique is contraindicated where there is significant lower respiratory tract disease or where there is ascites. Care should be taken if there is significant organomegaly or proventricular dilatation.

Injectable anaesthetics

There are many inherent disadvantages associated with the use of injectable anaesthetic agents in avian species. The most notable drawbacks include the difficulty involved with delivering a safe and effective volume, significant species variation, cardiopulmonary depression, and prolonged and violent recoveries (Ludders and Matthews, 1996). The advantages of injectable anaesthesia are few and mostly related to cost and ease of administration. The author strongly discourages the use of injectable anaesthetics, as the disadvantages significantly outweigh the advantages in all but the most severe situations (such as field conditions where inhalant anaesthesia is not available). If the decision is made to use injectable anaesthesia, the clinician should understand that most of the positive attributes associated with inhalation anaesthesia cannot be exploited. When using any of the injectable anaesthetic agents, it is advisable to intubate the patient and monitor its physiological state as if it were undergoing general inhalation anaesthesia.

Preanaesthetics

One of the major differences found in avian anaesthesia is in the preinduction and induction phase of the process. While preanaesthetics are commonly used in dog and cat procedures, they are rarely used in avian procedures. This is because in most avian cases they are simply not needed and often will simply add to the stress level of the animal being treated. As with injectable anaesthetics in general, the use of preanaesthetics is not normally warranted in avian anaesthesia.

Parasympatholytic agents

The use of routine parasympatholytic agents in avian species is counterproductive in most circumstances. Parasympatholytic agents (atropine and glycopyrrolate) in avian species exacerbate thickening of salivary, tracheal and bronchial secretions and increase the risk for airway obstruction. Dosage rates are: atropine 0.02–0.08 mg/kg i.m., 0.01–0.02 mg/kg i.v.; glycopyrrolate 0.01–0.02 mg/kg i.m., 0.01–0.02 mg/kg i.v.

Tranquillizers

Tranquillizers such as diazepam and midazolam are benzodiazepines that have excellent muscle-relaxant properties. They lack analgesic properties whether used alone or in combination with primary anaesthetic agents such as ketamine. Diazepam can be used to tranquillize a bird prior to mask induction with an inhalant anaesthetic, thus reducing the stress involved with the procedure (Ludders and Matthews, 1996). Many clinicians find this a useful preanaesthetic and have been very successful using this drug in birds that are difficult to control due to their elevated stress levels. This technique will effectively decrease the circulating levels of norepinephrine and epinephrine, which can help to reduce the problem of catecholamine-induced cardiac dysrrhythmias.

An important feature of diazepam, in contrast to midazolam, is its shorter duration of action, which leads to a faster recovery. Midazolam is more potent than diazepam and does not adversely affect mean arterial blood pressure and blood gases in select avian species. Dosage rates are: diazepam 0.2–0.5 mg/kg i.m., 0.05–0.15 mg/kg i.v; midazolam 0.1–0.5 mg/kg i.m., 0.05–0.15 mg/kg i.v.

Alpha-adrenergic agents

Xylazine, medetomidine and other related alpha$_2$-adrenergic agonists have both sedative and analgesic properties. They can have profound cardiopulmonary effects, including second-degree heart block, bradyarrhythmias and increased sensitivity to catecholamine-induced cardiac arrhythmias. When used alone in high doses, xylazine is associated with respiratory depression, excitement and convulsions in some avian species (Ludders and Matthews, 1996). When used in combination with ketamine, the sedative and analgesic effects of xylazine are enhanced. One positive aspect of this class of drug is that an overdose or slow recovery can be treated with an alpha-adrenergic antagonist reversal agent such as yohimbine or atipamezole.

General anaesthetics

Ketamine

Ketamine hydrochloride, a cyclohexamine, produces a state of catalepsy and can be given by any parenteral route. When used alone, ketamine is suitable for chemical restraint for minor surgical and diagnostic applications, but it is not suitable for major surgical procedures (Ludders et al., 1989b). Given intramuscularly, ketamine produces anaesthesia in 3–5 minutes with a duration of 10–30 minutes. The recovery period is from 30 minutes to 5 hours. The dosage varies among species but in general it is inversely proportional to body weight on a per kilogram basis.

Higher doses of ketamine do not provide a better plane of anaesthesia; they simply prolong its duration while decreasing its margin of safety. Ketamine is generally used in conjunction with other drugs such as diazepam or xylazine to improve the quality of the anaesthesia by providing more muscle relaxation or increased analgesia.

Ketamine can also be given intravenously to larger birds, rapidly inducing anaesthesia, which lasts from 15 minutes to several hours. It may be combined with diazepam to smooth induction and recovery and to enhance muscle relaxation. The usual dose of ketamine in this combination is 30–40 mg/kg and diazepam is 1.0–1.5 mg/kg. As with the intramuscular route, there is substantial variation in the amount of anaesthetic required by different species. It is important to inject the drug slowly and to give it in small increments separated by a few minutes. Too much ketamine given too quickly can result in apnoea and even cardiac arrest.

Ketamine may also be used in combination with xylazine. A 100 mg/ml concentration of ketamine may be mixed with a 20 mg/ml concentration of xylazine on an equal volume basis. Administered intramuscularly, this combination induces an anaesthetic level adequate for diagnostic procedures or minor surgery. The combination is given based on the ketamine dose and may be given intravenously.

To extend the duration of anaesthesia, the dose of ketamine can be repeated. The duration of anaesthesia and recovery time are dose dependent, but analgesia appears to be incomplete even at high doses.

Propofol

Propofol is a substituted phenol derivative developed for intravenous induction and maintenance of general anaesthesia. Its major advantage is rapid onset and recovery and thus it has very little residual or cumulative effect. Its major disadvantages are dose-dependent cardiovascular and respiratory depression (Machin and Caulkert, 1996) and that it gives a very short period of anaesthesia. Propofol dosage rates are 10 mg/kg slow i.v. infusion to effect; up to 3 mg/kg increments for supplemental doses.

Analgesia

Recognition of pain is not easy in prey species such as parrots, as they will often not show overt signs. In parrots, pain evaluation studies have been hampered by parrots' ability to recognize and respond to repeated painful stimuli before receiving the stimulus. Similarly, excessive vocalization may be normal rather than a sign of pain!

The clinician is therefore advised to ask the following questions:

• Would the lesion be painful to a human?
• Is the lesion damaging to tissues?
• Does the bird display behaviour(s) that may indicate pain, e.g. change in temperament (aggressive or passive), restlessness, reduced grooming, reluctance to perch, lethargy, reduced appetite, constipation, dyspnoea, lameness, biting/chewing at surgical incisions or wounds, tonic immobility?

If the answer to any of these questions is 'yes', then it should be assumed that the patient is in pain and analgesic drugs should be used. An excellent overview of this subject is provided by Hawkins and Machin (2004).

Injectable anaesthetic drugs such as alpha-adrenergic agents (see above) and ketamine (see later) have analgesic properties. Opioids, local anaesthetics and non-steroidal anti-inflammatory drugs are more commonly used for pain relief in parrots.

Opioids

Opioids are commonly used as a premedication in small mammal medicine both for presurgical analgesia and to reduce the amount of anaesthesia necessary to achieve a surgical plane. In pigeons, the kappa opioid receptors account for the majority of the opioid receptor sites; thus butorphanol, a kappa agonist, may be a better analgesic than mu opioid agonists (Mansour *et al.*, 1988). In addition, it has been demonstrated that butorphanol reduces the concentration of isoflurane needed to maintain anaesthesia in cockatoos (Curro *et al.*, 1994). Butorphanol dosage rates are 1.0 mg/kg i.m., 0.02–0.04 mg/kg i.v.

Local anaesthetics

Local anaesthetics have been shown to provide excellent results when used as preventive analgesia in avian species. However, they do not provide relief from the stress involved with the restraint and handling of the conscious avian patient.

It has been established in humans and animals that it is easier to prevent pain than it is to treat pain. In fact, it has been demonstrated that the repeated stimulation of the neurons in the dorsal horn of the spinal cord can cause them to become hypersensitized. The morphology of these neurons actually changes and they become 'wound up'. As a result, the response to successive incoming signals is changed. This neuronal hypersensitivity continues even after the noxious stimulus stops and can last 20 to 100 times longer than the original stimulus (Woolf and Chong, 1993). The technique of administering a preoperative local anaesthetic to block the transmission of noxious stimuli can prevent or attenuate the 'wind-up'. This procedure is especially effective for painful procedures such as amputations, fracture repairs and coelomic surgeries. However, care must be taken not to induce seizures or cardiac arrest with an overdose. If necessary, the volume can be diluted to make it a more convenient volume for administration.

In summary, local anaesthetic agents should be used primarily as an adjunct to general anaesthesia in helping to prevent 'wind-up'. In general, due to the high levels of stress involved with handling and restraint, they should not be used in conscious birds for local anaesthesia, except in rare circumstances where the patient is not overly stressed and the procedure is uncomplicated (e.g. a broken toe nail). Lidocaine dosage rates (i.m. and s.c. only) are 1.0–4.0 mg/kg, diluted at least 1:10.

Non-steroidal anti-inflammatory drugs

Non-steroidal anti-inflammatory drugs (NSAIDs) act by inhibiting cyclo-oxygenase, thus reducing the synthesis of prostaglandins. Prostaglandin synthesis is mediated by one of two isoforms of cyclo-oxygenase: cyclo-oxygenase 1 (COX-1) and cyclo-oxygenase 2 (COX-2). Prostaglandins formed by COX-1 are constantly present during normal physiological events. Prostaglandins formed by COX-2 are active only intermittently. As a category, NSAIDs inhibit both COX-1 and COX-2, but a preference is given to drugs that act more strongly on inhibition of COX-2. Preoperative administration of NSAIDs can decrease tissue sensitization that occurs as a result of surgical trauma and can also reduce the amount of time necessary for postoperative opioid therapy. Much of the information about dosages for birds has been established empirically (Figure 8.4).

Drug	Dosage
Acetylsalicylic acid	5.0 mg/kg orally, q8h or 325 mg/250 ml drinking water
Carprofen	2.0–4.0 mg/kg orally, q12h to q8h
Flunixin meglumine	1.0 mg/kg i.m. q24h
Ibuprofen	5–10mg/kg orally q12h to q8h
Ketoprofen	2.0 mg/kg i.m. or s.c. q24h to q8h
Meloxicam	0.1 mg/kg orally q24h
Phenylbutazone	3.5–7.0 mg/kg orally q8h
Piroxicam	0.5 mg/kg orally q12h

8.4 Dosages for NSAIDs.

Patient monitoring

Monitoring the avian patient during anaesthesia is the most critical aspect of the process. The bird must be maintained and properly monitored while appropriate responses to its physiological state are performed in a timely fashion.

Apnoea and hypoventilation are the most commonly experienced problems noted during anaesthesia. Because of the bird's small functional residual capacity, periods of apnoea are critical: without sufficient airflow through the lungs, gas exchange does not occur and the physiological acid–base balance maintained by the respiratory system is made ineffective.

Respiratory system

Both the respiratory rate and tidal volume should be monitored during anaesthesia to help to assess the adequacy of ventilation. These parameters can be supervised by observing the respiratory rate and pattern and auscultating the coelomic cavity. There is no formula involving respiratory rate and tidal volume that can be used successfully to determine the correct ventilatory status of the patient. The only way to assess ventilation in the patient accurately is through some measure of arterial carbon dioxide.

One study in Grey Parrots indicated that capnography can be used to monitor arterial CO_2 effectively and that the end-tidal (ET) CO_2 consistently overestimates arterial CO_2 by approximately 5 mmHg (Edling *et al.*, 2001). When using capnography in avian patients, a side-stream capnograph should be utilized and the dead air space associated with the endotracheal tube must be minimized. The capnograph can be connected to the breathing circuit through an 18 G needle inserted into the lumen of the endotracheal tube adaptor (Figure 8.5).

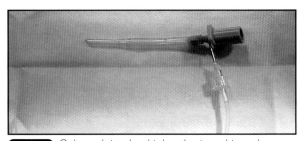

8.5 Cole endotracheal tube shortened to reduce dead air space. The endotracheal tube adaptor has been modified to allow the attachment of a side-stream capnograph. This has been accomplished by mounting an 18 G needle into the lumen of the adaptor, with the needle bevel facing the patient.

Positive pressure ventilation by means of a mechanical ventilator or by manual compression can be used successfully to maintain the avian patient during inhalation anaesthesia. To prevent volotrauma to the air sacs during positive pressure ventilation, airway pressures should not exceed 15–20 cm H_2O. When using IPPV techniques, the ventilations should be adjusted per minute and/or per minute volume either mechanically or manually according to the $ETCO_2$, striving to maintain the patient within normal physiological range. As a guideline, an $ETCO_2$ of 30–45 mmHg indicates adequate ventilation during inhalation anaesthesia in the Grey Parrot (Edling *et al.*, 2001).

Circulatory system

There are several non-invasive methods to monitor the circulatory system of the avian patient, such as auscultation, pulse rate and an electrocardiogram (ECG). In addition, monitoring the pulsations of blood through a peripheral artery can assess heart function. An 8 MHz Doppler flow probe is an effective means to monitor pulse rate and rhythm. This is an excellent method for assessing peripheral circulation, as strength of 'pulse' is directly correlated with the signal volume. Standard bipolar and augmented limb leads can be used to monitor and record the ECG, which reports the electrical activity of the heart. The ECG equipment used must be able to detect and accurately record the high heart rates (up to 500 beats per minute) associated with avian species.

A new technique, employing an oesophageal probe, can be used to obtain ECG readings: the probe is inserted into the oesophagus of the patient and attached to the standard ECG leads via an adaptor. This technique achieves accurate readings without the use of limb leads. It is difficult to measure arterial blood pressure directly in psittacine birds, due to their small size, the invasiveness of the procedure and the cost of the equipment. This procedure is generally only performed in laboratory settings and when working with large avian species such as ratites. Chapter 20 discusses ECG techniques and interpretation.

Central nervous system

The central nervous system can be assessed in avian patients by directly observing jaw tone, cloacal reflex, eye reflex, pedal reflex and muscle relaxation. One study indicated that the ideal anaesthetic level had been reached when the patient's eyelids were completely closed and mydriatic, the pupillary light reflex was delayed and the nictitating membrane moved slowly over the entire cornea; in addition, the muscles were all relaxed and all pain reflexes were absent (Korbel *et al.*, 1993). Although these are reliable indicators of anaesthetic depth to experienced clinicians, there is a fine line between the presence of these central nervous system assessments and the absence of reflexes altogether, which is a life-threatening situation.

Oxygenation

Ensuring that the patient has an adequate P_aO_2 is very important to the successful outcome of anaesthesia. An intubated bird on 100% oxygen during inhalation anaesthesia is usually well oxygenated but, even in well oxygenated birds, problems such as apnoea, ventilation–perfusion mismatch and tracheal obstructions can significantly alter the partial pressure of arterial oxygen. Mucous membrane colour can be used to monitor change but is not effective in a critical patient. The only method for determining a patient's arterial oxygenation status accurately is arterial blood gas analysis. Studies using pulse oximetry indicate that, while this is a valuable tool for assessing mammalian oxygen saturation, it is not consistently accurate in avian patients, though it can be used successfully to monitor trends (Schmitt *et al.*, 1998). It is very important that the anaesthetist be careful not to interpret satisfactory oxygenation, through the use of a pulse oximeter, as adequate ventilation. P_aO_2 is not a reliable indicator of the ventilatory status of a bird or any other animal. Birds can be well oxygenated and at the same time extremely hypercapnic (Edling *et al.*, 2001).

Temperature

Hypothermia is the most common problem associated with prolonged anaesthesia: it decreases the requirement for anaesthetic, causes cardiac instability and prolongs recoveries. Maintaining the correct body temperature is one of the most critical aspects of successful anaesthesia. The flow of dry anaesthetic gases through the respiratory system, removing feathers for sterile skin preparation, surgical skin preparation, blunted physiological responses and the small body mass in relation to surface area are among the many factors that quickly serve to decrease the patient's body temperature. Hypothermia is also significant post-surgically, because hypothermic patients must use critical energy reserves to generate heat by shivering.

There are many methods for maintaining a patient's body temperature during anaesthesia, including circulating-water blankets, warm-air blankets, heated surgery tables, warm towels and warm intravenous fluids. With warm-air blankets, the patient's eyes must be kept well lubricated, as these devices tend to dry the eyes. Although very effective, warm-air blankets tend to get in the way of the surgical procedure, especially in the smaller avian patients. Many clinicians use several of these methods simultaneously to help to ensure that the patient's core body temperature is maintained within normal parameters.

The most effective method for providing heat during anaesthesia is with a radiant energy source (Phalen *et al.*, 1997). This simple and cost-effective method consists of a radiant heat lamp 'aimed' at the body of the patient. It does not hinder access to the patient, but it does add considerable heat to the operating arena, sometimes making it uncomfortable for the surgeon and technicians. It should be remembered that many of these techniques are so successful that a fatal *hyper*thermia is also a possibility. Body temperature can be reliably monitored with a long flexible thermistor probe inserted into the oesophagus to the level of the heart. Temperature monitoring through the use of cloacal probes can be accurate but is dependent on body position and cloacal activity over time.

Recovery

Recovering the avian patient is usually a rapid process once the anaesthetic gas has been turned off. The birds should be disconnected from the anaesthetic circuit, which should be flushed with oxygen before the patient is reconnected to it and the recovery continued with the patient on 100% oxygen. Most birds will experience muscle fasciculations as they become lighter. If the bird is being auscultated at this time, the heart sounds will become less audible due to the muscle movement (Edling, 2001). Care should be taken not to interpret this incorrectly as a deep plane of anaesthesia. This is especially important during surgical procedures. As the bird becomes lighter, more apparent movements will become evident, such as wing flutter and leg withdrawal. When the patient starts to exhibit jaw movement, it should be extubated (to keep it from severing the endotracheal tube) and held lightly in a towel in an upright position. The mask used for induction, without the latex glove, should be used to provide oxygen. (Wrapping the towel too tightly will not only inhibit breathing but can also produce excessive retention of body heat, leading to hyperthermia.) The patient should be held in this fashion until it can hold itself upright. At this point it should be placed in a dark padded box and the box should be placed in a heated oxygenated cage. This will allow the bird to recover fully in a less stressful environment. Most patients will appear fully recovered from inhalation anaesthesia within 15–30 minutes.

Anaesthetic emergencies

Emergency situations arising from anaesthesia are no longer as common as in the past. Psittacine birds can be successfully maintained under inhalation anaesthesia for 2 hours or more with a low prevalence of morbidity and mortality. This is primarily due to the practitioner's ability to monitor and maintain the patient within its normal physiological parameters.

Although emergencies are not common, anticipated emergency drugs should already be drawn into syringes and readily available for use. Time is critical in emergency situations and trying to find and calculate drug doses during these stressful circumstances can make the difference between a happy outcome and a tragedy. In long procedures, emergency procedures, procedures involving potential significant blood loss or in birds with a history of cardiovascular problems during surgery, it is advisable to place an intravenous (basilic, jugular, medial metatarsal) or interosseous catheter (ulna, tibiotarsus) after induction but prior to the start of surgery. This will allow immediate access to the bird's circulatory system and can save valuable time in case an emergency arises. It also allows for constant infusion fluid therapy, which is a very useful tool during any surgical procedure. Figure 8.6 describes common emergency treatments.

A. AIRWAY	If not already done, the bird should be intubated Where tracheal obstruction is suspected, air sac cannulation should be performed
B. BREATHING	Mechanical ventilation should be provided If not available, IPPV may be provided by *gentle* pressure on the circuit's rebreathing bag or by gently compressing the bird's body such that the keel is moved up and down Doxapram 5–10mg/kg i.v.
C. CIRCULATION	Intravenous or intraosseous access should be provided (Chapter 6) A bolus of Hartmann's (10 ml/kg) can be given followed by infusion at 10 ml/kg/hour External cardiac massage is *not* possible in birds
D. DRUGS	In cardiac arrest: epinephrine 0.1 mg/kg i.v., intraosseous or intracardiac or via endotracheal tube, diluted 1:10 with Hartmann's prior to use If brachycardiac due to supraventricular bradycardia: atropine 0.01–0.02 mg/kg i.v. Other anti-dysrhythmics according to ECG indication

8.6 Anaesthetic emergencies: a clinical approach.

9

Diagnostic imaging

Nigel H. Harcourt-Brown

Radiology

Radiology is used in all branches of clinical veterinary science. Most of the radiographic techniques used on dogs and cats are applicable to birds. Whole-body radiographs should be used as part of the routine examination of most ill birds.

Any small-animal radiography set will be able to produce good avian radiographs. It is very uncommon to have to use a voltage of more than 60 kV. A large amperage is useful as it will allow fast exposure times, but perfectly adequate radiographs can be produced with 20 mA and exposure times of up to 0.2 seconds. Exposure times of > 0.2 s will produce blurred images on the radiograph. Because of this, image-intensifying screens are necessary. Fine-definition screens that are used for the extremities in humans are very useful for cats and small dogs as well as birds. Fine-definition screens require a higher amperage than fast screens but a lot less than non-screen film. Fast screens lose too much fine detail to be useful for avian radiography.

The choice of film and processing chemicals is decided by the type of screen to be used in the cassette. Mammography film used with appropriate screens and cassettes will give extremely good detail but processing temperature is critical and the screens are easily marked with scratches and dust. The machine needs a large amperage to avoid having to increase the exposure time so much that cardiovascular and other soft tissue movements blur the detail that the mammography film provides.

Positioning the patient

It is important to consider what is wanted from the radiograph. A bird that only needs to be screened for the presence of metal in its gizzard requires a different technique to the bird that is lame. For accurate diagnosis it is usually important to have two correctly positioned views, the second view taken at 90 degrees to the first. To allow perfect positioning and to keep within the law in the UK, some form of restraint is necessary that allows the radiographer to stand away from the patient whilst the X-rays are emitted. It is possible to restrain conscious parrots using various positioning devices and these allow whole-body radiography if used sensibly. Most parrots are best restrained using a general anaesthetic and this allows perfect positioning using sandbags and ties.

Lateral (Figure 9.1) and ventrodorsal (VD) views (Figure 9.2) of the whole body of the bird are very useful as a general overview of the body and are often the next step towards a diagnosis after the clinical examination. As well as both views it can be useful to use two different voltage values (5 kV apart) for each view. This will give the best set of radiographs for accurate diagnosis. Ties, sandbags and zinc oxide tape are useful for positioning. For the lateral view the wings should be extended dorsally so that they do not overlie the body. Birds that are not used to flying are often unable to extend the shoulder joint fully. Too much dorsal extension of the wings places a strain on the humerus, which could result in a fracture. The legs should be held in caudal extension.

Interpretation of radiographs

Respiratory system

The trachea can be seen lying next to the neck and entering the body, where it terminates at the syrinx. The syrinx leads into the primary bronchi, which are not normally seen. The lungs are visible on both lateral and VD views in a normal bird. Laterally the normal lung looks like a sponge, due to the parabronchi being seen end-on (Figure 9.3).

The lungs overlie each other on this view. The VD view shows each lung on either side of the vertebral column and on this view the lungs have the appearance of a thumbprint, as the parabronchi tend to run across the lung (Figure 9.2). The air sacs are visible around the heart and abdominal viscera as dark, air-filled spaces. The clavicular air sac can be seen just below the shoulder joint, again dark against the denser surrounding muscle because of the air contained in it.

Pneumonia and air sacculitis can be seen on both views. With pneumonia, the fine detail of the lung is lost and the organ becomes blurred. It is possible to see abscesses in the lung as areas of increased density, either a solid mass or as a halo of density.

In cases of air sacculitis, the air sacs can become radio-opaque if filled with pus or fluid but usually there is air within the air sac and the walls are thickened, which causes a loccular appearance that is typical of aspergillosis (Figure 9.4). Birds that are dyspnoeic with a swollen abdomen may have large amounts of fluid in the air sacs or peritoneal cavities. Common causes are congestive heart failure, tumours, or serositis. This fluid should be drained by paracentesis prior to anaesthesia. Ultrasonography is useful for these cases (see later) as the presence of fluid can be assessed prior to drainage.

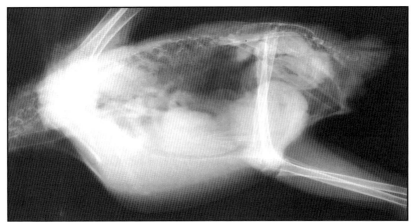

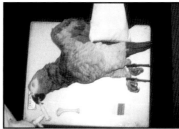

9.1 A lateral radiograph of a normal adult male Grey Parrot. This bird has no grit in its gizzard. It has been starved for 12 hours and its crop is empty. The bones may be identified by looking at Figure 2.4.

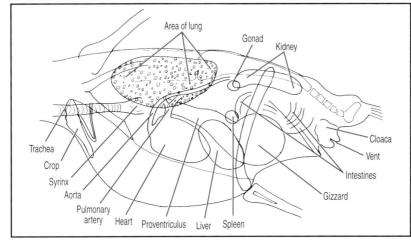

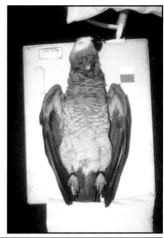

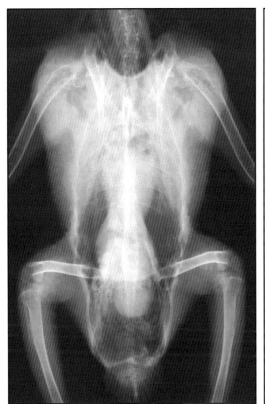

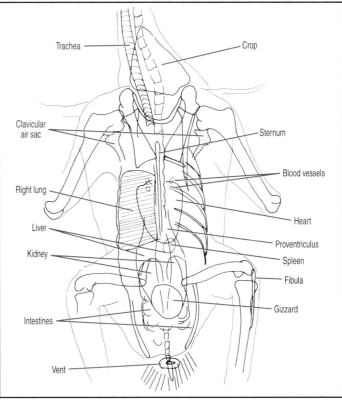

9.2 A ventrodorsal radiograph of a normal adult male Grey Parrot. The parrot is correctly positioned, as the sternum lies directly above the vertebrae. The bones can be identified from Figure 2.4. On this view the parabronchi appear as a series of parallel lines, like a thumbprint. Compare with Figure 9.3, where on the lateral view they have a sponge-like appearance.

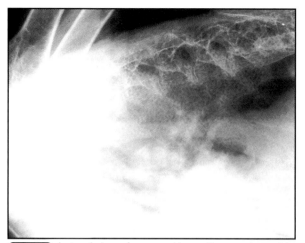

9.3 Lateral view of a normal lung. The parabronchi are seen as black dots within the lung field, as they are being viewed end-on. An exposure of 5 kV more would show the syrinx and trachea more clearly but would show less lung detail.

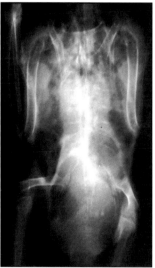

9.4 Clinical signs of dyspnoea and weight loss in a Hispaniolan Amazon. Loss of parabronchial (thumbprint) detail and 'fluffy' opacities can be seen in the lung field. All the air sacs can be seen clearly, due to thickened air sac walls. The interior of each air sac was full of *Aspergillus* fungus. The clavicular air sac is overdistended and obvious as it runs across the cranial part of the body and enters each humerus.

Cardiovascular system

The heart is visible on both views; the main arteries appear as a pair of twin dots above and lateral to the heart on the ventrodorsal view. On the lateral view these blood vessels are much more recognizable. Enlargement of the heart, calcification of the major arteries and oedema within the lungs can be seen when present. Transudate/oedema due to congestive heart failure is impossible to differentiate radiographically from effusion from a visceral tumour, purulent air sacculitis, serositis and occasionally an enlarged liver. Ultrasonography is very useful for this.

Coelomic contents

The liver can be seen best on the VD view. If the bird has eaten recently and has a full proventriculus and gizzard, or has a pathological dilatation of the proventriculus, the liver is spread laterally to occupy more space in the abdominal air sac. This must be differentiated from pathological enlargement of the liver. On a VD view the proventriculus also overlies the left side of the liver and on occasions makes it difficult to know whether the liver is enlarged or not.

The proventriculus is seen most clearly on the lateral view (Figure 9.5). It can be distended normally with food but will enlarge and distend pathologically with a number of conditions. Barium will often help to differentiate these conditions (Figure 9.6). Most pathological distensions slow or stop the passage of food through the gut. Increased time for the passage of ingesta is only an indication that the bird is ill and is not necessarily diagnostic of any particular disease.

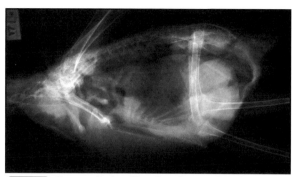

9.5 Proventricular dilatation disease (PDD) in a Grey Parrot. The proventriculus and gizzard are over-distended. Some cases are best highlighted with barium.

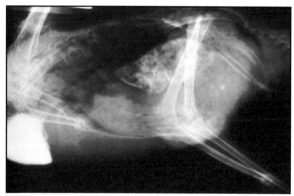

9.6 This bird was thin and regurgitating its food. A plain radiograph showed abnormal density in the coelomic region. Liquid barium sulphate (2 ml) was introduced using a gavage tube passed down the oesophagus, through the crop and into the thoracic inlet so that barium was given directly into the start of the proventriculus. This has outlined the almost invisible mass of sunflower seed in the dilated proventriculus.

The gizzard is visible on both lateral and dorsoventral views. If the parrot is given grit this will be easily seen within the muscular grinding gizzard. (The gizzard is less obvious in birds that do not have access to grit.) Grit outlining the gizzard can be very useful in determining the nature of enlarged abdominal contents: if the liver is enlarged, the gizzard is moved caudally; if the kidneys or oviduct is enlarged, the gizzard is moved cranially. The grit can reflux into the proventriculus in a normal anaesthetized bird. Lead is sometimes ingested and in this case it will collect in the gizzard. Birds that have lead in their gizzard will *always* be suffering from lead poisoning and should be treated. Lead is much more radio-opaque than grit. Galvanized wire will cause zinc poisoning if retained in the gizzard. Other metallic objects may or may not be poisonous (Chapter 20).

The intestines are seen as a mass in which only small amounts of detail are visible. They may or may not contain gas. The cloaca can be demonstrated most obviously on the lateral view and can be seen to contain urates in some individuals.

The spleen is usually only visible on the lateral view but can also be seen on the VD view if very enlarged, when it adds to the confusing mass of liver overlying kidneys. A slightly oblique VD view is often useful. Parrots with splenomegaly should be considered as candidates for *Chlamydophila* infection but chronic bacterial infections, tuberculosis and lymphoma will cause similar splenic (as well as liver and kidney) enlargement.

The kidneys are seen on a lateral radiograph but overlie each other. They can be differentiated into their various divisions on the VD view but are overlain and somewhat obscured by the intestines. Sometimes they are very distinct on the VD view and they may well be enlarged and more dense in these cases. They can also contain urates, which are radio-opaque.

Occasionally the gonads of either sex are obvious just ventrocranial to the kidney on the lateral view.

Extremities

The head and neck and the thoracic and pelvic limbs should each be evaluated separately. Although the whole wing or leg can be examined on a single 'shot', the necessary detail will be revealed better if the affected area is viewed with the beam coned down and at an appropriate exposure. The exposure will vary for different areas of the limb in the same bird. Positioning is important. With the use of fine-definition screens, a lot of useful soft tissue detail is visible on limb radiographs.

Growing bones

Although bone growth occurs at a similar position to that of the mammalian growth plate, the growing bird has cartilaginous epiphyses. No growth plates are visible but the distal tibiotarsus and proximal tarsometatarsus look as if they have them, due to the presence of the tarsal bones. The same is seen in the carpometacarpus. Metatarsals II, III and IV and the two metacarpals of the hand can be seen as separate entities in the first third of growth (see Figures 11.10 and 11.11).

Medullary bone

The medullary cavity of the long bones of female birds becomes filled with special bone in the breeding season (Chapter 2; see Figure 18.4).

Osteopathology

The appearance of osteomyelitis in birds differs from that in mammals because of the caseous nature of avian pus. Abscesses form in the medullary cavity and slowly enlarge. The bone is distorted around the abscess and may either form a bubble-like appearance or disappear (see Figures 11.6 and 11.16).

Septic arthritis is different, as the joint fluid keeps the pus more liquid. The surface of the joint is eroded and the joint space expands. The edge of the lesion is not clear cut and has a more roughened outline (see Figure 11.17).

Bone tumours are uncommon and cause osteolysis, increased soft tissue density and often a periostitis. These changes do not cross a joint (see Figure 11.15).

Osteoarthritis gives the same periarticular changes as are seen in mammals. Trauma causes single joint involvement. Age-related osteoarthritis affects pairs of joints, usually the knee.

In young growing birds the first sign of nutritional osteodystrophy is bone deformity. Bones tend to bend, trabeculae occur in unusual places and double cortices occur where the bone has bent and the periosteum has changed position (see Figures 11.12 and 11.13). Advanced cases show loss of density and folding fractures. In adult birds advanced osteoporosis causes loss of bone density, gross irregularity of the cortices of long bones and multiple fractures. Early or mild osteoporosis is difficult to diagnose with certainty. In humans at least 30% of bone density has to be lost before it can be seen radiographically; the same is probably true for birds. Comparison with the surrounding soft tissue and great confidence in both the radiographic technique and the processing are required to make diagnosis of osteoporosis. It can be useful to have a normal bone that can be placed on each cassette next to the bird as a standard reference.

In skeletally normal birds, fracture and subsequent callus formation are similar to mammals. Malunion of fractures is usually atrophic and shows as rounding of the ends of the fracture with no periosteal proliferation.

Contrast techniques

Air

Air is infrequently introduced as a contrast medium, as it is present in a number of areas as a norm. In healthy birds it can be seen in areas such as the clavicular air sac or the abdominal cavity. In some cases of pathology, such as rupture of the cervicocephalic air sac or compound fractures, air can be found in abnormal situations. Air can be introduced into the alimentary tract with a piece of tubing or an endoscope and will show the extent of the crop, proventriculus or gizzard. It is also possible to introduce air into the oviduct and intestine through the cloaca, using an endoscope, with similar results.

Barium

Oral barium sulphate is useful, either as a diluted liquid or mixed with liquid baby food. A standard liquid barium preparation is diluted half and half with water and given directly into the crop with a crop tube. An empty gut is ideal but frequently this is not possible. Occasionally a parrot will require a barium meal to be followed through the alimentary tract over a period of several hours. Administering a general anaesthetic to a bird with a crop containing liquid causes a risk of an inhalational pneumonia. Repetitive anaesthesia compounds this risk, especially in birds with proventricular dilatation disease (PDD), as gut transit times are very much reduced and the crop may contain barium for hours.

For cases where the rate of passage is more important than the positioning, a specially constructed box can be used (Figure 9.7). The cassette is positioned in the rear wall and the bird stands on the perch in front of it. This allows repeated exposures without handling the bird and the barium can be followed through the alimentary tract. This technique is limited to

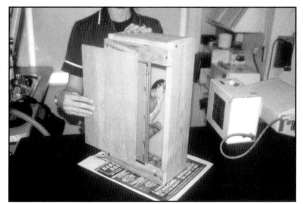

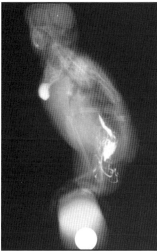

9.7 Barium meal radiograph of a Black-headed Caique perched in the box (which is half open for illustration purposes). This bird was well but had a swelling on its lower abdomen, which the barium shows to contain intestines. The radiograph was taken 35 minutes after the administration of barium. However, it did not show that half the hernia was occupied by a large fatty liver; this required better positioning under general anaesthesia.

a lateral view only. In cases where good positioning and a VD view are needed, the bird will have to be anaesthetized and positioned correctly.

The first radiographs are taken 5 minutes later, by which time a normal parrot should have barium in its crop, proventriculus, gizzard, and even into the duodenum. A lot of ill parrots will take 30 minutes to move the barium this far. The barium will outline the alimentary tract and will give an indication of the rate of passage of ingesta. The direction in which the intestines are displaced will differentiate radiographically amorphous abdominal distension, which is especially common in the Budgerigar. Cases of PDD may require the barium to be introduced by tube or endoscope through the thoracic inlet into the proventriculus, as peristalsis may be so weak that the barium may not leave the crop.

Iodine media
Intravenous Iohexol will safely give an arteriogram or venogram, or outline the heart internally. It is also safe for producing an intravenous pyelogram, which will increase the contrast of the kidneys with the surrounding tissue as well as filling the ureters. A Blue-fronted Amazon given 1 ml of Iohexol intravenously will have a good flow of contrast through the ureters 5–10 minutes after administration.

Fluoroscopy
Fluoroscopy has been used to study the movement of the bowel and, if available, is very useful for diagnosing PDD. The normal peristalsis is replaced by very abnormal movements between the proventriculus and gizzard.

Ultrasonography

Ultrasound scanning is available in many general practices. A 7.5 MHz sector or micro-curved probe can be used to examine parrots of 200 g body weight upwards; the probe must have a small contact surface. Ultrasound is very useful in cases where the coelomic cavities are filled with fluid; it will allow accurate diagnosis as to which cavities are filled with fluid and allow the fluid to be safely removed by paracentesis. The best ultrasound views are obtained with the probe positioned midline and caudal to the sternum. The bird can be restrained manually and is best held in an upright position if it contains fluid. Birds that do not have lots of transudate can be anaesthetized and laid in dorsal recumbency. It may be necessary to remove some feathers but there is usually a featherless tract midline. Ultrasound gel must be used and it is useful to wipe the skin with alcohol before putting probe and gel in contact with the skin. It is possible to 'see' the liver, intestines, kidneys and heart (Figures 9.8 and 9.9). Even the heart's valves can be seen; the right atrioventricular valve is muscular.

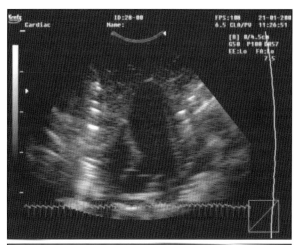

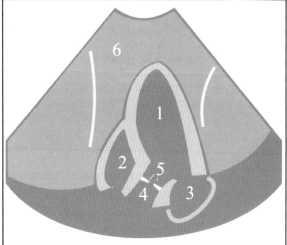

9.8 Normal heart of a Grey Parrot: (1) left ventricle; (2) right ventricle; (3) left atrium; (4) aorta; (5) aortic valves; (6) liver. Image (courtesy of Dr Michael Pees) obtained using a paediatric micro-curved 7.5 MHz probe.

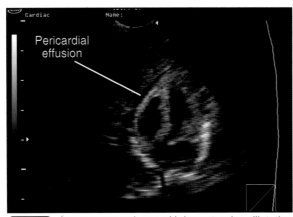

9.9 Amazon parrot heart with hypertrophy, dilatation and some pericardial effusion. (Image courtesy of Dr Michael Pees.)

Reference values for the assessment of cardiac function have been evaluated using healthy Grey, Senegal and Amazon parrots as well as cockatoos (Pees *et al.*, 2004). The left ventricle was the easiest structure to examine and measure reliably; the parameters obtained provided valuable information about the contractility and performance of the heart. Smaller structures, including the right ventricle, were more difficult to assess.

Other more sophisticated scanning techniques have been reported. Computed tomography (CT) and magnetic resonance imaging (MRI) scans are expensive and not widely available. Their advantages over normal radiography are the excellent soft tissue differentiation and the fact that there is no superimposition of overlying structures. These techniques could be used more frequently if they become affordable.

Endoscopy

Endoscopy is always a compromise. Small endoscopes are able to fit into small spaces but carry less light and tend to produce poorer quality images. Usually the finer the endoscope the shorter it is, the more expensive it is and the more easily broken. As a general rule, larger rather than smaller endoscopes should be used for any given procedure as this will always give the best view. Endoscopes fall into two categories: flexible and rigid. It is unusual to use a flexible endoscope to examine a parrot.

A rigid endoscope is a telescope with an outer casing of stainless steel tube. Internally the majority of rigid endoscopes have a rod–lens system: there are lenses at each end with a series of glass rods that help to transmit the image. The lens system is such that it gives a wide angle of view and infinite depth of field. Although everything is in focus, the novice will find that the 'fish eye' lens effect makes size and distances difficult to judge. Within the stainless steel casing, as well as the rod–lens system, there are optical fibres that carry the light to the tip of the endoscope. The light is produced by a separate light source that is connected to the endoscope by a light-carrying cable.

Rigid endoscopes useful for birds are much less expensive than flexible endoscopes; they are smaller in diameter (1.2–4.0 mm) and shorter (10–20 cm) and usually give a far clearer image. There are three

different angles of view: 0 degrees, which allows the operator to look straight ahead, and 30 and 70 degrees – the deviation from the central axis. The 0 degrees view is the easiest to use at first because it looks straight ahead, but 30 degrees is useful as it can be rotated longitudinally to give a wider field of view as well as allowing a view of biopsy forceps, which are introduced down a sheath surrounding the endoscope. The 70 degrees view is not useful for avian endoscopy.

Endoscopes will only view the interior of a cavity. In the respiratory system, which includes the air sacs, the cavity already exists. In order to examine the interior of the alimentary tract and oviduct it is necessary to inflate the organ. Attaching the last 30 cm of a giving set to the sheath of the endoscope will allow the operator to inflate the organ by blowing down the tube. This method is very sensitive and prevents over-inflation of the viscus.

The endoscopic techniques reviewed below require familiarity with normal anatomy to allow accurate diagnosis. It is worth examining as many cadavers as possible endoscopically prior to examining live patients. It is also useful to examine post-mortem specimens endoscopically prior to full examination.

Laparoscopy

Laparoscopy is of great diagnostic importance in ill birds. It is possible to examine and even perform a biopsy on the external parts of nearly all the internal organs (Figures 9.10–9.13). It is possible to see the gonad in all but the most immature parrots. This has revolutionized captive breeding of the sexually monomorphic majority of Psittaciformes and although recently this has been superseded by DNA techniques it is still useful in some circumstances, especially as contamination can make DNA obtained from feathers potentially unreliable (Ciembor *et al.*, 1999). Figures 9.10–9.13 illustrate laparoscopic examination of the gonads, carried out in this case on a Timneh Grey Parrot. Figures 9.14–9.17 illustrate sex determination in other species.

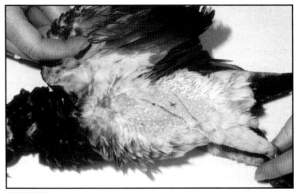

9.10 The site for routine laparoscopic examination is through an incision between the last two ribs; the left side is used for examining the gonads. The last two ribs can be found between the caudal border of the pectoral muscle (cranial line) and the cranial border of the iliotibial muscle (caudal line). The ribs can be palpated under the skin if the bird is not too fat. This and the photographs in Figures 9.11–9.13 are of a Timneh Grey Parrot cadaver. It has been positioned with the wing and leg extended away from the incision site (marked with an X), which is how the live anaesthetized bird would be positioned for this technique.

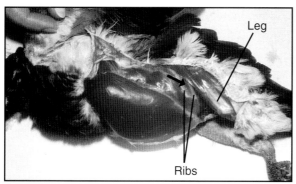

9.11 The same bird skinned, showing the last two ribs and the pectoral and cranial iliotibial muscles. The incision is usually made between the last two ribs ventral to the uncinate process, with short, sharp scissors (Stevens tenotomy scissors are very satisfactory). It is better to use blunt dissection as this limits bleeding. Never close the scissors inside the body; intestinal repair is almost impossible. The incision site is marked by →. An incision positioned more dorsally will cut the internal thoracic artery and vein, which run on the inside of the ribs. Whilst this is unlikely to be fatal, the bleeding will obscure the view and be a possible focus for infection.

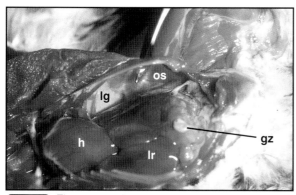

9.12 The cadaver has been placed in dorsal recumbency and the sternum and associated muscles have been removed. The viscera have been left relatively undisturbed but the peritoneal cavities surrounding the heart and liver have been destroyed. The tip of the scissors has penetrated into the caudal thoracic air sac. The oblique septum (os) is intact. Portions of the lung (lg), heart (h), and liver (lr) can be seen laparoscopically from this position. The gizzard (gz) is caudal to the liver.

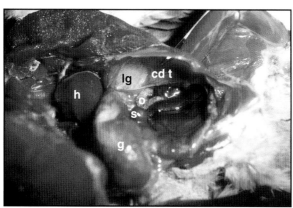

9.13 The oblique septum has been cut and the viscera have been reflected to show the ovary (o). This dissection shows the heart (h), cranial thoracic air sac, caudal thoracic air sac (cd t), lung (lg), gizzard (g) and spleen (s).

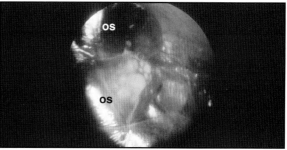

9.14 This is the view that is seen when the endoscope is first advanced through the incision in the wall of the abdomen into the caudal thoracic air sac. The oblique septum (os) separates the air sac from the abdominal viscera. In small parrots, such as this Maximilian's Pionus Parrot, a well developed ovary can be seen through the oblique septum. However, it is usually necessary for the endoscope to go to the other side of the oblique septum to see the structures within the abdominal air sac clearly. The tip of the endoscope is advanced until it 'pops', sometimes audibly, through the oblique septum.

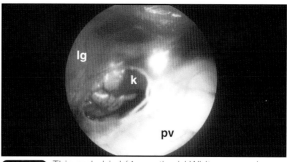

9.15 This male bird (4-month-old White-capped Pionus Parrot) has had a hole made through the oblique septum using a 4 mm 0 degree endoscope. Retracting the endoscope will give the view seen here: the lung (lg) and proventriculus (pv) are obvious, the adrenal gland, kidney (k) and immature testis can be seen through the hole. Usually, the endoscope would be advanced through the hole for a clearer view. In both these views the caudal edge of the lung can be seen. The parabronchi are seen as lines in the lung, and ostia are obvious holes.

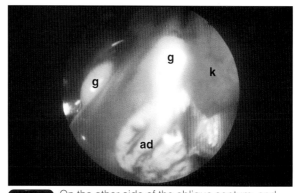

9.16 On the other side of the oblique septum, and attached to the body wall, is a triad of structures: the cranial division of the kidney (k), which is dark red; the adrenal gland (ad), which is always vascular and yellow; and the gonad (g). This view of the bird in Figure 9.15 shows both testes. The far testis is clearly visible and is typical of an immature parrot's testis; the closer testis is blurred as there is body fluid on the tip of the endoscope. The fluid can be removed by touching the endoscope's tip on an adjacent viscus, in this case the kidney. This usually clears the tip of any fluid, blood etc. without the need to remove the endoscope from the bird.

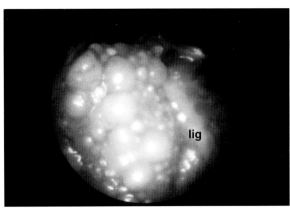

9.17 Once the ovary has matured it hides the adrenal gland. This Yellow-headed Amazon has a half-developed ovary. As the ovary becomes more active the follicles become larger and have a more vascular appearance. Immature ovaries can appear similar to the testes in shape and colour but usually have a granular appearance and are often comma-shaped. The suspensory ligament of the oviduct (lig) can usually be seen as it runs over the surface of the cranial division of the kidney.

Laparoscopy requires anaesthesia. The bird must be starved to allow its intestines to empty. It is uncommon for birds to regurgitate food after anaesthesia, but they can if they have a full crop. More importantly it is very difficult to see their internal organs if the alimentary tract is distended with food. Parrots weighing more than 200 g usually require fasting for 12 hours. Aviary birds should be put in cages overnight, as there is often enough food on the floor of the aviary for them to scavenge and fill their gut. Small ill birds should be starved for a much shorter period (or not at all) and fed soon after recovery.

At the end of laparoscopy, the holes in the body are so small that it is usual to close only the skin wound. The hole in the oblique septum closes within a few hours.

Endoscopic approach to organs: which side to 'scope?

Left side	Right side
Spleen	
Ovary and oviduct	
Gizzard	
Pancreas	Pancreas
Left testis (larger of the two)	Right testis
Left liver lobe	Right liver lobe
Left kidney	Right kidney
Left lung	Right lung

The proventriculus and intestines can be examined from either side but each side shows a different part; for example, a right side approach shows the medial proventiculus, while the left side shows the lateral proventriculus.

Cranial and caudal air sacs are paired and so full examination requires endoscopy of both sides. If there is unilateral pathology (e.g. aspergillosis) it is possible to examine a surprising amount of the air sacs and viscera of the affected side by inserting the endoscope into the other side and approaching across the midline.

Endoscopy equipment

The *light source* needs a halogen or xenon lamp and a fan to cool the bulb. The light source must not be moved when the bulb is hot. The *light cable* is a fibre light guide that runs from the light source to the endoscope.

Endoscopes: The commonest diameters are 4.0 mm (human cystoscope) and 2.7 mm (human arthroscope). Both have a set of lenses at each end connected by a series of tiny glass rods that run the length of the 'scope and enhance the passage of light. Both are available as 0 degrees and 30 degrees. The 4.0 mm is more robust, and cheaper to buy and mend; it carries more light and gives a better field of view. All the endoscopy pictures in this chapter are taken using a 4.0 mm scope (without a sheath).

The 2.7 mm endoscopes are smaller (and therefore more fragile) and shorter, and they are more expensive; they have a different perspective and tend to carry less light that 4.0 mm 'scopes. They are often used within a sheath that, although it increases the overall diameter, allows forceps to be introduced within the sheath for biopsy etc.

The 1.2 mm endoscopes have proximal and distal lenses connected by optical fibres rather than rods. This allows some degree of flexibility in the endoscope – enough to prevent the scope from breaking continually. The view is not as good as with a 2.7 or 4.0 mm but this is offset by the diameter, allowing examination of tiny cavities; for example, it can be used to look down the trachea of Budgerigars and Cockatiels and through the lung of most parrots (Figure 9.25). This 'scope also comes with a sheath and biopsy forceps, but again this increases the overall diameter.

Endoscopic biopsy

An endoscope may be used without a sheath (to give the minimum diameter), with the biopsy forceps being inserted alongside the 'scope through the same incision; or the endoscope is used with forceps that are designed to run within the sheath (e.g. 2.7 mm forceps in a sheath using 5 Fr gauge biopsy forceps).

Diagnostic laparoscopy

Diagnostic laparoscopy is carried out through the same initial site as sex determination but the endoscope is used to look at a much wider range of structures. Some organs are seen better from the right side of the body and certainly all the air sacs should be inspected. Therefore, after examination of the left side, the bird should be turned over and a similar procedure carried out on the right side. Examination of the entire abdominal cavity will enable many diagnoses to be made: e.g. avian tuberculosis, aspergillosis (Figures 9.18 and 9.19), air sacculitis, air sac parasites, visceral gout. Visual appraisal will allow a presumptive diagnosis; biopsy and/or culture will confirm it.

Endoscopically guided biopsy is a useful technique (Figures 9.20 and 9.21). This may be done using a wide-bore sheath, which allows the biopsy forceps to be introduced alongside the endoscope; or the biopsy forceps may be introduced through a different incision and approach the organ from a different angle.

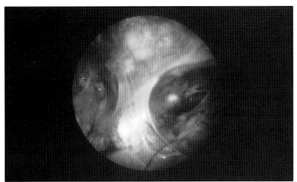

9.18 Diagnosis of aspergillosis is often difficult, and endoscopy can be very helpful as is shown in these two endoscopic views (see also Figure 9.19) of a Green-winged Macaw. Examination of the air sacs frequently reveals them to be thickened with fungal plaques or caseous lesions dotted all over their surface. Normal air sacs usually appear to be avascular but blood vessels can be seen easily in cases of chronic air sacculitis. Swabs taken from the air sac or, better still, biopsies of lesions, allow confirmation of aspergillosis by culture or histology.

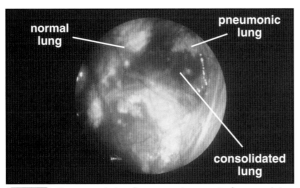

9.19 Pneumonia is often seen in parrots for a variety of reasons. In this Green-winged Macaw it is possible to see areas of normal lung, consolidated lung and pneumonic lung. The white spots on the lung are plaques of fungus and the caseous material that *Aspergillus* spp. produce. There is an air sacculitis and the greyish mass between lung and air sac proved to contain large amounts of the fungus.

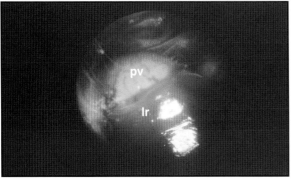

9.20 The liver (lr) may be seen from both sides. It is contained in its peritoneal cavities. It overlies the proventriculus (pv) and is best seen via an approach on the right side, as the proventriculus is less prominent. The hepatic peritoneum is adherent to the air sac that overlies the proventriculus. Liver biopsy usually requires the peritoneum to be removed from the liver by an initial bite of the biopsy forceps. The liver in this view is normal.

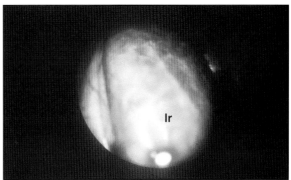

9.21 In comparison with Figure 9.20, this Grey Parrot had a grossly abnormal liver (lr). As well as weight loss and inappetence, it had a fasting bile acid level of 340 µmol/l and a hepatomegaly on radiography. This view has been obtained from within the hepatic peritoneal cavity and shows an abnormally coloured liver with a very rounded edge. It was easy to take diagnostic biopsies. An air bubble within some blood can be seen at the bottom of the picture.

It is possible to examine some of the lumbosacral plexus in larger parrots, which is useful in cases of hindlimb paresis. The cranial and middle divisions of the kidney are not tightly placed against the pelvis, and the endoscope can be inserted between kidney and pelvis.

Examination of the interior of the upper alimentary tract

This should be a part of the routine clinical examination when signs of regurgitation and even inappetence are present. In parrots, it has to be carried out under general anaesthesia.

The interior of the oesophagus, crop, proventriculus and gizzard is easily inspected if they contain no food, but even after 12 hours' starvation the gizzard is rarely empty and usually contains a small amount of green fluid and some grit. It is necessary to insufflate the alimentary tract to view it. A piece of tubing is attached to the inlet to the sheath and the other end is placed in the operator's mouth. The operator can then blow down the tube, which allows sensitive and hands-off control of the insufflation. Samples are easily obtained for examination by suction, either up the sheath around the endoscope using a syringe attached to the sheath, or by using a suitably sized urinary catheter inserted down the instrument channel.

The oesophagus and crop can be examined (Figures 9.22 and 9.23). Before insufflation they lie in folds; once insufflated, they are thin-walled structures through which other organs may be seen, such as the trachea. It may be necessary to hold the oesophagus closed (using finger pressure) over the endoscope whilst insufflation is being carried out. The crop is a bilobed bag and the entrance and exit are offset. The exit to the crop leads to the proventriculus, whose lining has longitudinal streaks. The koilin lining of the gizzard is usually covered with bile-stained vegetable material and is only seen if the gizzard is irrigated.

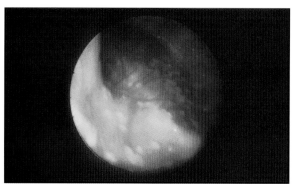

9.22 In parrots with vitamin A deficiency, such as the Grey Parrot illustrated here, the mucus glands that are found in the lining of the crop and oesophagus become hypertrophied. They are very obvious as the crop is insufflated. The rest of the crop appears normal and it is usual to see blood vessels in the wall of the crop.

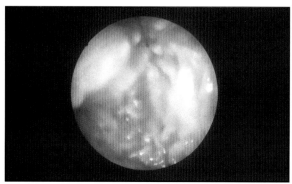

9.23 This parrot's crop has been insufflated to examine the cause of its inappetence and regurgitation. The crop is lying in thickened folds with creamy-coloured mucus on its surface. The endoscope's tip was rubbed on the surface and a smear made. Gram's stain showed typical yeasts. Culture from a crop washing, obtained using a urinary catheter and sterile normal saline, produced a heavy growth of *Candida albicans*.

Examination of the cloaca

Where there is a problem with defecation, or where there is infertility, examination of the cloaca and its surrounding structures is very helpful. With infertility cases this should be carried out after a laparoscopic examination of the external surface of the gonads and reproductive tract. The cloaca should be examined first with an auriscope and any faecal material washed out. Then the endoscope should be inserted carefully into the cloaca, the vent held shut around the endoscope and insufflation gently carried out. The oviduct can be entered and its caudal portion examined in a bird in breeding condition; however, care must be taken as the oviduct is very tortuous and fragile (see Figure 2.13).

Examination of the upper respiratory tract

The caudal part of the nasal passages can be examined through the choana in most parrots. On opening the mouth, a 2.7 mm 30 degree 'scope can be inserted through the slit-like choana in the palate and used to view the caudal nasal passages and caudal nasal conchae, found on each side of the midline nasal septum. It is possible to see nasal and sinus discharges as well as foreign bodies and abscesses.

Opposite the choana is the larynx, the entrance to the trachea. Its internal surface is smooth and easily traversed by the endoscope. In parrots, the trachea reduces in size as it runs to the syrinx (Figure 9.24). Because of this it is usually necessary to use an endoscope without its sheath. A Grey Parrot is often just big enough to allow a 2.7 mm 'scope to view the syrinx. Larger cockatoos and macaws can be examined with a longer 4 mm endoscope. Small-diameter semi-rigid endoscopes (1.2 mm x 25 cm or 1.0 mm x 20 cm) can be used to examine the airway from larynx to air sac in birds as small as Cockatiels and even Budgerigars.

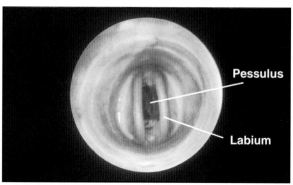

Pessulus

Labium

9.24 View of the distal trachea and syrinx of a Festive Amazon. The complete rings of tracheal cartilage can be seen. The syrinx arises in the trachea with paired labia, beyond which is the pessulus, a wedge-shaped piece of cartilage that divides the airway into left and right primary bronchi.

It is essential to use general anaesthesia to avoid injury to the bird and endoscope. Anaesthesia is induced using a mask and then the bird can be quickly examined from larynx to syrinx (Figure 9.25) and even further. It is helpful to deliver anaesthetic in oxygen through a small tube into the mouth whilst this is happening. If long-term maintenance of anaesthesia is necessary, an air sac tube should be placed (Chapter 8).

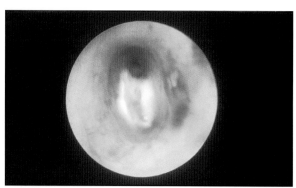

9.25 The syrinx of this Grey Parrot has a plaque of caseous material due to aspergillosis.

Foreign bodies are easily seen and diagnosed but are uncommon except in Cockatiels, which often become obstructed with a millet seed. The trachea in most Cockatiels is <2 mm in diameter and therefore difficult to examine endoscopically. Transillumination of the trachea will often reveal the seed.

10

Avian soft tissue surgery

Neil A. Forbes

Introduction

Avian surgeons require experience and regular surgical work, even on dogs and cats. Sympathetic handling of soft tissues is mandatory in a successful avian surgeon. Avian surgery requires care because the small body size and increased metabolic rate of birds magnify errors. Surgery on parrots can require microsurgical techniques and equipment. For avian surgery to be safe and effective, haemorrhage, tissue trauma and duration of anaesthesia must all be minimized and good postoperative care (including analgesia and fluid therapy) must be provided.

Preparation

The patient should be assessed in relation to energy and nutritional status, as well as circulatory fluid or blood deficit, and any abnormalities should be corrected. Intraoperative and postoperative hypothermia and hyperthermia, pain, sepsis and shock must be controlled (Chapter 8). For external surgery, preoperative starvation should be sufficient to ensure an empty crop (Budgerigar 1 hour, parrot 3 hours). The time taken for a crop to empty varies with the species, its weight and state of health, and the nature of the crop contents. Internal surgery, especially of the intestines, requires longer fasting. However, smaller species can become hypoglycaemic quite quickly and a long period of starvation can be dangerous.

Heat sources

Irrespective of the anaesthetic agent used, in typical theatre temperatures a bird tends to lose 2.8–3.3°C (5–6°F) in the first 30 minutes of any anaesthesia. Heat loss must be prevented so as to minimize intra- or postoperative losses. Heat loss can be reduced by using a low-flow vaporizer and reducing the rate of anaesthetic gas flow, humidifying inspired gases and reducing heat loss from the body core (using bubble-wrap or an exposure blanket). Supplementary heat should also be provided by heat pads, 'snuggle pads' (fluid-filled pads heated in a microwave oven), radiant heat, heated circulating water mats or hot air circulated over the patient. Hyperthermia is potentially more dangerous than hypothermia and core body temperature should be monitored, especially during longer surgical procedures.

Skin preparation

To minimize body heat loss and hypothermia during avian surgery, a minimum area of plumage should be plucked. Sufficient feathers (never flight feathers) are removed to enable adequate sterile access to the operative site. Adjacent feathers may then be retracted from the surgical field and held in place with adhesive tape.

Excessive wetting of the skin should be avoided, in particular with labile fluids such as alcohol (in view of heat loss due to latent heat of evaporation). In the author's practice, skin preparation is performed using iodine-based alcoholic tincture disinfectant. An aerosol surgical adhesive is applied to the skin, and a sterile transparent drape is applied.

Equipment

Surgical drapes

The accurate visualization of respiration is essential for monitoring depth of anaesthesia. The use of sterile clear plastic surgical drapes, maintained on the skin with an aerosol surgical spray adhesive, is advantageous.

Sterile cotton buds

These are invaluable for applying 'point pressure' to control haemorrhage, as well as for moving tissues in an atraumatic manner.

Magnification

Some form of magnification is essential for all patients weighing less than 1 kg. It is advisable to avoid equipment that requires cables to a separate immobile light source; these may hinder the surgeon's mobility, and also trailing cables in time become damaged. The ideal is bifocal surgical lenses, attached to a rechargeable halogen light source (hence no trailing cables) and with a variable focal distance, but the cost is significant. For those new to this field a very adequate start would be with a 'voroscope' (now supplied with ultra-bright diode bulb and rechargeable 12-hour battery packs) or with a modified hobby loupe, with the disadvantage that the latter would require a separate light source and cable.

Optical loupes have a fixed focal distance and relatively limited depth of field. The stronger the lenses selected, the shorter is the focal distance and the closer the clinician will be to the surgical tissues. This should be considered in relation to table and standing or sitting height. An ergonomic operating position is important. A seated position for avian surgery is recommended, in order to achieve greater hand movement control. It is essential that good magnification and, in particular, bright powerful illumination are available in order to see within the body cavities.

Microsurgical instruments
These instruments are not necessarily expensive and in any event few are required: the essentials include fine-pointed scissors, needle holders, artery forceps, atraumatic grasping forceps (e.g. Harris ring tip forceps) and a retractor (e.g. Alm). Only the tips should be miniaturized; the handles should be of normal length, and preferably counterweighted (though this tends to increase the cost significantly). The key is that delicate structures should be able to be handled safely in an atraumatic manner. Care of such instruments is important: they are delicate and will not last long if abused.

Counterweights do minimize digital fatigue, but this is not relevant unless there is a considerable surgical case load. Where possible handles should be round in outline, so that instrument tip movement can be accomplished by a finger-rolling action, rather than the more normal wrist movement. Spring-loaded locking instruments will also greatly assist in reducing finger fatigue.

Suture materials
The finest material, with the least number of sutures, should be used. A material that does not permit capillary action and that causes minimal tissue reaction (i.e. monofilament nylon or polydioxanone, but not braided polyglactin) should be used. The duration of maintenance of suture strength must be appropriate to the speed of tissue healing. Tendons, ligaments and fascia heal slowly (50% strength in 50 days) and should be repaired using polydioxanone or nylon. Suture sizes for birds vary, but generally range from 2 metric (3/0) to 0.7 metric (6/0). Birds tolerate bandages and dressings poorly. In areas where some additional support is required over a suture line, hydrocolloidal skin dressings may be sutured in place. Such a dressing will promote healing, whilst also providing protection to the area.

Haemoclips
Haemoclips (and applicators) are essential for clamping intra-abdominal vessels that are difficult to ligate because of their position. Care and practice are required for the safe and effective application of clips.

Radiosurgery

Radiosurgery is invaluable, but training and care are required. Correctly used, radiosurgery will not cause excessive tissue damage or delayed wound healing but will facilitate incision in the absence of significant haemorrhage, as well as accurate control of any bleeding points (using the bipolar forceps). The control of haemorrhage is essential to prevent significant blood loss and to facilitate uninterrupted visualization of the surgical field, thus reducing surgical time and increasing precision of surgery.

Radiosurgery employs high-frequency alternating current to generate energy. There are two electrodes: active and indifferent. The active electrode should remain cool. The Surgitron (Ellman International Inc., Hewlett, New York) and other radiosurgical units use radio-frequency current (as opposed to an electrical current), which is received at the indifferent plate, so that direct contact between the patient and the plate is not required. This removes any risk of heat generation at the contact point between patient and indifferent plate, which can otherwise lead to patient tissue necrosis.

The two points of the bipolar forceps constitute the two separate electrodes, so there is no need for a ground plate. Bipolar forceps are invaluable for controlling point haemorrhage, even in the presence of a liquid blood-filled field. Cautery with the monopolar head is ineffective in a wet (e.g. blood) field. Intraoperative sterile switching from monopolar to bipolar is essential to facilitate effective mono- and bipolar use.

The optimum frequency for incisions is 3.8–4.0 MHz. This frequency provides a precision focus of the energy in a minimal area. Excessive sparking or lateral heat should not occur; if it does, the power setting is too high. If the power is too low, the electrode drags and this in turn increases the lateral heat and tissue damage, which is undesirable (this can also occur when trying to cut through fat). Any excessive tissue damage will delay postoperative tissue healing.

A fully filtered waveform is ideal, as this minimizes lateral heat. The smallest possible electrode size (in order to minimize lateral heat and hence collateral tissue damage) is always used. For the same reason the electrode should be in contact with the tissue for the minimum time possible. Once tissue is cut, the operator should not return to the same tissue with a single wire within 7 seconds, or 15 seconds if it is a loop electrode. Fully rectified, fully filtered (90% cutting, 10% coagulation) current should be used for cutting skin and biopsy collection. Fully rectified (50% cutting, 50% coagulation) current should be used for dissection with haemostasis, whilst partially rectified (10% cutting, 90% coagulation) current should be used for coagulation.

Surgical lasers

Laser surgery is now more readily available and affordable. Tissues may be cut or ablated (vaporized) using contact mode (which gives the least co-lateral damage – typically 300–600 μm) or non-contact mode (when lateral damage tends to be slightly greater but visualization is improved). Using either technique, blood vessels of up to 2 mm in diameter may be incised in the absence of any haemorrhage. Laser surgery can be used endoscopically. There is no doubt that the application of surgical lasers will have an increasing role in avian surgery during the next few years (Bartels, 2002). The main advantages are the reduction of oedema, postoperative swelling, lateral damage, reduced healing times and less postoperative pain, enabling more extensive surgeries (e.g. orchidectomy) to be performed.

Microsurgery

Surgeons must become familiar with magnification. Slight instrument movements are exaggerated when magnified, but the surgeon's natural ability to control such movements is improved by magnification. Increased manual control is essential, which requires a sitting position with forearm support.

- Assess all risks and possible complications prior to surgery so that they are manageable when they occur.
- Never commence surgery unless wholly familiar with the anatomy.
- Use cadaver surgery for anatomical familiarization and in order to become experienced at tissue handling and evaluating what traction and trauma can be placed on delicate structures without causing lasting damage.
- Prior to anaesthetic induction, ensure that all the equipment that is required for a procedure is available and sterile (small infrequently used instruments are those most likely to have been misplaced).
- The operating table must be stable against movement of people or machinery in the vicinity. Staff should be advised not to touch or knock the table during surgery, as even slight patient movements result in significant surgical risks.

Surgery of the skin and adnexa

Feather cysts

Feather cysts are unerupted feathers which give rise to significant inflammatory swellings. They have recently been reclassified as 'plumafolliculoma' and are considered to be neoplastic. They occur most commonly at the sites of insertion of primary or secondary flight feathers. They may occur subsequent to feather infection or trauma (including plucking of flight feathers). Feather cysts are common in canaries and are considered to be hereditary.

Under anaesthesia cysts may be lanced and cleaned out, in the hope that the feather will then grow back normally. Such an approach should initially be used for tail and primary flight feathers. The other option is to remove the entire cyst surgically, together with the dermal papilla (the point of development of the feather; in flight feathers this is situated in the periosteum on the ventral aspect of the wing).

Uropygial gland

The uropygial or preen gland (Chapters 2 and 16) may suffer from ductal blockage, gland abscessation or neoplasia. Blockage is often overcome by application of digital pressure, resulting in a jet of thick waxy and oily secretion. Abscesses are treated by curettage and topical and systemic antibiosis.

Infection and neoplasia can be difficult to differentiate, as both result in a significant inflammatory response. A biopsy sample should always be taken in doubtful cases. Adenoma, adenocarcinoma and squamous cell carcinoma may occur. Preen gland neoplasia requires careful surgical excision and bipolar radiosurgery is invaluable. The gland itself has a significant blood supply and is bordered ventrally by fibrous connective tissue that attaches firmly to the dorsal surface of the pygostyle and caudal vertebrae. Surgical removal must extend to the connective tissue layer, which is relatively avascular in comparison with the gland itself. The two sides of the gland are separated by a central septum. In many species, in early cases it is possible to remove one side of the gland alone. The skin overlying the gland should be preserved in order to enable postoperative closure.

Self-trauma over and around the preen gland is a common feature in psittacines. Application of a collar during healing, environmental enrichment (releasing the bird into an extensive aviary in the company of other parrots) and surgical removal of the preen gland have all proved efficacious on occasions. If a collar is applied to a parrot for any reason (Chapter 16), it is preferable to hospitalize the parrot for 24–48 hours to give it time to get used to the collar. If this is not done, typical clients will be upset at the bird's initial distress and will remove the collar themselves.

Soft tissue wounds and injuries

Birds typically have very thin skin, with minimal soft tissue structures (in particular on the extremities). Desiccation and devitalization of subcuticular tissues following loss of skin integrity is common. A decision must initially be taken as to whether a skin deficit may be closed by first intention as opposed to second intention healing. Closing the skin, or covering it with hydrocolloidal or vapour membrane dressings to prevent desiccation, is essential in all cases. Tissue damage, necrosis, organic contamination or significant bacterial or fungal infection will preclude first intention healing (Redig, 1996). In the majority of cases, debridement and irrigation will facilitate primary intention healing.

The commonest site for skin deficit is the cranium, subsequent to trauma whilst in flight. In these cases single pedicle or bipedicle cervical grafts may be used, to move loose skin from the neck up over the deficit. Free skin grafting tends not to be successful, but pedicle grafts often are. Care should be taken with respect to the orientation of the graft such that the feather direction is in keeping with the surrounding plumage.

Skin closure may be achieved with vertical or horizontal mattress sutures (as opposed to single interrupted sutures) where the potential for wound site tension is a risk. Psittacine wounds are generally best protected or covered, though parrots are often reluctant to accept bandaging. Granuflex may be sewn in place over a wound to stimulate healing as well as simultaneously providing protection to the wound, in particular by limiting tension across a healing wound. On occasion, neck restraint collars may need to be used in order to prevent self-trauma whilst wounds heal (Chapter 16).

Neoplasms

Birds suffer from a range of cutaneous, subcutaneous and internal neoplasms (Chapter 20). These should be approached in a similar manner to that in other species. Masses may be aspirated for cytological examination, biopsies may be performed, or masses removed and submitted for histopathology.

Lipoma

A benign tumour of fat tissue is a common finding in many psittacine species, particularly Budgerigars. Lipomas are most commonly situated over the bird's breast. Birds presented may have a ventrally displaced tail (counterbalancing the additional weight in the cranial aspect of the body caused by the lipoma). Nutritional manipulation should be considered prior to surgery. Birds on seed-based diets should have their diet changed (Chapter 12). The addition of L-carnitine to the diet may assist in the non-surgical resolution of lipomas (De Voe *et al.*, 2003). Budgerigar lipoma surgery should be undertaken with care. Lipomas frequently have a singular blood supply of significant size and, whilst removal is not difficult, great care and attention must be paid to haemostasis. There is a high chance of fatality in any bird losing blood in excess of 1% of its body weight (i.e. 0.5 ml for the average Budgerigar) during the course of surgery.

Xanthoma

Xanthomas are non-neoplastic masses that typically occur on extremities, in particular where there has been trauma or haemorrhage. They are defined as intradermal deposits of cholesterol clefts with an associated inflammatory reaction. Confirmed xanthomas have also been removed from the infraorbital sinus and from the lumen of the trachea. The exact appearance varies; they are often seen as yellowish plaques under the skin, diffuse thickening or lobulated masses, which will on occasions ulcerate. Xanthomas tend to be highly vascularized and invasive by nature. Reduction of the dietary fat content (converting the bird from seed- or nut-based diets) may assist but surgical removal when initially diagnosed is usually recommended. If the skin cannot be closed following removal, the deficit may be covered with tissue glue or, if applicable, the distal limb (e.g. the extremity of the wing, which is the commonest site) may be amputated. Histology is always indicated, as this is also a common site for fibrosarcoma.

Abscessation ventral to the mandibles

Squamous metaplasia of the submandibular salivary glands, a common sequel to vitamin A deficiency, is encountered most commonly in aged parrots who have been on a long-term nut- or seed-based diet. The lesion appears as a white nodular swelling between the rami of the lower beak and is typically sterile. The swelling should be lanced and the contents surgically removed (haemorrhage can be a complication), together with the surrounding membrane. The bird should receive antibiotics (5–10 days), plus weekly vitamin A injections for 3 weeks. Owners should be warned that such abscesses can recur over subsequent months. The diet should be altered to include more highly coloured fresh fruit and vegetables, especially sweet corn (maize) and apricots.

Hyperinflation of the cervicocephalic air sac

This condition is seen as generalized or localized subcutaneous emphysema. The aetiology has not been elucidated but is commonly considered to involve trauma or chronic respiratory disease or irritation. Several surgical approaches to the condition have been described. The author's preferred technique is to burn an aperture through the overlying skin, to release the air. The concept is to delay healing in the skin (subsequent to the burn) so that the air sac is able to heal internally before the skin wound closes. The procedure may need to be repeated, in particular if there is underlying pathology or respiratory irritation (e.g. a bird living in a tobacco smoke-contaminated environment). If the lesions recur a stent may be placed in the skin to facilitate long-term leakage of air or, failing that, the air-filled dilation may be dissected back to its apparent source (this may be a hole in the notarium), which may be closed by overlaying and suturing with muscle.

Gastrointestinal and reproductive tract techniques

Tongue

Due to the manner in which psittacine birds use their tongues and chew at solid hard abrasive and fragmentary objects, penetrations, lacerations and foreign bodies do occur in the tongue. Any recurrent or non-healing lesion of the tongue should be fully investigated with this in mind. Differential diagnosis includes infections with *Cryptococcus neoformans* and mycobacteria. Other differentials for tongue pathology include candidiasis, trichomoniasis or bacterial granuloma. Non-infectious differentials include hypovitaminosis A (cysts or abscesses), lymphoreticular neoplasia, cystadenoma and squamous cell carcinoma.

Proximal oesophagus

Oesophageal stricture formation may occur after infections (trichomoniasis, capillariasis, candidiasis), tube-feeding trauma, thermal or caustic trauma, foreign body ingestion or iatrogenic surgical trauma. Where strictures occur, the eliciting cause must be determined and addressed. If necessary, a pharyngostomy tube (see later) may be placed during supportive and medical care. If a stricture remains it may be relieved by serial mechanical dilation, using oesophageal balloon dilators or cuffed endotracheal tubes, or by passing tubes or cannulae of increasing size periodically over a period of several weeks.

Ingluviotomy

This procedure is commonly indicated for:

- Retrieval of foreign bodies that are not accessible via the mouth
- Retrieval of proventricular or ventricular foreign bodies (using micro-magnets glued in place within plastic tubes, or lavage or endoscopy)

- Placement of an ingluviotomy or proventriculotomy tube
- Collection of biopsies.

Crop calculi or ingluvioliths may also form and require such removal. A whole range of materials may be found, including rolled-up hay, newspaper or other nest material; these may be hard and inert or may be susceptible to putrefaction, leading to toxaemia.

The bird is placed in dorsal or lateral recumbency and is intubated, with the head elevated above the level of the crop. A probe is placed through the mouth into the crop, to delineate the position of the organ. The skin is incised over the left lateral crop wall, close to the thoracic inlet. The crop wall is localized and isolated. The incision site is selected to avoid large blood vessels and so as not to interfere with post-operative feeding or tube placement. Stay sutures are placed in the crop and an incision one-third to one-half of the length of the skin incision is made (it will stretch to equal that of the skin). Crop closure is achieved with 1.5 metric (4/0) to 0.7 metric (6/0) synthetic monofilament absorbable material using a single or double continuous inversion pattern, followed by separate skin closure.

Treatment of crop burns

Hand-reared parrots may suffer crop burns when fed excessively hot or inadequately mixed food (which is too hot). The bird may present with delayed crop emptying or a wet skin patch over the crop, often 4–7 days after the incident. Necrosis may also occur in adult birds following the consumption of caustic substances. Necrosis of the crop wall and skin leads to fistula formation. Surgical repair should be delayed 4–5 days until necrotic material can be clearly differentiated from viable tissue. It is essential that nutritional support and prevention of secondary infections (bacterial or fungal) be maintained. Pharyngostomy feeding may be necessary (see later). By the time a fistula has formed, the crop wall will have adhered to the skin. Following anaesthetic induction and intubation, the skin is surgically separated from the crop wall. The crop wall is then closed, using a double inversion pattern 1.5 metric (4/0) to 0.7 metric (6/0) synthetic monofilament absorbable material, followed by a separate skin closure.

Crop or oesophageal lacerations

These may occur following traumatic tube feeding or external trauma. Tears are often not seen at the time of trauma but are recognized later, when a significant build-up of foetid toxin-producing food material has occurred subcutaneously. These patients tend to be very sick, and surgical procedures should be kept as brief as possible. A significant active inflammatory reaction will be present. Surgical exploration, closure of the crop wound, drainage, pharyngostomy tube placement (if required) and significant support in terms of fluid therapy, analgesia, anti-inflammatory and antibiotic therapy will be needed, prior to surgical skin closure some days later once infection is controlled and the bird is a stronger surgical patient.

Crop biopsy

Crop biopsy is the safest and least invasive ante-mortem diagnostic technique for psittacine proventricular dilatation syndrome (PDD) (Chapter 13). This method has 68% sensitivity with a 100% specificity (Doolen, 1994). The collection site should be in the left lateral (non-dependent) area of the crop. The sensitivity is further maximized (up to 76%) by selecting a section of crop wall where a clearly visible blood vessel terminates and by harvesting a large full-thickness biopsy (0.5–1.0 cm × 0.5–1.0 cm).

Pharyngostomy, oesophagostomy or ingluviostomy tube placement

Tube placement is required in situations where the mouth, proximal or distal oesophagus or crop needs to be bypassed. Such conditions may include orthopaedic conditions of the beak and head, or trauma, infection, neoplasia, severe parasitic infestations or strictures affecting any part of the gastrointestinal tract between the mouth and the proventriculus, or a bird may simply be so weak that it is unable to feed itself.

1. The bird is anaesthetized, intubated and placed in lateral recumbency.
2. A metal feeding tube is placed through the mouth and tented up in an appropriate position in the cervical oesophagus (cranial to the crop).
3. The skin is prepared and a small incision is made over the end of the feeding tube.
4. An appropriately sized rubber or plastic feeding tube (which can be connected to a feeding syringe) is passed via the incision into the oesophagus, and advanced in a caudal direction.
5. The tube is passed via the crop and distal (thoracic) oesophagus into the proventriculus.
6. A skin suture is placed around the tube.
7. Tape is placed on either side of the feeding tube as it exits the skin incision and is sutured to the skin.
8. The capped feeding end is then enclosed in a bandage wrapped around the neck or attached to the bird's back.

Regular small meals (smaller than if feeding into the crop) are administered and care is taken to flush the tube clean after each use. Such a tube may be left in place for several weeks if necessary.

Coelotomy

The caudal thoracic and abdominal air sacs receive fresh air from the trachea. It is important to appreciate that coelotomy is impossible without opening the posterior air sacs. This has a profound effect both on the effectiveness of inhalant anaesthesia and on intraoperative heat loss. Once a coeliotomy incision is made, openings around the surgery site may be packed off, or plugged with abdominal organs. Alternatively, parenteral anaesthetic agents may be used. During any coeliotomy procedure, the bird's head should be raised at 30–40 degrees to prevent any surgical irrigation fluid from entering the lung field.

Left lateral coelotomy

This is the most useful approach and is used for access to the gonads, left kidney, oviduct, ureter, proventriculus and ventriculus.

1. The bird is placed in right lateral recumbency. The uppermost wing should be reflected dorsally, whilst the left leg is restrained in a dorsocaudal direction.
2. The skin web between the abdominal wall and the left leg is incised to facilitate further abduction of the left leg.
3. A skin incision is created from the sixth rib to the level of the pubic bone on the left abdominal wall (Figure 10.1).
4. The superficial medial femoral artery and vein will be visualized traversing dorsal to ventral across the lateral abdominal wall ventral to the coxofemoral joint (Figure 10.2). These vessels should be cauterized with the bipolar forceps prior to transection.
5. The musculature (external and internal abdominal oblique and transverse abdominal muscles) is tented up away from the coeliomic contents and incised with sharp fine scissors whilst protecting the internal viscera. The incision is extended from pubis to the eighth rib, the caudal two to three ribs (i.e. numbers 7 and 8) being transected.
6. Bipolar forceps are placed around each rib, from the caudal aspect, such that the forceps close over the anterior border of the rib in order to cauterize the intercostal vessels (Figure 10.3) prior to transecting the rib (with large scissors).
7. A small retractor (e.g. Heiss or Alm) is then inserted between the cut rib ends to enable full visualization of the abdominal cavity. The Lone Star retraction system (see Figure 10.7) is invaluable for such surgeries.
8. On completion of the intercoelomic surgery, the incision is closed using 1.5 metric (4/0) to 0.7 metric (6/0) absorbable monofilament synthetic material in a continuous or interrupted pattern in two layers. The intercostal muscles are apposed and no attempt is made to rejoin the transected ribs.

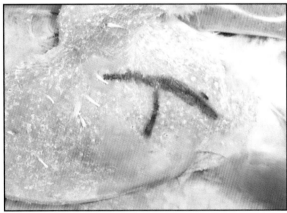

10.1 Cadaver of Grey Parrot, plucked, with left leg abducted dorsally. The site of skin incision for left lateral coeliotomy (from sixth rib to pubis), with a potential ventral flap (if required), is marked.

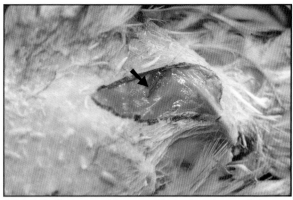

10.2 Cadaver of Amazon illustrating the medial femoral artery (arrowed) and vein prior to cauterization.

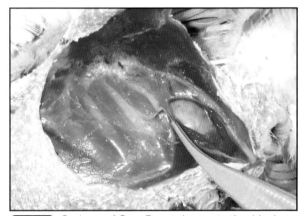

10.3 Cadaver of Grey Parrot demonstrating bipolar radiosurgery cauterization of the intercostal vessels.

Salpingohysterectomy

Removal of the avian ovary is challenging and often dangerous, as it is firmly attached to the dorsal abdominal wall. Instead, in order to prevent further egg laying, *all* of the oviduct and uterus may be removed. A review of ovariectomy techniques is discussed by Echols (2002). The ventral suspensory ligament of the oviduct and uterus is broken down with blunt dissection (Figure 10.4). A significant blood vessel that enters the infundibulum on the medial aspect from the ovary should be clamped off with two haemoclips (Figure 10.5), prior to transection. The dorsal suspensory ligament of the uterus should be identified extending from the dorsal abdominal wall to the uterus. In this ligament are a number of blood vessels, which should be coagulated or clipped. The uterus and oviduct are then exteriorized. Moving dorsocaudally towards the dorsal abdominal wall, care should be taken in resecting the dorsal suspensory ligament. If resection is continued too far, there is a danger of resecting one or more ureters. Placing a cotton bud into the cloaca will assist in delineating where the uterus should be clamped (Figure 10.6). The latter is achieved by applying two clips to the uterus and transecting on the uterine side of these. All haemorrhage is controlled prior to closure of the abdominal muscle wall and the skin, each with a simple continuous suture pattern.

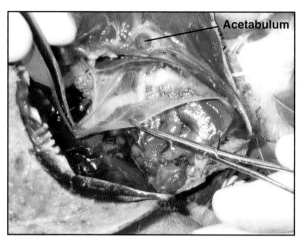

10.4 Cadaver of Grey Parrot following blunt dissection of the ventral oviductal ligament. For this and the following views, the hip joint has been disarticulated to allowed photography.

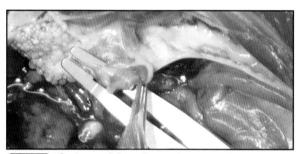

10.5 Cadaver of Grey Parrot demonstrating haemoclip application to blood vessels supplying the medial aspect of the infundibulum.

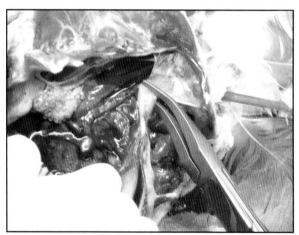

10.6 Cadaver of Grey Parrot demonstrating haemoclip placement at the junction of the oviduct and cloaca.

Caesarian section

Caesarian section may be considered as an alternative where a hen is suffering from egg binding (Chapter 18), if the egg and hen are of high financial or conservational value, or the condition is not responsive to medical support or ovacentesis and eggshell implosion. Depending on the position of the egg, a caudal left lateral or midline incision is made. The oviduct is incised directly over the egg, avoiding any prominent

blood vessels. After egg removal, the oviduct is inspected and the cause of binding is determined and rectified. If correction is not possible, salpingohysterectomy may be indicated at a later date but would be inappropriate at this time. The oviduct is closed with single interrupted or continuous pattern sutures using 1.5 metric (4/0) or finer absorbable material.

Uterine torsion

Egg binding (Chapter 18) may arise subject to a range of aetiologies. If the condition does not respond to medical support, and in particular if there is a markedly swollen coelom, torsion of the oviduct should be considered as a cause (Harcourt-Brown, 1996a). In such cases the oviduct will have suffered a torsion, through which no eggs can pass. A number of eggs in varying states of decay may be present in the proximal oviduct. For torsion to occur, typically there will have been a traumatic breach in the dorsal oviductal suspensory ligament through which the oviduct will have passed. Many such patients are in poor condition and represent poor surgical cases. Once the bird has been stabilized as much as possible, a ventral midline surgical approach is used to access the oviduct. On occasions the torsion may be reduced (often surgical drainage of the oviduct is required first) and the breach of the suspensory ligament repaired. Alternatively, a salpingohysterectomy may be performed.

Orchidectomy

Orchidectomy may be performed via the left lateral coelotomy approach. The testicles (like the ovaries) are attached to the dorsal abdominal wall, adjacent to the aorta, and connected only by a short testicular artery. The left testis is identified, the caudal pole is elevated and a haemoclip is placed under the testis (Figure 10.7). The testis is then surgically cut away from the clip, after which a further clip is applied from the caudal direction, between the testis and the existing clip, into a more craniad position and so the process is continued until the testis can be totally

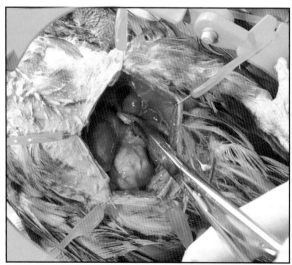

10.7 Cadaver of Amazon after exposure maximized by use of Lone Star Retractor, showing haemoclip application to the caudomedial aspect of the left testis.

removed. If any testicular tissue is left, there is a possibility of regeneration. Access to the right testis will be more difficult, requiring blunt dissection through the air sac wall, or via a fresh incision on the contralateral abdominal wall. A similar removal process may then be performed on this testis.

Neutering

As described above, ovariectomy is a very risky procedure and orchidectomy is marginally less so. The indications for neutering may be to prevent breeding (for which vasectomy is safer in a male bird and salpingohysterectomy is a preferred option in a female, though ova may still on occasions be released into the abdomen) but such a cause is rare. More often in the past, neutering has been recommended to control persistent egg laying in females or aggression and hypersexuality in males. Currently the view is that surgery can be avoided by reducing the energy density of the diet (converting from seeds and nuts to a pellet-based diet with fresh fruit and vegetables), hormone therapy (Chapter 18) and the institution of behavioural modification training.

Proventriculotomy

Proventriculotomy for access to the proventriculus or ventriculus is most commonly indicated for the removal of foreign objects that are not retrievable through the mouth or from the crop using rigid or flexible endoscopes. Proventricular biopsy is no longer recommended as the diagnostic method of choice where PDD is suspected, in view of the unacceptable risk (McCluggage, 1992). Although the technique has been described, ventriculotomy is generally avoided in view of the highly muscular walls (the physiological muscular activity readily pulling sutures out of the muscle wall), the inability to form an inversion closure and the increased vascularity compared with the proventriculus. Ventricular foreign bodies can be accessed via an incision in the isthmus between the proventriculus and the ventriculus.

Access is gained via the left lateral coeliotomy approach; sufficient exposure is necessary to enable visualization of the suspensory membranes and to avoid the proventricular vessels along its greater curvature. The ventriculus (gizzard) is identified as a muscular organ with a white tendinous lateral aspect. Blunt dissection is used to break down the ventricular suspensory attachments. Two 2 metric (3/0) stay sutures are placed in the white tendinous part of the ventriculus, and sutured to structures outside of the abdomen, to maintain the ventriculus firmly in the abdominal opening (exteriorization is possible in some species) (Figure 10.8). Depending on the size of the patient, it is advantageous to pack off the abdomen (behind the ventriculus) with saline-soaked gauze swabs to minimize the effect of any leakage. The triangular portion of liver that covers the isthmus is identified. Using a sterile cotton bud, the liver is elevated, revealing the optimum incision site into the isthmus (the junction between the proventriculus and the ventriculus) (Figure 10.9), to facilitate biopsy or access to the ventriculus for foreign body removal. An initial stab incision is made, which is extended with iris scissors. Suction should be available

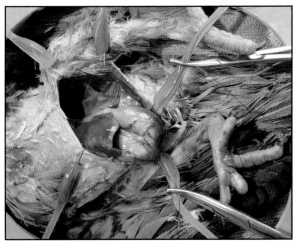

10.8 Cadaver of Amazon after exposure maximized by use of Lone Star Retractor, showing exteriorization of the ventriculus by placement of stay sutures in ventricular fascia.

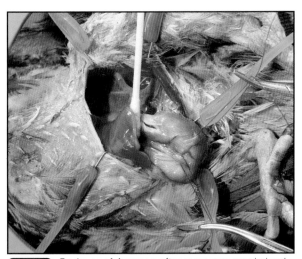

10.9 Cadaver of Amazon after exposure maximized by use of Lone Star Retractor, indicating proventriculoventricular isthmus with incision site for access to ventricular lumen.

to remove enteric contents in a controlled manner. An endoscope may be passed into gut via the incision in both cranial and caudal directions to verify that all foreign objects have been removed. The incision is closed in two continuous layers (opposed then inverted) using 1.5 metric (4/0) to 0.4 metric (8/0) synthetic absorbable monofilament material, after which the liver is tacked in place over the proventricular incision site. The body of the proventriculus has a poor ability to hold sutures, and tears readily as sutures are tightened. Care should be taken to place sutures a sufficient distance from the wound edge so that they do not tear through, but not so far that undue pressure has to be used to close the wound, as this will also lead to tearing.

Suture placement in normal gut surgery includes the submucosa, in view of its greater collagen content. However, the avian proventriculus has minimal collagen and so greater care is required. The placement of collagen patches over a traditional ventricular closure does not reduce the incidence of wound breakdown.

As birds have no mesentery, enterotomy (see below) carries a higher risk of postoperative peritonitis. The liver may take the role of the mesentery in overlying the closed isthmal incision. The ventricular suspensory ligaments are not repaired. Closure is as described above. Care should be taken to minimize collateral damage during incision and repair of the isthmus. It has been demonstrated in turkeys that the entire neural network situated within the isthmus must remain intact for normal gastroduodenal motility to occur.

Neoplasia of the proventriculus and ventriculus is uncommonly reported in psittacine birds.

Yolk sacculectomy

In neonate chicks, the presence of an infected or unretracted yolk sac necessitates surgical removal. Chicks that eat early after hatching and those affected by reduced gut motility are believed to have a higher incidence of unretracted yolk sac but it is also a common abnormality in artifically incubated birds, where it may be accompanied by other abnormalities. Yolk sac infections are often associated with umbilical infections, enteritis or septicaemia. Clinical signs include anorexia, lethargy, constipation, diarrhoea, weight loss and abdominal distension. Non-invasive diagnosis is readily achieved by ultrasonography. Signs are typically not detected early enough for medical therapy alone to be effective.

Following induction of anaesthesia, the bird is placed in dorsal recumbency. A small incision is delicately created cranial to the umbilicus. This incision is extended around the umbilicus and the umbilical stump is excised. The yolk sac is exteriorized and the duct ligated. Care is taken to avoid rupture or spillage of the yolk sac contents. The abdominal incision is closed in two layers. Chicks that are unwell prior to surgery must be given a guarded prognosis. Full retraction of the yolk sac in a normal chick enables absorption of all energy and protein content of the sac; this is not possible in chicks with unretracted sacs.

Enterotomy

Enterotomy is an infrequent procedure typically necessitated following trauma to the gastrointestinal tract, iatrogenic surgical damage, intussusceptions, torsions, adhesions, enteroliths or areas of necrosis. The procedure carries a guarded to grave prognosis. If colon is prolapsed via the cloaca (Figure 10.10), an intussusception must be present. Such cases require an immediate midline (with or without flap) coeliotomy and reduction of the intussusception, which may contain a length of devitalized gut. An enterectomy will be required to remove any devitalized gut. Intussusception has also been seen secondary to linear foreign bodies or following enteric infections.

If the bird is particularly shocked or weakened, then rather than resecting and rejoining the gut at one surgery, it may be prudent to create a stoma or a loop jejunostomy or colostomy, with reattachment several days later (VanDerHeyden, 1993). Midline flap incisions give optimal access. Microsurgical instrumentation and techniques are mandatory. Blood

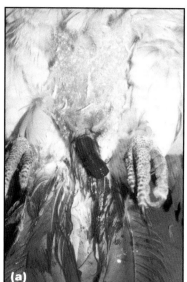

10.10

(a) Grey Parrot presented with a mass protruding from its vent. After gentle cleaning it looked like intestine. (b) The intestines were examined via a midline abdominal incision. An intussusception was found and successfully reduced.

(a)

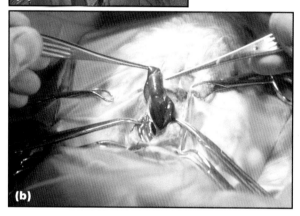

(b)

vessel appositional clamps (e.g. Acland clamps) are invaluable to achieve intraoperative intestinal occlusion atraumatically whilst simultaneously maintaining the tissue sections in apposition during suture placement. These vascular clamps are designed to avoid tissue slippage, whilst maintaining low pressure to avoid tissue damage. The clamps may be used individually, or preferably attached to a bar or rectangle, so that both ends of the tissue are adjacent to each other. When passing needles through fine tissue, it is important that the needle is encouraged to follow its natural curvature; otherwise an excessive needle hole is created. The arcing instrument action achieved by finger rolling of round-bodied instruments minimizes this problem.

Intestinal anastomosis

Anastomosis of the intestine may be performed with an end-to-end technique using 0.7 metric (6/0) to 0.2 metric (10/0) material with a simple appositional method. If the gut is < 2 mm in diameter, 6–8 simple interrupted sutures are used (similar to a blood vessel anastomosis). If the gut is > 2 mm in diameter a continuous pattern should be used. The advantages of a continuous pattern is that it reduces surgery time, yields improved apposition and so reduces risk of leakage, reduces tissue irritation and achieves improved endothelialization.

Care should be taken not to overtighten a continuous pattern, as this would cause a purse string and compromise food passage across the repair site. Sutures are initially placed at 12 o'clock and 6 o'clock, then in the caudal section of gut and finally in the anterior aspect. If the sections of gut being joined are of unequal size, or where end-to-end anastomosis is technically difficult for other reasons, a side-to-side or side-to-end technique may be used. If using a side-to-side technique, the end sections may be closed with sutures or haemoclips. One section of gut is offered up to the side of the other and the back of the anastomosis is sutured, prior to the aperture being created and then the front being sutured. If necessary, the front repair sutures may be pre-placed.

Ventral midline coeliotomy

This approach gives poor visibility of the majority of the coelom but it will facilitate surgery of the small intestine, pancreatic biopsy, liver biopsy or cloacopexy and is used in diffuse abdominal disease such as peritonitis, egg binding and cloacal prolapses. The bird is placed in dorsal recumbency, the midline is prepared and the legs are abducted caudally. The skin of the abdominal wall is tented and an initial incision is made using scissors or the single wire radiosurgical electrode. Care is required to prevent iatrogenic visceral damage. The risk is minimized by creating the incision caudally over the cloaca, rather than over the small intestine. The incision is extended with fine scissors. This approach can be extended along the costal border cranially and to the pubis caudally to create a flap on one of both sides of the midline to increase access. This approach is particularly useful for access to the caudal uterus and cloaca.

Cloacal conditions

Cloacal conditions are common in pet birds, with varied aetiologies such as cloacitis caused by papilloma, neoplasia, uroliths, mycobacteriosis, parasites, cloacal prolapse associated with oviductal or urethral obstruction, other oviductal disease or behavioural abnormalities (hypersexuality and lack of dominance).

Organs prolapsed through the cloaca

Apart from partial cloacal prolapses, or prolapsed cloacal masses (papilloma, neoplasia or mycobacterial granuloma – see Chapter 5 for differential diagnosis), total prolapses can occur where the colonic, urethral and oviductal junctions may be everted. Alternatively, the oviduct or intestine may be prolapsed (Figures 18.5 and 10.10). Differentiation of the tissues involved is important and is achieved by assessing the size of the structures present (Best, 1996). Birds presented with such prolapses are typically extremely shocked. Fluid therapy, analgesia and anti-inflammatory therapy are all mandatory. If a colonic or uterine prolapse is present, inevitably there must be an intussusception. Pushing the offending organ back through the cloacal opening and placing a purse-string suture will not lead to a satisfactory outcome. Such action must be followed by a coeliotomy and reduction or removal of the intussuscepted material.

Cloacal papilloma

Cloacal papillomas are particularly common in South American species (e.g. macaws (Figure 10.11) and Amazons). All such birds should undergo a choanal and cloacal examination for papilloma as a routine part of any clinical examination. One or more cotton buds are passed into the cloaca and then gently retracted so as to evert the cloacal lining. Chapter 13 gives details of additional health considerations for cloacal papilloma. Cloacal, colonic or oviductal prolapses may resemble neoplasms, particularly if the prolapsed tissue is necrotic. Histological examination of cloacal tissues is advised.

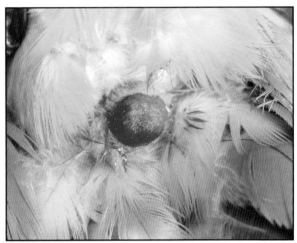

10.11 Blue and Gold Macaw illustrating a cloacal papilloma.

Many different treatments have been suggested, including repeated alternate-day applications of silver nitrate, inclusion of 2% capsicum in the diet, autogenous (high antigen-loaded) vaccination (Krautwald-Junghans *et al.*, 2000), cryosurgery, radiosurgery and yag laser therapy.

Cloacotomy yields the best access and enables complete surgical removal of papilloma (Dvorak *et al.*, 1998). The bird is placed in dorsal recumbency. A ventral midline incision is made with scissors through the skin, vent sphincter muscle and cloacal mucosa into the proctodeum (see Figure 2.12). Haemorrhage is controlled with radiosurgery bipolar forceps. Following surgery to remove the papilloma, the cloacal mucosa is closed using 1.5 metric (4/0) synthetic absorbable material with a simple continuous pattern. The vent sphincter is apposed with 1.5 metric (4/0) synthetic absorbable material in a horizontal mattress fashion and the skin is closed with simple continuous pattern using similar material.

Bladder mucosal stripping has been used extensively in mammals as a treatment for carcinoma (Wishnow, 1989). Cloacal mucosal stripping has been reported in one Amazon. Although the bird tolerated several episodes of mucosal stripping, it did not prevent the papilloma from reforming (Antinoff and Hottinger, 2000). Vent strictures can occur following any extensive cloacal surgery and can be addressed with regular stretching using an aural speculum. Even mild strictures can prevent a bird laying an egg. In light of the current knowledge as to the aetiology, contagious nature and long-term patient prognosis of these cases, excessive efforts to achieve a complete surgical resolution now seems questionable.

Cloacoliths

Cloacoliths are firm rough-surfaced aggregations of urates. They are uncommon and the pathogenesis is unclear. This author has experienced them most frequently in carnivorous birds, especially in those that have recently undergone extended nesting or brooding behaviour, such that they may not have voided faeces as frequently as normal. Birds present with repeated straining, often passing scant traces of blood. The condition is readily diagnosed on digital exploration of the cloaca. The bird is anaesthetized; the cloacolith may be fragmented with artery forceps and removed piecemeal. Analgesics and antibiosis should be administered. There is often an area of severe inflammation in the ventral wall of the cloaca. The patient should undergo cloacal endoscopic examination 10–14 days after treatment to ensure that there is no recurrence.

Cloacopexy

Cloacal prolapse is a common indication for a cloacopexy. It tends to occur in hypersexual birds, usually cockatoos. Behavioural modification is important, in particular gaining dominance over the bird and reducing its psychological and nutritional drive towards sexual activity.

A cotton bud is advanced into the cloaca and used to tent the cloaca within the abdomen, to confirm its position. A horizontal incision is made over the most anterior portion of the cloaca, being careful not to incise the thin-walled cloaca. The fat pad that is present on the ventral aspect of the cloaca is removed. In severe cases, two sutures are placed: one around the eighth rib on each side, then each is passed through the full thickness of the cloaca on the same side and each suture is tightened, such that the cloacal wall is apposed to the rib. To achieve this a needle is passed from the external surface of the abdominal wall, via the intercostal space between ribs 7 and 8, into the coelomic cavity. The needle is exteriorized via the coelomic opening (adjacent to the cloaca). The needle is passed through the cloacal wall, then passed back into the abdomen and back through the abdominal wall (inside to out), just caudal to the eighth rib. Two further sutures are placed through the cloacal wall and incorporated in the abdominal wall closure.

Although surgical procedures exist for the control of cloacal prolapses, recurrence is common, particularly if the behavioural abnormalities are not addressed. Cloacoplasty is often performed simultaneously with cloacopexy.

Cloacoplasty

Cloacoplasty (reducing the diameter of the cloacal aperture) is also recommended where there is atony of the vent sphincter. The internal margin of the vent (lateral or dorsal section) is excised for up to 60% of the circumference, to provide a cut edge for healing. The edges are then sutured from side to side to reduce the diameter of the cloacal aperture. This condition often occurs in hypersexual cockatoos that masturbate. If the underlying behavioural or sex hormone abnormality is not resolved, the cloaca is likely to stretch again.

Abdominal hernia

Abdominal hernias are seen most commonly in obese female psittaciforms, especially cockatoos and Budgerigars. They are often related to breeding, hormonal influences or other reasons for space-occupying coelomic masses. High-energy diets lead to obesity and also serve as a drive to egg production (increasing liver size and follicular activity, respectively). Prior to any consideration of surgery, the bird must be converted from a seed-based diet to a more balanced (pelleted) or fresh food diet; exercise must be enforced (e.g. 30 minutes walking daily) and the weight reduced significantly.

Avian abdominal hernia is dissimilar to mammalian umbilical or inguinal hernia but similar to abdominal wall rupture. Instead of a specific hernia ring, there is a thinning and gradual separation of muscle fibres. Surgery to pull the sides of the deficit together is not effective. It is recommended that the bird should undergo salpingohysterectomy at the time of hernia repair. Following this, a tuck may be taken in the abdominal musculature. The owner should be warned that this may not be effective and that additional surgery may yet be required.

Additional surgery may involve the surgical placement of a non-absorbable mesh material across the expanse of the present or potential deficit. Such surgery should be contemplated only if trauma and skin abrasion are occurring over the herniated mass, after obesity has been corrected. An extensive bilateral flap ventral midline approach is used. Surgical mesh or a collagen sheet can be attached bilaterally to the pubis and to each eighth rib, as well as the sternum. Surgical meshes are generally well tolerated but intense attention to sterility during surgery is mandatory. If surgery can be avoided by dietary change and weight loss, this is preferable. On occasions, herniation will occur secondary to abdominal lipoma, cystic structures, neoplasia or other space-occupying masses.

Tracheotomy

This procedure is most commonly indicated in the treatment of syringeal or tracheal aspergilloma or retrieval of a tracheal foreign body. The technique is more commonly practised in psittacine birds than in raptors as in the former the distal trachea narrows significantly, which makes endoscopic treatment of such lesions more difficult.

Air sac intubation should be performed prior to undertaking tracheal surgery. A hypodermic needle may be usefully placed across the trachea distal to any foreign body to prevent the material passing caudally. The bird is placed in dorsal recumbency, with the head directed towards the surgeon. The front of the bird should be elevated at 45 degrees to the tail, so as to facilitate interoperative visualization into the thorax. A skin incision is made adjacent to the thoracic inlet. The crop is identified, bluntly dissected and displaced to the right. The interclavicular air sac is entered and the trachea is elevated. The sternotracheal muscle (attached bilaterally to the ventral aspect of the trachea) is transected. Stay sutures may be placed into the trachea, in order to draw it in an anterior direction. In most species it is impossible to exteriorize the syrinx completely.

A tracheotomy may now be performed, cutting half of the tracheal circumference, through the ligament between adjacent tracheal cartilages (using a number 11 scalpel blade). Foreign material may be scraped out using a Volkmann's spoon, and foreign bodies (e.g. seed) may be removed via a tracheotomy but they can be moved craniad using a suitable catheter as a probe or a forceful blast of air from a hypodermic syringe and out through the glottis. The incision is repaired with single interrupted sutures (0.7 metric (6/0) maximum of two or three sutures only) placed to include two rings either side of the incision. If additional access is required, the superficial pectoral muscles may be elevated and an osteotomy of the clavicle performed. On closure the two ends of the clavicle are apposed but not rejoined. The muscle is replaced and sutured into position. The crop is sutured back into place, to create an airtight repair over the interclavicular air sac, using a continuous suture pattern and absorbable suture material. The skin is closed in a routine manner.

Trachectomy

In cases where a severe tracheal stenosis occurs, typically following trauma (most commonly associated with recent intubation, especially in macaws) or infection, tracheal resection and removal of the affected tissue can be performed. Depending on the site of the lesion, most species can cope with losing up to five tracheal rings. In such cases close apposition of cartilages following surgery, using a suture material that elicits minimal tissue reaction (e.g. polydioxanone) is used in order to minimize the risk of intraluminal granuloma formation. Trauma to tracheal tissues during surgery must be minimized. It is preferable to place sutures in the trachea at the time of resection, to facilitate apposition and anastomosis. Two to four sutures are used (depending on patient size) and are all pre-placed before any are tied.

Biopsy

Lung biopsy

Lung biopsy samples may be collected endoscopically via the air sac or surgically (the method favoured by this author). Fine-definition radiographs may usefully assist the surgeon in locating an area of lung tissue with apparent abnormalities from which biopsy is most likely to yield a useful result. The bird is laid in lateral recumbency, the leg extended caudally and the wing abducted dorsally. The fifth rib (of eight) is located, typically at the caudal extremity of the scapula. A skin incision is made over the rib from the scapula to the level of the uncinate process. The incision is continued down on to the rib. The lung tissue may be visualized either side of the rib. A section of rib (0.5 cm) overlying the lung is removed and a biopsy sample is harvested using iris scissors from beneath the position of the rib (Figure 10.12). The skin alone is closed afterwards.

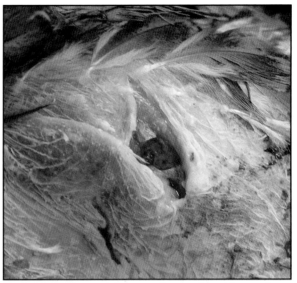

10.12 Cadaver of Amazon showing lung biopsy site caudal to scapula and medial to fifth rib.

Liver biopsy

With the patient in dorsal recumbency, a 2–3 cm incision through skin and then abdominal musculature is created parallel to and 0.5 cm caudal to the caudal edge of the sternum, just lateral to the midline. The liver will be identified beneath the sternum (see Figure 2.10). The liver is examined for any apparent lesions. If a specific lesion is present, a biopsy sample from that site is indicated. If no discrete lesion is apparent a wedge biopsy sample is collected from the caudal border of both the left and right lobes of the liver. In both situations two pairs of fine artery forceps are used to triangulate and isolate a wedge of liver tissue (1 cm wide and 0.75 cm deep) (Figure 10.13). The segment of liver is removed and the forceps are removed approximately 1 minute later. Alternatively, a monopolar loupe electrode may be used to harvest a biopsy sample. In such cases, the power is activated prior to making contact with the tissues, ensuring a sufficient margin between the incision and the tissue to be examined. Cauterized tissue yields poor histopathological results.

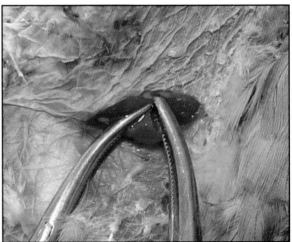

10.13 Cadaver of Amazon showing triangulation of liver with fine haemostat forceps. The incision site is 1 cm left lateral of midline, 0.5 cm caudal to sternum.

Pancreatic biopsy

A number of pancreatic diseases have been reported but there has been little research into the clinical significance of amylase and lipase levels (Fudge, 1997), although a fourfold increase in amylase level may be suggestive of pancreatic pathology. Currently histopathology is the diagnostic tool of choice (Speer, 1998). Clinical signs associated with avian pancreatitis include anorexia, abdominal discomfort (colic), weight loss, polyuria, polydipsia, abdominal distension, polyphagia, or pale bulky faeces, though many cases are asymptomatic.

The bird is anaesthetized, intubated and placed in dorsal recumbency. A small (1–2 cm) craniocaudal incision is made in the mid-abdominal region. Care is taken not to damage underlying viscera. The pancreatic lobe in the duodenal loop of the small intestine is readily located and exteriorized. The dorsal and ventral pancreatic loops are separated by the pancreatic artery (which must not be damaged). Although lesions may be apparent in other areas of the pancreas, the distal-most aspect of the organ is harvested. To achieve this safely, the distal edge is lifted and the underlying tissues examined for the presence of the artery, prior to careful biopsy removal. If specific lesions are present, these should be sampled for biopsy if in the ventral or dorsal lobe (but not the splenic lobe), so long as the procedure can be achieved without damaging the arterial supply to the remaining panreatic tissue. The incision is closed in a routine manner.

Renal biopsy

Renal biopsy is a frequently used technique in the diagnosis of kidney disease. The technique is simple and carries few risks if undertaken endoscopically.

Other procedures

For abdominal air sac placement, see Chapter 8. For sinus surgery, see Chapter 14. For egg binding (dystocia), see Chapter 18.

Devoicing

Devoicing of birds is considered by the Royal College of Veterinary Surgeons to be a mutilation and is illegal in the UK. Even in countries where it is not prohibited, it is a risky procedure with uncertain short- and long-term outcomes: many birds continue to vocalize despite surgical devoicing.

Postsurgical care

Postsurgical care greatly affects the outcome of the procedure. Prevention of self-trauma, a rapid recovery, sufficient analgesia, and fluid, thermal and nutritional support, as well as the minimization of stress, are vital.

11

Orthopaedic and beak surgery

Nigel H. Harcourt-Brown

Equipment for hard tissue surgery

The surgeon's preference predicts much of the choice and use of surgical instruments. Many pieces of equipment are used for different techniques by different surgeons. The following is the author's preference.

Magnification

Most of the parrots that are presented for orthopaedic surgery weigh between 100 g and 1 kg. For many surgical techniques it is helpful to use magnification. There are several ways of achieving this. A cheap method is to buy a magnifying lens surrounded by a circular fluorescent light, which can be used like an operating light. Care must be taken to avoid the exposed tissues from drying out – rehydrate regularly with warm sterile normal saline dripped on to the desiccating tissues. Some practices have an operating microscope, which can be very useful but they are large and expensive. Optical loupes are the best compromise: they are small, presenting no storage problems; they are convenient to use; and they are reasonably priced. Panoramic loupes with 3× magnification work well but there are many brands. Some loupes are integrated with lighting (Chapter 10).

Instruments

Most orthopaedic (or hard tissue) surgery requires small instruments to gain access through the soft tissue as well as to manipulate the hard tissue. Those listed below are especially useful:

- Backhaus paediatric towel forceps, 7.5 cm
- Bard Parker scalpel handle, No. 9
- Stevens tenotomy scissors, straight pointed 10 cm
- Metzenbaum scissors, straight 15 cm
- Iris scissors, fine-pointed straight 11.5 cm
- DeBakey tissue forceps, 15 cm straight, atraumatic 1.6 mm jaws
- Gillies dissecting forceps, 15 cm 1-into-2 teeth
- McIndoe tissue forceps, 15 cm non-toothed serrated jaws
- Microjeweller's forceps, No. 5
- Halstead mosquito artery forceps, 11.5 cm straight jaws
- Halstead mosquito artery forceps, 11.5 cm curved on flat jaws

- Halstead mosquito artery forceps, 11.5 cm curved on flat jaws 1-into-2 teeth
- Fosters needle holders, 12.5 cm
- Ryder (micro) needle holders, 15 cm
- Allis tissue forceps, American pattern 15 cm
- Alm retractor, 10 cm
- Mini Travers retractor
- Mini West retractor
- Rongeurs, e.g. mini Friedmann, and bone cutters are available in small sizes. Both these instruments should be used carefully with small deliberate bites. Avian bone is very brittle and shatters easily; large bites of tissue are much more likely to do this.
- For bone manipulation:
  - Dandy arthroscopy hook
  - Dental excavators: Ash Patt 125/126 and Ash Patt G2
  - Dental periosteal elevators: No. 9 and Clappison CA/OA
- A small Volkmann's spoon
- Small Hohmann's retractors of various widths are also useful.
- Small vice (chuck) for pins up to 2.5 mm diameter
- It is not necessary to use a power tool to drive pins into parrot's bones, but drilling small holes can be difficult. A 2 ml syringe with a 23 G needle can be used to 'drill' small holes by rotational movements. If the needle blunts or bends, replace it. The Stratec minidrill can be very useful as it will accommodate drill bits down to 1.1 mm in size and will drill them through small pieces of bone without breaking the bone. Various attachments include saws and pin drivers.
- IMEX positive profile threaded half-pins: 0.9, 1.2, 1.6, 2.0 mm (all 75 mm long)
- IMEX positive profile threaded full-pins: 2.0 mm
- IMEX mini clamps and external rods
- Kirschner wires: 0.8 mm to 2 mm
- Chemical metal or methylmethacrylate
- Cerclage wire 0.4 mm (24 G); 0.6 mm (22 G); 0.8 mm (20 G).
- Suitable suture material: 1.5 metric (4/0) and 1 metric (5/0) polydioxanone; 2 metric (3/0) and 1.5 metric (4/0) polyglactin 910; and 3 metric (2/0) and 2 metric (3/0) coated, braided polyester.

Examination of the lame parrot

It is uncommon for bruising or a sprain to cause lameness that lasts long enough for the bird to be brought to the veterinary surgeon. This diagnosis should only be made if other causes of lameness have definitely been ruled out. It is important not to jump to conclusions or think that a single problem is the whole answer. The bird may have an obvious injury or cause of lameness but the rest of the bird should always be examined. Long-term captive birds are often nutritionally deficient and newly imported birds or young birds that have been recently purchased can be affected by infectious diseases that can make the bird clumsy and more likely to injure itself.

The bird should be watched whilst a history is being taken from the owner. Abnormal behaviour should be noted: is the wing placement normal, or does the bird favour one leg? Owners frequently refer to a bird having a dropped wing, which just means that its wing is hanging in the wrong position. After the history has been taken, the veterinary surgeon should move closer and examine the bird in its cage, again watching its behaviour.

The bird should now be caught carefully. It is often useful to remove some perches. A routine clinical examination should be carried out and then the affected limb should be examined. In general, any lame bird should be examined under general anaesthesia. Almost always further investigations are required.

- Induce general anaesthesia and then re-examine the whole bird.
- If both legs are affected, palpate the vertebrae, especially at the vertebral synsacral junction; it is useful to wet the feathers to examine this joint.
- Examine and compare the affected limb with the normal limb.

If the bird has a wing problem:

1. With the bird in dorsal recumbency, extend both wings fully by holding the second or third primary, feeling for differences in resistance between the two wings.
2. Release the wings and see how much the wing's elasticity pulls the wing into flexion. The affected wing will resist extension and will not return to flexion as easily as the unaffected wing. (This is a sensitive test. Many caged parrots do not fly much, so they may well have reduced wing spread but it should be equal on both sides.)
3. Examine the long bones again, feeling both wings at once.
4. Examine each joint.
5. If it is not obvious which wing is affected, take note of the plumage. Uneven feather wear can point to a problem in one wing and not the other.

The legs can be examined in a similar manner:

1. Extend both legs together by pulling on the claw of the third digit.
2. Release the legs. Again, either resistance or failure to return to normal position is significant.

3. Palpate the long bones and the joints.
4. Examine the plantar aspect of the feet. Long-term pressure causes the skin to lose its texture, the digital pads flatten and the scutes lose their form; the skin can even become thin enough to see the subcutaneous structures. Unilateral changes suggest that the bird is lame on one leg, usually the leg that has the least affected plantar surface. The longer that the bird has been affected by lameness or illness, the more obvious are the changes.

The next step is radiography: whole body ventrodorsal and lateral views, then specific limb radiographs. Comparable radiographs of the contralateral limb are often useful, if only to help the owner to understand what the normal view looks like. It is also useful to make a 'library' of normal views of common species, which can be used in a similar manner. Two views should always be attempted, which may be difficult for elbow and carpus. However, there are cases where the bird will have to be held, using lead gloves with the radiologist near to the primary beam. Birds with joint injuries may need radiographs with the joint under strain.

Fractures and their treatment

Parrots are less likely to be presented with fractures than are falconers' or wild birds. Fractures that are caused by fights and bites are often affected by skin damage and bruising. The skin can have its blood supply disrupted, becoming affected by dry gangrene; it will die. This possibility should be reflected in the prognosis. The larger the area of damaged skin, the greater is the possibility of skin death. Bruises in birds may be bloody but quickly turn green, which is 'normal'.

Many of the techniques used in small animal orthopaedics can be used for birds but there must be some modifications to take into account the bird's much smaller size and the fact that the bones are quite brittle, with a thin cortex and large medullary cavity if compared with those of mammals.

There have been many descriptions of fracture repair. The following procedures are not the only methods that could be used for each fracture but will give satisfactory results in the majority of cases and should be possible in most veterinary practices. Some techniques, such as intramedullary polydioxanone (PDS) rods, shuttle pins, plates and screws, are not discussed.

Osteoporosis

This is usually seen in productive adult birds on a poor diet. It is very likely that there has to be considerable bone loss before osteoporosis is visible on radiographs. In one human study, 40% of bone density had to be lost before changes could be seen on the radiograph. In birds, the usual signs are poor contrast between bone and soft tissue and a loss of cortical bone. When osteoporosis is seen to be a contributory factor to a fracture:

- Do *not* fix the fracture on day one
- Support the fracture as necessary and supplement the bird's calcium and phosphorus intake (Chapter 12)
- Give some access to vitamin D or sunlight (Stanford, 2004a,b).

Radius and ulna fractures

It is common for the ulna to be fractured, usually when the bird's wing hits something hard whilst flying or flapping. Even though it is on the trailing edge of the wing and much larger than the radius, the ulna can be fractured on its own. This can be seen in any size of parrot, often macaws. If the radius is undamaged, the ulna will heal using cage restraint. Strapping is not necessary and would increase the risk of the formation of a synostosis (see later). The bird should be kept in a cage for 4 weeks, with enough room to stretch its wings for grooming etc. but not enough to flap them. The ulna usually heals very well (Figure 11.1).

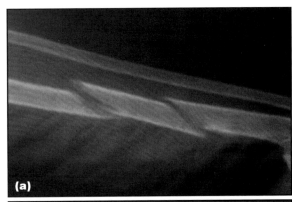

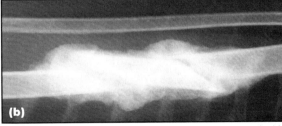

11.1 (a) A Blue and Gold Macaw was presented with a slightly 'dropped' wing and was reluctant to fly. This comminuted fracture of the ulna healed with cage restraint. (b) Four weeks later the fracture showed the typical signs of normal callus formation and no synostosis.

Even though the radius is a smaller bone, it is less commonly fractured on its own in parrots. If the fracture is mid shaft with little displacement, cage restraint will be sufficient. If the fracture is close to the elbow, the biceps tendon distracts the proximal fragment and moves it sufficiently to prevent healing. Distal fractures can also displace significantly. In both cases the bone should be supported by an internal intramedullary Kirschner wire. This should be inserted in a retrograde manner, exiting the pin from the carpal region and running the blunt end of the pin to the other end of the medullary cavity. The surgical approach should be decided by palpation: the short fragment tends to protrude through the muscles – follow this down to the distal fragment. The pin must not enter the elbow joint

and the carpus should be flexed whilst the pin is placed. The pin should be cut short, bent over and covered by the skin. Postoperatively the bird should be kept in its cage until the pin is removed in 4–6 weeks. As with a fractured ulna, immobilization of the wing tends to cause problems and is not necessary.

Some birds fracture both radius and ulna. In small birds (e.g. Budgerigars) there is often so much swelling that this supports the fracture sufficiently for it to heal with just cage restraint. It is also possible to immobilize the wing with strapping (Figures 11.2 and 11.3). Immobilization will allow the bones to form callus but can also encourage the radius and ulna to fuse together whilst healing. This fusion (synostosis) prevents the wing

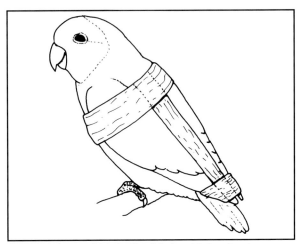

11.2 In small birds, like this lovebird, adhesive bandages should be wrapped around the body and cranial part of the wing; another strip should be wrapped around the distal primaries. The two bands of tape should be connected with a third strip of tape that is bound in with them. This prevents the tape around the wings from riding up the body and coming off. Attention should be paid to the position of the legs, and no attempts should be made to strap them in place as well. It will take some time for the bird to come to terms with this strapping and it should be kept as an in-patient until it has learnt to stand up.

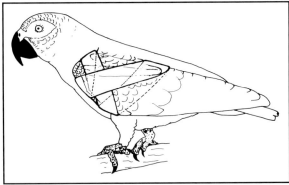

11.3 Larger birds can have a single wing strapped. A figure-of-eight bandage pattern is used to restrain the wing. It is not necessary to use adhesive bandage. The strapping covers the carpus and the elbow, illustrated here as dotted lines on the bandage. Although the bird will cope with this strapping very easily, it should be kept as an in-patient until it is happy about the strapping. It may also require a collar to prevent it from removing the strapping.

from functioning correctly and it is very difficult to reverse. If possible, a fracture of both radius and ulna requires surgical intervention. Occasionally both bones require stabilizing but often repair of the radius, using an intramedullary pin, combined with cage restraint is sufficient. If the wing is allowed to move (but not bear weight) a synostosis is unusual.

It is worth bearing in mind that the ulna has the secondary flight feathers attached to its dorsal surface. Although it can be stabilized with an intramedullary pin, it is probably best stabilized by external fixation using positive profile threaded half-pins (see tibiotarsus fractures for the technique). Coles (1996) suggested using a layer of foam covered by VetLite (a thermosetting casting material) moulded to the wing and held in place with sutures looped around the shaft of the secondary feathers and then passed through the foam and VetLite before knotting. Bear in mind that the ulna has a considerable caudal curvature that should be maintained.

Tibiotarsal fractures

In most pet parrots, the tibiotarsus is the major weight-bearing long bone. It is commonly fractured, usually by external trauma. In these cases it usually results in a simple fracture just distal to the fibular crest. Some birds catch their identity rings on a protruding wire, causing a spiral comminuted fracture of the distal third of the tibiotarsus. Both these fractures require internal fixation and some anti-rotational stabilization; the latter fracture is more challenging. An intramedullary pin combined with external fixation is the best method of stabilizing these fractures in all but the smallest parrots.

Repair of a mid-shaft fracture of the tibiotarsus

A number of techniques have been described for fixing this fracture. The quickest, easiest and most reliable is an intramedullary pin (i/m pin) tied into an external fixation frame connected to proximal and distal full-pins (Figure 11.4).

1. Under general anaesthesia prepare the surgical site by plucking the feathers, rather than cutting them. It is best to tense the skin and pluck out feathers in small numbers going against their direction of growth.
2. Sterilize the site with chlorhexidine in industrial methylated spirit (IMS).
3. Use sterile plastic drapes: they are lightweight and cover the bird with a sterile non-strike-through layer that is transparent enough to watch the bird breathing etc.
4. For this technique it is necessary to have access to both lateral and medial aspects of the leg.

It is possible to place the i/m pin normograde from the proximal tibiotarsus. This technique is quite difficult to perform and most surgeons find it quicker and easier to open the fracture site via a craniomedial approach between the cranial tibial and medial gastrocnemius muscles (see Figure 2.7b). These muscles are held together by superficial fascia only. Once through the skin, the fascia is cut and the gastrocnemius can be easily dissected away from the cranial tibial muscle.

The cranial tibial muscle is attached to the shaft of the tibiotarsus but usually the fracture has stripped the muscle from the shaft, making the surgical approach easier. An arthroscopy hook or small Hohmann's retractor helps to raise the proximal fragment and gain access to the medullary cavity.

1. Use an i/m pin with one point. Find the proximal fragment, which has usually overridden the distal (Figure 11.4a).
2. Insert the trochar pointed end into the medullary cavity of the proximal fragment (Figure 11.4b). Run the pin up the cranial surface of the medullary cavity so that it leaves the tibiotarsus outside the knee joint. Flex the knee during this procedure.
3. Reduce the fracture. The blunt end of the pin is placed into the distal fragment. Using a blunt end, rather than a pointed end, tends to prevent the pin leaving the medullary cavity and penetrating the intertarsal joint (Figure 11.4c). It is very easy to push a pointed pin through the

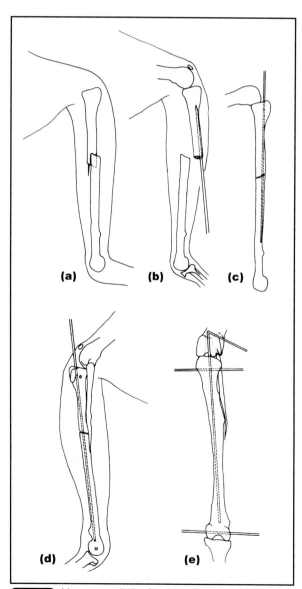

(a)　**(b)**　**(c)**

(d)　**(e)**

11.4 How to repair the fracture of the tibiotarsus of a Grey Parrot.

articular surface of the distal tibiotarsus transfixing the tibial cartilage and some of the flexor tendons that run through it (see Figure 2.7a). This would cause temporary or even permanent disability of the foot.

External fixation with two full-pins will prevent rotation at the fracture site and also prevents comminuted fractures from overriding. Kirschner wires of 1.6 or 1.2 mm diameter are suitable. Positive profile threaded pins are currently only available down to 2 mm in size.

1. Insert the proximal pin from the lateral aspect (Figure 11.4d).
2. Palpate the fibula. Place the pin cranial to the fibula and proximal to the fibular crest. This avoids the arteries, veins and nerves that run between the fibula and tibiotarsus. The fibula and tibiotarsus are not tightly connected at the knee joint. Normal knee movement will be prevented if the fibula is transfixed, usually resulting in a fracture of the fibula. Placing the pin too close to the knee joint will allow it to penetrate the joint capsule and cause a continuous leak of joint fluid. If this occurs, remove and replace the pin a little more distal.
3. The distal full-pin should be drilled from the lateral to medial condyle (Figure 11.4d); careful placement will not affect other structures. Do not place the distal pin through the shaft of the distal tibiotarsus: it will strike the i/m pin and will usually be forced cranially. The pin can then trap the common digital extensor tendon against the supratendinal bridge (Figure 11.5).
4. Repair the muscle layers and skin using 2 metric (3/0) polyglactin 910. This suture will fall off within 2 weeks.
5. The i/m pin should be bent laterally (Figure 11.4e) and tied into an external fixation rod. Larger parrots (Grey Parrot and bigger) can have small clamps with connecting rods. For smaller birds a plastic tube or Penrose drain filled with methylmethacrylate or chemical metal can take the place of a rod. It may help to place a length of redundant stainless steel pin inside the Penrose drain.
6. The medial connecting bar should be as short as possible. If it is too long it will traumatize the body wall.

The leg should be bandaged for a few days to limit postoperative swelling and then it is unbandaged. It is critical to attend to the pin/skin interface on a regular basis. A fibrinous crust will form around the pin and force the skin away from the pin. If this is not removed it will grow and allow infection to track down the pin and into the tissues below, causing the pin to loosen. The crust should be removed with dilute chlorhexidine skin scrub, cotton buds and a small probe.

The repair should be subjected to a staged disassembly. If there are two full-pins and an i/m pin, both full-pins are removed at about 3–4 weeks and the i/m

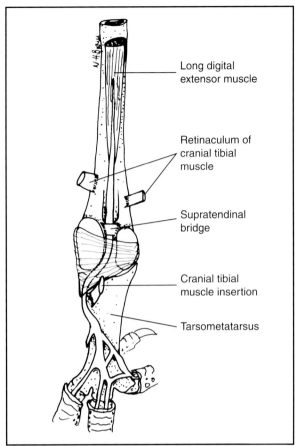

11.5 The cranial intertarsal joint has two tendons of insertion that run across it. Superficially the cranial tibial muscle is held in place by a retinaculum; a neurovascular bundle runs through the retinaculum too. Deeper to this the long digital extensor tendon runs close to the bone and is held in place by the supratendinal bridge and a fibrous portion of the joint capsule. Fractures in this region are severely complicated if there is any injury to these two structures, or if they are involved in bony callus. Caudally the joint is closely associated with the tibial cartilage and the digital flexor tendons (see Figure 2.7).

pin cut short, leaving enough length to pull it out when there is radiographic union in another 2–4 weeks. The bird must wear a collar (Chapter 16) or it will preen out the i/m pin. Cutting the pin too short will make it difficult to remove. Leaving the pin will cause problems such as arthritis and tendinitis.

It is possible to repair a midshaft tibiotarsal fracture using only external fixation with positive profile threaded half-pins. For maximum stability at the fracture site, there need to be three pins above and three pins below the fracture site and the pins should each penetrate two cortices. Drawbacks to this technique are that it is very difficult to reduce the fracture and also to maintain the line of the bone. If this technique is used the half-pins should be held in removable clamps and then postoperative radiographs should be taken. If the proximal and distal fragments are misaligned, the clamps can be loosened and then readjusted.

If the tibiotarsus is badly aligned it will affect the bird's ability to bear weight, promoting bumblefoot of the good foot.

Spiral comminuted fracture of the distal third of the tibiotarsus

These fractures are complicated by a lack of soft tissue and so the fractured bone has usually penetrated the skin. Breeding birds often hide in the nest box after their leg is broken, which means that the fracture may not be found for several days. Desiccated bone or bone that has protruded from the fracture site should be cut off; trying to clean desiccated infected bone, even with antibiotic therapy, seldom prevents osteomyelitis. Occasionally the fracture occurs between the medial and lateral anchor points of the retinaculum of the cranial tibial muscle, or worse still the supratendinal bridge (Figure 11.5). This worsens the prognosis, as the repair must be perfectly aligned so that a minimum of callus forms. Postoperatively the intertarsal joint must not be prevented from moving, or adhesions will permanently cripple the bird.

As with a midshaft fracture, the easiest way of fixing a distal tibiotarsal fracture is usually with an i/m pin and two full-pins. The fracture 'envelope' should be disturbed as little as possible. The surgical approach is usually medial, as this area is covered by skin only (see Figure 2.7).

1. Place the i/m pin in a retrograde manner, exiting it through the proximal fragment as described above.
2. Reduce the fracture and slide the blunted end of the pin to the extremity of the medullary cavity. Use a pin that has a sufficient diameter to fill the medullary cavity of the distal tibiotarsus completely. Avoid entering the intertarsal joint.
3. Place the full-pins in the cranioproximal tibiotarsus and across the distal condyles.

Open fractures carry a poor prognosis. The use of long-term antibiosis is required: marbofloxacin is first choice; clindamycin can be useful as well.

Radiography

Radiography at 2-week intervals is advisable, especially if there is possible infection (Figure 11.6). A staged deconstruction should be undertaken. It is usually best to remove the i/m pin first but the veterinary surgeon should be guided by the bird's behavioural requirements, clinical signs and radiography.

If the tibiotarsus is fractured so that only the epicondylar area is intact and there is no medullary cavity, it is possible to repair it using a modified cross-pin technique (see Figure 11.9). This will cause difficulties while the pins are in place, as many parrots walk on the caudal tarsometatarsus as well as their foot.

Fractures of the humerus and femur

Fractures in these bones are often comminuted or spiral. Both have the potential to shorten the bone by overriding. External fixation pins are vital to preserve the length of the bone. An intramedullary pin keeps the line of the bone as well as adding extra stiffness to the repair.

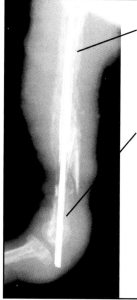

Periostitis. The periosteum is raised from the cortex and produces a thick line of fuzzy bone. This is usually caused by infection and can be confirmed by a leucocytosis with a left shift.

Osteomyelitis. In most cases fibrin is deposited in caseous masses as part of the inflammatory reaction and this shows on the radiograph as black round areas where there is no bone deposition. The cortex is also absorbed, giving an irregular appearance. There is usually little sign of secondary callus.

11.6 A compound (open) fracture of the distal tibiotarsus of a cockatoo has become infected. By 20 days postoperatively, there was a periostitis of the proximal bone and osteomyelitis of the distal part of the fracture. The leg was hot, swollen and painful. The distal fragment was so small that two small-diameter flexible pins were placed through the outer edges of the condyles in a similar manner to Rush pins. The pins eroded through the skin and this was the cause of an ascending infection. The pins were left in place and the wounds in the intertarsal skin were kept clean. The bird remained on antibiotic therapy until the pins were removed at 6 weeks post-operatively, and this was continued for 2 further weeks until radiography showed no signs of active inflammation and infection. The periosteal bone reduced to nearly normal over the next few months.

Humerus

The humerus has a large pneumatized medullary cavity. Fractures will lead to emphysema. In comparison with wild birds, fractures of the humerus in parrots are uncommon.

The technique for repairing a midshaft humeral fracture is to use an intramedullary pin combined with two to six threaded half-pins (depending on the fracture and the size of the bird and bone) (Figure 11.7).

1. Place the bird in sternolateral recumbency so that the broken wing can be extended and flexed during surgery. The surgical approach is dorsal.
2. Pluck the surgical site, removing the small feathers from the elbow to well above the shoulder, and sterilize.
3. Make a skin incision over the fracture site and do not manipulate the skin too much. There is very little soft tissue covering the distal third of the humerus. There is a large nerve dorsal to the bone (see Figure 19.2). There is also one ventral to the bone that must also be avoided. The vascular supply is also ventral (see Figure 2.6).
4. It is impossible, and undesirable, to fill the medullary cavity with the i/m pin; use a 1.6–2.0 mm Kirschner wire, trochar pointed at one end. Elevate the proximal fragment and place the i/m

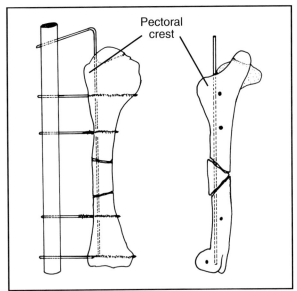

11.7 Pin placement to repair a fractured humerus in a parrot.

pin retrograde, keeping the pin close to the craniolateral surface so that it avoids the shoulder joint.

5. Reduce the fracture and push the blunt end of the pin to the distal end of the medullary cavity. Do not enter the elbow.

6. Once the fracture is reduced, it is important to get the correct alignment for the humerus. Flexing the wing into its normal resting position against the body places the humerus in its correct alignment. Plastic drapes are very flexible and make this technique easy.

7. Decide the site of the external pins and clear the skin and any underlying soft tissue from the bone. A drill guide must be placed on to the bone to avoid the thread catching surrounding soft tissue. The external pins must be drilled into the cortex slowly.

8. Place one proximal half-pin at the level of, and caudal to, the pectoral crest (the most prominent and palpable part of the proximal humerus). This allows penetration of two cortices and keeps the pin away from the joint. The most distal half-pin should be placed across the condyles. Connect the proximal and distal pins using clamps and a rod.

9. In large parrots and macaws it may be necessary to add more pins at this stage (Figure 11.7). It is possible to place a drill guide through the pin-hole in the clamp to prevent soft tissue injury during pin placement.

Femur
The femur is not pneumatized in parrots and has a very large medullary cavity. Mid-shaft femur fractures can be stabilized either by using several i/m pins (stack pinning) or preferably by a single i/m pin tied into two positive profile threaded full-pins placed at each end of the bone. The surgical approach is lateral between the lateral iliotibial muscle and iliofibular muscle (see Figure 2.7a).

These muscles separate easily but due care must be given to the nerves and blood vessels that are covered by these muscles. The intramedullary pins are placed in a retrograde manner, exiting through the proximal femur. The hip joint must be in extension to prevent the pins from fixing the femur to the antitrochanter (see Figure 2.7a). The distal threaded half-pin is placed across the condyles and the proximal pin is placed so that the tip emerges on the medial side of the femur distal to the hip joint. In large birds with comminuted fractures it is better to use several half-pins, but there is an increased risk that pins placed in the mid-shaft region will become incorporated into the surrounding muscles, whose movements will cause the pins to loosen.

Fractures of the proximal humerus and femur
These should be reduced and stabilized with one or two pins combined with a figure-of-eight compression wire (Figure 11.8). The technique is as follows:

1. Drill the hole in the lateral wall of the distal fragment.
2. Place the wire (22 or 24 G orthopaedic), making sure that it forms a loop that goes to the medial part of the medullary cavity.
3. Place one or two pins (0.8–1.2 mm Kirschner wires) normograde or retrograde on the lateral aspect of the medullary cavity.
4. Reduce the fracture and run the pin(s) into the distal fragment's medullary cavity, making sure the pins are long enough to end distal to the wire.
5. Incorporate the pin(s) outside the bone in the proximal loop of wire and tighten both sides of the figure-of-eight. This should pull the pins to the lateral wall as well as reduce the fracture.
6. The protruding end of the pin should be bent over caudally or cranially and embedded in the bone.

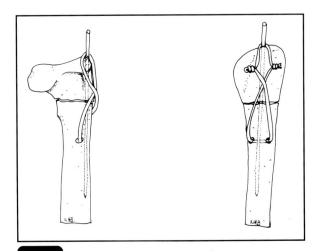

11.8 Repair of a proximal femoral fracture.

Fractures of the distal humerus and femur
Even quite short fragments can be fixed with external fixation tied into an i/m pin. If the distal fragment consists of only the condyles and therefore no medullary cavity, the fracture can be fixed using external fixation with modified cross-pins and half-pins (Figure 11.9). This is only possible in larger parrots but can be

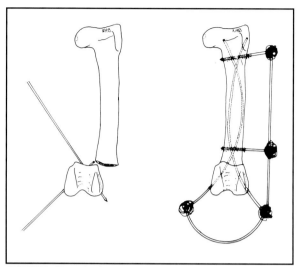

11.9 Repair of a distal femoral fracture. The technique can be adapted for other bones.

a useful technique. The fracture is reduced with two flexible Kirschner wires so that they emerge from the epicondyles and do not affect the movement of the joint. Two threaded half-pins are drilled across the proximal and distal shaft; a third could be placed across the condyles in a large bird. The pins should be connected to an external pin with clamps or cement (Figure 11.9). The curved portion of the supporting bar should not interfere with the movement of the knee.

Coracoid

Flying 'headlong' into something will often cause this fracture. If the bird strikes a solid object with its shoulder, the coracoid is likely to break. The bird is obviously lame on its wing but has no long bone fractures. Careful radiography will show the fracture. In larger parrots it is possible to palpate the bone by placing a finger on the inside of the thoracic inlet and using the wing to lift the pectoral girdle up and down: the finger in the thoracic inlet will detect crepitus. Cage restraint for a month is usually sufficient to allow the bone to heal. Stabilization of the fracture has been described using an i/m pin but the surgical approach is challenging.

Carpometacarpus

This bone is rarely fractured. Figure-of-eight strapping (see Figure 11.3) will allow many fractures to heal. Other techniques have been described, such as i/m pins or suturing foam and VetLite over the fracture site. However, many cases fail due to loss of blood supply or infection. Amputation is usually the salvage technique.

Tarsometatarsus

This bone is uncommonly fractured in large birds but such fractures can occur during a fight with another bird or when the identity ring has been caught on a protruding wire. It is possible to reduce the fracture using full-pin fixation; the tarsometatarsus has a medullary cavity in large parrots. The bird must be able to use the foot as freely as possible or the callus will incorporate the flexor and extensor tendons causing permanent disability.

The tarsometatarsus is more commonly fractured in birds the size of Budgerigars and Cockatiels. Bony injuries above or below the intertarsal joint can be treated using a Granuflex (Duoderm) semipermeable hydrophilic dressing splint. The leg should be held with the bones in apposition and correctly aligned; this usually requires an anaesthetic. Strips of Granuflex can be used in three layers to make a close-fitting malleable splint. This is then strengthened with narrow strips of zinc oxide tape, and making a firm 'cast'. It is necessary to include the foot, especially in fractures below the intertarsal joint. Some of the digits are left sticking out to allow the bird to grip and to prevent adhesions between the callus and digital tendons.

Digits

Many fractures will be stabilized by the large ventral flexor tendon running in the thick fibrous tunnel and need no further treatment. Digits II and III can be strapped together to provide support. A piece of non-adherent bandage (e.g. Skintact) should be used in between the digits as padding. This technique is not usually possible with digits I and IV. A splint made of Granuflex and zinc oxide tape will provide semi-flexible support. Serious fractures, which are often compound, will require amputation.

Dislocations

Dislocations are usually the result of trauma. Some (e.g. intertarsal joint) are so severe that there is very little chance of a functioning limb; some (e.g. interphalangeal joints) are trivial, as they may easily be reduced. Dislocations in the pectoral limb may be difficult to replace and have a fully functional wing but this is less of a problem in pet parrots than it would be for a hunting falcon or a bird for rehabilitation. The following specific dislocations are reparable.

Elbow

A bird with a dislocated elbow has a swollen joint and difficulty using its wing. It cannot extend the joint and so the wing is often held at a strange angle. Diagnosis requires palpation under general anaesthesia and two radiographic views.

The elbow is a complex joint: when extended, it locks to make the wing a nearly rigid structure; when flexed, it allows the forearm to pronate and supinate. There are lateral and medial collateral ligaments that incorporate some tendons of origin and insertion of the wing muscles. There is also a ligament on the cranial aspect of the joint that ties together the humerus, radius and ulna. If this ligament is broken, the prognosis is poor as the relationship between the radius and ulna is changed. Unfortunately, because of its position, it is usually difficult to know if the ligament is damaged.

The elbow is rarely injured in parrots. Fracture/dislocations where there is a condylar fracture with little or no ligament damage should do well if the humeral condyle is replaced with a pin and wire or even a small screw. Traumatic joint disruption with little ligament injury will do well if replaced immediately and if the joint's movement is limited by cage restraint for 2–3 weeks. However, these cases are in the minority and the prognosis for elbow dislocation is usually poor with the bird being unable to fly. The joint should be replaced and obvious ligament damage repaired. The author's preference is either 1.5 metric (4/0) polydioxanone or 2 metric (3/0) polyglactin 910 or, if a permanent suture is required, 2 metric (3/0) braided polyester. It is possible to immobilize the elbow completely by placing two or three half-pins in both ulna and humerus and connecting them with three external rods in the shape of a triangle.

Carpus

Ligament damage of the dorsal aspect of the joint is usually reparable, but on the ventral aspect of the wing it is much less likely to be repaired well enough for the bird to fly properly. Occasionally injury on the ventral aspect causes the artery to be occluded as it runs between the bones and the ventral aponeurosis, resulting in dry gangrene of the distal wing. It is possible to see aviary birds that have had complete dislocation of the carpus that has been left with no treatment. Some of them fly surprisingly well within the confines of their aviary. Surgical repair or strapping the affected wing are both possibilities.

Hip

The hip is the most commonly dislocated major joint. The bird will be seen as lame and it will have difficulty in raising its leg to stand and grip the perch. The hip should be examined radiographically, as many dislocated hips have an avulsion fracture of the femoral head with a piece of femoral head left attached to the ligament in the acetabulum. For dislocations with an undamaged femur, the joint should have an open reduction with surgical repair of all the surrounding soft tissue. The bird should be kept in a box-like cage for 3–4 weeks (solid sides will limit climbing) and the prognosis is usually good.

Birds with an avulsion fracture of the femoral head, a repetitive dislocation or a longstanding dislocation should have a femoral head arthroplasty using a craniolateral approach to the joint. It is possible to place a piece of caudofemoral muscle (see Figure 2.7a) through the joint in the manner of a biceps femoris sling but it does not seem to be vital that this is done. Cage restraint for 10 days is needed. The prognosis after this surgery should be good (MacCoy, 1989).

Knee

Dislocation of the knee will involve rupture of the cruciate ligaments. It is possible to replace them with a synthetic suture by drilling holes through the distal femur (lateral to midline) and tibiotarsus (midline to medial) using a hypodermic needle and threading the suture through the centre of the needle. The suture should be passed back through the distal femur (medial to lateral). It can then be tied tight on the lateral aspect of the joint, taking care not to involve the fibula, and the bird should be kept confined to its cage for a month.

Another successful method is to place a pin from outside the knee joint up the medullary cavity of the femur, and another pin from outside the knee joint down the medullary cavity of the tibiotarsus. The dislocation is reduced and the pins are held together using a clamp or methylmethacrylate. Although this has only been described in young birds, it could work well for adults (Bowles and Zantop, 2002).

Digit

The interphalangeal joints seem to be easy to dislocate and easy to replace.

Growing birds

Figures 11.10 and 11.11 show radiographs of a normal 42-day-old Green-winged Macaw. Bone growth occurs from each end of the bone. The epiphyses are not calcified and so joints are 'invisible'. The metaphysis is weak but is relatively thick so that it maintains strength; the diaphysis is narrower but it is strong because it has a well developed cortex (Harcourt-Brown, 2004). The metacarpals partially fuse and are also joined to the distal carpals; at this stage of development they are mostly cartilaginous.

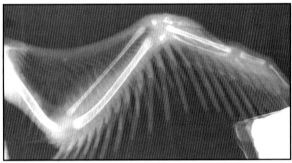

11.10 In the growing bird, the humerus is not pneumatized. The elbow joint consists of cartilage. The proximal radial and ulnar carpal bones are forming. The distal radial carpal bone is also visible and will fuse with the large and small metacarpal bones to form the carpometacarpus.

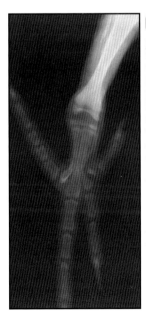

11.11 Metatarsals II, III and IV fuse and are joined by the distal row of tarsal bones to form the tarsometatarsus. The gaps between the proximal metatarsal bones remain as holes through which arteries run from the main artery, which is cranial, to supply the caudal part of the limb. The distal tibia fuses to the proximal row of tarsal bones to form the tibiotarsus. At 42 days in this Green-winged Macaw, these fusions are incomplete and this causes the area to look as if there are two epiphyseal lines above and below the intertarsal joint.

Limb deformity and juvenile osteodystrophy

Bony deformity is commonly seen in captive-bred parrots (Figure 11.12). It is mostly caused by rearing birds on a diet deficient in calcium and/or vitamin D (Chapter 12).

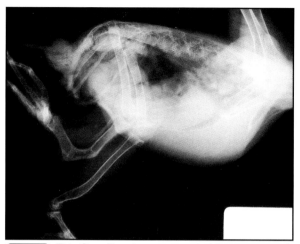

11.12 This Grey Parrot was presented for surgery as it had an obvious deformity of its right leg (more caudal of the two). The deformed left leg, synsacrum, and pelvis (as well as both radii and ulnae) were not noticed by the owner. The bird had also had a chronic nasal discharge since it was first seen in the nest box at about 2 weeks old.

The bone most commonly affected is the tibiotarsus, primarily because this is the major weight-bearing bone. In their nest cavity, birds being reared by their parents form a mutually supporting huddle; as they get older they are confined by the size of the nest chamber and they do not become fully active until they are skeletally mature (Harcourt-Brown, 2004). Hand-reared parrots are overactive whilst growing; they are not confined within a relatively small nest cavity and are usually unsupported by their siblings. They are often encouraged to over-exercise by the person feeding them. Osteodystrophy is very common in hand-reared Grey Parrots. In one study, 44% of apparently normal birds were affected (Harcourt-Brown, 2003).

Badly affected growing birds may be presented because they cannot stand and their legs stick out on either side: the colloquial term is 'splay legs'. These birds can have multiple fractures but usually they are affected by weak bones that bend and crumple. Sometimes the bones can be affected by longitudinal rotational deformity. If mildly affected, the birds will reach skeletal maturity and their deformity is not obvious until the bird has radiography for some other reason.

Badly affected birds require surgical correction or euthanasia. It must be borne in mind that young birds that are affected with a nutritional osteodystrophy may well have other nutritional deficiencies (see Chapter 12 for treatment).

The bird should be anaesthetized for examination and radiography. Ventrodorsal and lateral views will allow assessment of the whole of the bird's body and its limbs. The legs should be assessed for rotational deformity:

- Hold both legs by the femur (one in each hand) so that each leg is comparably elevated and positioned. This allows the rest of the leg to be assessed by looking at the position of the intertarsal joint and feet and comparing one leg with the other. Then assess by individual palpation
- Stretch out both wings to see if they extend fully and whether their conformation appears to be normal. The line of the secondary and primary feathers will be deformed in many birds with bent wings.

Treatment of deformed bones

If the bones are still growing there should be diet and husbandry changes (Chapters 12 and 18). Early mild cases seen whilst the bird is still growing can be cured by hobbling the legs together with a soft bandage, or placing the bird in a deep cup-shaped depression that forces the legs together. Reduced lighting is useful to control the bird's activity.

Once the bones have stopped growing, the treatment is surgical. Deformities of the vertebral column, ribs and pelvis do not require treatment and seldom affect the bird. Even quite severe deformity of the pelvis does not seem to prevent normal egg laying. Deformed wings in pet birds or even breeding birds seldom require surgery.

However, the tibiotarsus is the most commonly affected bone and its deformity usually has serious consequences for the bird. Apart from the obvious consequences of disability, lameness forces the bird to place more weight on the 'good' leg, which causes a serious pressure sore on the plantar aspect of the foot; this can become infected (bumblefoot). A grossly affected tibiotarsus (Figure 11.12) requires surgical correction of the deformity.

1. The deviation is usually in two planes. Feel for the site of maximum deviation; this is usually a useful place to site the soft tissue incision. In badly bent legs the bend has forced the rest of the soft tissue away so the layer under the skin is usually bone covered by periosteum.
2. The area around the bone should be freed of soft tissue using a dental periosteal elevator.
3. The osteotomy usually needs a small bone cutter but a small saw can be used to make the initial cut in the bone. Make the cuts parallel to the surface of the joint or at right angles across the shaft. Remove the redundant triangular wedge of bone; save it temporarily in case there is need for a bone graft. If there has to be double osteotomy (Figure 11.13) it is good practice to maintain a blood supply to the isolated piece by preserving soft tissue attachments.
4. Place an i/m pin retrograde, exiting at the knee.
5. Reduce the fracture(s). Place two full-pins through the proximal tibiotarsus and distal condyles; align femur and tarsometatarsus, which corrects longitudinal deformity; place external clamps and bars.

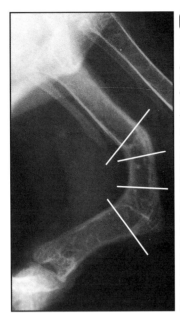

11.13 The knee is seen as a lateral view, the intertarsal joint as a craniocaudal view. This bird required a double osteotomy and the leg had to be realigned so that the foot could be used correctly. In a normal leg the femur and tarsometatarsus are in the same alignment when the leg is flexed. The lines of cut for the osteotomy should be pre-planned: the most proximal and distal cuts should be parallel to the adjacent joint's surface. As much length as possible should be saved.

Staged deconstruction probably starts at 4 weeks postoperatively. A bone graft is not usually necessary. The length of the bone compared to its muscles is now increased and the leg is usually held in forced extension (Figure 11.14). This will return to normal over the next few weeks. Occasionally the parrot will chew its foot. This is probably neurogenic and is probably due to stimulation of the deep fibular nerve as it runs beside the tendon of insertion cranial tibial muscle within the retinaculum (see Figure 2.7a). Reshaping the bone changes the position of this tendon within the retinaculum. This also resolves over a few weeks but the bird may need a collar.

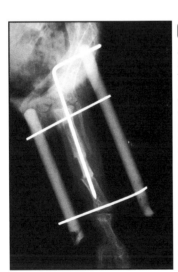

11.14 The bird was disabled after surgery for about 2 weeks. He was able to place his leg and use his foot normally within 6 weeks. There were no significant complications once the muscles had 'lengthened'. The external rods were made from 5 mm semi-rigid plastic tubing filled with Chemical Metal. Staged deconstruction of the fiaxtor started 4 weeks after surgery and was complete by 8 weeks.

It is possible to have several bones involved in osteodystrophic limb deformity. These may have to be corrected simultaneously, which can be a surgical challenge. If the bird has serious deformities in more than one limb it is probably better to opt for euthanasia. However, some birds can have useful lives after several corrective operations.

Other causes of fractures

Other causes of fractures include bone tumours (Figure 11.15), which are rare in parrots, and avian tuberculosis (Figure 11.16).

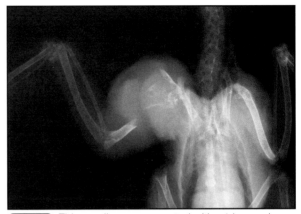

11.15 This rosella was presented with a 'dropped wing'. There was firm soft tissue swelling that was not painful. There was a palpable fracture of the humerus. Radiography shows typical signs of a bone tumour: bone lysis and deposition. The changes do not cross the joint even though the proximal humerus is severely affected.

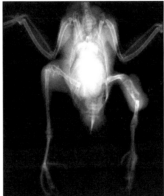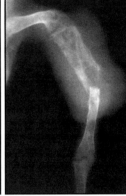

11.16 A kakariki presented for examination with a fracture of its tibiotarsus. Radiography revealed multiple areas of lysis in more than one bone. There was bone loss but no deposition. The areas of lysis looked like osteomyelitis. Smears made from the tissues revealed the presence of acid-fast bacteria. It is common for avian tuberculosis to be present in several sites, often with surprising symmetry. Histology revealed that this bird had granulomas in its intestines and was shedding the organism: this is usual. Note also the hepatomegaly.

Sequelae to fractures

Atrophic malunion

This may be seen when a fracture has had inadequate support. If a pet parrot is managing well, as is often the case with wing fractures, it is probably best left alone. If the malunion is in a leg bone, it is worth considering surgery. The atrophic bone ends should be stimulated by elevating the periosteum and using rongeurs to roughen the bone end. Parrots have no accessible cancellous bone. Bone grafts may be obtained by removing part of the carina from the bird during surgery:

1. Dissect the pectoral muscles from one side of the carina.
2. Cut out and remove a section of bone.
3. If possible, leave the most ventral edge intact so that the pectoral muscle can be reattached easily.

This thin rectangular slab of bone can be used whole as an on-lay graft or can be munched up with rongeurs to pack into irregular defects. This technique never feels as satisfactory as using a cancellous bone graft in a dog but it does appear to make a difference to healing in some cases (Rodriguez-Quiros *et al.*, 2001). It is possible to use cancellous bone as a graft; it can be harvested sterilely from the long bones of ratites at the time of slaughter for meat (Matthews *et al.*, 2003).

Osteoarthritis

For osteomyelitis and periostitis see Figure 11.6.

Osteoarthritis is more frequently diagnosed as the pet parrot population ages. The knee joint appears to be most commonly affected; it is usually bilateral. Other joints can be affected but this often seems to be as a result of old trauma as it is usually unilateral and in some cases there is evidence of a previous injury. Meloxicam at 1 drop daily for a Grey Parrot seems perfectly safe in the long term (months). Carprofen has also been used in birds and shown to work as an analgesic.

Septic arthritis

This is an uncommon condition in pet parrots but can be extremely serious (Figure 11.17). It can occur because of a penetrating wound but it can also occur after a bruise or injury, presumably with haematogenous spread of bacteria. The presenting signs are lameness with heat and swelling of the joint. If radiography shows no bony involvement, the diagnosis can be confirmed with aspiration of joint fluid for cytology plus culture and sensitivity. Some joint fluid should be placed into a nutrient broth prior to culture. If nutrient broth is unavailable, a swab with joint fluid on it should be placed in transport medium and incubated for 12–24

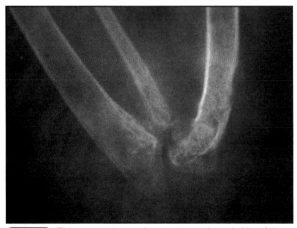

11.17 This parrot has advanced septic arthritis of the elbow joint. The head of the radius has eroded, as have the ulna and the humeral condyles. Infection has also tracked up the tendon sheath, causing an erosion of the caudal humerus. There are periarticular changes around the radius. The medullary cavity of the humerus was also involved in inflammatory changes.

hours before culture (this will increase the chances of growing the organism). Irrigating the joint with the appropriate antibiotic combined with a long course of systemic antibiotic gives a chance of a cure. If there are signs of bone loss from the articular surfaces of the joint, the prognosis is very poor to hopeless.

Amputation

Wing

Serious wing injury requires amputation. The wing can be amputated through the humerus by means of a similar technique to that used in dogs and cats, except that a piece of muscle should be inserted into or over the pneumatized medullary cavity and sutured in place. This tends to prevent air from leaking out during healing. To hold the muscle in or over the medullary cavity, a hole can be drilled into the bone using a 23 G needle on a 2 ml syringe and the suture is passed through this as well as the muscle. It is beneficial to preserve the metapatagium and some of the other secondary feathers to cover and insulate the bird.

Distal amputations need to be through the proximal part of the carpometacarpus or major digit rather than the carpus or distal radius and ulna. Great care must be exercised to prevent a prominent bony mass on the end of the amputation that will continually be banged and injured. Attention must also be given to the large feathers, which need to remain in their correct alignment. It may be necessary to amputate the alula too. Finally, for the bird to be able to extend its wing after surgery, attention must be given to attaching the long extensor tendons to the bone at the amputation site, otherwise the wing will stayed flexed (see Figure 2.6).

Toes

Parrots often amputate their own injured toes but sometimes it should be a surgical procedure.

1. Clean the digit carefully and sterilize.
2. Incise the skin distal to the amputation site and dissect back.
3. Dissect free the extensor and flexor tendons, taking care to preserve their tendon sheath.
4. Finally, cut the phalangeal bone – do not amputate through the joint. The digital arteries, veins and nerves are lateral and medial and will need tying off but take care not to remove the blood supply to the soft tissue that will provide the repair.

To close the wound:

1. First join the extensor and flexor tendons over the end of the cut phalangeal bone.
2. Cover the tendons with their sheaths, which should be sutured to the joined tendons too.
3. The skin should have been left longer than the bone, to give a good covering of soft tissue, but it is impossible to obliterate dead space with subcutaneous sutures. Mattress sutures placed through the skin will do this.
4. The incision edge should be closed with simple interrupted sutures.

The suture material of choice for all layers is usually 1.5 or 1 metric (4/0 or 5/0) polydioxanone on a round-bodied needle. The digit should not be covered with a dressing and the bird must be kept in clean surroundings. The skin sutures should be removed after 3 weeks, which will often require a general anaesthetic. More rapidly dissolving sutures do not seem to remain long enough to allow the scaly skin to heal.

Foot

In most cases, amputation of the leg will lead to an intractable bumblefoot on the remaining limb. However, it is possible to amputate the foot and most of the tarsometatarsus and fashion a weight bearing structure that will prevent this.

Most larger parrots walk on the caudal aspect of their tarsometatarsus. If the cranial tibial muscle's insertion is intact and the gastrocnemius muscles are attached to the hypotarsus (see Figure 2.7), scaly skin can be used to cover the proximal tarsometatarsus and the parrot will be able to walk on the caudal aspect of this stump. The flap of skin should not be made too large, as there is a risk that it may lose its blood supply and die.

It is worth bearing in mind that the majority of parrots tend to favour using their left foot (much as people are usually right-handed). Foot amputation is a salvage technique and a last resort. It should not be undertaken if other options are available. Inexperienced avian surgeons should seek guidance before going ahead with amputation of a whole foot.

Beak

The beak is modified skin supported on the maxillary and mandibular bones (see Chapter 2 and Figure 2.3). Many of the problems affecting the parrot beak and their treatment are related to its structure. The beak can heal by first or second intention and can also be incised and sutured.

Much as hydrophilic dressings (e.g. Granuflex or Duoderm) are useful as 'bandages' for encouraging skin growth, Coe-Pak can be used to promote the healing of the beak. This product is used in humans after oral trauma surgery to cover pins, wire and open wounds. It allows granulation tissue to form and encourages epithelialization. Coe-Pak does not stick to the beak, or to soft tissue, and so it is easily removed; it sets to the texture of bubblegum. If Coe-Pak is to be used to cover a defect, 0.8 mm Steinmann pins are driven through the beak and looped round on either side. Usually three are used and then they can be connected with orthopaedic wire (23 G). As wounds healing by secondary intention produce fibrin and clots of pus and blood, the Coe-Pak should be changed regularly to allow removal of fibrin clot and other debris; if it is not removed this mass will prevent wound closure. After the beak has healed the wires are removed, the holes are coated with fucidin ointment and healing takes place in a few days.

Traumatic injuries to the beak are common. Most parrots fight by biting the beak (and feet) of their opponent. Most fights are mock battles, with lots of sparring and no resulting injury, but in serious territorial fights (usually between sexually active birds) the beak can have a hole made into it or right through it. Occasionally in these serious fights the mandible can be cut in half or the maxilla can be amputated.

Injury to the maxilla

The rhamphotheca and its underlying soft tissue is supported by a layer of bone (see Figure 2.3). Penetrating injuries usually push these three layers into the space beneath the bone. It is best to see these cases soon after the injury, certainly within 24 hours. Under general anaesthesia the beak should be cleaned and surgically sterilized with chlorhexidine in spirit. The sterilizing fluid must not be allowed to enter the maxillary sinus.

1. Use a dental excavator to elevate the keratin of the beak and bend it out of the way (Figure 11.18). Avoid breaking it off.

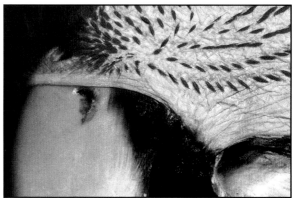

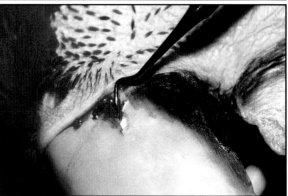

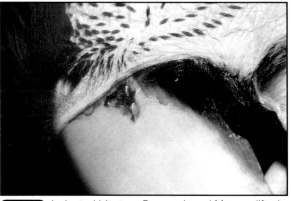

11.18 Indented bite to a Green-winged Macaw, lifted with dental excavator and returned to normal position. It healed within 3 weeks.

2. Reach beneath the keratin and elevate the soft tissue, dermis and finally the bone, bringing it into alignment with the rest of the maxilla.
3. Lay the dermis back, smoothing out any wrinkles.
4. If possible, replace the horn.

Small defects need coating with some fusidic acid ointment (do not use one containing steroid) and the bird should be given a course of antibiotic: 5 days on marbofloxacin would be ideal.

Large defects should be dealt with in the same manner but have to be covered with Coe-Pak postoperatively, to prevent desiccation and further infection. This requires placement of pins and wires (Figures 11.19 and 11.20).

Infected or longstanding injuries need thorough irrigation with normal saline and removal of all infected or dead tissue. Antibiotic should be instilled into the interior of the mandible and the bird should receive a long course of systemic antibiotic. The wound will need to heal by second intention. It must be covered with Coe-Pak, which must be changed every 7–14 days so that the wound can be cleaned and the fibrin plug removed.

Occasionally the whole maxilla is bitten off. Although euthanasia may be the option of choice, it is possible to save a bird even though it will never regrow its beak. The stump should be cleaned, painted with antiseptic and covered with Coe-Pak to encourage it to heal. Although the beak does not regenerate, it will heal and become a fibrous pad that will allow the bird to cope. Some manage to eat seed; others need a pelleted diet.

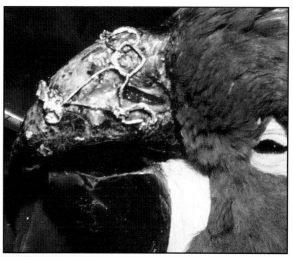

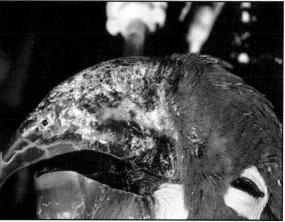

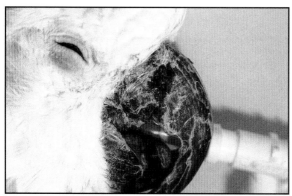

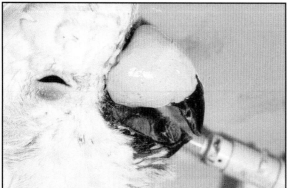

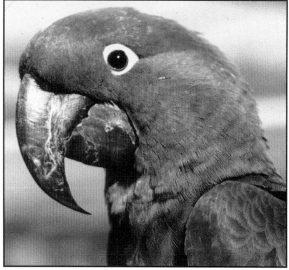

11.20 This Hyacinth Macaw was bitten by another macaw. The entrance wound was big (2 cm diameter) and went through to the other side (exit hole about 1 cm diameter). The beak, soft tissue and bone were moved into the correct position on both sides but an area of 1 cm x 1 cm was missing. Three pins were placed through the beak and joined with wire. The wound was covered with Coe-Pak, which was changed regularly. At first it was changed every week. As the healing progressed and the plug of fibrin became smaller, the interval between changes was increased. The wound filled with granulation tissue and contracted before finally epithelializing. The final picture was taken about a year later.

11.19 A larger defect that was still viable was repositioned and covered with Coe-Pak. Two changes were enough. The bird was given a 10-day course of antibiotic and made a complete recovery. Two wires were passed through the maxilla and were used as a scaffold to keep the Coe-Pak in place.

133

Injury to the mandible

This is often injured by being bitten. It may be bitten into two pieces but more often there is an injury that leads to a loss of keratin and the death of bone and soft tissue. This results in the mandible breaking into two parts. Various techniques for repair have been described involving wires and acrylics but these seldom seem to work well. The acrylic loosens and the fracture site loosens as the bird uses its beak; the repair cannot stand the strain of bottom beak grinding against the top. Most birds are able to cope with two hemi-mandibles and will easily remove the shells on sunflower seeds as well as being able to eat fruit and pellets.

One case has been described (Leijnieks, 2004) where the separate halves of the beak were joined using a plate that was bent to the shape of the mandible and bolted to the jaw. The space between the beak and the bar was filled with acrylic. The bar projected above the beak so that the force of the upper beak was distributed by the plate. The injury healed.

Deformities of the beak

Congenital deformity of mandible

In most birds the mandible can be seen as smooth horn overlying smooth bone. There is usually no sign that these are two pieces of bone. In some birds there is a distinct line in the horn in the middle of the mandible that looks like a raphe. In some birds the bones are separate and appear to have developed as such, rather than being broken in two. These birds are usually in good bodily condition and seem to be perfectly able to feed and groom. It would be possible to use surgery to fuse the mandibles in young growing birds.

Cleft beak and palate: This is an uncommon congenital deformity. The beak is separated on the lateral aspect. Repair is best done early. It is possible to split the unfused edges of the beak and then join them together with everting sutures. Care should be taken to repair the part of the defect near the nostril, as this seems to be the most difficult to make normal. The defect also allows the mandible to spread and so a temporary horizontal mattress suture is applied to pull the walls of the mandible into a more normal position.

Acquired deformity

The commonest acquired deformity of the beak is seen in macaws and it starts during rearing. It is likely that a bruise to the base of the beak slows its growth: the beak bends towards the injured side. It is possible to prevent this by feeding on alternate sides. Once the deviation has started, it can be corrected in the early stages by repeated manual pressure or by taping the beak between feeds so that the maxilla is pulled back across the mandible. In spite of this, it is common for macaws to be presented with a twisted beak when they have fledged, i.e. they are skeletally mature (Figure 11.21).

Adult birds with twisted beaks tend to be presented because of overgrown horn that further exacerbates the deformity. Regular reshaping of the horn, using a Dremel drill, can redirect the beak's growth. This is adequate in many mild cases but can take 12–18

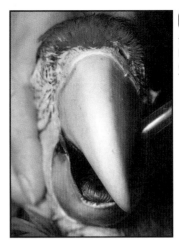

11.21 This Scarlet Macaw has finished growing but it has a significant deviation of the maxilla. This must be corrected.

months, with four or five interventions, to achieve a beak that wears normally (Chapter 6).

There are two other techniques that can correct maxillary deformity. According to Tully (personal communication), it is possible to use a dental composite manufactured for temporary crowns and bridges (Protemp™ 3 Garant™: 3M ESPE AG Dental Products, Seefeld Germany; 3M ESPE Dental Products, St Paul, Minnesota, USA) that cures cold, fast and hard. The mandible is covered with a thick mass of composite that is then shaped, using a hand-held grinder, into a groove that guides the maxilla (Figure 11.22). A

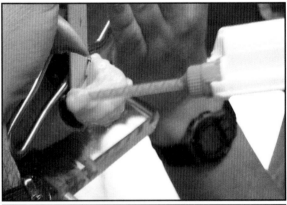

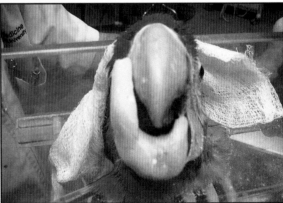

11.22 This Scarlet Macaw has been restrained manually and its head is held in a special clamp. Dental composite is applied whilst the beak is held open with a suitable gag. The composite is allowed to cure and is then shaped to guide the maxilla into a normal position. Some individuals would require anaesthesia for this procedure.

lateral flange is also useful. The aim is to make the guide exert a constant mild force that pushes the upper beak into the correct position and shape. In young birds this can happen within a few weeks. Once the mandible is straight, the composite is removed by grinding it down until it fragments.

A significant deviation in a skeletally mature bird may need to be corrected using trans-sinus pinning (Speer, 2003a). A medullary pin is placed through the skull, just caudal to the craniofacial hinge. On one side the pin is bent into a circle to prevent it pulling out. The other side of the pin is bent at right angles and cut off at the same length as the upper beak. In young birds this end is curled and hooked under an elastic band placed around the upper beak. The band should be 'super-glued' in place (Figure 11.23). This exerts gentle tension that will pull the beak into the correct position within a few days to a couple of weeks.

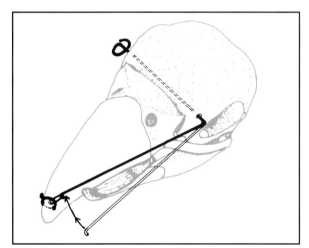

11.23 The wire extending beside the beak is attached to the ramphotheca with an elastic band in young birds. This gives gentle but continuous pressure, pulling the beak towards the wire. In adults, the bar is put under tension by attaching it with wire to the ramphotheca, which exerts greater force. This technique can take months to pull the maxilla straight in adults.

Older birds require much longer to redirect beak growth. The upper beak should be held on to the pin by a piece of cerclage wire. The tension of the wire will redirect the growth of the beak over several months. The deviation seems to correct quickly at first but the final redirection takes considerably longer.

A similar technique has been described that will correct maxillary prognathism, an uncommon problem that is usually seen in young, and occasionally adult, cockatoos (Speer, 2003a). The upper beak is usually deformed and bends at too great a curvature, ending up inside the mandible rather than outside. A triangular frame is used; the base is formed by a pin running through the skull (Figure 11.23). The apex of the triangle is used to attach an elastic band to the tip of the ramphotheca (upper beak). Constant firm tension pulls the beak slowly into position. This can take months and requires regular adjustments to the tension in the band.

Choanal atresia

This term describes a condition where the nasal passages do not open into the choana (Greenacre *et al.*, 1993). The birds are nearly always juvenile Grey Parrots with a profuse bilateral nasal discharge that was first seen in the nest box (Figure 11.24). The birds have usually been removed for hand rearing and treatment. Under general anaesthesia it is impossible to flush into the nostril and see the fluid (1% enrofloxacin solution) flow out of the choana, as would be expected. The technique described by Harris (1999) relieves this condition and can be modified. The blunt end of a 1.6 mm Steinmann pin should be advanced through the nostril and guided caudomedially, ventral to the conchae. Aiming the pin for the choana, a depression can be felt. The pin can be pushed through this without too much force and will emerge through the choana. A 5 Fr feeding tube is pushed over the end of the pin and drawn back so that it runs through the choana and exits the nostril. Because this condition is bilateral, the operation is performed on both sides and the tube is tied together behind the head with the tube sitting in the commissures.

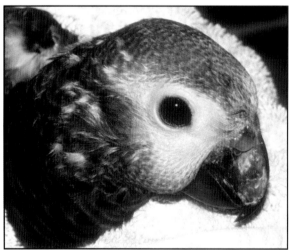

11.24 Choanal atresia in a Timneh Grey Parrot. The rhamphotheca in this subspecies is normally pale but the flaking horn is caused by the constant nasal discharge. The infraorbital sinus is distended: digital pressure on this sinus causes mucus to come out of the nostril and tear duct.

12

Nutrition and nutritional disease

Michael Stanford

Introduction

Chronic malnutrition is a common clinical presentation in captive parrots. Provision of a nutritionally adequate diet should therefore be of paramount concern to both aviculturists and veterinary surgeons. Unfortunately, due to the lack of scientifically controlled nutritional studies in psittacine birds, this can be very challenging. Most pet parrots have multiple nutrient deficiencies or excesses, rather than problems with a single dietary component.

Traditionally, diets were based on anecdotal information from aviculturists and the limited field observations of zoologists. More recently, by establishing research populations of captive parrots, scientists have been able to produce valid quantitative information about the nutritional requirements of these birds. Despite this, parrot diets are mostly based on standard nutritional requirements for poultry – and will be for the foreseeable future.

Recent research indicates that the optimal diet for pet parrots is one based on a complete balanced formulated product with limited seed and human food supplementation (Hess *et al.*, 2002). It has been shown that parrots fed diets consisting of < 50% balanced formulated food risk deficiency of several vitamins and minerals, particularly vitamin A, vitamin E and calcium. However, the majority of psittacine birds are still fed 'parrot seed' mixes, promoted by the pet trade, that are usually both nutritionally inadequate and of poor quality. Aviculturists tend to be resistant to change.

Although nutritional problems are common in all psittacine birds, Grey Parrots, cockatoos, Budgerigars and Cockatiels are the most frequently represented. This is probably because they are the parrots most likely to resist changes to their diet. They are also those most likely to become obsessed with individual food components within it.

Functional digestive anatomy

Parrots are habitually thought of as seed eaters but they are actually classified as florivores that consume plant-based diets (Klasing, 1998). They are further subdivided into granivores (seed eaters), frugivores (fruit eaters) and nectarivores (nectar eaters). Granivores consume not just grains but also hard dry fruits such as beans and nuts. Fruit consumption by frugivores is restricted to fleshy fruits rather than nuts or legumes. In addition, many individual species will consume foods from more than one plant category. Figure 12.1 indicates the food preferences of commonly presented psittacine birds and shows suitable substitutes in captivity (see also Figure 1.1). The table demonstrates that one 'parrot mix' will not cater for the needs of individual species and care should be taken when planning diets. Foods of plant origin are more diverse in their nutrient value than those of animal origin and this is shown in the different nutritional strategies in different psittacine species. The anatomy of the digestive tract reflects the feeding strategy of particular psittacine species.

Species	Feed group	Common dietary components in wild	Recommended diet in captivity
Budgerigar	Granivore	Native grass and chenopod seeds	Formulated diet or good quality boxed fresh seed mix with sprouted seeds as supplement Avoid seed sold from open containers Do not feed *ad libitum* due to problems with obesity
Cockatiel	Granivore	Seeds (prefer fresh but mature hard seeds of native grasses)	Formulated diet or mixture of fresh budgie seed with sprouted seeds as supplement Avoid larger fatty seeds such as sunflower commonly found in 'cockatiel mixes'
Ringneck Parakeet	Granivore	Seeds mainly but also some flowers and fruit	Formulated diets or fresh budgie seed with sprouted seeds as supplement Avoid larger fatty seeds such as sunflower
Maximilian's Pionus Parrot	Florivore	Seeds, flowers, grain, fruit pulp	Formulated diet or pulse-based diet with fruit
Red Lory	Nectarivore	Primarily nectar, fruit, pollen and seeds, insects	Formulated nectar mix with additional fruit

12.1 Feeding preferences of wild parrots, with a suggested substitute for captive birds (see also Figure 1.1). (continues) ▶

Species	Feed group	Common dietary components in wild	Recommended diet in captivity
Grey Parrot	Florivore	Seeds, fruit, flowers, nuts Preferred food: stone palm fruit	Formulated diet with limited vegetable supplementation Provide UV-B light for adequate vitamin D_3 metabolism or calcium supplement in seed-fed Greys, as very prone to hypocalcaemia
Orange-winged Amazon	Frugivore	Fruit	Formulated diet or pulse mixture supplemented with fruit Avoid seed – very prone to obesity and fatty liver disease
Sulphur-crested Cockatoo	Omnivore	Seeds with plant roots and insect grubs	Formulated diet Avoid high-fat seed diets.
Blue and Gold Macaw	Florivore	Seeds, fruits, leaves, nuts	Formulated diet with 10% vegetable supplementation Avoid excessive use of nuts as treats
Scarlet Macaw	Frugivore–granivore	Fruit, nuts, leaves, shoots, bark	Formulated diets with 10% vegetable supplementation Avoid excessive use of nuts as treats

12.1 (continued) Feeding preferences of wild parrots, with a suggested substitute for captive birds (see also Figure 1.1).

Nutritional requirements

Despite distinct differences in functional digestive anatomy and lifestyle between commercial poultry and captive psittacine birds, the nutritional requirements for poultry derived by the National Research Council (NRC, 1994) are still considered to be the standard for predicting the nutritional requirements of parrots. An adaptation was adopted by the Association of Avian Veterinarians (AAV) in 1996 as a guideline for developing formulated parrot diets, recommending maintenance needs for adult birds (Figure 12.2). Scientific nutritional research has revealed that parrots have a lower requirement for calcium, proteins and fat than do production poultry,

which is only to be expected in a non-production animal. To date, controlled studies have shown that parrot requirements for vitamins and minerals (with the exception of calcium) are similar to those of poultry.

The nutritional requirements of poultry vary with their physiological state and (despite lack of research) it is reasonable to assume that this would also be the case with parrots. It is already known that during the breeding season many species of parrot supplement their diet with invertebrates in order to increase their dietary calcium and protein (Gilardi, 1996). Growth, moulting and reproductive activity would all be expected to affect the requirements for nutrients, as would severe disease.

Nutrient	Recommended requirement for maintenance
Protein	12.00%
Lipid	4.00%
Energy	3000.00 kcal/kg
Vitamin A	5000.00 IU/kg
Vitamin D	1000.00 IU/kg
Vitamin E	50.00 ppm
Vitamin K	1.00 ppm
Thiamine	5.00 ppm
Riboflavin	10.00 ppm
Niacin	75.00 ppm
Pyridoxine	10.00 ppm
Pantothenic acid	15.00 ppm
Biotin	0.20 ppm
Folic acid	2.00 ppm
Vitamin B_{12}	0.01 ppm
Choline	1000.00 ppm
Vitamin C	No requirement demonstrated in adults
Calcium	0.5%

Nutrient	Recommended requirement for maintenance
Phosphorus (available)	0.25%
Phosphorus (total)	0.40%
Sodium	0.15%
Chlorine	0.35%
Potassium	0.40%
Magnesium	600.00 ppm
Manganese	75.00 ppm
Iron	80.00 ppm
Zinc	50.00 ppm
Copper	8.00 ppm
Iodine	0.30 ppm
Selenium	0.10 ppm
Lysine	0.60%
Methionine	0.25%
Tryptophan	0.12%
Arginine	0.60%
Threonine	0.40%

12.2 Nutritional requirements of psittacine birds (adapted by Association of Avian Veterinarians from National Research Council poultry requirements, 1994).

Moulting

Healthy parrots moult once a year (Chapter 2) and this is nutritionally very demanding. Moulting is principally hormonally controlled, induced by extrinsic factors, but birds will stop moulting if adequate nutrition is not provided. This results in dull, old and damaged plumage, a frequent sequel to which is feather plucking or picking, as brittle feathers cause irritation.

Feathers contain approximately 25% of total body protein, 15% of which is contained in the sheath. The bird usually consumes the sheath as the feather develops and this may be a useful recycling of dietary protein for parrots. Production of new feathers usually increases protein requirements by 4–8% and this increase is specifically for the amino acids methionine, cysteine and lysine. Deficiencies in any of these amino acids will lead to plumage and moulting disorders.

Moulting is also energetically expensive as energy is required for the formation of new feathers, increased protein metabolism and loss of heat due to reduced feather cover. The increased energy requirement varies between 3 and 20%, depending on the stage and degree of moulting.

There has been no reported need for additional vitamins, minerals and fatty acids during the moulting cycle, but it has been shown that water requirements double for many species of bird.

Wild birds adapt to moulting by eating more and by being more selective about what they eat. They also become less active, in order to conserve energy. In captivity, diets should provide these additional needs during a moult.

Reproduction

Protein is required for oviduct growth and egg protein formation, and the increased protein requirement during the breeding season depends on clutch size, frequency of clutch production and the protein composition of the eggs. Birds producing single-egg clutches do not require significantly more protein, but birds producing multiple-egg clutches require an increase of 2% total dietary protein. Egg-laying birds do not require an increase in any specific amino acid.

Dietary lipid requirements increase during egg production as fat is deposited in the yolk to sustain the embryo during incubation. The yolk has been shown to contain no lipid when the bird hatches (Deeming, 2001).

Laying females have an increased requirement for calcium; their diet must also not contain excessive phosphorus. The increase in calcium requirement is not excessive compared with production poultry: Cockatiels will produce eggs with normal shells on 0.85% calcium (compared with 0.5% for maintenance). In poultry the increased calcium is used to form medullary bone in the marrow cavity of the long bones 10 days prior to laying eggs. Medullary bone provides around 40% of the calcium required for the eggshell in laying hens in less than 24 hours (Driggers and Comar, 1949). It is also important to ensure that vitamin D_3 levels are adequate for correct calcium homeostasis.

There is probably an increased requirement for vitamin E and other antioxidants during the breeding season. This is important particularly in male birds, in order to preserve sperm, and vitamin E deficiency should always be suspected in cases of infertility. Vitamin E is increasingly thought of as an important dietary component for efficient reproductive behaviour in poultry and this would be expected to be the case for breeding parrots too (Surai, 2002).

Females require considerably more energy during the breeding season for oviduct and egg formation, whereas males do not have an increased energy requirement above maintenance for sperm formation.

Many manufacturers produce formulated diets specifically for the breeding season, which supply these increased requirements. The diets should be fed around 4 weeks prior to expected egg production.

Growth

Parrots are altricial birds, with rapid skeletal development compared with precocial species. However, they are among the slowest growing altricial birds, with lower energy requirements from hatching until weaning than might be expected for this group (Starck and Ricklefs, 1998). Energy and protein requirements are highest at hatch and then steadily decrease until weaning. The protein requirement for growth in Cockatiels has been estimated at 20% and it is essential that the food protein contains adequate lysine, methionine and cysteine for feather development. Many formulated rearing mixes do not appear to contain adequate sulphur amino acids and, because of this, feather development in chicks is often poor. Wild parrots are known to supplement their diet with invertebrates, including insects, in order to obtain additional protein (Morse, 1975).

Relatively rapid skeletal growth in psittacine chicks results in an increased requirement for calcium but, surprisingly, this is not excessive (1% appears sufficient). Failure to provide sufficient vitamin D prevents adequate calcium absorption, leading to osteodystrophy in growing chicks (especially Grey Parrots).

Evaluating diets

A full dietary history should constitute part of the routine investigation for any psittacine bird presenting for clinical examination. Evaluation of the type of food fed, the amount fed and any supplementation is essential. It is also vital to analyse what the parrot actually eats, rather than just what it is offered, as parrots in captivity can be very selective feeders, often becoming addicted to individual dietary components (e.g. a Grey Parrot obsessed with sunflower seed). It is important to consider how long an individual has been deficient and whether or not it is a productive bird. In young birds, the diet of the parents should be evaluated for deficiencies.

Full chemical diet analysis is prohibitively expensive in most cases but should always be considered for larger collections, especially for those with poor breeding performance. An economical practical alternative is the Zootrition System developed by the Department of Wildlife Nutrition at Bronx Zoo (www.zootrition.com). This is a commercial computer program that analyses diets via the nutrient composition of each individual component in order to produce a full analysis of the complete diet. The same program will then compare the results with the nutritional requirements for poultry or parrots where this information is known.

Protein and amino acids

Dietary proteins can be divided into two groups: the essential amino acids, which must be supplied in the diet; and the non-essential amino acids, which can be synthesized from dietary precursors. The essential amino acids are arginine, glycine, histidine, isoleucine, leucine, lysine, methionine, phenylalanine, proline, valine, trypotophan and threonine.

The protein maintenance requirement for parrots has been determined at 10–15%. This positively correlates with body size but can vary with both age and physiological state. Young birds need 20% protein for optimum growth, but nectarivorous species such as Red Lories have a lower protein requirement due to reduced gastrointestinal loss of protein in comparison with other psittacine birds.

Traditionally, the aetiology of renal disease and gout was thought to be high-protein diets but recent studies have failed to prove this. Cockatiels, although prone to gout, showed no evidence of renal disease when fed a 70% protein diet. However, a rapid change from a low-protein to a high-protein diet has been implicated in the development of renal disease (Koutsos et al., 2001a).

Energy

The basal metabolic rate of parrots depends on the climate of their country of origin, with temperate species (mainly from Australia and New Zealand) having a rate 20% higher than those from the tropics (McNab and Salisbury, 1995). Energy requirements vary with age, environment, activity, physiological processes, reproductive behaviour and species. For example, in the Budgerigar energy requirements for flight are 20 times basal needs. Figure 12.3 estimates the metabolizable energy requirements of adult parrots in various situations. If food is provided *ad libitum* parrots usually eat enough to satisfy their energy needs, but obesity is common if diets with high energy content are fed or if selective feeding is permitted.

Environment	Estimated energy requirement (kJ/day)
Indoor cage	$647 \times BW^{0.73}$
Indoor flight	$739 \times BW^{0.73}$
Outdoor aviary (summer)	$853 \times BW^{0.73}$
Outdoor aviary (winter)	$946 \times BW^{0.73}$
Free living	$959 \times BW^{0.73}$

12.3 Estimation of metabolizable energy requirements of parrots under different housing conditions based on body weight ($BW^{0.73}$) (Koutsos et al., 2001b).

Lipids

High-fat seed diets have traditionally been associated with clinical obesity in captive parrots. Although the aetiology of fatty liver disease is still uncertain excessive dietary fat is a contributory factor. Some fat is required, to enable the absorption of fat-soluble vitamins and to provide an immediately available energy source, for which 2% is thought to be adequate.

The lipid composition of seeds varies considerably and seeds eaten in the wild are rarely available in traditional parrot mixes. A high-fat seed such as sunflower, which is found in the majority of parrot mixes, often results in a diet with a fat content > 20%.

Water

Water should always be freely available. The daily water requirement of adult parrots is approximately 2.4% of body weight. This varies with environmental temperature, species and diet. A rise in environmental temperature of 10°C has been shown to increase water intake 12-fold in Quaker Parakeets, whereas Budgerigars can survive without water at room temperatures (Macmillen, 1990). The provision of fruit in the diet has been shown to decrease water consumption significantly, whereas the feeding of formulated diets increases it. This variability in water intake makes it impossible to standardize intake of vitamin supplements through the water supply. Also, stability in water cannot be controlled, as many vitamins are destroyed by the presence of zinc or copper in domestic water supplies and some are light sensitive. The provision of medicines and nutritional supplements through the water supply is therefore not ideal (Hess et al., 2002).

Water should preferably be supplied from a filtered source, free from bacterial contamination, and in clean containers located in an area not easily contaminated by faecal or food material. Water bowls should be kept clean and disinfected regularly, as contaminated water is a common source of infections (e.g. yersiniosis caused by rodent fouling). Automatic drinking equipment is now available for parrots and this reduces contamination problems. Acidification of water by addition of organic cider vinegar (1 drop per 200 ml of drinking water) has been shown to discourage crop yeast growth.

It is common practice for parrot owners to offer drinks such as tea, coffee or soft drinks as an alternative to water but this should be discouraged, as parrots are very susceptible to caffeine toxicity. Tannins have been used to treat iron storage disease and so decaffeinated tea may be useful in susceptible birds such as Hawk-headed Parrots.

Vitamins

Vitamins are essential molecules that act as cofactors for enzymes and also as hormones. Psittacine birds are unable to synthesize most of the vitamins they require and so these have to be supplied in the diet. Over-supplementation with multi-vitamin mixtures is common in aviculture and can lead to either hypervitaminosis or secondary hypovitaminosis. This is particularly true for vitamins A and D (Koutsos et al., 2001b).

Fat-soluble vitamins (A, D, E and K) can be stored for long periods and so parrots can withstand long periods of depletion before deficiency signs manifest. This can also lead to problems with toxicity, especially of vitamins A and D in over-supplemented birds. Toxicity of vitamins E and K are less common, as both vitamins have a low toxicity. Fat-soluble vitamins compete for the same lipid-binding sites, which means that the correct vitamin balance is vital as an excess of one fat-soluble vitamin can lead to a deficiency in another. Carotenoids (provitamin A) also compete with the fat-soluble vitamins for binding sites and so a dietary excess of fat-soluble vitamins may also lead to carotenoid deficiencies (Surai, 2002).

Water-soluble vitamins (B complex and C) cannot be stored and must be supplied constantly in the diet. Toxicities of these vitamins are rare, as excesses are excreted in the urine.

Vitamins are the least stable of dietary components and are affected by storage temperature, high humidity and exposure to ultraviolet light. Vitamin instability, together with varying water intake, suggests that it is not advisable to administer vitamins in the water supply. It is better to attempt to provide sufficient in the diet. This is simple with a formulated diet, where vitamins can be added during the manufacturing process, but there are concerns that many of the formulated diets have vitamin levels above those recommended. Vitamin requirements in psittacine birds are unknown but are thought to be similar to those of poultry (see Figure 12.2).

Minerals

There are 13 minerals that are essential for the optimum health of parrots but, with the exception of calcium, research is lacking into specific mineral activity and requirement. Relatively high levels of the macrominerals calcium, phosphorus, magnesium, sodium, potassium and chloride are essential, whereas the trace minerals zinc, copper, iodine, selenium, iron and manganese are only required in low concentrations (Klasing, 1998). The availability of minerals depends not only on their concentration in food but also on many other factors, such as the chemical form of the mineral (for example, selenium has four valent forms, each with different chemical activity) and the level of other minerals in the food (for example, high phosphorus levels will reduce calcium absorption). The active absorption and excretion of minerals in the intestine is tightly regulated to prevent toxicities or deficiencies.

Practical feeding

Commercially available parrot diets can be divided into two broad groups: traditional seed-based mixes and modern formulated diets. The appearance of the common diets used in aviculture is shown in Figures 12.4 to 12.7. Both diet groups are frequently supplemented with a combination of soaked pulse mixtures, vegetables and fruit. In addition commercial vitamin and mineral supplements are often added. Figure 12.8 indicates the general advantages and disadvantages of common parrot feeding protocols. Figure 12.9 indicates the basic nutrient content and usefulness of individual food materials commonly used for feeding captive psittacines.

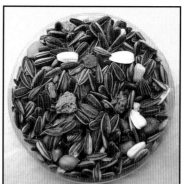

12.4 Traditional seed diet. This is a mixture of seeds with a high proportion of sunflower seed. Unfortunately this is still the most common diet used for parrots despite known multiple nutrient excesses and deficiencies. Seed diets are often of poor quality, and bacterial and fungal contamination is common. Even though this diet is 90% sunflower seed it is sold as a complete diet.

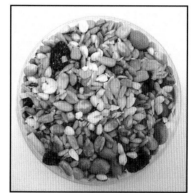

12.5 Dehusked seed diet. The dehusking improves a seed diet by removing the chance of problems from bacterial and mycotic contamination; however, the diet is still poor nutritionally and the dehusking process further reduces the nutrient content of the mix.

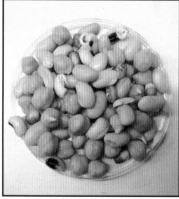

12.6 Pulse diet. This diet is popular with aviculturalists. Although far superior to seed mixes and with better protein content, there are still nutrient deficiencies (in particular, calcium). Pulses are probably best thought of as a supplementary diet to formulated mixes, to provide interest.

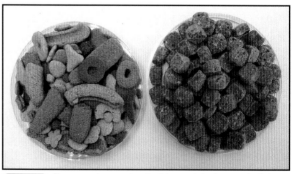

12.7 Two modern extruded formulated parrot diets. Kaytee Exact (left) has nuggets in different shapes and colours to provide interest for the bird. Harrison's High Potency mix (right) is organic and free from artificial preservatives.

Diet regime	Potential deficiencies	Potential excesses	Imbalances	Other factors	Comments
Seed only	Vitamin A, B_{12}, D_3, E and riboflavin Calcium, iodine, iron, copper, zinc, sodium, manganese, selenium Lysine and methionine	Fat (up to 65%) increased by selective feeding of favourite seeds	Calcium/phosphorus Vitamin E/selenium Amino acids	Fungal and bacterial contamination of diets very common	Use not justified though still widely promoted and used in aviculture
Seed supplemented with fruit and vegetables	Vitamin E, D_3 and B_{12} If fed non-pigmented fruit/vegetables, vitamin A would also be deficient Calcium, iodine, iron, copper, zinc, sodium, manganese Lysine and methionine	Sugars and fibre High fibre levels can reduce biotin availability High fat	Calcium/phosphorus Amino acids	Fungal and bacterial contamination of both seed and vegetable matter very common	Not justifiable though still widely used Very dependent on quality of vegetables supplied
Seed supplemented with both fruit/ vegetables and vitamin/mineral mix	Failure to ensure birds consume vitamin and mineral supplements would lead to same problems as all-seed diets	Sugars and fibre High fat Possibility of hypervitaminosis	Amino acids Difficult to ensure hypovitaminosis and hypocalcaemia not a problem	Fungal and bacterial contamination of diet common	Most common diet used in aviculture but impossible to supplement diets adequately with powder mixes accurately Not recommended
Formulated extruded diet	No deficiencies expected as long as manufacturer follows AAV recommended nutrient requirements	Many formulated diets appear to have nutrients in excess of requirements	None expected if diet formulated correctly	Hypervitaminosis may be problem in future as true requirements found	Author's recommended diet for all psittacine birds at present time Care should be taken to choose diet without excessive levels of vitamins Can be supplemented with pulses or pigmented vegetables to 10% of total diet
Pulse mix diet with vitamin/mineral mix	Low calcium Failure to ensure birds consume vitamin and mineral supplements would lead to similar problems as with seed-based diets	High carbohydrate	None expected.	Excellent supply of protein	Traditional aviculturist diet Probably best reserved as supplementary diet now formulated diets are available Requires experience and time consuming to prepare
Homemade diet	Would depend on nature of food material used Variability of content a problem	High salt High fat Potential toxins such as caffeine	Use of homemade foods will reduce consumption of main food source, creating potential deficiencies	None perceived but useful as training aid	Not commonly used but increasingly with tame pet birds the use of human food material could be potential problem

12.8 Advantages and disadvantages of common parrot feeding protocols.

Food item	Protein (%)	Fat (%)	Energy (cal/g)	Vitamin A IU/g	Vitamin E (mg/kg)	Ca²⁺ (%)	P (%)
Apple	0.4	0.1	0.42	0.27	5.31	0.0	0.00
Banana	1.2	0.3	0.95	0.35	2.69	0	0.03
Grape	0.4	0.09	0.57	0.27	–	0.01	0.02
Orange	1.1	0.1	0.37	0.47	2.4	0.05	0.02
Pear	0.31	0.1	0.4	0.31	5.01	0.01	0.01
Pomegranate	0.95	0.3	–	0	5.5	0.0	0.01

12.9 Nutritional analysis of common dietary components. Data supplied by Zootrition program (www.zootrition.com). (continues) ▶

Food item	Protein (%)	Fat (%)	Energy (cal/g)	Vitamin A IU/g	Vitamin E (mg/kg)	Ca²⁺ (%)	P (%)
Mango	0.7	0.19	0.57	30.01	10.51	0.01	0.02
Kiwi fruit	0.99	0.44	–	1.75	11.2	0.03	0.04
Plum	0.6	0.1	0.36	4.91	6.1	0.01	0.02
Passion fruit	2.61	0.4	0.36	12.5	–	0.01	0.06
Honeydew melon	0.6	0.1	0.28	0.8	1.0	0.01	0.02
Mango	0.51	0.27	–	38.94	11.2	0.01	0.01
Pea	5.42	0.4	–	6.4	3.9	0.03	0.11
French bean	18.81	2.02	–	0.08	–	0.19	0.3
Carrot	1.03	0.19	–	281.29	4.6	0.03	0.04
Broccoli flowers	2.98	0.35	–	30.0	16.6	0.05	0.07
Sweet corn	3.22	1.18	–	2.81	0.9	0.0	0.09
Spinach	2.8	0.8	0.25	58.93	17.1	0.17	0.05
Pepper, red	1.0	0.4	0.32	64.01	8.0	0.01	0.02
Potato, new	1.7	–	0.7	–	0.6	0.01	0.03
Tomato	0.7	0.3	0.17	10.67	12.2	0.01	0.02
Courgette	1.8	0.4	0.18	10.17	–	0.03	0.04
Mung bean	3.04	0.18	–	0.21	0.1	0.01	0.05
Chickpea	21.33	5.4	3.2	0.99	28.8	0.16	0.31
Black beans	21.60	1.42	–	0.17	2.1	0.12	0.35
Sweet potato	1.21	0.29	0.87	65.51	45.6	0.02	0.05
Almond, blanched	20.42	52.53	–	0.0	202.60	0.25	0.53
Brazil nut	14.09	68.23	6.82	0.0	71.83	0.17	0.59
Coconut meat	3.33	33.49	–	0	7.3	0.01	0.11
Macadamia nut, dry	8.3	73.72	–	0	4.1	0.07	0.14
Pine nut	14.01	68.6	6.88	0.19	136.51	0.01	0.65
Sunflower seed	22.78	49.67	–	0.5	502.72	0.12	0.71
Safflower seed	16.18	38.45	–	0.5	–	0.08	0.64
Walnut	14.68	68.53	6.88	0	38.3	0.1	0.38
White millet	11.61	3.51	–	–	–	0.03	0.43
Canary seed	17.00	8.4	–	–	–	–	–
Peanuts, shelled	25.8	49.24	–	0	91.30	0.09	0.38

12.9 (continued) Nutritional analysis of common dietary components. Data supplied by Zootrition program (www.zootrition.com).

Seed diet

Seed-based diets have until recently been the foundation of most aviculturist diets and the resistance of owners to change can be extremely challenging. The pet trade continues to recommend and sell seed mixes, usually based on sunflower seed, as 'complete' parrot diets. The seed mixes are normally balanced using a biscuit supplement containing vitamins and minerals to create a complete diet – but only if the parrot eats the whole ration. As selective feeding is common, the majority of birds presented to veterinary practices will eat a nutritionally inadequate diet. Parrots will survive on seed mixes, but they are chronically malnourished and unhealthy, with poor reproductive performance.

Studies have indicated that seed diets are deficient in many nutritional components, especially essential amino acids (chiefly methionine and lysine), calcium, vitamin A, vitamin D and iodine (Hess *et al.*, 2002). Seeds are also high in fat and most have an inappropriately low ratio of calcium to phosphorus. Although it is possible to fortify seeds with minerals, vitamins and essential amino acid coatings, it is difficult to create a balanced diet as seeds are rapidly dehusked when eaten. Supplementation via water sources is unreliable. Many respected formulated diet manufacturers also produce 'complete' seed mixes in their product range, which is confusing for the purchaser.

Seed quality in the pet trade is generally poor and is usually classified as unfit for human consumption. This means that the nutritional content of seeds in the mix is also poor. In addition, the seed may be contaminated with bacteria and fungal spores (Figure 12.10) that are potential pathogens, especially when fed to malnourished birds. Mycotoxins are also a common problem in poorly stored seed mixes. Seeds should really only be considered as a complementary diet; they should be stored in airtight bins and, if seeds are fed, they should always be of human food-grade quality. Such seeds, however, have usually been dehusked, which can further reduce their nutrient composition.

Three simple practical tests can be used to demonstrate poor seed qualities to the client:

- Culture a small sample of the diet. A profuse growth of fungus and bacteria will usually be produced within 24 hours
- Open a sample of sunflower seeds to examine the kernels. Poor quality sunflower seed will contain shrivelled, dry kernels as well as evidence of powdery fungus in many cases
- Examine the germination of the seed mixture. Usually the germination rate will be < 10%, demonstrating poor quality.

Formulated diets

Figure 12.11 indicates the constitution and key features of several popular formulated diets, based on information provided by the manufacturers and compared with NRC nutrient requirements. A typical unsupplemented parrot seed and pulse mix is included for further comparison.

Studies suggest that the optimal maintenance diet for pet parrots is a complete formulated diet (at least 50% of total food consumed) with some additional fruit and vegetables (McDonald, 2002a). It should be noted that not all commercial products are of comparable quality and so care should be taken before recommending particular products.

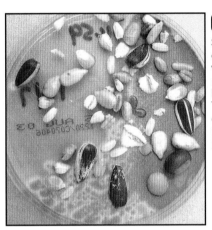

12.10 Seed mix contaminated with *Aspergillus fumigatus* (24-hour growth). This is a common pathogen in parrots.

Manufacturer	Diet	Protein (%)	Lipid (%)	Vit A (IU/kg)	Vit D (IU/kg)	Vit E (mg/kg)	Calcium (%)	Comments
NARC nutrient requirement		12	4	5000	1000	500	0.5	
Harrisons International Bird Foods	Adult Life Time High Potency	15 18	5.5 15	8616 11,000	1077 1650	300 400	0.6 0.9	100% organic with no insecticides, herbicides or fungicides Free of artificial preservatives or colours
Mazuri	Small bird maintenance Parrot maintenance Parrot breeder	15.6 16.4 20.0	7.0 7.0 7.5	12,000 12,000 9000	1800 1800 1500		0.9 0.85 1.20	Natural antioxidants
Kaytee	Exact original Exact rainbow	15.0 15.0	6.0 6.0	10,000 10,000	1000 1000	100 100		Different colours and shapes to provide interest
Pretty Bird	Daily Select Macaw hi energy Amazon/cockatoo African	14.0 16.0 14.0 14.0	5.0 10.0 8.0 8.0	17,500 19,000 17,500 17,500	800 700 800 800	200 300 200 200		Nuggets are different colours and shapes to provide interest
Hagen	Tropican Lifetime Granules	15.0	10.0	16,000	500	220	0.7	
ZuPreem	Avian Breeder Avian Maintenance	20.0 14.0	10.0 4.0					Five different shapes and colours to provide interest No artificial flavours or preservatives

12.11 Nutritional analysis of popular formulated diets, based on information from the manufacturers. The pulse and seed diets were analysed using the Zootrition program. (continues) ▶

Manufacturer	Diet	Protein (%)	Lipid (%)	Vit A (IU/kg)	Vit D (IU/kg)	Vit E (mg/kg)	Calcium (%)	Comments
Roudybush	Psittacine Breeder Psittacine Maintenance	20.0 11	3.0 7	10,130 7880	1400 800	– –	0.9 0.4	
Seed mix	Based on 60% sunflower seed diet with pine nuts, oats and peanuts and safflower	22.79	51.89	470	–	413.73	0.11 (phospho-rus 0.77%)	Must use human food-grade seed mix to prevent exposure to pathogens High fat and severe deficiencies in vitamin A and D. Low calcium and protein. Must be supplemented
Pulse diet	Based on mix of equal parts black beans, mung beans chickpeas and black-eyed peas with 10% apple and carrot	23.45	2.53	4310	–	568.00	0.13	Economic, fit for human consumption. Good source of protein Low calcium. Can lead to obesity in inactive birds due to high carbohydrate levels. Must be supplemented. Time consuming to prepare leading to owner non-compliance

12.11 (continued) Nutritional analysis of popular formulated diets, based on information from the manufacturers. The pulse and seed diets were analysed using the Zootrition program.

Formulated diets are manufactured by either a pelleting process or an extrusion procedure. The latter binds components at high temperature, pasteurizing ingredients to reduce bacterial contamination and dust. In addition, the process increases the palatability and digestibility of many dietary components. Pellet diets are produced at lower temperatures and are considered inferior, due to (i) the increased risk of bacterial contamination and (ii) only moderate palatability. Formulated diets use the extrusion process to combine dietary ingredients, providing a nutritionally complete nugget. This means that parrots cannot select individual components, thereby preventing imbalances.

Although there is a lack of published information on the nutritional requirements of parrots, it is the author's opinion that a formulated diet (based on the nutritional requirements for poultry) should constitute the bulk of a captive parrot's diet. It is expected that, in the future, formulated diets will be produced to reflect different nutritional requirements of different parrot species as they become known. Diverse diets should also be devised for different stages of the parrot's life cycle.

Pulse diets

Diets based on soaked pulses were first advocated by forward-thinking aviculturists who were unimpressed with the breeding results obtained when feeding traditional seed diets. The high protein content is the main advantage of pulses over other seeds. Dried pulse mixes are also usually of human food-grade quality, unlike more traditional parrot seed mixes. All pulses should sprout after soaking. They should be pre-soaked for 24 hours and washed to decrease the toxin content of the beans. This process also increases digestibility and palatability. Fermentation must be avoided by storing the mixture in a fridge and washing thoroughly prior to feeding.

The disadvantages of pulses are their high carbohydrate and low calcium levels. A vitamin and mineral mix should be added to pulse diets to correct deficiencies, as with seed mixes. Although they have been used successfully for many years in aviculture, good formulated diets would be expected to replace pulse mixes completely in the future, as they are more convenient and have a better nutritional balance. Despite this, pulse mixes are still considered useful, interesting complementary foods for captive psittacine birds. South American species, which tend towards frugivore behaviour, are usually keen to eat pulse mixes but African species are more reluctant.

A typical pulse recipe might be as follows:

1 Soak a mixture of mung beans, soybeans, black-eyed beans, haricot beans and chick peas for 24–48 hours until germination occurs.
2 Avoid high temperatures, as this may create ideal conditions for fermentation.
3 The soaked mixture can be kept for up to 48 hours in a fridge if kept moist and covered.
4 Rinse mixture well in running water every 24 hours to remove potential toxins and fermentative bacteria.
5 The addition of sweet-flavoured fruit and vegetables, such as carrot or apple, will improve palatability.
6 Vitamin and mineral supplements must be added to the pulse mix to improve nutrient content. The addition of oyster shell grit as a source of calcium is useful.

Fruit and vegetables

Aviculturists generally supplement diets with a combination of fruit and vegetables to add variety and interest. It is also generally believed that this will supply essential vitamins or minerals, although frequently this is not the case. Figure 12.9 indicates the nutritional content of several commonly used vegetables and fruits. The following points should be borne in mind:

- Fruits produced in temperate conditions are nutritionally poor for parrots and usually should only be considered as a sugary drink. Tropical fruits have a better protein and fibre content and so their incorporation into diets is more rational.
- With formulated diets thought to be nutritionally complete, the addition of fruit and vegetables dilutes the important nutritional components, thereby unbalancing the diet.
- Vegetables, especially pigmented varieties, are nutritionally useful.
- Prime grade 1 products should always be used in order to avoid feeding material contaminated with potential pathogens such as *Aspergillus* moulds.
- The use of organic fruit and vegetables is to be recommended wherever feasible.
- Formulated diets should be supplemented with 10% pigmented vegetables or tropical fruits to provide interest.
- Avocado should *not* be fed to captive parrots, as some strains contain toxins that cause death within several hours (Hargis *et al.*, 1989; Chapter 20).

Vitamin and mineral supplementation

Vitamin and mineral supplementation is widespread in aviculture, despite lack of knowledge of the nutritional requirements of parrots and dietary composition. The correction of dietary deficiencies via vitamin and mineral supplementation is fraught with difficulties. It often leads to both toxicities and deficiencies, since it is not possible to quantify accurately the levels of vitamins and minerals taken by individual birds using water-based or food-based supplements. Many commercial formulated diets already appear to contain excess levels of fat-soluble vitamins, especially vitamins A and D, and further supplementation could be dangerous. Prior to supplementing any diet, an attempt should be made to detect which nutrients are genuinely lacking. Figure 12.12 indicates the vitamin content of several commercial vitamin and mineral products. These

products should be added to parrot diets based solely on seed or pulse mixes but would not be expected to be required for birds fed on formulated diets.

Grit is a good source of minerals, especially calcium. In the smaller granivores, such as Budgerigars, grit helps digestion by enhancing the grinding action of the gizzard. The lack of grit for Budgerigars has been implicated in cases of megabacteriosis. Grit should be supplied regularly in small amounts as either mineralized grit or oyster shell. Iodine deficiency is a common nutritional problem in Budgerigars and can be easily prevented by the supply of commercial 'pink' iodine blocks. The provision of grit is recommended for the large psittacine birds, though no requirement has been demonstrated (Chapter 15). Several species of psittacine birds have been shown to practise geophagy, with clay and quartz material found in the gizzard. This has been shown to have a detoxifying effect on the diet and is probably a useful source of minerals for the birds (Gilardi *et al.*, 1999).

Converting to formulated diets

The majority of captive psittacine birds should be expected to have nutritional problems (MacWhirter, 1994). Corrective dietary manipulation is therefore mandatory but can be difficult to achieve, as parrots frequently become addicted to individual food items (monophagism) and are resistant to change. Owner education is of paramount importance: many are totally unaware that parrots in the wild eat a variety of foods, not just seeds. There is also resistance amongst aviculturists against formulated diets, as they are felt to be both uninteresting for the birds to eat and expensive.

Many birds require treatment of primary diseases before dietary changes can be implemented but improved nutrition should always be considered once normal appetite has returned. It should be explained that many deficiencies will take a long time to recover; for example, vitamin A deficiencies take several months to improve, as the abnormal epithelial cells have to be replaced. There are a number of strategies that can help the clinician to achieve a successful dietary conversion.

Product	Vitamin A (IU/g)	Vitamin D (IU/g)	Vitamin E (IU/g)	Ca²⁺ (mg/g)	P (mg/g)
Daily Essentials (Bird Care Company)	2660	2660	666	–	–
Calcivet (Bird Care Company)	–	25000 IU/l	–	440 g calcium borogluconate (40%/l)	–
Feather Up (Bird Care Company)	266	266	–	–	–
Ace-High (Vetark)	2530	20	122	9.9	4.9
Avimix (Vetark)	1177	118	54	142	5.0
Nutrobal (Vetark)	500	150	20	200	4.5
Zolcal (Vetark)	–	25000 IU/l	–	400g calcium borogluconate (40%/l)	–

12.12 Analysis of popular vitamin and mineral supplements, based on information supplied by the manufacturers.

- Weigh bird and monitor weight gains or losses during conversion period, as it is possible to starve birds to death (for example, hepatic lipidosis cases will deteriorate if the bird is starved).
- Introduce new diet dispersed through previous mix, gradually increasing the percentage of new diet fed.
- Do not feed *ad libitum* but 2–3 times daily for 60 minutes.
- Add the new diet to favourite foods.
- Encourage the owner to eat the new diet in front of the bird. Place the bird in sight of other parrots that are already eating the formulated diet.
- Conversion is easier if there are several birds involved especially for the smaller parrots.
- Soak formulated foods in sweet juices (e.g. fresh orange juice) to encourage consumption.
- Hide food in favourite toys or in the substrate used on the cage floor.
- Feed the new diet outside the cage.
- Feed the new diet on alternate days, gradually increasing the number of days fed.
- Hospitalize the bird for dietary conversion if the owner is adamant that the bird will not change.
- Birds resistant to formulated diets can be stomach tubed for several days so that they acquire a taste for the food.
- Advise owners that complete dietary conversion may take up to 6 months.
- Advise breeders to wean their young birds on to formulated diets.
- Advise owners that visible improvements in their bird's plumage and general condition may take up to 12 months.

Nutritional disease

Up to 75% of diseases seen in parrots have at least a partial nutritional basis and a full dietary history should always be obtained. The most common nutritional diseases seen in practice are covered in detail below.

Integument

Chronic malnutrition commonly presents as deterioration in the integument and plumage. Since research has shown that the plumage of wild birds is affected only when malnutrition has reached severe levels, such signs in a pet parrot are a cause of real concern, confirming the generally poor quality of current nutrition. A thorough examination of the plumage can give an indication of the health and nutritional history of the bird. Deficiency in nutrients will result in structural feather defects and colour changes (Figure 12.13).

It is useful to ascertain when the bird last moulted, as feather growth rates and feather quality can be affected by nutritional deficiencies and severe malnutrition can increase the moulting interval. It must always be considered that feather abnormalities can have a variety of aetiologies (Chapter 16). All these changes are potentially reversible but owners should always be advised that improvements will take up to 18 months as new feathers will need to be produced.

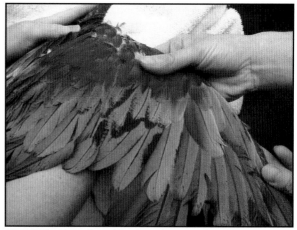

12.13 Alteration of feather pigments in a Green-winged Macaw. The black discoloration is due to exposure of the basal melanin pigments due to loss of carotenoids.

Obesity and fatty liver disease

Psittacine birds, especially Budgerigars, Cockatiels and single pet parrots, are prone to obesity as they are frequently fed high-fat seed mixes *ad libitum* without adequate opportunity to exercise. Fat becomes deposited in the subcutaneous tissues, resulting in an increased incidence of lipomas.

Fatty liver disease is common in captive parrots, especially South American species, and in cockatoos, Cockatiels and Budgerigars. Cholesterol is distributed in the body as high-density or low-density lipoproteins. High serum concentrations of low-density cholesterol lipoproteins are not desirable, as they create a predilection for fatty liver disease and atherosclerosis. The aetiology of fatty liver disease is uncertain but it has been demonstrated that feeding diets with a high saturated fat content will increase serum low-density lipoprotein cholesterol concentrations (Bavellar and Beynen, 2003). Affected birds present with abdominal enlargement; diarrhoea is a common symptom, due to chronic malabsorption. There is usually also evidence of increased respiratory effort, due to enlarged hepatic size. Enlarged livers and increased abdominal fat (Figure 12.14) are usually visible on radiographs.

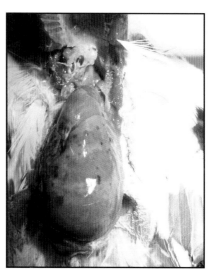

12.14 Fatty liver disease. There is gross enlargement of the liver and obvious fatty change. Histology indicated lack of normal hepatocyte architecture and replacement by adipose tissue.

Atherosclerosis can develop, with fatty infiltration of the arteries. The intima becomes replaced with fibrous tissue – a condition that is irreversible and can lead to sudden death in pet birds. Atherosclerotic vessels are sometimes radio-opaque, due to calcification. The use of hypocholesterolaemic agents has been investigated in parrots but no significant effect was seen on serum cholesterol concentrations in initial studies (Bavellar and Beynen, 2003).

Central nervous system

Ataxia and convulsions (seizures) are common clinical presentations in Grey Parrots and are usually caused by hypocalcaemia, frequently combined with vitamin D deficiency. This is discussed in detail below. Vitamin E deficiencies also cause neuropathies, but these have rarely been reported in psittacine birds.

Nutritional problems associated with vitamins

The common nutritional problems associated with vitamins are shown in Figure 12.15. The most prevalent vitamin problems involve the fat-soluble vitamins, especially vitamins A, D and E. Water-soluble vitamins are widespread in commercial diets and so deficiencies are unlikely. They may, however, occur during a time of general food deprivation. Deficiency symptoms for different water-soluble vitamins are essentially similar, including perosis, anaemia, poor feathering and dermatitis.

Vitamin A and carotenoid chemistry

Vitamin A is important for normal vision, reproduction, immunity, cellular differentiation, growth and embryonic development. A variety of carotenoid precursor forms of vitamin A are found in plants. Parrots are believed to convert these to vitamin A by intestinal enzyme activity. The requirement for maintenance in the Cockatiel has been shown to be 2000 IU/kg (Koutsos *et al.*, 2001a). Despite this, many formulated diets have levels in excess of 10,000 IU/kg.

Vitamin A deficiency is widely regarded as the most common vitamin deficiency suffered by captive parrots being fed a seed-based diet. Due to the extensive use of unsupplemented seed diets in aviculture, vitamin A deficiency is probably still the most common nutritional

Fat-soluble vitamin	Deficiency signs	Toxicity signs
Vitamin A	Keratinization of mucous membranes Squamous metaplasia of epithelial membranes Poor feathering and altered coloration Poor reproductive performance Chronic infections, especially respiratory Renal disease Poor correlation between blood vitamin A concentrations and vitamin A status of bird; liver biopsies preferable	Keratinization of mucous membranes Chronic infections, especially respiratory Increased vocalization Behavioural changes Poor reproductive performance Evidence of other fat-soluble vitamin deficiencies
Vitamin D	Decreased eggshell thickness Decreased eggshell production Decreased hatchability and increased embryonic death Osteodystrophy Clinical signs of hypocalcaemia Assay 25-hydroxycholecalciferol to evaluate vitamin D status of birds	Calcification of soft tissues Renal insufficiency Bone demineralization
Vitamin E	Poor reproductive performance Myopathies in young birds Measure serum alpha-tocopherol to assess vitamin E status	Uncommon but excess amounts might lead to deficiencies of other fat-soluble vitamins
Vitamin K	Cerebral haemorrhage in Fig-parrots (these birds are rare in captivity; in the wild they obtain vitamin K from eating termites)	Uncommon but excess amounts might lead to deficiencies of other fat-soluble vitamins

Water-soluble vitamin	Deficiency signs
Vitamin C	Not documented. Parrots synthesize vitamin C in the liver
Thiamine B_1	Seizures, opisthotonus, sudden death Rare in psittaciforms
Riboflavin B_2	Poor feathering, weakness and diarrhoea
Pyridoxine B_6	Unreported in psittacine birds
Pantothenic acid and biotin	Dermatitis and perosis, poor reproductive performance, poor feathering and ataxia
Folic acid	Poor feathering, anaemia and perosis High levels in plant materials, so deficiencies rare
Choline	Poor growth and fatty liver disease Widespread in foodstuffs, so deficiency rare

12.15 Nutritional problems associated with vitamins in parrots. Toxicities with water-soluble vitamins are unreported in psittacine birds.

disease seen in veterinary practice. Recent work with formulated diets has indicated that toxicities are also prevalent. The clinical signs for toxicity and deficiency are similar so a definitive diagnosis is difficult. Care should always be taken prior to supplementing any diet with vitamin A, as an excess of vitamin A in the diet can also cause deficiencies of other fat-soluble vitamins. Liver biopsies are more reliable than blood samples as an indicator of the vitamin A status of a parrot. The normal range is 2–5 IU vitamin A/kg.

Deficiency signs: Vitamin A deficiency affects the differentiation of epithelial cells forming the protective linings of the respiratory, urogenital and gastrointestinal tracts (Figures 12.16–12.19). These become stratified and keratinized and therefore less functional. Affected birds have an increased susceptibility to infection, resulting in the clinical signs of respiratory disease and diarrhoea. The birds show hyperkeratosis and colour changes to the feathers. There is damage to the integument, best seen in the feet. The structure of the

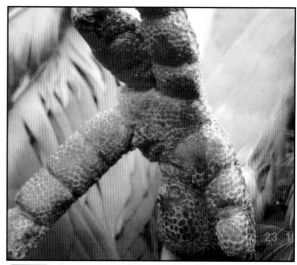

12.18 Appearance of the feet in a Blue and Gold Macaw with vitamin A deficiency. There is a loss of the epidermal architecture, making the bird predisposed to secondary foot infections.

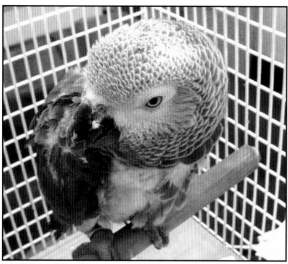

12.16 Classic appearance of a seed-fed parrot with vitamin A deficiency. The bird is poorly feathered and has respiratory symptoms.

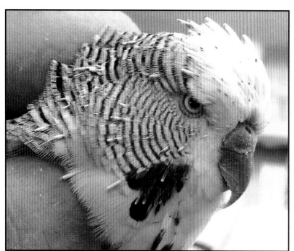

12.17 Severe hyperkeratosis due to vitamin A deficiency in a Budgerigar. The sheaths are retained and painful if manipulated.

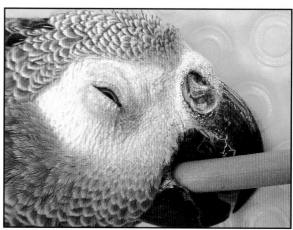

12.19 Rhinolith formation due to vitamin A deficiency causing metaplasia of the epithelial lining of the sinus. Compare the normal nostril in Figure 3.10a.

choanal slit papillae is lost. Poor reproductive performance is also common, with low hatchability and fertility. Young birds fail to grow. The epithelial cells of the tear glands may also be affected, usually characterized by a tacky discharge that sticks the eyelids together. Eventually vision will be lost, due to degeneration of both the rods and cones in the retinal tissue.

Toxicity signs: In the wild, parrots are not exposed to high levels of vitamin A as they rely on dietary conversion of carotenoids. In captivity, it was believed that up to 10 times the level recommended for poultry was safe for parrot diets, but this has recently been disproved. Toxicity leads to similar damage to the epithelial cells, producing almost identical clinical signs of respiratory, alimentary disease and poor reproductive performance (Bauck, 1995). In addition, abnormal vocalization patterns have been reported. Vitamin A toxicity has also been implicated in iron storage disease and pancreatitis in nectar eaters. Dietary excess of vitamin A can also cause a secondary deficiency of other fat-soluble vitamins D, E, and K.

Carotenoids

Carotenoids are a group of naturally occurring compounds that act as pigments in plants. They are classified into two groups: carotenes and xanthophylls. Carotenes (alpha- and beta-carotene) are important in parrot nutrition as they can be converted into vitamin A. Recent studies have indicated that Cockatiels can be maintained with diets containing as little as 2.4 mg beta-carotene/kg, reducing the risk of hypervitaminosis A (Koutsos *et al.*, 2001b). Xanthophylls are responsible for the bright colours of many bird orders. Carotenoids are now considered increasingly important as antioxidants and stimulants of the immune system in poultry (Surai, 2002).

Vitamin D

Clinical problems associated with vitamin D metabolism affect all psittacine birds, especially Grey Parrots. It is vital to consider calcium homeostasis as a whole, taking into account UV-B (315–280 nm) radiation levels, dietary calcium and vitamin D when evaluating disorders of calcium metabolism.

The vitamin D_3 metabolism of birds has been extensively reviewed. It has been established that the domestic chicken secretes 7-dehydrocholesterol (provitamin D) on to the featherless skin of the skin and feet. Conversion of the provitamin D to cholecalciferol (vitamin D_3) occurs by a UV-B-dependent isomerization reaction. Cholecalciferol is a sterol prohormone, which is subsequently activated by a two-stage hydroxylation process. Cholecalciferol is initially metabolized to 25-hydroxycholecalciferol in the liver, which is transported to the kidney via carrier proteins and converted to either 1,25-dihydroxycholecalciferol or 24,25-dihydroxycholecalciferol, the active metabolites of cholecalciferol in the domestic fowl. Research in psittacine birds has suggested a similar metabolic route. The measurement of serum 25-hydroxycholecalciferol is the best assessment of the vitamin D status of an individual. There appear to be species differences but any parrot with serum 25-hydroxycholecalciferol concentrations below 15 nmol/l should be considered vitamin D deficient.

Vitamin D levels in Grey Parrots have been shown to vary depending on dietary supply of vitamin D and on ambient UV-B light levels in a similar way to poultry (Stanford, 2003a). Most parrots are fed a diet deficient in vitamin D and calcium; additionally, they are usually kept indoors, thereby creating a UV-B deficiency. It is, therefore, not surprising that vitamin D deficiency and hypocalcaemia are commonplace.

UV-B light is an important consideration often overlooked in captive parrot husbandry. Parrots denied access to adequate natural UV-B light in the 315–280 nm spectrum could have it supplied artificially, using UV-B fluorescent bulbs (see Chapter 3). Poultry do not have a dietary requirement for vitamin D if they receive adequate UV light. Practically this equates to only 30 minutes of UV-B light daily (Klasing, 1998). Excess exposure to UV-B does not produce vitamin D toxicity, as the epithelial cells switch to produce inactive chemicals, which can be safely excreted once vitamin D requirements have been met (Holick, 1981).

The symptoms of vitamin D deficiency are discussed in the calcium section below but include juvenile osteodystrophy and convulsions (seizures) due to hypocalcaemia.

Vitamin D_3 is toxic if supplied in excessive levels in the diet, as it causes mobilization of calcium from the bone, causing hypercalcaemia, soft tissue calcification and finally renal failure. Vitamin D toxicity has been induced in macaws at lower dietary levels than in other species (1000 IU/kg). Several of the formulated diets contain levels of vitamin D_3 that are apparently in excess of requirement, so care should be taken. Poultry fed excessive vitamin D_3 use the egg as an excretion vehicle, leading to embryonic death. It is perhaps more sensible to supply a formulated diet with vitamin D_3 concentrations close to the poultry requirements but then supply adequate UV-B light to prevent toxicity problems.

Dietary supplementation with cholecalciferol is unlikely to cause toxicity signs, as it requires hydroxylation into active metabolites and this is tightly controlled by parathyroid hormone.

Vitamin E

Vitamin E is an important antioxidant in poultry and, in recent years, has received increasing attention in relation to reproduction. It has been found to be vital for male fertility, as it stabilizes sperm membrane structures. The presence of vitamin E in yolk prevents oxidation of embryonic tissues. Since 1990 vitamin levels in poultry diets have been increased by 300% (Surai, 2002).

Despite lack of research in parrots, vitamin E deficiencies have certainly been responsible for poor reproductive performance, especially in macaws. Analysis of egg yolk for vitamin E levels is useful in cases of poor fertility, poor embryonic development and weak chicks and it is thought that this will be an important area of research in psittacine medicine in the future.

In young birds vitamin E deficiency causes signs of myopathy due to encephalomalacia, but adult birds are not similarly affected. Vitamin E does not appear to be toxic.

Poor packaging or storage of parrot diets failing to avoid contact with air, light and moisture leads to rapid breakdown of vitamin E (McDonald, 2002a).

Vitamin K

The short intestinal tract in parrots would suggest dietary dependency for vitamin K, compared with intestinal manufacture by bacteria as in mammals. Despite this, vitamin K deficiencies and toxicities are rare in psittacine birds. It is thought that Fig parrots, which naturally nest in termite mounds, may have an increased requirement when kept in captivity. Whilst nest building, these birds consume vast quantities of termites containing vitamin K-forming bacteria, and they may have lost the ability to absorb and convert vitamin K from plant sources.

Nutritional problems associated with minerals

The nutritional problems associated with minerals in parrots are indicated in Figure 12.20. The most common problems are associated with disorders of calcium metabolism. The Grey Parrot is especially prone to clinical signs attributable to problems with this mineral.

Essential mineral	Deficiency signs	Toxicity signs
Calcium	Secondary nutritional hyperparathyroidism with hypocalcaemic fits and osteodystrophy Deficiency of vitamin D or excess phosphorus in the diet exacerbates problem Important common condition of Grey Parrots	Toxicity signs rare in parrots but may increase as more formulated diets with high vitamin D_3 levels are fed If high dietary levels are combined with excessive vitamin D, signs of soft tissue calcification can be seen radiographically Renal disease is sequel to chronic ingestion of high calcium diets
Phosphorus	Unlikely, as phosphorus common in most food stuffs Clinically would present with poor reproductive performance in females	Common in seed-fed diets as most seeds contain excessive phosphorus Clinically exacerbates signs of secondary nutritional hyperparathyroidism
Iron	Unusual severe chronic deficiency would lead to non-regenerative anaemia	Iron storage disease rare in psittacine birds with the potential exception of nectar eaters fed diets with high vitamin A content Clinically present as severe hepatopathies
Iodine	Traditionally common in Budgerigars Clinically present as hypothyroidism with pronounced goitre Easily prevented with commercial mineral blocks	Rarely reported in psittacine birds fed high levels of iodine supplements Clinical signs same as for deficiency
Selenium	Selenium deficiency rare in companion birds compared with poultry Poor growth rates and feathering have been reported. In severe cases myopathies can occur	Increasing evidence that levels above 5 ppm may cause embryonic death and poor reproductive behaviour Potentially in diets where selenium used as economic alternative to vitamin E
Zinc	Rare in psittacine birds. In poultry low zinc levels affect immune system and bone growth	Unusual from dietary source but potentially common from chewing toys and galvanized wire Clinically present with haemorrhagic enteritis and regurgitation Probably over-diagnosed due to large normal range. Must correlate blood values with radiographic findings and clinical signs

12.20 Nutritional disease attributed to problems with mineral metabolism.

Calcium

Calcium is the most prevalent mineral in the avian body. The dietary requirements depend on age and physiological state. Compared with adults, growing chicks have a high calcium requirement for rapid skeletal development. The laying hen has a high requirement for eggshell production.

As in mammals, calcium metabolism is tightly regulated by the action of parathyroid hormone, vitamin D and calcitonin, but the system is much more responsive in birds. For example, a chicken injected with pure parathyroid hormone will become hypercalcaemic within 8 minutes of injection, whereas in mammals this can take up to 24 hours. Many diets fed to parrots in captivity are deficient in both calcium and vitamin D, thereby creating a secondary nutritional hyperparathyroidism. Vitamin D requires adequate UV-B light in the 315–280 nm spectrum for conversion to the active metabolites and many captive parrots are kept indoors. Vitamin D plays a particularly important role in the absorption of calcium when feeding diets with low calcium content. Many birds fed a diet deficient in vitamin D and calcium suffer disorders of calcium metabolism, with symptoms ranging from osteodystrophy in young parrots to hypocalcaemic seizures and poor reproductive performance in adults. Grey Parrots have been shown to have an increased incidence of clinically significant hypocalcaemia and osteodystrophy (Figures 12.21 to 12.23) compared with other psittacine species. Bone deformity is particularly common in captive-bred hand-reared Grey Parrots (Harcourt-Brown, 2003). This may reflect an increased requirement for UV light.

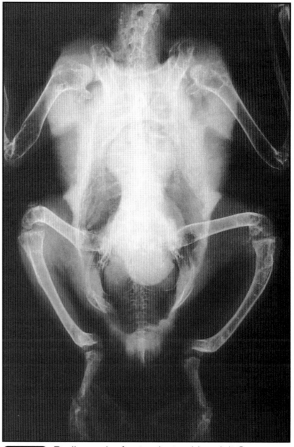

12.21 Radiograph of osteodystrophic adult Grey Parrot.

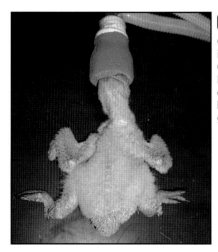

12.22

Osteodystrophy in a 5-week-old Grey Parrot. The bird was euthanased on humane grounds.

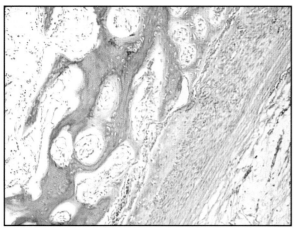

12.23 Histology of tibiotarsus from an 8-week-old Grey Parrot with juvenile osteodystrophy. There is a lack of normal mineralization and replacement of osteoid with fibrous tissue.

It is generally considered more useful to measure serum ionized calcium levels in parrots rather than total calcium levels when investigating disorders of calcium metabolism (Stanford, 2003b). Calcium exists as three fractions in the avian serum: the ionized salt; calcium bound to proteins; and complex calcium bound to a variety of anions (citrate, bicarbonate and phosphate). Ionized calcium is the physiologically active fraction of serum calcium, with a role to play in bone homeostasis, muscle and nerve conduction, blood coagulation, and the control of secretion of hormones such as vitamin D_3 and parathyroid hormone. The ionized calcium level would be expected to be maintained within a narrow range in the normal individual compared with the total calcium level, and any major change in the serum ionized calcium level is likely to be of pathological significance. The protein-bound calcium fraction is physiologically inactive and any increase would not be considered to have a pathophysiological significance. This calcium fraction is bound mainly to albumin and so any physiological or pathological condition affecting serum albumin will affect total calcium concentration, giving an imprecise result. The binding reaction between the calcium ion and albumin is strongly pH dependent so that any acid–base imbalance will affect

the ionized calcium level, though the total calcium level will be unaffected. An increase or decrease in pH will respectively increase or decrease the protein-bound calcium fraction. Most veterinary pathology laboratories still report total calcium serum concentration, which is the sum of all three calcium fractions. Blood samples for ionized calcium assays should be taken into heparin and analysed as soon as possible after venipuncture (Chapter 7).

Affected chicks often present with bowing of the tibiotarsus (Figures 12.21 and 12.22) and pathological fractures. In severe cases, radiography often reveals deformities and pathological fractures of the spine, tibiotarsi, radii and humeri, which frequently require surgical intervention (Chapter 11), or even euthanasia. Histopathology of the parathyroid glands of young Grey Parrots with radiographic evidence of osteodystrophy reveals enlargement of the glands due to chief cell vacuolation (Figure 12.24). This is evidence of secondary nutritional hyperparathyroidism due to vitamin D deficiency.

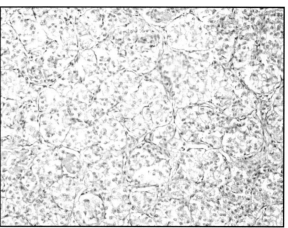

12.24 Histology of the parathyroid glands from an 8-week-old Grey Parrot with juvenile osteodystrophy. There is hypertrophy of the gland with vacuolation of the chief cells consistent with nutritional secondary hyperparathyroidism.

Adult Grey Parrots suffering from chronic hypocalcaemia present with neurological changes ranging from twitching to convulsions (seizures). The condition usually responds to injections of vitamin D and calcium supplementation in the short term. In cases of chronic hypocalcaemia, it may take several days for the clinical symptoms to resolve and for blood levels of ionized calcium to return to normal. Recurrence can be prevented by the supply of a formulated diet containing adequate calcium and vitamin D. Consideration towards providing increased UV-B radiation above the bird would also be useful. It has been shown that it is possible to alter serum ionized calcium, vitamin D and parathyroid hormone concentrations by varying dietary calcium and vitamin D in Grey Parrot diets. Exposure to increased UV light also has a significant effect on calcium metabolism in this species (Stanford, 2004).

Abnormally shaped and thin-shelled eggs are a common presentation in laying psittacine birds fed a diet deficient in either vitamin D or calcium. Embryos from hens fed a diet deficient in vitamin D_3 are weak with poor bony calcification, resulting in chicks that are unable to pip their shells and therefore often die at the end of incubation. The increased calcium required by laying birds is usually supplied by medullary bone, which can release up to 10% of the total body calcium within 24 hours, but calcium-deficient hens do not have this store (Figure 18.4). Calcium deficiency has also been implicated as a contributing factor to egg binding.

Iron

Haemochromatosis is common in frugivores and insectivores such as toucans but is rare in psittacine birds, with the exception of the lorikeet family. The high levels of vitamin A found in commercial nectar diets have been implicated in the development of iron storage disease in these birds (McDonald, 2002b). To avoid this condition, nectar diets containing < 100 ppm iron and with vitamin A concentrations of < 5000 IU/kg should be fed to lorikeets wherever possible. Tannins reduce iron absorption and might be used in nectar diets. The condition presents clinically with loss of weight and hepatomegaly. Diagnosis can be confirmed by iron analysis of liver biopsies, as blood values are unreliable. Treatment is difficult, as it involves repeated phlebotomy or chelation therapy (Chapter 20).

Selenium

Although most research involving selenium involves aquatic birds, selenium toxicity is receiving increasing interest amongst aviculturists experiencing poor breeding performance. Selenium is an antioxidant similar in activity to vitamin E and for economic reasons selenium is used in place of vitamin E in formulated diets. Selenium toxicity produces poor reproductive performance in poultry, with increased embryonic death, reduced hatchability, increased teratogenesis and reduced fertility. It would be expected to be a differential in any investigation of poor psittacine reproduction if the diet fed contained more than 5 mg/kg selenium (Klasing, 1998).

Zinc

Zinc toxicosis has been reported in a number of parrots, but its diagnosis may be exaggerated due to the large serum zinc range (17–44 µmol/l) in normal birds. There are also taxonomic differences for normal zinc concentrations. Any potential diagnosis should be correlated with both clinical signs and a serum zinc level > 50 µmol/l. Clinical signs include acute gastroenteritis, haemorrhagic droppings and regurgitation. Toxicity is rarely of dietary origin but usually due to ingestion of zinc from galvanized toys or cages. Treatment involves chelation therapy and removal of the toxic source of zinc (Chapter 20).

Iodine

Chronic iodine deficiency is only commonly seen in Budgerigars fed a poor quality seed diet without adequate supplementation. Packaged seed mixes and formulated diets tend to be supplemented with iodine. Affected birds develop a thyroid hyperplasia or goitre and are clinically obese due to the resulting reduction in metabolic rate. This is a non-specific finding in many seed eaters fed *ad libitum* and a more reliable clinical sign is a change of voice due to pressure on the syrinx from the hyperplasic thyroid glands. Affected birds also develop a characteristic click on inspiration. Definitive diagnosis is difficult, due to the problems associated with dynamic thyroid testing in psittacine birds; presumptive diagnosis is based on clinical signs, dietary history and response to treatment. The condition can be treated by the introduction of Lugol's iodine to the drinking water (Chapter 21), or by the use of the commercial 'pink' iodine mineral blocks.

Iodine deficiency is less common in larger parrots, but hypothyroidism has occasionally been implicated in feather disorders in macaws. Currently, thyroid testing is inadequate for these birds, making diagnosis difficult. 'Trial' treatments are considered hazardous, due to the risk of inducing iatrogenic hyperthyroidism.

Diets for growing birds

Hand rearing parrot chicks following artificial incubation of eggs is common practice in the captive-bird trade, in order to increase the production of healthy tame birds (Chapter 18). Incorrect hand rearing can lead to acute nutritional imbalances, as the growth of parrot chicks is so rapid (growing birds can increase their body weight by up to 20% daily). Traditionally, homemade rearing diets are based on human commercial baby foods, which are imbalanced for parrot chicks. Recently, formulated parrot rearing diets have become available, dramatically improving results. Although scientific studies are lacking for rearing foods, formulated foods produce more consistent results than homemade diets. The key features of common formulated rearing diets are indicated in Figure 12.25.

Diet	Vitamin A (IU/kg)	Vitamin D (IU/kg)	Vitamin E (IU/kg)	Calcium (%)	Protein (%)	Fat (%)	Comments
ZuPreem Embrace	–	–	–	–	22	9	For Old World parrots such as Cockatoos
ZuPreem Embrace plus	–	–	–	–	19	13	For New World parrots
Harrisons Neonate	11,000	1000	300	0.8	26	14	Easily digestible Designed for first 2–3 weeks

12.25 Nutritional analysis of popular formulated rearing diets. (Information provided by the manufacturers; dash indicates information unavailable.) (continues) ▶

Diet	Vitamin A (IU/kg)	Vitamin D (IU/kg)	Vitamin E (IU/kg)	Calcium (%)	Protein (%)	Fat (%)	Comments
Harrisons Juvenile Formula	11,000	1650	450	0.8	18	11	Designed to be fed up to weaning. Author has found juvenile formula useful supportive diet for ill psittacine birds
Kaytee Exact Macaws	–	–	–	–	22	8	
Pretty Bird	–	–	–	–	22 19 19 19	10 12 12 8	Four products to attempt to cater for all species
Roudybush Squab Formula	10,000	1400	–	1.45	50	9.5	Attempt to recreate crop milk for feeding from day 1
Roudybush Formula 3	10,000	1400	–	0.9	21	7	
Harrisons Recovery Diet	5000	1000	300	0.8	35	19	Designed for avian patients to provide nutrients easily; given by syringe or crop tube

12.25 (continued) Nutritional analysis of popular formulated rearing diets. (Information provided by the manufacturers; dash indicates information unavailable.)

Parent-reared birds have improved growth rates compared with hand-reared chicks and it is proposed that this is due to the parents providing protective molecules or commensal microflora to the chicks. They would also provide more regular meals. Hand rearing from birth is a time-consuming and difficult task and a sensible compromise is to leave the parents to rear the chicks for 3–4 weeks and then hand rear to weaning. Feeding behaviour in young parrots is learned, so it is simple and advisable to wean chicks on to formulated diets rather than seed mixes. Many manufacturers produce weaning diets, which aid this transition to solid food.

Feeding nectarivores

Lorikeets are unusual parrots in that they consume predominately plant nectars. They are kept in captivity because of their bright coloration. They have specific nutritional needs, which makes them difficult to keep outside zoological collections. Their tongues have numerous papillae and bristles, which effectively increase the surface area for nectar collection by capillary action. Although nectar is essentially just a sugar solution, whilst drinking it these birds consume large quantities of pollen, which is an excellent supply of protein. They have a lower protein requirement than other parrots (1–3% dry matter), due to reduced intestinal loss of nitrogen. Parents feeding a mainly insect-based diet supply the higher protein requirement of young nectarivores.

In captivity the birds are usually fed one of a number of commercial nectar substitutes. It has been suggested that most of these have excessive levels of vitamin A, despite available data suggesting low requirements in psittacine birds (McDonald, 2002b). These diets may be the cause of vitamin A toxicity in lorikeets, particularly haemochromatosis (iron storage disease), which is reported in this group. A nectar mix containing < 5000 IU vitamin A/kg diet is advisable.

As nectar mixes are ideal media for bacterial or fungal growth, excellent hygiene is vital and food dishes should be cleaned and disinfected daily. Nectar mix should be made fresh for each feed and refrigerated prior to use.

Nutrition of unhealthy parrots

Anorexia is a common symptom in diseased birds. The nutritional requirements of ill parrots differ from those of healthy birds in that they need increased energy, fat, protein, vitamin and minerals in their diet. Commercially prepared juvenile hand rearing formulae can be used to supply these additional nutrients to diseased adult birds. Also, as anorexia is common, these foods have the advantage that they can be tube fed. This field is gaining more interest and there is a recovery diet specifically produced for ill parrots.

Practical diets for captive parrots

The aim of this chapter has been to present the current scientific data on parrot nutrition in order to enable the reader to recommend an appropriate diet. The key points of captive parrot nutrition are as follows:

- Diets should be based on a formulated parrot food forming at least 50% of total diet
- Avoid seed-based diets and temperate fruits contributing more than 10% of total diet
- Only use human-quality foodstuffs, to prevent exposure to pathogens
- Dark-pigmented vegetables are nutritionally superior to fruits
- Use organic produce wherever possible
- Consider UV-B supplementation

- Take great care with vitamin and mineral supplementation. Formulated diets do not need additional supplementation.

The following are suggested practical diets for large and small parrots.

Large parrots

- Feed a formulated diet with nutritional contents that meet the known requirements for psittacine birds.
- To provide interest, supply organic vegetables, fruits and pulses as recommended by the formulated diet manufacturer. This element should not be more than 10% of the total diet.
- Do not supplement further with seeds, vitamins or minerals.
- Provide grit.
- Provide some UV-B light (315–280 nm) either artificially or naturally. It should be noted that glass and most plastics filter out UV-B radiation.
- Always supply clean fresh water. The addition of organic cider vinegar (one drop per 200 ml) helps to prevent overgrowth of common potential pathogens.

Generally this diet should be adequate for maintenance but in situations when birds have increased requirements (moulting, breeding and growth) it is useful to vary the diet by:

- Increasing protein
- Increasing fat
- Increasing vitamins A, D and E
- Increasing calcium and phosphorus.

Manufacturers now produce specific diets in an attempt to supply these increased needs (Figure 12.11).

Small psittacine birds

Budgerigars and Cockatiels tend towards granivorous feeding behaviour and are frequently difficult to convert to formulated diets. A suitable dietary compromise is as follows:

- Feed a branded clean boxed seed mixture consisting of the smaller clean millet seeds
- Sprout some of the seed and ensure this is constantly available to the birds. Sprouting seeds must always be rinsed thoroughly and refrigerated to prevent fermentation
- Always provide an iodine block and grit
- Always supply fresh water.

Useful addresses

The formulated diets discussed in the chapter are not always easily available through the pet trade but can all be purchased mail order through the internet:

Harrisons Bird foods www.harrisonsbirdfoods.com
Kaytee Products Incorporated www.kaytee.com
Mazuri Diets www.mazuri.com
Pretty Bird International www.prettybird.com
Rolf C. Hagen Corporation www.hagen.com
Roudybush foods www.roudybush.com
ZuPreem Diets www.ZuPreem.com

The vitamin and mineral supplements discussed can be obtained through pet retail outlets or at the following internet sites:

Bird Care Company www.birdcareco.com
Vetark Products www.vetark.co.uk

13

Systemic infectious disease

Michael Lierz

Viral diseases

Pacheco's disease

Aetiology and pathogenesis
Pacheco's disease is caused by a psittacine-specific β-herpesvirus with different strains showing differences in their pathogenicity. It is not transmissible to other avian species. It belongs to the same group of herpesviruses that cause inclusion body hepatitis in other avian species, but does not share common antigens. It is excreted mainly in faeces but also in other body fluids. A vertical transmission of the virus is also suggested. Infection may be airborne or oral. The incubation period is short, being approximately 7 days. The virus primarily infects lymphatic tissue, epithelial cells (skin, hepatocytes) and nerve cells but also reproduces in several organs, leading to multiple small foci of necrosis, mainly in liver, spleen and kidneys. As with other herpesviruses, latently infected birds (carrier birds) are common and the virus can persist for life. In situations of stress or immune depression the disease can recur, even years after infection. Latently infected birds shed the virus irregularly, often for years whilst appearing in good health. Macaws and Amazons seem to be more susceptible to the disease than other psittacine birds. In pet bird practice the disease is uncommon but in quarantine stations (wild-caught birds) or import facilities big losses are described, which can be transmitted to breeding establishments on fomites or by carriers.

Clinical signs
Clinical signs are rare as most birds die suddenly. In surviving cases the birds are depressed and pass watery droppings with green to bronze urates. Central nervous system (CNS) signs can occur.

Diagnosis
Sudden death in quarantine stations or in newly imported birds is always suspicious.

On post-mortem examination (PME), a finding of multiple necrotic foci in the liver and spleen of a bird with good body condition suggests herpesvirus infection (Pacheco's disease; Figures 13.1 and 13.2). Similar findings in a bird with poor nutritional status are more likely to be due to salmonellosis or tuberculosis (see Figure 13.12). Both chlamydophilosis and yersiniosis can cause similar pale necrotic areas on the liver, but necrosis from *Chlamydophila* is usually in irregular

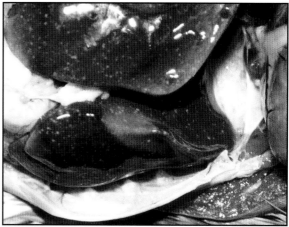

13.1 Multiple necrosis of the liver due to an infection with Pacheco's disease. Note the very small white spots, mostly of the same size. Compare with Figure 13.12 (tuberculosis). A direct smear with Ziehl–Neelsen stain may help a quick diagnosis. Salmonellosis may also cause multiple spots on the liver (see Figure 13.2) and must be considered for differential diagnosis.

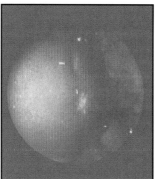

13.2 An endoscopic view of a liver with multiple necrotic foci. Such foci seldom protrude above the surface of an organ. Differential diagnoses would be Pachecho's disease and salmonellosis. Tuberculosis is usually different (see Figures 13.12 and 7.32).

patches and yellow (not white), while *Yersinia* will induce granulomas on the intestinal wall as well as the liver.

Liver, spleen and kidneys are enlarged (also on radiographs). When birds do not die during leucocytosis, a leucopenia follows. The diagnosis must be confirmed by a virological examination (tissue samples, swabs) and isolation of the virus. Histological examination of the liver and spleen shows intranuclear inclusion bodies (Type Cowdry A). The detection of antibodies is subject to false negative results, as the birds are presented peracute or die before developing antibodies. Latently infected birds produce only low levels of virus-neutralizing antibodies.

Therapy and prophylaxis

Treatment is too late for most ill birds. Parenteral application of aciclovir can be tried. Contact birds can be treated orally. The treatment might avoid a clinical disease but not a latent infection.

Vaccines are available in the USA but not in Europe. The killed vaccine is based on an isolate from a parrot. According to the manufacturer, it should be used in birds on arrival in quarantine and in other birds at least 4 weeks prior to a stress situation or breeding season. Basic immunization is performed with two subcutaneous injections with a 4-week interval. A single booster dose is given annually. As different strains of Pacheco's disease virus have been demonstrated, it is suggested that this vaccination with one single isolate does not protect against all serotypes of the virus. Collection-specific vaccines (isolation of the virus from an affected collection and producing a vaccine from this) has given questionable results.

Pox

Aetiology and pathogenesis

There are a number of different strains of avipoxvirus that are more or less host specific. It is presumed that psittacine birds do have their own specific avipoxvirus, but crossing family or species barriers might be possible. Avipoxviruses are enveloped and very stable, especially in dry environments (up to several months). The pathogen is sensitive to most disinfectants but requires a long disinfection time (up to 90 minutes).

Avipoxvirus is mainly shed in sloughed crusty skin or diphtheritic mucous membranes. The pathogen is unable to invade healthy epidermis and needs damage to the epithelial barrier (e.g. a wound or insect bite). After initially multiplying in the epidermis (primary viraemia), the virus spreads to liver and bone marrow for a second replication (secondary viraemia). After the secondary viraemia the virus invades the rest of the organs, leading to the death of the bird. In most cases of the disease secondary viraemia does not occur; pox in parrots is often a localized disease affecting the skin and mucous membranes only.

This disease will cause latently infected birds. Whether it produces lifelong carriers is questionable but this cannot be excluded.

Clinical signs

This disease is most frequently seen in imported birds. Different clinical forms are described. Most commonly a skin and a diphtheritic form is seen in psittacine birds. Tumours, CNS or septicaemic forms as described in other avian species are rarely seen but should be kept in mind.

The diphtheritic form develops as a yellow crusty coating in the oral cavity, which seldom affects the crop and oesophagus. Bleeding occurs if this coating is removed. In some cases this coating is so thick that the bird is unable to swallow and risks suffocation. The diphtheritic form of pox should be a differential diagnosis for trichomoniasis and candidiasis. Occasionally the disease spreads to the heart muscle or mucous membranes of the intestine, causing severe illness.

In many cases the skin form of pox develops as well or is seen without the diphtheritic form. First signs are small brown thickenings on the unfeathered skin. These develop into crusty areas, causing greasy and wet skin wounds. Usually the skin form is a self-limiting infection, but secondary infection with bacteria or fungus complicates the clinical signs. In some cases the skin form is often limited to the eye only, and keratitis, uveitis and scarring of the eyelids are seen.

Diagnosis

Skin lesions or diphtheritic material can be used to confirm the diagnosis by demonstrating avipoxvirus DNA in a PCR test (which also allows differentiation of different strains). Skin biopsies of affected areas can be examined by histology. Eosinophilic intracytoplasmic inclusion bodies (Bollinger bodies) are pathognomonic for the disease. In addition the virus can be demonstrated by electron microscopy. Isolation of the virus is possible in cell culture and on the chorioallantoic membrane of chicken embryos. Detection of antibodies against avian pox is not reliable as the antibody response to an avipox infection can be poor.

Therapy and prophylaxis

There are no antiviral drugs for these avipoxviruses but the disease is usually self-limiting within 3–4 weeks. Secondary infections must be treated using antibiotics and antimycotics. Lesions of the skin and mucous membranes can be disinfected by using iodine (povidone–iodine and glycerine as a 1:4 mixture). Many psittacine birds have a vitamin A deficiency; the administration of vitamin A aids recovery of these birds. In mild cases the lesions normally heal completely, but severe cases will become scarred. Biting arthropods (e.g. mosquitoes, mites) must be controlled to reduce the spreading of the disease in a collection of aviary birds.

Vaccination is not possible at present, due to the lack of a psittacine vaccine. The use of vaccine produced for other species (canaries, pigeons, turkeys, chickens) is very questionable and will not protect the host, as the psittacine avipoxvirus is a different strain.

Paramyxovirus infection

Under the Diseases of Poultry (England) Order 2003, Newcastle disease and avian influenza are notifiable diseases (Chapter 22). Those who suspect the presence of either of these diseases in a bird or carcass that they own or have charge of *must* inform the local Department for Environment, Food and Rural Affairs (DEFRA) Divisional Veterinary Manager (DVM). The same applies to a person who examines or inspects any bird or carcass or who analyses any samples taken from any bird or carcass and suspects these diseases.

Aetiology and pathogenesis

Avian paramyxoviruses are divided into nine different serotypes. In psittacine birds PMV-1 and PMV-3 are of importance. Both are shed in all bodily secretions and are stable in the environment.

PMV-1 causes Newcastle disease in poultry, but all avian species are considered susceptible to this disease. In some countries it can be seen regularly in psittacine birds but in Europe it is rare, due to the vaccination programmes in poultry. In most countries it is a notifiable disease in poultry. The virulence of PMV-1 differs between strains. The strains are divided into lentogenic (no virulence), mesogenic (some virulence) and velogenic (very virulent) for chickens. This pathogenic potential can be different in other avian species: lentogenic strains in poultry can be velogenic for psittacine birds. This should be borne in mind when vaccinating psittacines with live attenuated vaccine from poultry, especially as in some countries mesogen strains of PMV-1 are used for vaccine production. Latent infections are possible and a considerable problem in the epidemiology of the disease. PMV-1 can be airborne and spread by inhalation but will also infect via the oral route. Target cells for the virus are epithelial cells in the respiratory and digestive tract as well as in the kidney and CNS.

PMV-3 has been isolated from different psittacine birds and mainly affects grass parakeets, Cockatiels and lovebirds. The PMV-3 virus affecting these birds can be differentiated from the PMV-3 virus affecting turkeys by monoclonal antibodies.

Clinical signs

PMV-1 infections can be peracute, with no clinical signs before death, but in most cases respiratory and intestinal symptoms develop. The birds are depressed and stop eating. Later CNS signs such as torticollis, loss of equilibrium, opisthotonus (Figure 13.3) and tremors occur.

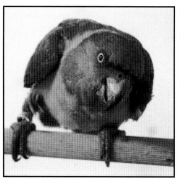

13.3 Oblique positioning of the head is often a first CNS sign accompanying a paramyxovirus infection.

Within a collection it is usual to see the full range of clinical signs: a few birds will show CNS signs; other birds die without any clinical signs. According to the pathogenicity of the strain, PMV-1 can also cause a latent infection or only mild symptoms. In such cases the birds are depressed for a few days without further symptoms. PMV-1 is a zoonosis and is able to cause severe conjunctivitis in humans.

PMV-3 infections are comparable to PMV-1 infections but in most cases not as severe. Mostly only mild CNS symptoms occur. In collections the death rate, especially of young birds, is increased. PMV-3 should always be considered in grass parakeets with CNS signs (circling and torticollis). These birds do not recover. On PME, pancreatitis is regularly seen.

Diagnosis

Tissue samples or cloacal swabs can be used for virus detection and isolation. By isolation, a positive result is often possible after a few days, as a negative result can only be reliable after several passages of the sample (about 4 weeks). Some strains from psittacine birds need to adapt to the chicken cell culture or chicken embryo host, which are used for isolation of the pathogen. The isolated virus is confirmed as PMV-1 or PMV-3 by haemagglutination and haemagglutination inhibition tests. Diagnosis is also possible by agar gel precipitation test or PCR using tissue samples. In non-vaccinated birds the detection of antibodies using the haemagglutination inhibition test is possible for a faster diagnosis. This allows also the differentiation of PMV-1 and PMV-3.

Therapy and prophylaxis

There is no specific treatment. Supportive symptomatic treatment might allow some birds to survive the disease. Hyperimmune serum can be used in exposed birds, especially in valuable breeding birds. Using both methods there is a high risk of infecting other birds or spreading the virus to other collections. As the disease is also highly contagious for other birds, euthanasia is usually recommended. CNS signs do not improve.

Psittacine birds must be vaccinated with killed vaccines (poultry or pigeon vaccines), because of the risk in using attenuated live virus for vaccination (see above). Live vaccine has been suggested as an emergency vaccination as it causes a competitive inhibition to the field strain. In most countries the vaccination of PMV-1 is regulated by law. For turkeys a PMV-3 vaccine is available and might be used in psittacine birds as well.

Psittacine beak and feather disease (PBFD)

Aetiology and pathogenesis

Psittacine beak and feather disease (PBFD) is caused by a very small circovirus and is one of the most common and most important viral disease of psittacine birds. The pathogen is very stable in the environment and it is suggested that it remains infectious for years. In addition it is resistant to many disinfectants. Circovirus infections are known in other avian species but the PBFD virus seems to be pathogenic only for psittacine birds. Within the group of psittacine birds different PBFD virus strains are present and are probably species specific. The virus is shed in feather powder and faeces for several months after infection. Infections occur by inhalation of contaminated feather dust, oral intake of fresh or dried faeces, or crop secretions. Vertical transmission is also possible. The virus is spread very easily by people having contaminated feather dust on their clothes as well as via vectors such as air, food, food utensils and travelling boxes.

The virus prefers dividing cells. The target organs for the virus are primarily replicating immune tissue (cloacal bursa and thymus), but also skin and feather follicles as well as oesophagus and crop cells and bone marrow. Therefore, in addition to feather loss and malformation, PBFD can also be a fatal systemic problem featuring severe immunodeficiency.

The incubation period varies according to the age of the infected bird. In nestlings it might be only 2–4 weeks whereas in older birds it can be years. In general, psittacine birds younger than 3 years seem to be more susceptible to the disease but older birds will also develop signs. The disease appears to thrive in young birds with poorly developed immune systems. Once the bursa, and presumably thymus, is involuted the virus is less likely to cause clinical signs. Hand-reared birds are more frequently affected. Also, the older the bird, the longer is the period between infection and clinical signs. Finally, in birds with adult immune systems the majority mount an immune response to the virus and remove the virus from their body.

The course of the disease is very variable and latent infection birds shedding the virus are common. This explains why it is very difficult to eliminate the virus from an infected population and why many collections are now positive. Vertical transmission also occurs. PBFD is a very common disease in avian practice. Importantly not only is the 'typical' form with feather loss and deformities seen regularly, but also illness and death in nestlings and young birds are commonly caused by a circovirus.

Clinical signs

Different courses of the disease have been described, depending mostly on the age of the infected bird. However, up to now, the disease has always proved fatal.

Peracute: This is mostly in newly hatched birds (cockatoos, Grey Parrots). Breeders report an unexplained increased death rate in young chicks. Most birds die without showing any clinical signs, some are depressed and a few have pneumonia and diarrhoea. There are no diagnostic post-mortem signs.

Acute: This is mostly in nestlings during the period of feather growth up to a few weeks after leaving the nest box, or in some cases in young birds up to 1 year of age. The birds are depressed and have diarrhoea; due to the immunodeficiency other disease might be more obvious (pneumonia). The feathers are often affected and a pathognomonic sign is the loss of powder down, which is especially obvious in parrots with a black beak: instead of having a white powdery covering (see Figure 5.6), the beak becomes shiny and black (Figure 13.4). However, not all birds with a shiny black beak are infected with circovirus.

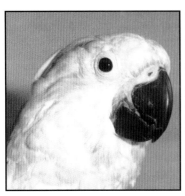

13.4 This Umbrella Cockatoo has a black shiny beak and dirty feathers. These are often the first signs of PBFD as the production of powder down ceases due to viral damage of the down feathers. (Compare Figure 5.6.)

Growing feathers might be malformed or feather colour changes might occur (e.g. Grey Parrots develop red body contour feathers; or Vasa Parrots, which are normally black, develop white feathers). In African parrots the most obvious sign is usually a severe heteropenia, which can also be accompanied by a general leucopenia and anaemia.

The acute form of PBFD is now the most common course of the disease. Unexplained problems in collections should always initiate a test for PBFD. Ill young parrots presenting a severe leucopenia are nearly always positive for PBFD. A negative sample from such a bird should never exclude this disease and further samples and different PCR tests must be initiated (see below). PME shows signs of anaemia and various secondary infections, especially aspergillosis.

Chronic: This is the best known form of PBFD and occurs mainly in older birds. The most obvious clinical signs are feather loss and feather deformity; this is usually worst in growing feathers and increasing from moult to moult. Again, the first sign in Grey Parrots and cockatoos is a glossy black beak (Figure 13.4). The feather changes are often followed by secondary infections due to the immunodeficiency. In later stages the beak and claws become very brittle and have a necrotic layer under the brittle outer horn. The disease is always fatal but this can be several years after the initial clinical signs.

The changes in the plumage can differ due to the damage of the feather follicle. Symmetrical feather loss starts with the tail feathers. Owners often assume that the bird is self-plucking. Importantly the feather loss (or damage) also includes head feathers (Figure 13.5) and this is a most important differential diagnosis: head feathers are not usually involved in self-plucking birds.

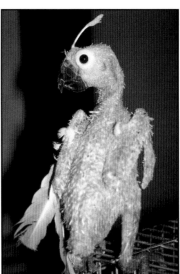

13.5 PBFD in a cockatoo. Note that all feathers, including head feathers, are involved in the disease process.

Growing feathers become curved (Figure 13.6) and the feathers break. As this occurs in blood feathers, the feather stump is covered with a dried bloody crust. Last but not least, the feather sheath of the growing feather persists and the colour of the feather might change (Figure 13.7). Budgerigars lose their major wing and tail feathers. Circovirus is one of the causes of the syndrome known by budgie breeders as 'French moult'.

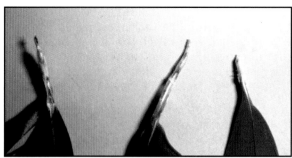

13.6 Round shape of feathers that have fallen off due to PBFD infection. (Compare Figure 2.2)

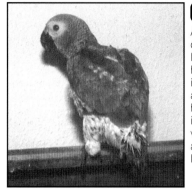

13.7

A Grey Parrot with circovirus infection. Its flight feathers have dropped out, its tail feathers are deformed, and it has pink feathers on its wings, neck and ventral abdomen. It also has a severe leucopenia.

Clinically inconspicuous form: This is mostly in older birds, shedding the virus. These birds are mainly responsible for contaminating collections and spreading the virus. This form is common in Budgerigars, Cockatiels and cockatoos.

Diagnosis

The disease is common in newly purchased hand-reared parrots, especially Grey Parrots. New owners of (expensive) birds that die because of this virus usually wish to make a claim against the source of the infected bird. It is vital that the diagnosis of circovirus infection is performed in a professional manner. The diagnosis must be confirmed by detection of the pathogen. Cultural isolation of circovirus has proved impossible so far. Reliable PCR tests have been developed to detect PBFD virus DNA and this is the method of choice.

All PCR tests are very sensitive and the tissues for testing must be harvested in a sterile manner to avoid contamination by psittacine circovirus from other sources. The virus is most easy to recover from growing tissues but there are many reasons why the test can lead to a false negative result. Feather pulp from growing feathers has been suggested to be the easiest source of virus and this is true, but not all growing feathers contain circovirus, especially in birds without feather lesions. Also, many Grey Parrots are presented with this disease at 3–6 months of age, when there are no growing feathers to sample. In such cases a blood sample should be taken, as the virus is usually present in circulating white blood cells. In cases where there is a massive leucopenia, this can also give a false negative result in the PCR examination.

The most useful source of test material in live birds under 12 months old is bone marrow. This can be obtained under general anaesthetic using a 23 G

$^3/_4$ inch needle on a 2 ml syringe so that it is 'drilled' into the medullary cavity of the tibiotarsus. The best approach is from the tibial plateau on the medial aspect of the knee.

If the bird is dead the cloacal bursa, thymus, bone marrow and liver are all useful sites. False negative results are always possible and must be borne in mind. It is economic to submit bursal tissue first but retain the other tissues frozen (and also a range of fixed tissues, including half the bursa) so that an unexpected false negative result can be checked by further PCR tests, and if necessary by light or electron microscopy.

In general the interpretation of PCR results for PBFD is difficult as false negative result can occur due to different circovirus strains in parrots; also not all PCRs used in the laboratories are able to detect all strains. In addition, the sensitivity of PCRs varies between laboratories. In cases where the clinical and other examinations strongly suggest a case of circovirus but a negative PCR result is given, additional samples or a different PCR or laboratory should be used to confirm the diagnosis. Other examinations (such as electron microscopy of the bursa of Fabricius or bone marrow) will also be helpful.

Histological examinations of skin biopsies that include a growing feather and bursa of Fabricius show characteristic changes (basophilic intracytoplasmic and intranuclear inclusion bodies) but this is not as reliable as the PCR test. Circovirus can also be demonstrated by electron microscopy. The most important differential diagnosis for PBFD is polyomavirus infection but this is usually less common.

Therapy and prophylaxis

Birds with clinical signs of PBFD have invariably died. Reports of successful treatments are rare. Para-immuninducer (Baypamun) has been tried, but as the main problem in parrots is the virus-induced immunodeficiency the use of such a drug is questionable. Recently interferon (derived from poultry) has been used. First reports are promising with 7 of 10 infected Grey Parrots showing regeneration of their bone marrow and becoming negative for circovirus (by PCR) after intramuscular injection daily for 90 days with 1 million units of avian interferon. This treatment should be investigated further. The use of commercial feline interferon at the same dose was not satisfactory (Stanford, 2004).

In spite of the above, sick birds in collections of breeding birds should be euthanased. Single pet birds might be treated with a supportive treatment and interferon, but they still represent a risk of spreading the disease via the owner. Feather loss might be acceptable, but beak and claw changes are painful and are usually the reason for euthanasia of chronic cases. The supportive treatment focuses on the stabilization of the immune system (vitamin A, probiotics) and the treatment of secondary infections (antibiotics, antimycotics).

In collections, infected birds should be removed. All cages, including all furniture, and clothes of the keepers must be disinfected with glutaraldehyde. As no vaccine is available, the most important prevention is hygiene and the quarantine of newly arrived birds. This is most useful if the collection is known to be free of

PBFD. Newly acquired birds should be tested (feather and blood, and in doubtful cases bone marrow). In the case of a positive result, the bird should be retested in 90 days. If the result is still positive, the bird should be removed. Cases that become negative, with no clinical signs, could have eliminated the virus or the first sample may have been contaminated.

Polyomavirus infection

Aetiology and pathogenesis
Polyomavirus infection was first described in Budgerigars (Budgerigar fledgling disease) but it has been found in other parrots, especially lovebirds, macaws and Eclectus Parrots. In Budgerigars, especially in youngsters, the disease is more likely to be fatal; in the others it is chronic or subclinical. The pathogen is very stable in the environment and is spread through persistent shedding from latently infected adult birds (mainly Budgerigars) and via fomites. The virus is excreted in faeces as well as skin and feather dust and can be transferred vertically. Latently infected adult birds transmit the virus to their immunoincompetent youngsters. The young birds may develop a tolerance to the virus and persistently shed the virus even if antibodies are present. These young birds are mainly responsible for spreading the pathogen to other flocks and infecting youngsters from healthy parents. Naive young birds may develop a severe disease and die. As with circovirus, the age of the bird at the time of infection is important.

Polyomavirus infection is the most important differential diagnosis for PBFD, especially in cases of feather deformities or in cases of a high nestling mortality in psittacine collections.

Clinical signs
The clinical appearance of the disease depends on the psittacine species affected and the age of the bird.

Peracute and acute forms: These are mainly reported from Budgerigar nestlings and can affect a collection severely, with up to 100% mortality. Other psittacine species can also be affected but usually less severely. Sudden death may occur in nestlings that are just about to leave the nest box. Younger birds are lethargic and weak and they tremble. The skin and sometimes the urates turn yellow (due to liver damage), and petechial bleeding in the subcutis and feather follicles can be observed. Polyomavirus infection must be considered whenever a breeder reports problems in hatching psittacine birds with increased losses or development problems in nestlings. Sudden death and CNS signs have been reported in adult parrots other than Budgerigars. Some birds have delayed crop-emptying times.

Chronic form: This form appears mainly in nestlings infected at more than 2 weeks of age, or who are protected by maternal antibodies. Budgerigars usually develop more severe clinical signs. Feather growth is affected and mainly large feathers (wing and tail) fall off first. This condition is another cause of 'French moult'. New growing feathers are deformed and curled and feather sheaths persist. The round curves, as seen in PBFD, are usually missing. The disease is progressive and also small contour feathers are involved later on. Down feathers are often without changes but as in PBFD they might be involved as well. Subsequently the birds are unable to fly and run mostly on the ground. The general state of health is often not disturbed. In some cases the feather changes resolve.

Inapparent infection: Latently infected birds, especially adult Budgerigars, are common. They shed the virus intermittently and have high levels of antibodies but do not develop clinical signs. In stressful situations (e.g. breeding, exhibition, new environment) they can develop feather changes and clinical signs.

Diagnosis
There may be massive problems in Budgerigar collections, with an increased mortality in nestlings, subcutaneous petechial bleeding and feather changes all giving suspicion for the diagnosis. Circovirus infection is the major differential. The diagnostic method of choice is the detection of polyomavirus DNA using a PCR test. Isolation of the virus is possible in cell cultures but will take some time. The inside of the cloaca (urodeum) should be vigorously swabbed. Feather material can be used, as can blood or tissue samples (spleen, liver). It is possible to have birds infected with both polyomavirus and circovirus. The detection of antibodies in the serum is possible using a virus neutralization test. It is used in Budgerigars but false negative results occur, especially in acute cases. Histological examination can demonstrate baso- or amphiphilic intranuclear inclusion bodies in feather follicles, kidney, liver and spleen.

Therapy and prophylaxis
No treatment is available. Single pet birds that cannot fly can be kept in cages adapted for climbing rather than flying. Secondary infections should be treated, mainly using antibiotics.

In outbreaks in a Budgerigar collection, breeding should cease for at least 3–4 months. During this time the pathogen can spread to all adult individuals in the collection, which produces protective levels of antibodies. Maternal antibody protects the future nestlings from the acute form of the disease, but feather damage can still occur. Young birds can carry the virus when sold, and newly arrived birds will be unprotected. For these reasons, this might only be an option for private bird keepers. In breeding facilities, as well as employing disinfectant and hygiene measures, attempts should be made to eliminate the virus by removing positive birds. Newly acquired birds should be kept in quarantine and tested repeatedly on cloacal swabs by PCR testing. As Budgerigars are a reservoir for the virus, they should not be kept with other psittacine birds.

No vaccine is available in Europe, but in the USA there is a killed vaccine based on a psittacine isolate. To avoid pathogens contaminating the vaccine, gentamicin and amphotericin B are included. According to the manufacturer, the vaccine should be used in newly acquired birds after arrival in quarantine and in other birds at least 8 weeks prior to the breeding season. Basic immunization is performed with two subcutaneous injections with a 4-week interval; thereafter a single dose is given annually.

Papillomatosis

Aetiology and pathogenesis
This appears to be a virally induced disease. The causative pathogen has not been proven, but it has been suggested that herpesvirus, rather than papillomavirus, plays a role in this disease. Recent investigations have demonstrated herpesvirus DNA in many psittacine papillomas but not in all. Typical findings are proliferative epidermal masses on the mucous membranes, especially in the cloaca. The disease tends to occur in aviaries in pairs of birds; it has been suggested that the disease is transferred during pair-bond feeding and copulation as well as feeding of young birds. In general, therefore, only a few pairs of birds in a collection will show clinical signs, but in rare cases the disease can become a massive problem.

Clinical signs
In most cases the cloaca is involved in the pathogenic process (Figure 13.8). Birds are usually presented with considerable faecal soiling of the feathers around the vent, or with inflamed tissue prolapsed through the cloaca. Sometimes droppings are bloody (Appendix 2) or the bird may struggle to pass the droppings. If the cloaca is everted, a diffuse inflammation is seen involving masses that are like blackberries in shape and size. In some cases papillomas are also present in the oral cavity (especially around the choana and laryngeal entrance); in others papillomas are present throughout the alimentary tract. Most birds with papillomatosis have cyclical signs. When they are unwell they can be inappetent, and may be dysphagic or dyspnoeic. Vomiting can also occur. After a period of illness, with or without treatment, the birds make a good recovery that lasts some months. For this reason it is difficult to decide whether treatment is effective.

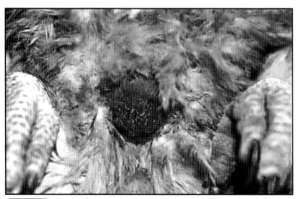

13.8 Papillomatosis mostly occurs at the cloaca, leading to bloody faeces or disturbed faecal passage.

Diagnosis
The clinical appearance of the papillomas (blackberry or cauliflower shape, and well supplied with blood) are typical for the disease. They often protrude through the cloaca but if small or pedunculate they may not be seen until the cloaca is everted. In the oral cavity the papillomas are usually less inflamed.

All birds with papillomas of the cloaca should have an endoscopic examination. This is useful for finding papillomas in the oral cavity, crop, proventriculus, gizzard and cloaca. The bright illumination of the endoscope and the ability to bring the mucous membrane into close view help to detect even small early lesions. Intestinal obstruction is uncommon but can be shown using contrast radiography. If 5% acetic acid is applied to the papillomas, they change colour from rose to white, which may be useful to demonstrate small lesions. To confirm the diagnosis and to differentiate the papillomas from neoplasms, a histological examination must be performed.

Therapy and prophylaxis
Secondary infections should be treated first, by plucking feathers and cleaning and antibiosis of the affected areas. Most large papillomas can be surgically removed with scissors or, better still, electrosurgery (Chapter 10). It is not possible to eliminate the disease and the majority of cases develop more papillomas, more frequently in stressful situations. Repetitive surgery causes scarring, and strictures of the cloaca are a problem. There have been many attempts to make autogenous vaccines from papillomas but, as no papillomavirus has been isolated, this technique does not work (though some have suggested that it does). The successful use of aciclovir has also been reported.

A number of retrospective surveys show that birds with papillomatosis have a higher incidence of tumours of the pancreas and bile ducts; these are fatal (Graham, 1991). Spontaneous regression of papillomatosis has been reported. Usually treatments are not successful, but affected birds can often be kept for years. In such cases, close contact with unaffected birds must be avoided. As there seems to be no vertical transmission, it is possible to hatch eggs from affected birds artificially and hand rear the youngsters, which should then be disease-free.

Proventricular dilatation disease (PDD)

Aetiology and pathogenesis
The cause of PDD has not yet been identified. It is suspected that a virus is shed in the faeces and ingested or inhaled. The length of the incubation period has not yet been determined but might be from at least 6 weeks up to years. Stress and changes in home and diet seem to precipitate the sudden occurrence of the clinical disease. PDD describes the main sign that is visible in an ill bird, but the pathology of the disease is located in the central and, most importantly, the peripheral nervous system. Degeneration of the ganglia is observed on histological examination. In addition lymphohistiocytic infiltrations, mainly in the autonomic nerve plexus of the proventriculus, are detectable. Due to the disturbance of the innervation, the muscle layer of the proventriculus becomes atrophic, leading to atony and dilation of the organ (Figures 13.9 and 13.10). In some cases the crop, parts of the intestine and the ventriculus might be involved as well.

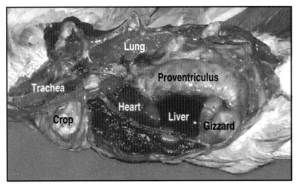

13.9 Proventricular dilatation disease in a Grey Parrot. The enlarged and blocked proventriculus is visible. Note the extremely thin wall of the organ: even the food is visible.

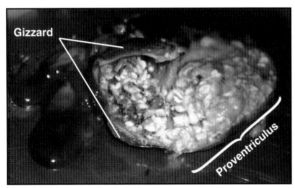

13.10 Proventriculus of a macaw with PDD. The organ wall is extremely thin and food is unable to pass due to the insufficient motility of the thin muscle layer. The gizzard was also dilated and its muscular layer much reduced (compare Figure 2.11 and see Figures 9.5 and 9.6).

Interestingly, only a few birds in a collection show the clinical disease at any one time, often without any obvious connection between the occurrence of these cases. This leads to the suspicion that birds can be carriers without developing a clinical disease. The disease has been seen in many psittacine species but Cockatiels, macaws (in which it is also known as macaw wasting disease), Amazons, Grey Parrots and cockatoos seem to be more susceptible. Often one member of a pair of birds dies and the other survives. The survivor is often a continual source of infection, and healthy birds that are placed with it might develop clinical signs of PDD. In collections, typically only a few birds develop the disease.

Clinical signs

In most cases an owner reports that the bird vomits seed after eating and/or that undigested seed is present in the faeces. Loss of weight, even when food ingestion is normal, is another sign of the disease and is caused by insufficient preparation of the food by the proventriculus. In some cases, depression and a crop dilatation can be detected. CNS signs can also occur, in rare cases even without clinically present intestinal symptoms. In such cases a dilated proventriculus can usually be seen on radiographs. Due to the maldigestion the affected bird becomes weak and finally dies. The time between first clinical signs and death can be short in younger birds but may be years in older birds.

Diagnosis

Radiographically the dilated proventriculus is clearly visible on the lateral view (Figure 9.6), best taken using contrast media. The time for the passage of the contrast medium is also lengthened. Detection of a dilated proventriculus is not confirmation of PDD, as other reasons might lead to the same signs. Fluoroscopy can be used to demonstrate incoordinate peristaltic movement between the proventriculus and gizzard, and this is pathognomonic for PDD. At PME the bird is emaciated and the proventriculus is full of food, often visible through an extremely thin, greaseproof paper-like wall.

Confirmation of PDD is difficult, as the pathogen is unknown. Histological evidence of ganglion degeneration and lymphohistiocytosis in the nerves is pathognomonic, so the diagnosis is usually confirmed at PME. In the live bird, biopsy of the proventriculus and crop has been used for confirmation but this carries a high risk, especially in the proventriculus as the organ wall is already very thin and a rupture might occur. In addition, only a positive histology result provides evidence, but the changes are not in all the nerves and so false negative results occur. In the clinic the diagnosis is made by excluding other possible causes of dilation of the proventriculus: foreign bodies, metal intoxication, bacteria, fungus and parasites. Several repeated examinations are necessary. Because the acid digestion of the proventriculus is affected and seed is stagnant, secondary bacterial and fungal infections often occur. If a primary bacterial or fungal infection is the cause of the signs, the condition will resolve rapidly with treatment. It should be noted that bacterial and fungal infections usually cause a thickening of the proventricular wall, which can be judged by an endoscopic examination. Fasting allows the proventriculus to empty in cases with bacterial or yeast infection, whereas with PDD this does not happen.

Therapy and prophylaxis

Treatment of the disease is not usually possible. For symptomatic treatment, cimetidine and metoclopramide or cisapride have been tried with variable success. Recently treatment using celecoxib, a cyclooxygenase-2 inhibitor, has shown promising results. The drug is supposed to suppress inflammation of the nerves and help them to function.

Due to the loss of motility, the proventriculus can be already obstructed by food that must be removed before starting any other treatment, though this may be impossible. Once the impacted seed has been removed, no more seed should be given. The food should be of high energy and easily digestible. Pellets or liquid food for hand rearing parrots are best. Human baby food can also be used. Liquid food can be given by gavage. It should be borne in mind that permanent gavage of liquid food by the owner is not recommended, due to stress on the bird. Hand-reared parrots that are used to being spoon-fed might be an exception. It is possible to insert a temporary feeding tube through the oesophagus into the crop or proventriculus. Administration of vitamin B complex and substitution of fluids are useful.

Euthanasia is an option.

Prevention of the disease within a collection is very difficult. Quarantine of new birds for several weeks and radiography to assess the proventriculus are recommended but these measures do not provide 100% safety, as the incubation period can be very long. As Cockatiels are susceptible to the disease, Cockatiel nestlings could be used as sentinel birds in breeding collections or in quarantine stations, but care should be taken not to introduce other diseases.

Bacterial infections

Septicaemia

Aetiology and pathogenesis

Bacteria are very common as pathogens and often they are secondary or involved in a whole disease process. 'Typical' diseases caused by a specific bacterium are rare. Whenever bacteria are involved in a disease, the diagnosis must be made by the isolation of the pathogen. The result of a bacterial examination must be interpreted carefully according to the possible symptoms and the sample of origin, as a normal bacterial flora exists in swabs (e.g. conjunctiva, nose, cloaca). To treat any bacterial infection it is important to run a sensitivity test, as resistance is common and the initial treatment may have to be changed in accordance with the results.

Many different bacteria cause clinical signs (e.g. *Staphylococcus*, *Streptococcus*) but these are rarely specific. Some might cause severe septicaemias, e.g. *Escherichia coli*, *Klebsiella*, *Pasteurella* and *Pseudomonas*. Bacteria infect via the oral route but can be airborne or enter through wounds; it is common for infected wounds to lead to septicaemic disease.

Clinical signs

Birds are suddenly very sick, are unable to stand on the perch and stop eating. Dyspnoea and diarrhoea are common. Birds often die within a short period (1–3 days). If pathogenic bacteria persist in a flock, an increased death rate of embryos is observed, especially if *E. coli* is involved as well.

PME of birds that die from septicaemia shows a swollen liver, often with petechiae on the liver (Figure 13.11) and heart. Pericardial effusion is often seen in conjunction with a *Pasteurella* infection.

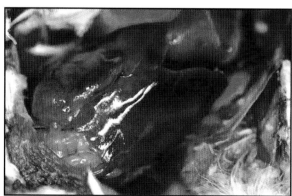

13.11 Petechial bleeding on the liver is often seen in cases of septicaemia. Isolation of the pathogen is necessary for confirmation of the diagnosis and sensitivity testing is required to protect other birds of the flock.

Diagnosis

The diagnosis of any bacterial infection is made by isolating the pathogen on an agar plate. As first choice, blood agars should be used as most bacteria grow on them. It is of advantage to use two plates for the same sample and incubate one of them in an anaerobic environment, in which some bacteria grow better. Identification of the isolated bacteria can be made by commercially available tests.

To detect the pathogen causing a septicaemia, the choice of the sample is important. In a live bird a blood culture is best. Organ biopsies (liver, kidney) are more complicated to obtain in a very sick bird. During PME, heart blood is the sample of choice; bacteria obtained from the liver have often invaded after death and are not the pathogen. Additionally, in the case of *Pasteurella*, a direct smear from heart blood stained with methylene blue may show bipolar stained rods, which allows a rapid diagnosis. This typical bipolar staining only occurs in direct smears, not from *Pasteurella* colonies from plates. Cytology of affected organs shows the direction if Gram-positive or Gram-negative rods are involved in the disease process, but has limited use in the selection of the antibiotic to be used (see below).

Therapy

It is important that the treatment should start after taking samples for bacteriology. As sensitivity tests need at least 2 days, an antibiotic treatment should be started immediately. The antibiotic of choice should not have been used recently in the same bird or in the same collection. The antibiotic should be quickly distributed to all tissues and should act against most bacteria (broad spectrum). Enrofloxacin is usually used as the first drug, but doxycycline or amoxicillin is also useful, especially for *Pasteurella* or *Yersinia*. Within the same practice, the antibiotic used first should be changed regularly to avoid resistance in clients' birds.

Salmonellosis

Aetiology and pathogenesis

More than 2500 serovars of the two different *Salmonella* species, *S. enterica* and *S. bongori*, are known. The incidence of salmonellosis and the species affected differs according to the year and area. New and unknown serovars are easily introduced by wild-caught imported parrots, and the pathogenicity of salmonellosis varies between and within serovars. Carriers are common. Some serovars, such as *S.* Enteritidis, are zoonotic and of special importance. Most parrots with salmonellosis are infected with *S.* Typhimurium. *Salmonella* is shed via faeces and eggs, and infection occurs orally or vertically. Pure infections of the intestine occur, but after penetration of the intestine wall several organs can be affected. Latently infected birds or vectors (rodents) are able to spread the pathogen to other flocks. *Salmonella* is sensitive to most disinfectants and is destroyed by temperatures above 60°C.

Salmonellosis is often supported by a weak immune system, disturbed intestinal flora and poor food quality, as well as contact with free-ranging birds. It is common in imported birds.

Clinical signs

Affected birds usually look unwell. In rare cases, especially in chicks, sudden death occurs. The disease is acute in imported parrots in quarantine, where hygiene is poor, stocking density is high and the birds are stressed. The birds are depressed, with dropped wings and green diarrhoea, and usually die after a few days. In these conditions morbidity and mortality can be high. Some of these birds recover and are carriers; they usually look unwell and have some diarrhoea. In single pet birds the chronic disease is more common. Diarrhoea is often the first sign, accompanied by loss of weight and CNS signs. Joints can be affected as well, so lameness might occur. Interestingly lameness also occurs without other symptoms, except ruffled feathers and slight weakness. In addition, the rate of embryonic death or newly hatched chicks with omphalitis might be increased.

Diagnosis

On radiographs, enlargements of liver, spleen and kidney are common. Soft tissue swellings at joints can also be detected. Multiple white spots (necrosis) in the liver and spleen can be seen on endoscopy or PME and an enteritis is common. Milky air sacs, ascites, salpingitis and inflamed ovarian follicles are other signs.

Diagnosis must be confirmed by the isolation of the pathogen from organs (biopsies) or joint fluid aspirates. Apart from direct smears of tissues on agar plates, it is important that samples are placed in pre-enrichment broth (peptone) followed by a *Salmonella* enrichment broth (Rappaport broth) and placed on *Salmonella*-selective agar (Rambach), as often the direct placement on agar is negative and only the enrichment broth leads to positive results. Isolation of *Salmonella* from faeces does not confirm the diagnosis of a clinical disease, as sometimes the organisms may be passing through the gut without making the bird unwell. Conversely, a single negative faecal result does not confirm that the bird is not infected, as the organisms are shed intermittently. The detection of antibodies using a serum agglutination is possible, but the reliability of the result depends on the *Salmonella* species; a limited number of antigens is commercially available. The most common anti-*Salmonella* antibodies can be detected using a polyvalent antigen. Unhatched eggs should always be examined for *Salmonella*.

If *Salmonella* is cultured, this finding must be reported to DEFRA, who will then require the organism to be identified by serotype and may need to investigate further.

Therapy and prophylaxis

Salmonella often exhibits multiple antibiotic resistance. A sensitivity test is vital. The first choices are enrofloxacin or tylosin. It must be borne in mind that antibiotic treatment reduces clinical signs and excretion of the pathogen but does not always lead to its elimination. Several (at least three) examinations are recommended at the end of treatment.

Affected joints should be irrigated with antibiotics. Probiotics might reduce the number of organisms within the intestine. Reduction of clinical signs of affected birds

often occurs, but affected joints seldom recover to full function. Chronic cases of salmonellosis can seldom be treated successfully. Recurrence of the disease is not unusual, as persistence of the pathogen, especially within a collection, is common. In affected flocks the positive birds are detected (and separated) quickly by testing them via serum agglutination.

The production of an autologous vaccine is possible and positive results have been obtained. After using such a vaccine, clinical signs disappeared and carriers stopped shedding *Salmonella*. However, using a vaccine makes it impossible to detect infected birds by means of antibody levels. Vaccination with commercially available vaccine might not provide positive results, though cross-antigenicity between types will allow some vaccines to protect against *S.* Typhimurium.

It is important that any new bird should be kept in quarantine and should be tested by serum agglutination and bacteriological examination of several faeces' samples. Some breeders suggest that spraying or dipping eggs in an antibiotic solution prior to incubation is useful.

If a *Salmonella* that is pathogenic for humans is isolated from a bird, the bird must be isolated and treated. As treatment does not mean elimination of the pathogen, the bird needs to be retested. In case of a repeated positive result, euthanasia should be considered. Such cases are presumably rare, but euthanasia of an affected bird should always be considered if children or old people are in the same household as the bird.

Tuberculosis

Aetiology and pathogenesis

Tuberculosis in parrots is caused by several mycobacteria, especially *Mycobacterium avium*, *M. genavense* and *M. intracellulare*. These pathogens have worldwide distribution, are extremely robust and survive for up to 7 years in the environment. Many disinfectants are ineffective, but some are useful (e.g. Lysoformin, or Virkon S). Skin tubercles caused by *M. tuberculosis* have occurred in pet parrots owned by TB-infected humans. Mycobacteria are introduced into a flock by latently infected birds or by vectors (contaminated soil). The pathogen is usually shed in faeces but also in other body fluids. Infection is usually oral, with the development of a primary tubercle within the intestine. The mycobacteria spread to other organs, especially liver and spleen, by haematogenous spread. Sometimes bone marrow or muscles are involved. In rare cases a percutaneous infection is possible, with the development of a local tuberculosis within the subcutis or a muscle. Airborne transmission has been described. The incubation period is usually long (up to 6 months).

Clinical signs

Tuberculosis is always a chronic disease; the birds are often ill with general malaise and ruffled feathers and are usually severely emaciated, despite the fact that they are still eating. Emaciation with diarrhoea in an older bird that otherwise looks surprisingly well is always suspicious. Many birds have a combination of several signs, such as diarrhoea with anaemia and icterus, CNS signs and lameness (often with a palpably swollen joint). Occasionally, birds die due to a ruptured liver, and sometimes lameness occurs without other signs. Skin tubercles can be seen as yellow knots below the skin but are rare. Eye infections with a swollen conjunctiva have been reported.

Diagnosis

Radiographs show massive liver enlargement and, in some cases, shadows of pea size within the bones and muscle (visible tubercles). Miliary yellow nodules are visible in the liver (Figure 13.12) and spleen during endoscopy or PME. Often they can also be found in other organs. Yellow cheesy material also occurs within the lung, interestingly often at the side oriented towards the ribs; at PME the lung must be taken out for a complete examination. Due to the liver enlargement, ascites might occur.

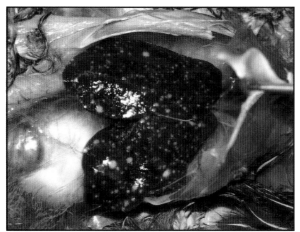

13.12 Tuberculosis of the liver. Note the typical formation of tubercles. They are of variable size, yellow, and protrude above the surface of the organ.

The clinical disease is often accompanied by a heterophilia and monocytosis with an increased level of bile acids and liver enzymes. Isolation of mycobacteria is possible but takes at least 4–6 weeks. Smears of tissue samples (obtained during endoscopy) or ascitic fluid can be stained (Ziehl–Neelsen) to detect acid-fast rods. In combination with the clinical signs, this confirms the diagnosis. Histological or PCR examination of tissue samples is also possible. A central necrosis with acid-fast rods, surrounded by typical cells (Langerhans cells, reticulohistiocytes), is typical for the tubercles. Detection of antibodies by whole-blood agglutination is possible but negative results are unreliable, as only a few subtypes (*M. avium*, serovars 1–4) are commercially available. Intradermal tests are unreliable.

Therapy and prophylaxis

Successful treatments of single cases of tuberculosis have been described but in general the treatment success is limited and euthanasia should be considered. Avian tuberculosis is a zoonosis that infects mainly immunocompromised humans (HIV-positive, or transplant organ recipients).

In collections, the whole flock should be in quarantine for 2 years. Every 6–12 weeks the birds are tested by whole-blood agglutination, and any positive birds are removed (negative results are unreliable). This is accompanied by hygienic and disinfectant measures. In large aviaries, waterfowl are frequently kept with parrots and can be a source of avian tuberculosis.

Clostridiosis

Aetiology and pathogenesis

Different *Clostridium* species are able to cause severe diseases. All that the species have in common is that they are anaerobic Gram-positive rods and are common in the environment. In mammals and other avian species *C. botulinum* causes botulism, *C. tetani* causes tetanus and *C. septicum* and *C. novyi* cause subcutaneous infections and gangrene, but all of these are very rare in psittaciforms.

Most importantly, *C. perfringens* can cause severe disease and losses in individuals and flocks. It is a ubiquitous bacterium, which is very stable in the environment and can survive for years. The strains of *C. perfringens* are differentiated by their toxins. A small number of *C. perfringens* organisms is considered normal in the intestinal flora or within the food but in cases of poor food preparation, especially liquid food (lories), the bacteria multiply considerably and produce toxin, which causes enterotoxaemia. Dry food discourages the growth of clostridia and so parrots that eat pellets or seed are rarely affected. Birds fed with fresh food (such as soaked pulses) are more at risk, especially if the pulses are placed in water for a long time or if washing after soaking is not done carefully. Liquid baby bird food should be made fresh for each feed.

Other gastrointestinal diseases (coccidiosis, viral infections), food change or stress might lead to an imbalance of the intestinal flora of a bird, putting the clostridia at an advantage. In general both causes of the disease are not clearly distinguishable and often overlap. Most importantly, poor hygiene, poor food, food change and other diseases are the main reasons for this disease.

Clinical signs

Enterotoxaemia is characterized by sudden death of the bird. In flocks, younger birds are affected first. In a few cases severe bloody chocolate-brown diarrhoea is visible. PME shows petechial haemorrhages on different organs, often on the myocardium, and sometimes a severe necrotizing enteritis (Figure 13.13) and a swollen liver. If the clostridia reproduce in the intestine, the disease can follow an acute or a chronic path. In the acute phase the onset is sudden; the birds are lethargic, with ruffled feathers. Faecal glued cloacal feathers are a sign of a severe diarrhoea. In most cases a bloody diarrhoea occurs and is seen only in birds with coccidiosis or clostridiosis. Often fibrinous material and diphtheroid membranes from the intestine are detectable as well. The birds mostly die after a few days. In chronic cases the appetite is still normal, but the birds are sleepy and inactive. They develop poorly, having a slight diarrhoea and losing weight continuously.

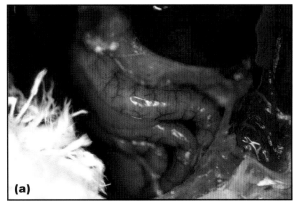

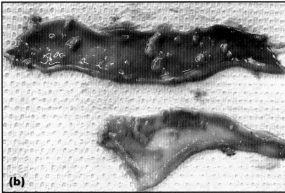

13.13 Clostridiosis. (a) Bloody enteritis with necrotic mucous membranes. (b) Necrotic enteritis due to clostridiosis (courtesy of HM Hafez).

At PME the main change is a necrotizing enteritis, sometimes with ulcers. The intestinal mucosa is detached and grey. Diphtheroid membranes may be present. Bacteria are able to leave the gastrointestinal tract usually after the toxin has damaged the intestinal wall. The bacteria and their toxins cause further changes such as pericarditis and air sacculitis, particularly in chronic cases.

Clostridiosis is potentially two conditions, caused by either toxin production in food or bacterial growth in the intestine. Both can usually develop, as clostridia from the food are also ingested, increasing the number within the intestine. Pure intoxication is possible as well as bacterial growth in the intestine without ingesting clostridia directly. In birds with imbalanced intestinal flora, small numbers of (until then commensal) clostridia are able to proliferate and cause the disease.

Diagnosis
During the clinical history, the owner reports food changes or provision of home-prepared liquid or soaked food. In some cases other gastrointestinal diseases are present and might be diagnosed separately (Chapter 15). In flocks the disease always affects several birds fed on the same food.

Faeces can be used for microbiological examination. Detection of many colonies of *C. perfringens* confirms the diagnosis; single colonies are clinically insignificant. In severe cases the detection of the pathogen from the liver is possible. Anaerobic incubation is important for the detection of clostridia. On blood agar

C. perfringens causes a double area of haemolysis, but it can be more easily detected on specific agars. In cases of enterotoxaemia, the detection of toxin from the serum is possible but expensive.

Therapy
First, the detection of the source of the disease must be located and eliminated. Food change might be necessary and dry food with low protein content is recommended. In addition, an antibiotic treatment with amoxicillin or tetracycline is important. Probiotics are useful to balance the intestinal flora. In cases with enterotoxaemia, treatment is often too late. In other cases it depends on the status of the damaged intestine. It takes at least 3–5 days to restore intestinal function. During this time fluid therapy and the control of electrolytes are important. In chronic cases a full recovery of the bird might not be possible. The application of antitoxin is possible in acute cases, but with questionable results as different toxins of *C. perfringens* exist.

Yersiniosis

Aetiology and pathogenesis
Yersiniosis is usually a disease found in flocks, where it can cause severe losses. It is rarely seen in individual birds. Different *Yersinia* species have been isolated from birds, but in psittacine birds *Y. pseudotuberculosis* is of importance. The virulence of the pathogen varies between the isolates. The pathogen can also be found in mammals, especially rodents, which play an important role in spreading the disease. Latently infected birds and contaminated food also bring the pathogen into a flock. Infection always occurs orally through food and water. The pathogen penetrates the mucous membranes of the intestinal tract. Alterations of the mucous membranes through other diseases or parasites facilitate this process. The incubation period varies from days to a couple of weeks.

Clinical signs
In flocks, up to 40% of the birds might be clinically affected, but more birds are latently infected. Birds with clinical symptoms usually die, mostly due to a septicaemia. A few days before death they are lethargic with ruffled feathers and diarrhoea. The sudden death of some birds occurs only for a short period but afterwards some chronically ill birds are present. They are sleepy, stop eating and lose weight with diarrhoea.

On PME of chronic cases, multiple granulomas can be detected from various organs, especially liver, spleen and intestine (this is an important differential for tuberculosis where there are acid-fast rods in a smear), and also from kidney, bone marrow and skeletal muscle. In addition a catarrhal enteritis is present.

Diagnosis
Histological examination (necrosis, bacteria and histiocytes, granulomas) are not specific for yersiniosis but, together with the clinical appearance of the flock, it supports the diagnosis. Confirmation requires isolation of the pathogen from faeces or tissue material. When sending the sample to a laboratory the suspicion

of yersiniosis must be mentioned, as certain procedures (e.g. cold incubation) are necessary to isolate the pathogen. In routine bacteriology the pathogen is usually overlooked.

Therapy and prophylaxis

Clinically ill birds are difficult to treat, as antibiotics usually do not enter the granulomas. Antibiotics should be used according to the sensitivity test but amoxicillin, enrofloxacin or tetracyclines are useful to start with and can be changed if necessary. All clinically affected birds must be separated from the rest of the flock to decrease the load of infectious material to the other birds; antibiotic in the drinking water helps with this. The isolated birds may be treated or euthanased. All other birds must be treated with an appropriate antibiotic (sensitivity test) to prevent further cases. The improvement of hygiene measures, rodent control and food is most important.

Psittacosis (Chlamydophilosis)

Aetiology and pathogenesis

Psittacosis is caused by the obligatory intracellular bacterium *Chlamydophila psittaci*, which is one of the most commonly distributed pathological bacteria in avian medicine. It can affect not only psittacine birds but also other avian species, mammals and humans. The organisms are shed in all kinds of body secretions, such as faecal, nasal and ocular fluids. Birds can be latently infected, distributing the pathogen through the psittacine population; these birds can be carriers for years, and stress (immunosuppression) can lead to a renewed excretion of pathogens.

Chlamydophila organisms survive as elementary bodies for several weeks in the environment and might be transferred by dust. In most cases the infection is airborne, with a first reproduction of the pathogen in cells of the respiratory tract; the bacteria are then distributed via blood to other organs. Excretion of *Chlamydophila* occurs as early as a few days after infection. The elementary bodies fasten to the target cells and change to initial bodies. The initial bodies do not have a complete cell wall (L-form), which explains why they are able to persist even if antibodies or cell-wall active antibiotics are present. These intracellular bodies reproduce and produce enzymes that lead to the destruction of the cell by a local endotoxaemia. The initial bodies reorganize to elementary bodies carrying a toxic surface factor. This surface factor is the 'real' pathogen, as the cell death does not explain the pathogenicity of *C. psittaci*. The surface factor can change, especially when the pathogen passes through different hosts. This explains the variation in pathogenicity in different avian species, as well as changes in the pathogenicity after passing through other species. The subtypes of *C. psittaci* have different pathogenicities and courses of disease in different avian species. This means that other latently infected birds can introduce the pathogen to a psittacine flock, causing severe problems.

Several factors influence the clinical occurrence of the disease. Firstly, the age of the bird is important:

younger birds are more likely to die than older birds. Species is important: for example, Grey Parrots are very susceptible and usually die, but Cockatiels and Amazons are far less susceptible and more likely to be carriers. Secondly, management plays the most important role. In particular, stress (e.g. exhibition, new bird in the collection, changes in the environment, poor food or water quality) might lead to a clinical disease in latently infected birds. Immune suppression or other accompanying diseases also influence the occurrence of a clinical manifest disease. Even though antibodies are produced, once the infection is over many birds are fully susceptible to a new infection.

Clinical signs

The clinical appearance of psittacosis varies and is without any pathognomonic signs. In most cases it is a latent infection without any clinical signs, though these might occur years after the initial infection. Importantly, these birds shed the pathogen for several months after infection and might be lifelong carriers. Mostly the clinical signs are of a very ill bird: ruffled feathers, depression, anorexia and in chronic cases loss of weight. Signs such as conjunctivitis (Figure 13.14), rhinitis and sinusitis with secretion of clear fluids may be detectable in the first place. Secondary bacterial infection makes these fluids purulent. Dyspnoea may be seen. These clinical signs are often accompanied by droppings with bright green urates or a watery green-yellow diarrhoea (Appendix 2), which is highly suspicious for psittacosis. In some cases CNS signs such as loss of equilibrium, opisthotonos, convulsions and tremor can occur.

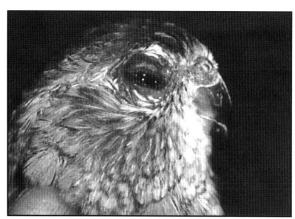

13.14 Conjuctivitis in a psittacine bird should always initiate an examination for psittacosis using a conjunctival swab for PCR.

On PME the most obvious sign is a very enlarged spleen. The serosa of the respiratory tract shows a yellow-white exudate, and in most cases a pericarditis (Figure 13.15a) and a very large liver, often with small necrotic foci (Figure 13.15b), are present. The surface of the sternum closest to the heart and liver is often yellow. Secondary infections are often present, accounting for some of the described postmortal changes.

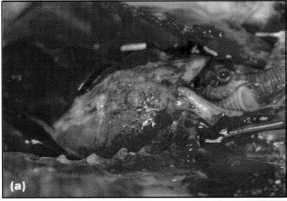

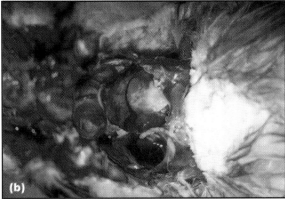

13.15 Some typical PME changes in birds with psittacosis: (a) pericarditis; (b) perihepatitis.

Diagnosis

Taking the clinical history, it is important to ask: for how long the bird has been owned; whether there were any changes within the collection (i.e. new birds, especially Amazons, Cockatiels and Budgerigars); and whether the bird had been in another carer's house (while the owners were on holiday) or had been to a bird exhibition.

Whole-body radiography often shows an enlarged spleen on the lateral view (Figure 13.16). This should always be suspicious for psittacosis and further diagnosis should be initiated. Enlarged liver and kidneys are usually also seen.

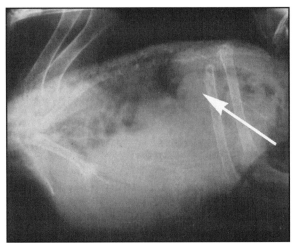

13.16 Lateral radiograph showing a clearly visible enlarged spleen (arrowed). This is suggestive of psittacosis.

Blood results are non-specific but a massive leucocytosis with increased numbers of heterophils, basophils and monocytes might occur. Levels of liver enzymes and bile acids are often increased but this is not a regular finding.

Conjunctivitis in psittacine birds, especially if newly purchased, always requires a conjunctival swab for further diagnosis. It is common for grass parakeets, Budgerigars and Cockatiels to develop a primary chlamydophilial conjunctivitis with no other signs. To confirm the diagnosis it is necessary to detect the pathogen or, more easily, its DNA. A quick first result in a PME can be obtained by a spleen or air sac smear stained according to Stamp (Chapter 7). Dealing with such samples must be performed carefully as the material is of zoonotic importance. Gloves, face mask and laboratory coat are important.

Chlamydophila dies quickly on transport and so a special transport medium must be used. Cell culture is necessary, as the organisms do not grow on cell-free media. False negatives are common. The safest method for detection of *Chlamydophila* is to find its DNA using a PCR. Conjunctival or cloacal swabs as well as tissue samples may be used.

There is a difference between diagnosing psittacosis in the ill bird and the carrier. When screening a collection, swabs can be pooled but the test should be repeated three times as *Chlamydophila* is shed irregularly. It must be borne in mind that to guarantee recovery of *Chlamydophila* during one experiment it was necessary to perform the test on three sets of swabs (conjunctival, choanal and faecal) taken on three different days. Because of this, some suggest using the same swab for the conjunctiva, choana and, finally, the cloaca (in that order). This covers all three sites for one fee. However, when the bird is ill with bright green urates (Appendix 2), a single faecal sample is invariably positive.

In practice an antigen ELISA is available but positive results should be confirmed by a more specific method (PCR). The antigen ELISA is useful to screen a psittacine collection via cloacal swabs to detect the positive (shedding) birds during a treatment regime to clear that flock.

The detection of antibodies (ELISA, Immunocomb) is also possible. However, if a bird is positive for antibodies, it does not mean that the bird is still a carrier. The presence of the pathogen in such birds needs to be confirmed by another method. If the antibody titre is high and the bird has clinical signs, it might be of diagnostic value but in such cases the pathogen can usually be demonstrated. The demonstration of antibodies is of interest in screening a collection, to know if the birds have faced the pathogen before and to screen for non-shedding carriers within that collection. Faecal samples should be avoided and are only of interest in screening collections (Chapter 7).

Therapy

In some countries the treatment of psittacosis is regulated by law. In general all birds in a collection must be treated. Application of drug to each bird is always preferable to medication in food or water. Sick birds should be quarantined and treated separately;

for all other birds water or food medication is possible. After treatment, three samples (pooled in a collection), taken with 5 days between, must be negative to confirm the success of the treatment. At the same time as the treatment, disinfectant and hygiene are of great importance.

Treatment success, even in clinically ill birds, often occurs but the elimination of the pathogen can be difficult. There is always the risk of latently infected but shedding birds.

As latently infected birds are common, quarantine and testing of newly acquired birds is recommended. Hygiene and the reduction of dust in the environment are important.

Treatment with chlortetracycline in food may be useful for collections. Treatment with doxycycline is governed by law in some European countries (e.g. Germany). Treatment with enrofloxacin, especially for a collection, within drinking water and mixed with corn as exclusive food for the duration of treatment, has been shown to be successful (Lindenstruth and Forst, 1993). The corn (cooked or from cans) is dried for a few hours and then the enrofloxacin solution (see Appendix 3) is absorbed into it. This method is well accepted by parrots; lories, however, should receive the drug within their liquid food.

C. psittaci has a natural resistance to sulphonamides, gentamicin, streptomycin, bacitracin, mycostatin and ristostatin.

Zoonotic risk
Psittacosis in humans is a chronic disease with pneumonia, fever and headache. It is able to cause a fatal myocarditis. The family doctor should be informed that infected birds are kept at home.

Blood parasites

Aetiology and pathogenesis
Blood parasites are uncommon in psittacine birds but may be seen in imported birds or in flocks. The most important are *Plasmodium* spp., *Leucocytozoon* spp. and *Haemoproteus* spp., all of which are transmitted through mosquitoes (e.g. *Anopheles*, *Culex*) that are also involved in the life cycle. The parasites may be found in both red and white blood cells but also have extraerythrocytic forms in different organs (liver, kidney, bone marrow, endothelial cells). They are differentiated by their appearance within the erythrocyte. Most infected birds are latently affected and blood parasites are detected by accident when checking a blood smear for other reasons.

Clinical signs
The clinical signs of affected birds are similar no matter which blood parasite is the causative pathogen. The primary sign is weakness and the bird is sleepy. Compared with other diseases, the bird's behaviour is normal with an undisturbed food and water intake. In the disease course a more or less severe anaemia occurs, apparent with white mucous membranes. Due to the lack of erythrocytes as transport cells for oxygen, a dyspnoea develops. In severe cases a swollen liver with increased liver enzymes and icterus can occur. During PME, subcutaneous bleeding and swollen organs (liver, kidney, spleen), often with a colour change, are detectable. *Leucocytozoon* can cause high mortalities in nestlings, *Plasmodium* often affects individuals and *Haemoproteus* seldom causes clinical signs.

Diagnosis
Diagnosis is always made from a Giemsa-stained blood smear. It is important to assess the erythrocytes (Figure 13.17). *Haemoproteus* develops only gametocytes, within the plasma of erythrocytes, which are filled with granules. *Leucocytozoon* also has only gametocytes in red blood cells, but they are located within the nucleus without any granules. *Plasmodium* has gametocytes with granules in the plasma of erythrocytes (comparable to *Haemoproteus*) but also develops schizonts in red blood cells visible as multiple nuclear structures. Within a blood smear both forms always appear.

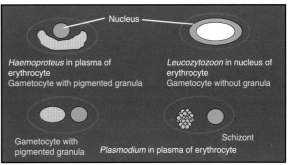

Nucleus

Haemoproteus in plasma of erythrocyte
Gametocyte with pigmented granula

Leucozytozoon in nucleus of erythrocyte
Gametocyte without granula

Gametocyte with pigmented granula

Plasmodium in plasma of erythrocyte

Schizont

13.17 Differentiation of the most common blood parasites (*Plasmodium* spp., *Haemoproteus* spp. and *Leucocytozoon* spp.) is easily achieved by accessing the erythrocytes in a Giemsa-stained blood smear. (M. Lierz, modified from Remple (1980).)

Therapy
The treatment of these blood parasites is difficult and is based on individual experience. Chloroquine is recommended for the treatment of *Plasmodium* spp., mepacrine hypochloride for *Haemoproteus* spp. and nitroimidazole derivatives for *Leucocytozoon* spp.

Other infections
Aspergillosis is described in Chapter 14. 'Going light' syndrome (megabacteriosis), trichomoniasis and giardiasis are described in Chapter 15.

14

Respiratory disease

Simon J. Girling

Anatomy and physiology

Avian patients have a markedly different respiratory anatomy from that seen in mammals. The trachea is generally 2.7 times longer than that seen in a mammal of comparable size, creating on average 4 times the dead space (King and McLelland, 1975). However, it is also wider in diameter, and reinforced with complete rings of cartilage, which means that greater flow rates and larger volumes of air may be inhaled and exhaled. In addition there is no diaphragm and the lungs themselves are semi-rigid in structure, and so do not increase appreciably in size during inspiration.

To enable air to move through the lung structure, birds have a system of air sacs that allow inspired and expired air to be shunted back and forth through the lungs so that gaseous exchange can occur. To create the negative pressure required for inspiration, birds rely entirely on the outward movement of the ribcage and downward movement of the sternum, so increasing the volume of the coelomic cavity. This has great significance when holding an avian patient, as overzealous restraint can lead to an inability to move the ribcage and sternum, causing asphyxiation. This situation is made all the more likely if the patient is already suffering respiratory system compromise due to disease.

Birds have a unique ability to extract oxygen on both inspiration and expiration. Fresh air passes through the lungs on the first inspiration and then moves into the caudal thoracic and abdominal air sacs. This is important, as pathogens (such as inhaled spores of *Aspergillus* spp.) often affect the caudal air sacs preferentially. On expiration, this air is then flushed back through the lungs and on into the cranial thoracic and cervical air sacs, allowing more gaseous exchange to occur. More fresh air is inhaled on the second inspiration, and the air remaining in the cranial thoracic and cervical air sacs is finally flushed out, again back through the lungs, on the second inspiration. The full avian respiration cycle occurs over two bouts of inspiration and expiration. For a more in-depth discussion of avian respiratory anatomy please see Chapter 2.

Diagnostic procedures

History

As with all diseases, thorough history taking is vital to aid a diagnosis. The association of clinical disease with the presence of new birds within a flock or in an owner's house is often suggestive of an infectious cause. Recent catastrophes within the bird's environment, such as local flooding, followed by breathing difficulties a week or so later may suggest fungal diseases such as aspergillosis. These pathogens grow rapidly in the damp and then, once drying out occurs, release massive amounts of spores, which are inhaled by the unfortunate parrot. Siting of the patient's cage is important, as certain rooms (e.g. the kitchen) may suggest a toxic cause to any respiratory disease. Nutrition is also important to consider, as rhinitis, sinusitis and aspergillosis are all seen more often in psittacine birds suffering from hypovitaminosis A.

Clinical examination

Standing back and carefully watching the breathing rate and depth before handling the patient is advisable, as this will often give a clue to the level of respiratory disease. Clinically severe signs including tail bobbing (regular flicking of the tail feathers in synchrony with respiration) suggest hyperpnoea, and evidence of dyspnoea and tachypnoea when at rest are obviously poor prognostic signs.

Examination of the external nares is important, and often overlooked. The nares should be the same size, free of any discharges and, depending on the species, may be surrounded by an area of smooth skin known as the cere. There is some variation in the presence of a defined cere as Eclectus Parrots and Amazons have feathers right up to and around the external nares, whereas Budgerigars, for example, have a pronounced cere (Chapter 5).

The proximal nasal passages may be examined through the nares and should be smooth, demonstrating a central flap of tissue called the rostral nasal concha. It is around this area that concretions of cellular debris and micro-organisms (rhinoliths) may form, leading to distortion of the external nares and the bones confining the nasal passages. It is also useful to examine the choanal slit: any discharges or swellings around the choanal slit may indicate upper respiratory tract disease. In addition, papillae on the palate surrounding the choanal slit may be reduced and this has been associated with respiratory disease, particularly psittacosis and vitamin A deficiency (Tully and Harrison, 1994).

It may not be easy to examine the sinuses during a routine clinical examination. Many avian sinuses lack a lateral bony wall to their structure and this is the case with the prominent infraorbital sinus, which sits beneath each eye. Inflammation of these sinuses causes lateral deviation of the skin in this area, producing a swelling, or a protruding eye, or in some instances making it appear that the eye is actually sinking into the head due to periorbital swelling. Gentle digital pressure ventral to the eye over the infraorbital sinus may produce discharge from the tear duct or nares. Occasionally, inflammation in the sinuses may affect the cervical air sac. Where inflammation does occur, the narrow entrance passages to the air sac may become inflamed and narrowed. This may act as a one-way valve to air flow through the sinuses and into this air sac, leading to its inflation, which is seen as a soft fluctuant swelling over the caudodorsal head.

Auscultation of the airways is possible but, due to the small size of many avian patients, clinicians should invest in a paediatric or infant stethoscope.

- The lungs may be auscultated over the dorsal thoracic area, as they are adherent to the ventral aspect of the thoracic vertebrae.
- Air sacs may be auscultated all over the body, but the caudal air sacs are the most useful to listen to for sounds of air sacculitis in the ventrolateral parts of the body.
- Respiratory wheezes and whistles may be heard with pneumonia or where focal lesions narrow the airways.
- Fluid sounds may be heard where respiratory secretions are produced, but even severe air sac pathology may not be audible.
- An increased respiratory rate, particularly with open-mouth breathing, may indicate respiratory pathology. Encouraging the patient to flap its wings two or three times will increase the oxygen demand and respiratory rate, allowing the clinician to auscultate any abnormal respiratory sounds more easily. It also allows an assessment of how quickly the patient's respiratory rate returns to normal after physical exertion.

Changes in 'voice', sometimes described by owners as the parrot gaining a sore throat, are often suggestive of tracheal and syringeal inflammation, a common condition seen in *Aspergillus* spp. infections.

Blood testing

Cell count
As part of a full investigation of respiratory disease, analysis should include as a minimum a full blood cell count. This is unlikely to diagnose a specific disease, though certain respiratory-associated diseases such as psittacosis and aspergillosis are known to elevate the total white blood cell count, often above 30×10^9/l (Aguilar and Redig, 1995). In acute cases this is mainly due to a heterophilia, but in chronic cases these elevations are often associated with a significant monocytosis.

Plasma proteins
Plasma protein electrophoresis is a powerful tool and may be used to help in the diagnosis of aspergillosis (Cray *et al.*, 1995; Cray and Tatum, 1998; Ivey, 2000; Girling, 2002). The most commonly recorded change is a significant increase in the beta globulin fraction, often 1.7 times the normal value (Cray *et al.*, 1995), with an increase in the gamma globulin fraction (Lumeij, 1987; Cray *et al.*, 1995; Cray, 1997). The trace outline is not on its own pathognomonic for aspergillosis, and there is species variation (even among parrots) as well as age variation between sexually immature and mature birds (Girling, 2002). In practice it has been found that birds with severe hypoalbuminaemia and low to normal beta and gamma globulins with *Aspergillus* spp. infection have a much reduced survival rate despite treatment (Reidarson and McBain, 1995). Figure 14.1 shows plasma protein electrophoresis results with aspergillosis.

Biochemistry
Plasma biochemistry testing may provide additional information to allow confirmation of respiratory diseases, such as psittacosis and aspergillosis, which both have a systemic (particularly hepatic) effect. Elevated aspartate aminotransferase (AST) and bile acid levels may indicate liver enzyme leakage and hepatic dysfunction, respectively, but AST may be found elsewhere in the bird, most notably the skeletal muscles. Glutamate dehydrogenase (GDH) is not a very sensitive test for hepatic necrosis but the only other source of GDH in the avian patient is the kidney tubular cells,

Parrot species	Albumin/ globulin ratio	Prealbumin	Albumin	Alpha globulins	Beta globulins	Gamma globulins
Grey Parrot	Decrease	No significant changes	Decrease	No significant changes	Increase (common split beta peak in healthy individuals becomes one combined peak)	Increase
Macaws	Decrease	No significant changes	Decrease	Increase in alpha 1 and 2 globulins	Increase	Increase
Amazons	Decrease	No significant changes	Decrease	No significant changes	Increase	Increase
Cockatoos	Decrease	No significant changes	Decrease	Increase in alpha 2 globulins	No significant changes	Increase

14.1 Significant changes ($P < 0.05$) in the plasma protein electrophoresis results seen in different species of parrot with aspergillosis, as compared with healthy parrots (Girling, 2002).

and when they release this enzyme it does not enter the bloodstream; rather, it exits the body via the urine. Elevated GDH (normal < 2 mmol/l) is therefore highly suggestive of hepatic necrosis, a condition seen particularly commonly in aspergillosis with aflatoxin release. In cases of hypothyroidism, with concomitant thyroid enlargement and respiratory distress, elevated levels of cholesterol may be seen as well as low levels of thyroxine.

Infectious agents

ELISA tests for *Aspergillus* spp. antibodies are prone to false negative results (Reidarson and McBain, 1995; Redig *et al.*, 1997). A solid-phase immunoassay has been created for the detection of antibodies to the *Chlamydophila* sp. organism (Immunocomb Biogel) which gives a semi-quantitative idea of antibody levels in psittacine blood. Interpretation may be complicated when low levels of antibodies are detected, as this may indicate previous exposure to the organism, or a current carrier state. In addition, antigen tests may be used on respiratory secretions or faeces, although false negative results may occur due to intermittent shedding of the organism. This is the same for the more sensitive polymerase chain reaction (PCR) tests for *Chlamydophila* antigen available through veterinary investigation laboratories (Chapter 7).

Diagnostic imaging

Radiography (Chapter 9) is an essential adjunct to the assessment of the severity of respiratory disease.

For upper respiratory tract disease, lateral, dorsoventral and oblique radiographs of the head may be used to assess sinus filling or masses. Positive contrast techniques using iodine-based contrast media diluted 1:5 with saline may also be used to assess whether sinuses and nasal passages communicate freely with each other. This is useful to indicate presence of blockages, granulomas, tumours, etc., but it should be noted that, in psittacine birds, the two nasal passages are completely divided from each other to the level of the choana normally. The sinuses should be flushed with sterile saline after this technique, as the iodine-based contrast may cause nasal irritation in itself.

For lower respiratory tract pathology, the ventrodorsal view is best for assessing air sac granulomas (Figure 14.2) and for lesions in the caudal lungs. The cranial lung fields are partially obscured by the overlying pectoral muscles and the heart. It is not possible to see interstitial patterns or air bronchograms. Atelectasis is not seen in birds, due to the semi-rigid nature of the avian lung. The lateral view is useful for determining the presence of air sacculitis, which may be seen as discrete lines crossing the radiolucent air sac areas.

In addition, with inflammation and granulomatous air sac conditions, a complaint known as 'air trapping' may be seen. This is where the inflammation/granuloma produces a one-way valve effect at the entrance of the air sac, allowing air to enter but not to exit. This leads to hyperinflation of the affected air sac, which is noticeable on radiography and occurs predominantly in the caudal air sacs (especially the abdominal).

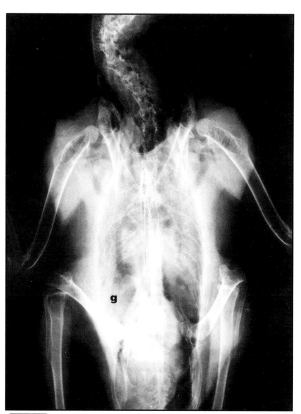

14.2 Ventrodorsal radiograph of a Blue and Gold Macaw showing air sacculitis and a fungal granuloma (g) due to *Aspergillus fumigatus.*

Magnetic resonance imaging (MRI) has been used to evaluate chronic sinusitis in psittacine birds (Pye *et al.*, 2000), where it has proved to be invaluable for examining the infraorbital sinus in particular.

Sinus flush and aspirates

The infraorbital sinuses may be sampled for microbial culture using a hypodermic needle and syringe, as the lateral wall of these is made of soft tissues only. It is important that the patient is sedated or anaesthetized for this technique, as any movement during the procedure could lead to puncture of the globe of the eye. The sinus is entered just above the jugal arch (Figure 14.3) and any exudate may then be aspirated for cytological analysis and microbial culture. Alternatively, a little sterile saline may be flushed into the sinus, and the flush collected from the choanal slit.

In addition the preorbital diverticulum may be sampled, again in the sedated or anaesthetized bird, by inserting a needle and syringe through the skin at the commissure of the beak, and under the jugal arch (Figure 14.3). Any fluid exudate may then be sampled, or a little sterile saline flushed through and collected at the choanal slit as before.

A nasal passage flush may be performed by applying a syringe of sterile saline to one nostril, inverting the patient and forcefully flushing the saline into the nasal passage. Some of this fluid may then be collected from the opposite nostril or choana, having flushed through the nasal passages, and may then be subjected to microbial culture and sensitivity and cytological analysis.

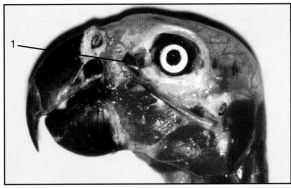

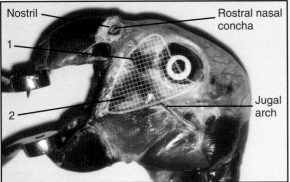

14.3 Grey Parrot dissected to reveal extent of main part of infraorbital sinus. The sinus (see delineated area) can be found extending medioventral to the globe. Two areas of the lateral wall of the sinus have been removed, dorsal and ventral to the bony jugal arch. These correspond to the potential access points to the sinus. The dorsal site (1) is best when using a needle and syringe to flush the sinus. The ventral site (2) is better for surgical exploration. It is possible to palpate both of these sites in the live bird. The sinus is 'larger' when the bird's mouth is open (see also Figure 2.16). When the bird's mouth is shut, the only access is midway between the nostril and medial canthus, just dorsal to the jugal arch.

Tracheal/lung wash

This may be performed using a sterile 3–4 Fr urinary catheter, passed through a sterile endotracheal tube to avoid contamination of the sample with oral commensal organisms. Alternatively, a transtracheal technique may be used whereby a sterile over-the-needle latex catheter is inserted between tracheal rings in the caudal trachea, avoiding oral contamination.

Once the catheter is in place, sterile saline may be introduced at a volume of 0.5–1 ml/kg, and rapidly aspirated. This may then be sent for microbial culture and sensitivity, as well as microscopic analysis for cytological examination. Cytology is useful. Large numbers of alveolar macrophages and heterophils, particularly with toxic changes, would indicate active infection.

In addition, air-dried smears should be made to allow examination of any cellular debris. These can be stained with standard (i.e. Giemsa-style) stains and Gram's stain for bacterial classification. Evidence of large numbers of one bacterium may suggest a causal organism, as will branching fungal septae or budding yeasts. Special stains may be used to attempt to identify *Chlamydophila* organisms within cells (Chapter 13). In addition, samples should always be sent for bacterial and fungal culture and sensitivity testing.

Endoscopy

Endoscopy is a vital component in the diagnosis of respiratory disease in psittacine birds. It is essential for physical examination of lesions detected using radiographic techniques, and for collecting samples for microbial culture and sensitivity testing. In addition, physical debulking of lesions such as granulomas/aspergillomas as part of a therapeutic regime is possible. Access is usually gained via the caudal thoracic air sac, but more caudal lesions may be approached via the abdominal air sac caudal to the pelvic limb (Chapter 9).

Lung biopsy

This procedure has some benefits, particularly where discrete lesions such as pulmonary granulomas are present, or where tracheal/lung washes have failed to provide a diagnosis but lung pathology is still suspected.

The lung may be accessed via the caudal thoracic air sac, as used in routine coelomic endoscopy, or via a dorsal intercostal approach over the third or fourth intercostal spaces (Chapter 10). Dorsal lung biopsy may be more useful, as much lung pathology is found on the dorsal aspects. A biopsy can be taken with 3 or 4 Fr endoscope-guided biopsy forceps, and retained in formal saline for histopathological analysis. Where possible, additional samples or swabs should be collected for microbial culture and sensitivity testing.

Respiratory disease

Respiratory disease may be broadly divided into:

- Upper respiratory tract disease, affecting the nares, nasal passages and sinuses to the level of the glottis
- Lower respiratory tract disease, affecting the trachea, syrinx, bronchi, lungs and air sacs.

As with many diseases in psittacine birds, the patient may successfully hide evidence of its condition until it is so advanced that the bird is obviously dyspnoeic. Success rates of treatment may be correspondingly poor.

The signs demonstrated by a bird with upper or lower respiratory disease are as suggested in Figure 14.4.

Upper respiratory disease
Oculonasal discharge(s)
Swelling below/around eye (or may appear as a 'sunken eye', particularly in macaws)
Cephalic air sac swelling on dorsal/caudal head
Blocked nares
Nares of different sizes
Swelling of cere/frontal area of head
Dyspnoea
Sneezing
Epistaxis
Head shaking
Clawing at nares
Choanal discharge
Naso-lacrimal punctum discharge
Respiratory stertor

14.4 Clinical signs that may be observed in cases of upper and lower respiratory disease in psittacine birds. (continues) ▶

Lower respiratory disease
Dyspnoea (particularly syringotracheal disease)
Tail bobbing
Loss of voice/change in pitch of voice
Coughing
Tachypnoea
Hyperpnoea
Cyanosis of mucous membranes
Exercise intolerance
Squeaks/rales when breathing
Non-specific weight loss
'Sick bird syndrome' (SBS)

14.4 (continued) Clinical signs that may be observed in cases of upper and lower respiratory disease in psittacine birds.

It should be noted that there are several non-respiratory system diseases associated with dyspnoea (Figure 14.5). The absence of a diaphragm in birds allows any disease applying pressure to the air sac system to reduce inspiratory volumes and cause dyspnoea.

Disease	Reason for hyperpnoea/dyspnoea
Any disease producing anaemia (e.g. haemorrhage, malnutrition, lead poisoning)	Lack of circulating oxygen-carrying capacity
Cardiovascular failure	Producing either ascites or cyanosis
Egg binding	Space-occupying lesion preventing inflation of caudal air sacs
Goitre (e.g. Budgerigar)	Thyroid hyperplasia at the level of the distal trachea causing narrowing of the tracheal lumen
Hyperthermia	Heat stress (gular fluttering may be mistaken for hyperpnoea)
Liver disease	Ascites (chronic liver insufficiency) or haemorrhage (from damaged liver or due to lack of clotting factors) causing pressure on the caudal air sacs reducing the inspiratory volume
Obesity	Space-occupying fat deposits applying external pressure to air sacs, reducing inspiratory volume
Peritonitis (e.g. yolk peritonitis)	Adhesions and ascites affecting air sac function
Renal disease	Protein-losing nephropathy resulting in ascites
Neoplasia	This may also cause ascites depending on its source or physical compression of air sacs and/or lungs

14.5 Non-respiratory diseases that may be associated with tachypnoea or dyspnoea.

Upper respiratory tract diseases

Rhinitis

Rhinitis may be caused by a number of factors. Aerosol sprays, tobacco smoke, excessively low humidity and the dander produced by some types of psittacine bird (such as Grey Parrots and cockatoos) may lead to irritant rhinitis, particularly in species such as Amazons. In young birds infection may be secondary to a choanal atresia (Chapter 11). Evidence of a nasal discharge may not be obvious, but staining of the feathers above the nares can be used as an indicator of disease. Serous discharges may also be associated with infectious bacterial pathogens such as *Mycoplasma* spp. or *Chlamydophila psittaci*. In addition, parasites such as the *Cnemidocoptes* sp. mite may cause severe trauma to the cere, leading to blockage of the nostrils and secondary bacterial or fungal rhinitis, as well as dyspnoea and mouth breathing. The latter condition is seen predominantly in Budgerigars.

With chronic conditions, the presence of a concurrent sinusitis is common. This is particularly the case with rhinoliths. This condition is often more likely to occur if the patient is suffering from nutritional hypovitaminosis A, which causes thickening of the respiratory epithelium and a reduction in the efficacy of the local immune system.

A rhinolith can cause progressive destruction of, initially, the soft tissue structures of the nasal passages, such as the operculum. This is followed by lysis of the bones forming the boundaries to the nasal passages, the rostral nasal conchae and usually extending into the sinuses as well. This will produce distortion of the external naris or nares, the frontal bones and the infraorbital sinus(es) (Figure 14.6). Micro-organisms often cultured from these rhinoliths include bacteria such as *Escherichia coli, Pseudomonas* spp. and *Klebsiella* spp. as well as fungi, particularly *Aspergillus* spp.

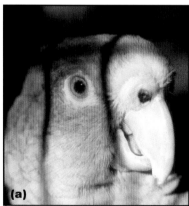
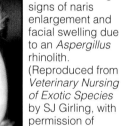
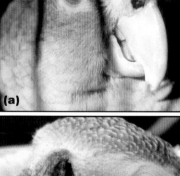

14.6

(a) Yellow-fronted Amazon showing signs of naris enlargement and facial swelling due to an *Aspergillus* rhinolith. (Reproduced from *Veterinary Nursing of Exotic Species* by SJ Girling, with permission of Blackwell Publishing.)
(b) Grey Parrot with chronic rhinolith in the external nares (courtesy of Aidan Raftery).

Treatment

Treatment of parasites such as *Cnemidocoptes* is with ivermectin, orally or by injection. Alternatively, a topical spot-on form of ivermectin may be made up to a 0.1% solution by veterinary order and applied once weekly on three occasions (Chapter 16).

With care, simple nasal plugs may be removed in the conscious restrained bird. A dental pick or blunted hypodermic needle may be used gently to remove the plug away from the naris. The naris may then be flushed with sterile saline containing appropriate anti-microbial medications (see next section for further details). For home treatment, topical drops, such as gentamicin eye drops in the case of Gram-negative bacterial infections, are useful. Care should be taken to avoid using drops that contain corticosteroids, as birds are very sensitive to the immunosuppressive side effects of even topical corticosteroids.

For larger, more extensive rhinoliths, treatment requires surgical debridement under anaesthesia. Follow-up treatment is required, as the normal anatomy of the nasal passages is generally destroyed or distorted, leading to frequent reinfection and mucus build-up. This may involve flushing the nasal passages (see below under Treatment of sinusitis) as well as systemic antimicrobial medication based on culture and sensitivity results. Regular flushing of the nasal passages with sterile saline for several weeks after treatment may also be necessary to remove mucus build-up. Humidification of the bird's local environment and attention to minimizing irritant aerosols and smoke in its environment are also helpful.

Sinus disease

Sinusitis

This is one of the most commonly seen respiratory problems in psittacine birds. The multiple blind-ending avian sinuses and nasal passages make successful treatment of sinusitis challenging. Clinically the patient may present with sneezing, nasal discharge, swelling around the eye(s) and discharge from the internal choanal slit. Alternatively, the eye may appear sunken, as has been reported in macaws. In psittacine birds the right and left infraorbital sinuses communicate, allowing infection within the infraorbital sinus of one side to lead to swelling and infection of the contralateral sinus.

Pathogenic bacteria that have been isolated from the sinuses include *Pseudomonas aeruginosa, Aeromonas* spp., *Escherichia coli, Nocardia asteroides, Mycoplasma* spp., *Mycobacterium* spp. and *Chlamydophila psittaci* (Van der Mast *et al.*, 1990; Tully and Carter, 1993; Baumgartner *et al.*, 1994; Hillyer, 1997). Fungi associated with upper respiratory disease include *Aspergillus* spp., *Candida* sp. and *Mucor* sp. (Redig, 1983; Dawson *et al.*, 1976). Often a serous sinusitis, initiated by primary pathogens such as *Chlamydophila psittaci* or *Mycoplasma* spp., can lead to a mucopurulent sinus discharge as secondary bacterial or fungal pathogens gain control.

Poor nutrition resulting in hypovitaminosis A may lead to hyperkeratosis of the lining of the sinuses and airways and a build-up of cellular debris that can block sinus drainage and harbour opportunistic bacteria (Figure 14.7) and fungi.

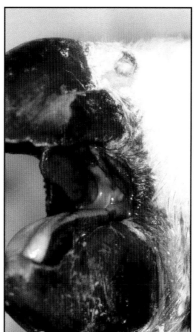

14.7 Grey Parrot with nasal discharge and choanal discharge demonstrating sinusitis and rhinitis as a result of nutritional (vitamin A) deficiency and *Pseudomonas multocida* bacterial infection. (Reproduced from *Veterinary Nursing of Exotic Species* by SJ Girling, with permission of Blackwell Publishing.)

Treatment: Treatment of sinusitis may be difficult, due to the often advanced nature of the condition and therefore the likelihood that chronic tissue damage has been caused. Flushing the nasal passages and sinuses with a saline solution mixed with antifungal agents (such as clotrimazole or itraconazole) or antibacterial agents (such as enrofloxacin or gentamicin) may be attempted. This can be performed in the conscious bird using a syringe applied to the external nares. In addition, the disinfectant F10 (Health and Hygiene Pty) diluted 1:250 with water may be flushed through infected sinuses (Chitty, 2002). The bird is held inverted and the solution is flushed through one nostril, with the excess flushing through the nasal passages and exiting via the opposite nostril and choanal slit. The same may then be performed via the opposite nostril (see Figure 21.6).

In some cases surgical debridement of the sinus may be required. This is relatively straightforward; as previously mentioned, the lateral wall to the infraorbital sinus and preorbital diverticulum is soft tissue. This may be incised and the contents of the sinus carefully debrided using a small cancellous bone curette or a dental pick. The incision may be left open to granulate, so allowing further topical flushing of the lesion.

Sinus cysts and neoplasia

An infraorbital cyst has been reported in an Umbrella Cockatoo (Stiles and Greenacre, 2001), and this author has seen the condition in a Budgerigar and a Blue-fronted Amazon. It may be diagnosed by fine-needle aspiration of the soft swelling below the eye which will reveal an acellular proteinaceous sterile fluid consistent with a cystic structure. Surgical excision is the treatment of choice where possible. Lymphoma in Amazons and melanoma in Grey Parrots have been observed in the infra-orbital region (N. Harcourt-Brown, personal communication).

Lower respiratory tract diseases

Tracheitis

Tracheal damage may be caused by a number of organisms, including parasites (Figure 14.8).

Viral diseases of the trachea are relatively uncommon in psittacine birds in the UK and are mainly seen in imported birds. Therapy is supportive. Attempts to treat Amazon laryngotracheitis with aciclovir have had varying degrees of success.

Parasitic causes of tracheal disease, such as the gapeworm *Syngamus trachea*, are uncommon in psittacine birds. *S. trachea* is associated with earth-floored aviaries; the parasite uses intermediate transport hosts (e.g. earthworms), which are consumed by the bird to allow infection to occur. Tracheal mites (*Sternostoma* spp.) are rare in psittacine birds.

Bacteria
Chlamydophila psittaci; Escherichia coli; Haemophilus; Klebsiella; Mycoplasma; Pasteurella; Pseudomonas; Staphylococcus; Streptococcus

Fungi
Aspergillus; Candida

Viruses
Herpesvirus (e.g. Amazon laryngotracheitis virus); Paramyxovirus; Avipoxviruses (e.g. Amazon poxvirus, Agapornis poxvirus)

Parasites
Syngamus (gape worms)*; Sternostoma* (tracheal mites)

 14.8 Pathogens commonly affecting the lower respiratory tract of psittacine birds.

Treatment

Treatment of both parasites may be performed using ivermectin orally, topically or subcutaneously. Care should be taken with gapeworm treatment, as the death of the worms can still lead to tracheal obstruction, pneumonia or asphyxiation.

Tracheal and syringeal obstruction

Partial or full obstruction of the trachea is a relatively uncommon condition in psittacine birds (Dennis *et al.*, 1999) and may be due to foreign body aspiration (Figure 14.9), fungal granuloma, stricture or neoplastic growths. Dyspnoea and changes in vocalization are usually seen, although in complete obstruction cases rapid asphyxiation is inevitable.

Treatment

In some larger species (e.g. macaws) or very small species (e.g. Cockatiel), it may not be possible to reach tracheal foreign bodies or syringeal granulomas via the glottis. These may be diagnosed using radiography, as well as clinical presentation of the patient (Chapter 9). In order to maintain the patient safely under gaseous anaesthetic and prevent hypoxia whilst removal of the obstruction is performed, the insertion of an air sac

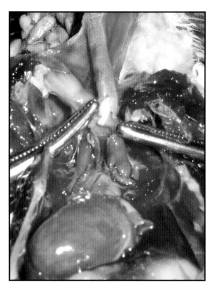 **14.9** Sunflower kernel lodged in the distal trachea of a Cape Parrot after regurgitation, resulting in subsequent asphyxiation.

tube is useful (Chapter 8). The tube may be left in place for several days whilst treatment for the tracheal lesion is performed, so allowing an unimpeded airway.

In some cases, a fine catheter with a 90 degree cut end may be used alongside a rigid endoscope to 'core' out any fungal growth, and aspiration by means of a syringe attached to the proximal end can aid removal via the glottis (see Aspergillosis, below). In cases that are beyond the reach of a catheter or too large to aspirate safely, a tracheotomy may be performed by incising between two complete cartilage rings (see Chapter 10 for surgical technique). The rings themselves must not be cut, as this can lead to a tracheal stricture as the wound heals, leading to dyspnoea and even obstruction of the tracheal lumen. (For a full discussion on how to treat syringeal aspergillomas, see Aspergillosis, below.)

Air sacculitis and pneumonia

These two conditions are sometimes seen together, as the two systems (air sacs and lungs) are of course closely linked. In general, air sacculitis is more commonly seen and is associated principally with fungal (chiefly *Aspergillus* spp.), *Mycoplasma* spp. and *Chlamydophila psittaci* infections, whereas pneumonias may involve many other bacterial pathogens as well.

Bacterial pneumonia and air sacculitis

Many bacteria have been associated with respiratory disease in psittacine birds (Figure 14.8). Some may be primary pathogens, such as *Chlamydophila psittaci*. Others may be more opportunistic in their behaviour, causing secondary infections as a sequel to respiratory tract damage from irritants such as smoke and toxic fumes.

Mycoplasma spp. and the cause of 'psittacosis', *C. psittaci*, are bacteria with a predilection for respiratory epithelium, as well as both being obligate intracellular organisms. They may produce a serous clear nasal discharge causing sneezing and upper respiratory signs, and they may produce an air sacculitis. *C. psittaci* often causes a systemic infection.

Treatment: The fluoroquinolone family (enrofloxacin and marbofloxacin) are particularly effective against most respiratory bacteria, including many *Mycoplasma* spp., *Pseudomonas* spp. and *Escherichia coli*.

Bacteria such as *C. psittaci* are also susceptible to fluoroquinolones such as enrofloxacin, but it has not been proved conclusively that enrofloxacin can fully eradicate the pathogen. The mainstay of psittacosis therapy is the antibiotic doxycycline, preferably as the injectable doxycycline hyclate intravenous human preparation, given intramuscularly. Alternatively, the licensed UK formulation of doxycycline hyclate is as an in-water powder medication.

Debulking of any bacterial granulomas present within the airways and air sacs is a useful adjunct to medical therapy by reducing the mass of infected material present and allowing access to the core of the infected areas for any topical or systemic medication. This is performed using rigid endoscopes with instrument sheaths that allow the guided use of biopsy cups and scissors, which can be employed in debulking the granuloma(s). The instrument sheath may then be used to allow the application of medications to the granuloma site(s) directly by threading a fine urinary catheter through the instrument port and attaching a syringe to flush medication through. The use of laser diode therapy for endosurgical debridement of fungal and bacterial granulomas has been described in parrots (Hernandez-Divers, 2002).

As well as systemic antibiosis and physical debridement, nebulization therapy (see later) is also extremely useful in treating air sac and lung infections.

Aspergillosis

This is the commonest cause of fungal pneumonia and air sacculitis; indeed Redig (1993) recorded aspergillosis as the commonest respiratory disease amongst captive non-domesticated birds. There are several species of *Aspergillus* associated with aspergillosis in psittacine birds, including *Aspergillus fumigatus, A. flavus, A. niger* and *A. terreus*. The disease is not contagious but is contracted from the local environment. Certain environments, particularly those containing large amounts of decomposing vegetable or fruit material (such as poorly cleaned floors of bird cages), encourage growth of *Aspergillus* spp. and spore release.

It is generally considered that aspergillosis is an opportunistic disease in birds, with some form of immunosuppression occurring at the time of infection. However, a primary infection can occur if the bird is exposed to overwhelming numbers of spores in its environment when the immune system may be breached without serious immunosuppression. An example of such a situation may be the inappropriate use of organic substrates, such as hay or straw, to litter the aviary or line a nestbox. These are commonly heavily contaminated with fungal spores and can produce rapid mould growth with further sporulation.

There are many features that may contribute to immunosuppression, one of the principal culprits being 'stress'. Birds most at risk are those that are subjected to inappropriate environmental conditions, or have recently been caught in the wild or transported long distances, and birds that are moved rapidly from one different environment to another, such as those moved from breeder to pet shop to a purchaser's home. Other factors that may predispose to the development of immunosuppression include: administration of corticosteroids and certain antibiotics (e.g. tetracyclines); nutritional disorders such as hypovitaminosis A; immune system naiveté in juvenile birds; and concurrent disease (particular viral conditions such as the circovirus infection).

Aspergillosis may present as a number of conditions, both chronic and acute. Clinical signs of chronic aspergillosis have been described by Redig (1993) as being non-specific, including change in behaviour, decreased weight and voice changes before severe respiratory signs become noticeable. It is frequently associated with a caudal air sacculitis, and lung granulomas may also be found (see Figure 14.2). The caudal air sacs are principally involved, as they are the area to which the first inspiration of fresh air travels. Any sizeable particles, such as fungal spores, are likely to drop out of the slowing air flow in the pause between inspiration and expiration and be deposited on the air sac lining.

Acute aspergillosis may be seen in the sudden death of an apparently healthy bird, and is frequently blamed on the systemic and chiefly hepatic destruction caused by the release of aflatoxins from the growing *Aspergillus* spp. In addition, an acute syndrome may be seen where the fungus starts to grow at the level of the syrinx. This can lead to obstruction of the airway in as little as 4–5 days, and presents as acute dyspnoea, but early signs include a change in the bird's voice, often described by owners as sounding like a 'sore throat'. Alternatively, if the granuloma starts within a bronchus, the onset can be more insidious as it gradually spreads to the trachea.

Treatment: Treatment of aspergillosis is very difficult, due to the drug resistance of the fungus and the inaccessible sites affected. Combination therapy is performed using both systemic and topical or nebulized medicants plus surgical debulking of any granulomatous material. Dietary improvement is vital.

Administration of amphotericin B is advised initially in cases of aspergillosis as an intravenous bolus (Redig, 1983). This is rapidly fungicidal, whereas it frequently takes several days for the fungicidal effect of the azole family to take effect. Care should be taken with dehydrated patients or those with existing renal disease or damage, as amphotericin B is potentially nephrotoxic. A bolus of intravenous fluids should therefore be given at the same time as this therapy.

Further systemic therapy includes agents such as the azole family (itraconazole, ketoconazole, fluconazole), which have become one of the mainstays of respiratory antifungal therapy. Itraconazole has been shown to be particularly effective against *Aspergillus* spp. infections (Forbes, 1992; Aguilar and Redig, 1995; Orosz and Frazier, 1995) (Figure 14.10) but it has been shown to be poorly tolerated by some psittacine birds such as the Grey Parrot and may indeed be toxic to this species (Orosz, 2000). It should be noted that all azoles produce varying degrees of hepatotoxicity, though itraconazole appears less hepatotoxic than ketoconazole (Orosz and Frazier, 1995).

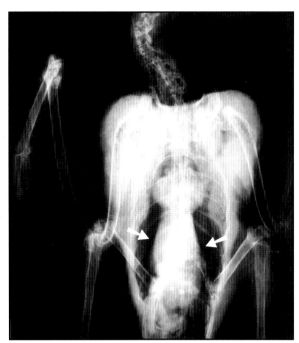

14.10 A ventrodorsal radiograph of the Blue and Gold Macaw seen in Figure 14.2 after 4 months of antifungal treatment (oral itraconazole), including one initial week of nebulization with F10. Note the disappearance of the fungal granuloma and the increased radiolucency of the caudal air sacs (arrowed).

The allylamine drug terbinafine hydrochloride may be used as an oral therapy in azole-sensitive psittacine birds, such as the Grey Parrot. It may be used in conjunction with topical nebulizable treatments such as F10 (see below) and this seems to be effective without significant toxicity (Dahlhausen *et al.*, 2000).

Endosurgical debulking of fungal granulomas is advisable where possible, to reduce the mass of pathogen and thereby increase the chances of a successful medical treatment, as mentioned above in the treatment of bacterial granulomas.

Tracheal/syringeal granuloma removal may be performed via endoscopy through the glottis in the anaesthetized bird. For this procedure to be successful it is necessary to place an air sac tube into the caudal thoracic or abdominal air sac, and to attach the anaesthetic circuit to this to allow the bird to breathe adequately. In the abdominal air sac position, caudal to the leg, the air sac cannula is more difficult to remove if the intention is to leave the cannula *in situ* for a few days after surgery to ensure unobstructed breathing. (Placement of air sac cannulas is covered in more detail in Chapter 8.) The granuloma may be removed with endoscopic biopsy cup forceps, or by using a canine urinary catheter with the distal tip cut off to leave an end opening, rather than a side opening. To the catheter is attached a 5 ml syringe, and the catheter is guided down the trachea through the glottis under constant observation via a rigid endoscope. The catheter may then be used to dislodge the bulk of the granuloma, whilst gentle suction is applied via the syringe to allow any dislodged particles to be removed proximally. If fragments of the granuloma are dislodged distally, they may be pushed through the primary

bronchus into which they fall and then into one of the associated air sacs. The fragments may either be removed via endoscopy through a lateral body wall approach, or be left and treated medically *in situ*.

Nebulization therapy is an essential adjunct in the treatment of aspergillosis (see below).

Alternatively, direct application of clotrimazole to an endoscopically visualized fungal plaque, such as a syringeal aspergilloma site after initial debulking of the granuloma surgically, can be effective in the ongoing successful treatment of the disease.

Reassessment: Birds affected by aspergillosis require regular examination to ensure satisfactory progress of the treatment. This will involve repeated endoscopic and radiographic examination of the trachea and coelomic cavity to assess regression of lesions. Continued reassessment of blood cell counts and plasma protein electrophoresis is also recommended, as resolution is suggested by a reducing monocytosis and heterophilia (where initially elevated) to normal ranges for the species concerned. In addition, the plasma protein electrophoresis results show normalization of albumin:globulin ratios and reduction of beta globulin levels to normal ranges. Reassessment of these parameters is advised every 3–4 weeks during the course of the treatment, assuming satisfactory clinical progress. More frequent reassessment is advised if the patient shows clinical deterioration. Courses of treatment for aspergillosis should be no less than 12 weeks, and frequently extend to 6–9 months or longer for advanced cases.

Nebulization therapy

Nebulization of medications in the treatment of respiratory disease is becoming one of the main planks of therapy protocols. It is particularly useful in cases of fungal respiratory disease such as aspergillosis, where the organism is highly resilient to many antifungal agents, and is growing in areas such as the air sacs, which are difficult for the therapies concerned to reach due to their poor blood supply. Commercial nebulizers are easily and cheaply obtained (Figure 14.11). There are some arguments about the importance of the droplet size produced by the nebulizer (Figure 14.12).

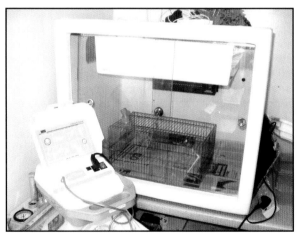

14.11 A nebulizer used in conjunction with a vivarium-style chamber to allow efficient nebulization of an avian patient.

Advantages

- Direct application of drug nebulized to site of infection
- Reduction or removal of systemic potential toxic effects of some drugs (e.g. amphotericin B nephrotoxicity)
- Humidifies local environment, preventing desiccation of respiratory epithelium and reducing tenacity of mucous secretions

Disadvantages

- Particle size of droplets produced by non-ultrasonic nebulizers varies. *Aspergillus* spores are 2–5 μm. Therefore, droplets ≤ 5 μm will penetrate the sites reached by spores
- Oil-based medications will not nebulize well
- If consolidation of the lung has occurred with blockage of airways, then nebulized drugs will not penetrate these areas, meaning that systemic antifungal agents are also needed

14.12 Advantages and disadvantages of using a commercial non-ultrasonic nebulizer in the treatment of respiratory tract infections.

Many medications may be nebulized, including antibiotics, antifungal agents, bronchodilators and anti-inflammatories (Figure 14.13). Treatment is usually repeated 3–4 times a day for periods of 15–20 minutes.

The commercial disinfectant F10 has also recently become popular in the treatment of respiratory tract infections, particularly aspergillosis in the UK. It contains biguanide and quaternary ammonium compounds (5.8%) and is viricidal, bactericidal, fungicidal and sporicidal, as well as being aldehyde-free (Chitty, 2002a). Used at a dilution of 1:250 it may be nebulized and appears clinically safe.

Bronchial spasm and pulmonary oedema

These conditions occur generally after exposure to inhaled toxins or irritants, such as fumes from over-heated non-stick frying pans, smoke, or other chemical fumes. These may result in oedema and sloughing of the lining to the trachea and bronchi, as well as true pulmonary oedema.

Treatment

Treatment is by conservative therapy and the use of nebulized or systemic short-acting corticosteroids, such as methyl-prednisolone. Extreme care should be taken with corticosteroid use as even one-off doses may cause severe immunosuppression, allowing opportunistic pathogens such as *Aspergillus* spp. a chance to cause infection. This, combined with the likely damage to the airway epithelium, makes the use of covering broad-spectrum antimicrobials advisable in these cases.

Other pulmonary diseases

Lung neoplasia has been reported infrequently in psittacine birds. There have been reports of a pulmonary carcinoma with metastases to the vertebral column and right humerus in a Moluccan Cockatoo (Jones *et al.*, 2001), a pulmonary fibrosarcoma with metastases to the liver in a Cockatiel (Burgmann, 1994) and a primary bronchial carcinoma with secondary metastasis to the right humerus in a Grey Parrot (André and Delverdier, 1999). It is interesting that, in all of these cases, respiratory disease was not the primary presenting sign, often being entirely absent. Rather, it was the disease caused by the secondary metastases that alerted the owner and clinician to a problem.

Medication	Drug efficacy	Concentration
Acetylcysteine	Useful as a mucolytic	2–5 drops per treatment in 15 ml saline (Clubb, 1986)
Amphotericin B	Useful for aspergillosis and some bacterial infections	1 mg/ml in 0.9% saline for 15 min q12h (Bauck *et al.*, 1992)
Enrofloxacin	Broad spectrum of chiefly Gram-negative and some Gram-positive (anti-staphylococcal and -streptococcal) activity, as well as efficacy against *Mycoplasma* spp. and *Chlamydophila psittaci*	100 mg in 10 ml saline for 15 min q8–12h
F10	Wide range of fungicidal (including aspergillosis), bactericidal (including *E. coli*, *Klebsiella* spp., *Pseudomonas* spp.), viricidal and sporicidal activity	4 ml in 1 litre of water for 20–30 min q8–12h (Chitty, 2002a)
Gentamicin	Gram-negative activity (including *E. coli*, and some *Pseudomonas* spp. activity)	50 mg in 10 ml saline for 15 min q8–12h
Tylosin	Useful for upper respiratory tract mycoplasmosis	100 mg in 10 ml saline for 1 hour q12h (Tully, 1997)

14.13 Drugs that may be administered by nebulization therapy for treating respiratory disease.

15

Gastrointestinal disease

Deborah Monks

Introduction

Primary gastrointestinal diseases may appear clinically similar to systemic diseases with secondary gastrointestinal effects. Thus accurate history taking, thorough examination and rational diagnostic testing must be employed to reach an accurate diagnosis and allow appropriate treatment. This chapter aims to present a discussion of psittacine gastroenterology, with emphasis on common presentations and diseases. Anatomy is described in Chapter 2.

Clinical signs

When a bird is presented with a gastrointestinal (GI) complaint, Figure 15.1 should be used to determine which areas of the GI tract are likely to be involved.

Obvious signs of GI dysfunction include vomition/regurgitation, dysphagia, inappetence, anorexia, crop enlargement, weight loss and abnormal droppings. Distinguishing between vomition and regurgitation is not of great value and these terms will be used interchangeably in this chapter.

Abnormalities of the droppings may be due to GI, urinary or reproductive tract problems (Appendix 2).

However, diarrhoea, undigested food (especially seeds) or malodour are likely to be indicative of GI problems. Dropping consistency will vary among different species and according to diet. Lories and lorikeets usually produce small amounts of faeces with a large volume of urine, while granivorous birds produce green/brown faeces with reduced urine component. Food colourings and some foods may discolour droppings. Brooding hens will usually have voluminous droppings, due to a reduction in dropping frequency. Anorexic birds will produce scant, dark green faeces.

Less obvious signs can include generalized ill-thrift, feather plucking or abdominal distension, but these are not specific for GI disease.

Although diarrhoea has been associated with *Chlamydophila psittaci* infection, clinical changes are usually observed in the urate rather than the faecal component of the dropping (Appendix 2). Nevertheless, psittacosis is an important zoonosis and testing must be considered whenever an ill parrot is presented (Chapters 7 and 13).

Any bird with systemic disease, depression or unexplained clinical signs should have a thorough investigation including radiography, haematology and biochemistry as well as GI-specific diagnostic tests.

Area	Dysphagia	Vomition/ regurgitation	Inappetence/ anorexia	Weight loss	Abnormal droppings	Ill–thrift	Feather plucking [a]	Abdominal distension
Oropharynx	+++		+++	+/++				
Crop	+++	+++	+++	++	+	+/++	±	
Oesophagus	+++	+++	+++	++	+	+/++		
Proventriculus		+++	+++	+++	+++	++	++	±
Ventriculus		+/++	+/++	++/+++	++/+++	++	+	±
Duodenum		+/++	++/+++	++/+++	++/+++	++	±	±
Pancreas		+/++	++	+++	+++	++	±	±
Intestine		+	+++	+++	+++	++/+++	+	+
Rectum					+++	+	±	
Cloaca					+++	+	+	

15.1 Clinical presentation by anatomical area. The likelihood of the clinical sign being caused by pathology of the specific anatomical area is indicated: +++ = common; ++ = frequent; + = infrequent; ± = uncommon. [a] Feather plucking related to a specific GI organ is often localized to an area over that organ.

Area	Physical examination	Wash/ lavage	Wash/ faeces/ impression smear		Culture and sensitivity	Faecal flotation	Blood analysis			Radiography		Endoscopy
			Wet mount/ cytology	Gram or other stain			Haematology	Biochemistry	Other	Plain/ Survey	Contrast	
Oropharynx	+++		+++ IS	‖ IS	‖					+	++	++
Crop	++	+++	+++ W/IS	‖ W/IS	‖					+	+	++
Oesophagus			+ W		‖					++	++	+++
Proventriculus		++	++ W	‖ W	‖		++	++	++	++	+++	+++
Ventriculus	+						+	+	+	++	++	++
Duodenum			+++ F	‖ F		+++	+	+		+	+	+
Pancreas			+++ F	‖ F			+++	+++		+	+	++
Intestine	+		+++ F	‖ F	‖	+++	++	++		++	++	+
Rectum	+.		+++ F	‖ F	‖	+	+	+		+	+	++
Cloaca	+++		+++ F/IS	‖ F/IS	‖		+	+		+	+	+++

15.2 Recommended diagnostics by anatomical area. The usefulness of each test is indicated: +++ = high; ++ = moderate; + = low. F = faeces; ‖ = if indicated; IS = impression smear; W = wash.

Diagnostic tools

Figure 15.2 can be used to determine which diagnostic tests may be useful (e.g. crop wash and cytology), according to the segment of GI tract affected.

A thorough history is crucial (Chapter 5). Droppings should be examined (Appendix 2). The bird should be assessed visually from a distance and then physically examined. A thorough examination of the oropharynx or vent may require anaesthesia (Chapter 8).

Microscopic examination

- *Wet smears*. Faecal smears and crop or proventricular 'washes' can be mixed with saline or counterstain (e.g. a drop of RapiDiff Solution 3 to provide background staining) and examined after placement of a coverslip. Motile protozoa, bacteria, yeast (both budding and with pseudohyphae), 'megabacteria', fungi and endoparasites can be identified (Figures 15.3, 15.4 and 15.5). Protozoan motility decreases

rapidly but immediate examination on a pre-warmed slide may improve diagnostic sensitivity. Brownian motion may be mistaken for protozoal or bacterial motility, though it does not usually result in net movement of organisms. Motile organisms tend to move appreciably within the visual field.

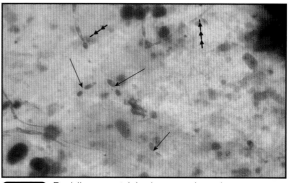

15.4 Budding yeast (single arrows) and pseudohyphal yeast (multiple arrows). Diff-Quik stain, original magnification 400× (high dry).

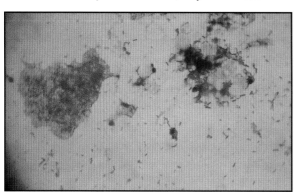

15.3 Dividing bacteria on a faecal smear. Diff-Quik stain, original magnification 400× (high dry). Faecal smears can demonstrate approximate bacterial morphology and numbers. Gram staining is advised when monomorphic populations of bacteria are identified.

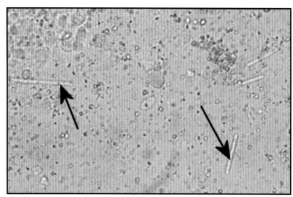

15.5 'Megabacterium', a yeast also known as *Macrorhabdus ornithogaster*, in an unstained wet smear. Original magnification 400× (high dry). The stained organism can be seen in Figure 21.10.

- *Gram stains* should be performed whenever monomorphic bacterial populations or increased bacterial numbers are demonstrated. Some practitioners routinely perform Gram stains and will identify 'megabacteria' and other yeasts from this stain rather than using wet smears.
- *Faecal Gram stains* are an area of current controversy (Figure 15.6).
- *Cytological examination* of exudates and impression smears may distinguish inflammation, infection or neoplasia. Wrights, Giemsa or May–Grünwald stains are commonly used, although 'rapid stains' (Diff-Quik, RapiDiff, Hemacolor) also give good results (Chapter 7).
- If mycobacterial infection is suspected, *Ziehl–Neelsen* stain should be used.

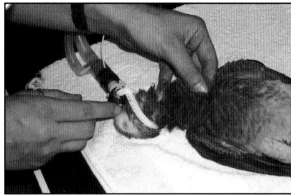

15.7 Placement of crop tube/catheter to perform a proventricular wash. Manipulation must be done very carefully to avoid iatrogenic damage.

In health

Advantages	Disadvantages
• Identify subclinical bacterial and yeast infections • Identify abnormalities in the distribution of Gram-negative and Gram-positive bacterial flora • Assess success of dietary conversion from seeds to pellets (Stanford, 2002)	• Lack of correlation between Gram stain and clinical health/disease in healthy patients • Time intense

In disease

Advantages	Disadvantages
• Early information about bacterial morphology. Allow more rational antibiotic choice while awaiting culture and sensitivity results • Not all bacteria present in the faeces will culture successfully – some may be damaged or have fastidious requirements. Gram stains will give information that can then be compared with culture and sensitivity results	• Lack of correlation between Gram stain and clinical health/disease in healthy patients • Time intense

15.6 Faecal Gram stains.

Proventricular washing

The procedure for performing a crop wash is discussed in Chapter 6. Proventricular washing can be useful in determining the aetiology of refractory proventriculitis. The procedure may be done 'blind' (Figure 15.7) or endoscopically guided. The use of an endoscope allows visualization of abnormal structures and sampling of focal lesions. Aspirated fluid is then examined microscopically.

Fasting prior to the procedure will improve visualization. The anaesthetized intubated patient is positioned in dorsal recumbency. The crop tube is placed as if for crop gavage, with one hand holding the proximal end of the crop tube (either metal or soft plastic catheter). Once in the crop, the tip of the needle is manipulated with the other hand and very gently advanced to the bird's right, dorsal to the clavicle and then caudally to the proventriculus. If resistance is encountered, the crop tube should be withdrawn and repositioned before again being gently advanced forward. Once in place, saline

(5–10 ml/kg) is injected and aspirated, avoiding overdistension of the proventriculus.

The pharynx may be packed with moistened gauze or cotton wool to prevent aspiration, though this is very rarely a problem. The packing is removed prior to anaesthetic recovery.

Tracheal intubation is necessary, to allow sufficient time for appropriate placement of the crop tube. Small birds have increased risk of complication, including trauma to the GI wall. In birds too small to intubate, the anaesthetic depth may vary dramatically with a mask-on/mask-off approach during crop tube positioning, and regurgitation and aspiration become more of a concern.

Other diagnostic tools

- A *cloacal sample* may be taken with a moistened, sterile swab, although samples taken from the urodeum or proctodeum may not be representative of the GI system (see Figure 2.12). Some organisms are only shed intermittently. *Faecal flotation* may increase the sensitivity of endoparasite detection compared to wet smears alone (Figure 15.8).
- *Impression smears* of abnormal masses, lesions or exudate can be performed (Chapter 7). Biopsy samples should be taken from lesions with ambiguous cytology and submitted for *histopathology*.
- *Culture and sensitivity* (aerobic and/or anaerobic) should be performed if abnormal bacterial populations are identified on cytological examination. Routine cloacal culture of healthy psittacine birds is not useful.
- *Haematology and biochemistry* are recommended in cases of systemic illness or to discriminate primary from secondary GI problems (Chapter 7). Elevations in amylase may be indicative of pancreatitis.
- *Radiography* is useful but distinction of GI versus extra-GI enlargement or displacement often requires *contrast studies* (Chapter 9). Organomegaly, gas or fluid distension and radio-opaque foreign bodies (e.g. lead or zinc) may be identified.
- *Endoscopy* can be performed on the oropharynx, crop, oesophagus, proventriculus, ventriculus and cloaca (Chapter 9).

Method	Technique	Finding
Direct smear	• Mix a small quantity of fresh faeces and a few drops of saline on a glass slide, and add a coverslip • Examine under low dry power (100× lens) for helminth larvae • Use high dry power (400× lens) for Protozoa. One or two drops of iodine placed at the edge of the coverslip may help to identify protozoal cysts	Motile protozoans Helminth larvae
Faecal flotation	Most solutions contain zinc sulphate, sodium nitrate, salt or sugar • Mix a moderate amount of fresh faeces with solution and place in a container on to which a coverslip is placed • Leave to stand for 5–10 minutes (or manufacturer's recommendations) • Remove the coverslip, place on a glass slide and examine Parasite morphology may alter if left in the solution for excessive times	Protozoan cysts Helminth eggs and larvae Protozoan cysts Coccidian oocysts Some trematode eggs

15.8 Detection of endoparasites.

Differential diagnoses by anatomical area

The beak is discussed in Chapters 11 and 16.

Oropharynx

Clinical signs of oropharyngeal disease include dysphagia, head flicking, yawning and inappetence. Ulceration, exudate, swellings, masses or foreign bodies may be present on oropharyngeal examination, which often requires general anaesthesia and endoscopic magnification. Good lighting is essential. It is important to examine the choana (Figure 5.10). Cytology of lesions is mandatory; biopsy should be considered if results are equivocal. Figure 15.9 presents a list of differential diagnoses.

A common cause of oropharyngeal lesions in large parrots is hypovitaminosis A. Papillomas and foreign bodies are less common, though occasionally foreign bodies will become lodged in the choana. Young Budgerigars are commonly diagnosed with trichomoniasis. Candidiasis is common, especially in younger birds.

Oesophagus and crop

The clinical signs of crop and oesophageal disease include dysphagia, head flicking, retching, vomiting, crop enlargement and anorexia. Figure 15.10 presents a list of differential diagnoses.

Physical examination, crop palpation and crop wash cytology are essential. Crop contents (fluid, ingluviolith or foreign body) should be determined, and any crop distension or crop wall thickening should be noted. Further information may be gained via endoscopic examination. Crop biopsy may be performed on unusual lesions, or to diagnose proventricular dilatation disease (Chapter 10).

Ingluvitis (crop inflammation) is common in psittacine patients. Bacterial infections are common in all species. Neonatal birds often have mixed bacterial and yeast infections. Trichomoniasis, with or without

---

Masses

Neoplasia
Papillomatosis
Granuloma/abscess
Hypovitaminosis A*
Poxvirus

Discharge/plaques

Bacterial
Fungal and yeast*
Parasitic (*Trichomonas**, *Capillaria*)
Choanal discharge secondary to sinusitis/rhinitis*
Viral, especially poxvirus

Choanal abnormalities

Blunting of papillae* (hypovitaminosis A*, chronic upper respiratory tract infection – bacterial/fungal)
Choanal atresia
Choanal foreign bodies

Other

Laceration/trauma
Toxic stomatitis
Oropharyngeal burns

15.9 Differential diagnosis of oropharyngeal disease. Asterisks indicate common conditions.

Exudative lesions

Trichomoniasis*
Candidiasis*
Bacterial infections*
Capillaria and other nematodes

Proliferative lesions

Trichomoniasis*
Capillariasis
Papillomatosis
Foreign bodies, especially neonates

Other

Crop burn/fistula*
Other trauma, including rupture with feeding tube in neonates
Crop impaction in neonates
Hypovitaminosis A
Ingluvioliths

Neoplasia

15.10 Differential diagnosis of crop and oesophageal disease. Asterisks indicate common conditions.

secondary bacterial infection, is most common in young Budgerigars. Hand-fed larger psittacine babies may present with crop burns (see Figure 5.16) or foreign bodies.

Delayed or absent upper GI peristalsis (delayed crop emptying) will result in 'sour crop' (fermentation of crop contents). Crop stasis is most common in birds being hand-fed but can be secondary to other problems.

Proventriculus and ventriculus

Vomiting, maldigestion, abnormal droppings and weight loss are suggestive of proventricular or ventricular dysfunction. Ill-thrift and mid-body feather plucking may also be seen. Figure 15.11 presents a list of differential diagnoses.

General

Viral: circovirus (PBFD)*; polyomavirus; reovirus; paramyxovirus; herpesvirus; internal papillomatosis

Intoxication: acute lead/zinc toxicity*; chronic lead toxicity*; plants

Other infections: megabacteriosis*; clostridiosis*; fungal parasites

Other: myoventricular dysgenesis; koilin dysgenesis; myoventricular calcinosis; vitamin E/selenium deficiency; mural lesions (granuloma, neoplasia)

Dilatation

Systemic disease: pancreatitis; hepatitis; peritonitis

Infection: megabacteriosis*; clostridiosis*; circovirus (PBFD)*; polyomavirus; parasitic

Neurogenic: acute lead/zinc toxicity*; chronic lead toxicity*; proventricular dilatation syndrome*

Other: foreign bodies; obstruction; myoventricular dysgenesis; koilin dysgenesis; nutritional/dietary problems; mural lesions (granuloma infection, neoplasia)

15.11 Differential diagnosis of proventricular and ventricular disease. Asterisks indicate common conditions.

After initial examination of crop wash and faecal cytology, plain radiography is performed. If abnormalities (e.g. dilatation, luminal or extraluminal masses or foreign bodies) are identified, then contrast radiography or GI endoscopy and/or proventricular washing should be performed. The use of barium sulphate will impede cytological and endoscopic examination for at least 12–24 hours. Haematology, biochemistry, *Chlamydophila* testing and lead levels are useful. The proventricular isthmus is a common site of proventricular infections and neoplasms.

Megabacteriosis is commonly diagnosed in Budgerigars. Heavy metal toxicosis is common in many species, especially the larger parrots.

Intestine

Intestinal disease can manifest as abnormal droppings, weight loss, ill-thrift or abdominal pain. Vomiting is rare and tends to occur with ileus or obstructive problems. Figure 15.12 presents a list of differential diagnoses. The most common diagnostic test is faecal cytology with culture and sensitivity.

Although intestinal ileus is often observed, it is a clinical sign and not a diagnosis (see below). Bacterial

---

Intestinal inflammation

Viral: herpesvirus; polyomavirus; reovirus; paramyxovirus; circovirus (PBFD)

Bacterial*: *Clostridium;* mycobacteria; Enterobacteraciae; *Chlamydophila;* others

Parasitic: Protozoa (*Hexamita, Cochlosoma, Giardia, Cryptosporidium,* coccidia); trematodes; cestodes; nematodes* (including ascarids)

Obstruction

Foreign body
Volvulus
Intussusception
Stricture
Parasites (especially ascarids)

Ileus

Toxicosis including lead/zinc*
Generalized ileus*
Proventricular dilatation disease*

Other

Internal papillomatosis
Hernia
Nutritional/dietary problems

Neoplasia

15.12 Differential diagnosis of intestinal disease. Asterisks indicate common conditions.

enteritis occurs frequently in all species. Candidiasis can occur secondary to antibiotic use. Proventricular dilatation syndrome may involve the intestine. Protozoal enteritis is less common.

Cloaca

Abnormal droppings (Appendix 2) and faecal accumulations around the vent and tail feathers, although not pathognomonic, are commonly seen with cloacal problems. Tenesmus, tissue prolapse and feather picking around the vent may also be seen. Figure 15.13 presents a list of differential diagnoses.

Masses

Cloacal papilloma*
Neoplasia (other than papilloma)
Cloacolith
Cloacal impaction (egg, urates, faeces)

Cloacitis

Bacterial
Fungal
Yeast

Cloacal prolapse (need to identify tissue)

Cloaca: neurogenic disorders; tenesmus (inflammation, infection, cloacolith, egg binding, foreign body); idiopathic; vent laxity, especially with hypersexuality*

Oviduct (Chapter 18)

Rectum: enteritis* (bacterial, parasitic, protozoal, fungal); intussusception*

15.13 Differential diagnosis of cloacal disease. Asterisks indicate common conditions.

Gross, cytological and parasitological examination of fresh faeces should be performed. The vent and cloaca should be examined under general anaesthesia. The proctodeum is usually easily accessible and portions may be everted with cotton buds for closer inspection. Examination of the urodeum and coprodeum usually requires cloacoscopy (Chapter 9). In conjunction with saline irrigation, cloacoscopy allows mucosal visualization, lesion localization and focal sampling. In the absence of cloacoscopy, swabs for cloacal cytology and culture may be taken blindly. It should be noted, however, that it can be difficult to know which cloacal chamber has been sampled.

Cloacal papillomas are most common in Amazons and macaws. Cloacal infections (cloacitis) and impactions can occur in any species.

Pancreas

Pancreatic problems may be broadly grouped into inflammatory/infectious disorders (pancreatitis), dysfunction (endocrine or exocrine) and neoplasia (Figure 15.14). Figure 15.15 presents a list of differential diagnoses.

Pancreatitis
Vomiting
Polyuria/polydipsia
Weight loss
Abdominal pain
Abnormal posturing
Depression
Changed urate colour
Exocrine pancreatic dysfunction
Weight loss
Bulky pale droppings
Undigested food in droppings
Endocrine pancreatic dysfunction
Weight loss
Polydipsia/polyuria
Neoplasia
Any combination of signs in the other categories

15.14 Clinical signs of pancreatic disease.

Pancreatitis/pancreatic necrosis
Viral: paramyxovirus 3; adenovirus; herpesvirus; avian influenza A
Bacterial (including chlamydophilosis)
Toxic (including zinc)
Other (including egg-related peritonitis)
Pancreatic fibrosis/atrophy
Pancreatic exocrine insufficiency
Diabetes
Other
Lipidosis
Haemochromatosis
Neoplasia

15.15 Differential diagnosis of pancreatic disease.

Diagnosis of pancreatic disease may be difficult. Usually, a combination of clinical signs and hyperamylasaemia is used to localize disease to the pancreas. Amylase is not pancreas specific, but elevations of three to four times the upper reference range may be consistent with pancreatic pathology (Doneley, 2001). Full haematological and biochemical testing should be performed to rule out other diseases. A pancreatic biopsy sample should be taken for a definitive diagnosis (Chapter 10). A biopsy is also indicated in the case of pancreatic masses or pancreatic disease refractory to medical management. The sample can be taken endoscopically or via a mid-line coeliotomy, with the latter giving better visualization (Figure 15.16).

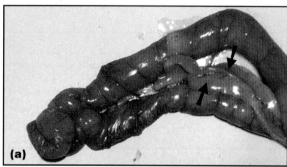
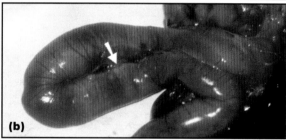

15.16 (a) Two of the three lobes of the pancreas are normally situated in the duodenal loop. Here, the dorsal and ventral lobes can be seen (arrowed) in the mesentery of the duodenum of a Grey Parrot. (b)The intestine from a cockatoo that had been passing large green droppings, became very unwell and died. The ascending and descending duodenum are scarred and adherent. The pancreas (arrowed) is atrophied and there is no functional pancreatic tissue remaining.

Risk factors for pancreatitis include high-fat diets and egg-related peritonitis. Anecdotally, Quaker Parakeets appear predisposed to pancreatitis. Australian grass parakeets often develop pancreatitis during paramyxovirus-3 infection. Pancreatic exocrine insufficiency is often secondary to neoplasia or chronic egg-related peritonitis.

Treatment of pancreatitis involves aggressive parenteral fluid therapy, supportive care and analgesia. The addition of pancreatic enzyme supplements to food may have an analgesic effect. Supplementation with N-6 and N-3 fatty acids in a ratio of 5:1 for 2–4 weeks may reduce pro-inflammatory fatty acid production (Doneley, 2001). Antibiotics are usually given. Fasting is not advisable in avian patients but the bird should be changed to a lower-fat diet. Initially, feeding with hand-rearing, juvenile or recovery diets should be performed. The bird may then be converted to a healthier diet as it improves (Chapter 12). High-fat foods should be eliminated.

Common GI conditions

Delayed crop emptying, crop stasis and sour crop

Delayed crop emptying or crop stasis is not a diagnosis. Impaired crop motility, regardless of the initial cause, will result in infection. A crop wash and microscopic examination should be performed; identified organisms may be normal flora, primary pathogens or opportunists secondary to stasis. If the underlying aetiology is not immediately apparent, a thorough investigation should be performed. Possible sequelae to crop stasis include fluid and electrolyte imbalance, dehydration, hypoglycaemia, toxaemia, septicaemia, enteritis and shock. Differential diagnoses are listed in Figure 15.17.

Infection

Viral: proventricular dilatation disease; circovirus (PBFD)*; polyomavirus; other
Bacterial*
Fungal (e.g. *Candida**)
Parasitic: trichomoniasis*

Mechanical

Enlarged thyroid gland due to iodine deficiency
Fractured coracoid

Other

Part of generalized ileus
Overstretched crop
Drug administration
Toxicity: lead/zinc*; pesticides; other
Inappropriate feeding of young birds: too hot; too cold; too thick; too fatty

Neoplasia

Internal papillomatosis
Other neoplasia

15.17 Differential diagnosis of crop stasis. Asterisks indicate common conditions.

Appropriate therapy requires symptomatic management of crop stasis and treatment of underlying or initiating factors. The crop contents should be evacuated and lavaged with warm saline. The bird must be handled carefully to avoid regurgitation. Despite the concerns of stress and mucosal trauma, repeated crop gavage may be preferred over general anaesthesia and ingluviotomy to empty a fluid-filled crop. If anaesthesia is performed, the cranial oesophagus should be packed to reduce the chance of aspiration. Treatment should include appropriate antibiosis and antifungal medication (guided by crop cytology results) and fluid therapy. The administration of prokinetic drugs is advisable. Initially, the bird should be fed electrolyte solution or very dilute feeding mixture, the concentration of which may be increased as improvement occurs.

Foreign bodies of the crop

Inadequately secured crop or feeding tubes and inappropriate substrate may be ingested, particularly by younger birds. Smaller items may move into the proventriculus within an hour, while larger items tend to remain in the crop. Immediate removal is necessary. Smaller blunt objects can be removed orally, either blindly or endoscopically guided. Otherwise, an ingluviotomy may be indicated (Chapter 10).

Crop burns and fistulas

Crop fistulas are usually caused by feeding excessively hot hand-rearing formula (see Figure 5.16). Lesions incorporating both crop and skin usually begin as an area of erythema and oedema, progress over 3–5 days to an area of necrosis, and end with fistulation. At this point viable and non-viable tissue can be distinguished and surgery is indicated. Preoperative care involves frequent feeding of small meals, cleaning of the developing fistula and antibiosis. The aim is to control infection and maintain body condition until surgery. Nystatin is used to prevent yeast overgrowth. Birds usually remain bright, though weight loss can occur. Lesions of the crop alone present as an area of subcutaneous swelling, caused by food leakage and infection. These birds are often severely depressed and require immediate surgery. If treatment is delayed, sepsis and death can result. Surgical techniques are described in Chapter 10.

Parasitism

Generally, parasitism is relatively uncommon in pet psittacine birds. Aviary birds are more frequently infected, due to increased access to the ground. This provides more chances for exposure to, and reinfection by, endoparasites, especially those with direct life cycles. Suspended aviaries are ideal for parasite control but the husbandry requirements of some species preclude their use. Otherwise, concrete flooring is hygienic, easily cleaned and may be covered with substrate to accommodate species' needs. Soil substrate makes endoparasite control much more difficult. There is an increasing trend for birds in zoos and collections for public display to be housed in large mixed-species naturalistic exhibits. Intermittent losses are often experienced in these situations due to the inability to treat individual birds at appropriate dose rates while controlling intermediate hosts and reducing environmental contamination.

Figure 15.18 presents a summary of frequently identified endoparasites and their treatment. To reduce the chances of reinfection, owners should be advised to clean and sanitize cages and aviaries thoroughly.

Trichomoniasis

The flagellate protozoan *Trichomonas*, common in young newly purchased Budgerigars, spreads via direct contact. Clinical signs include emaciation, vomiting, diarrhoea, depression, dyspnoea and 'wetness' around the beak. The upper respiratory tract may become involved in severe infections and aspiration can occur. Secondary bacterial infection is common and birds may become septic. Diagnosis is via wet mount examination of a crop wash with warmed saline. Trichomonads can burrow deep into the crop wall (Figure 15.19) and so it is worth repeating crop washes on suspect birds with negative results. Treatment is with either metronidazole or carnidazole.

Parasite	Treatments	Notes	Species commonly affected
Trichomonas[a] (Figure 15.19)	Metronidazole, carnidazole[b]	Spread via direct contact	Budgerigar
Hexamita	Metronidazole	Spread via direct contact. More common in lorikeets	Cockatiel, lorikeets
Giardia (see Figure 7.7)	Metronidazole, fenbendazole	Faecal–oral spread. Clean cage to inactivate cysts. Infrequent to rare	Budgerigar, Cockatiel
Coccidia	Trimethoprim/sulphonamide, toltrazuril	Faecal–oral spread. Infrequently diagnosed	Lorikeets, Budgerigar
Ascarids[a] (see Figure 7.39)	Fenbendazole, ivermectin, pyrantel	Direct life cycle. Not infective until larvate, which takes 2–3 weeks. Need good hygiene to prevent reinfection	Australian parakeets, Cockatiel, lorikeets, macaws
Capillaria (Figure 15.20)	Ivermectin, fenbendazole	Direct or indirect life cycle. Often resistant to multiple anthelmintics. Retest after treatment. Uncommon to rare	Wild-caught macaws
Proventricular spirurids	Ivermectin	Usually indirect life cycle – need intermediate host. Rare	Parrots, macaws, Australian parakeets
Cestodes	Praziquantel	Indirect life cycle. Rare except in imported birds	Wild-caught Grey Parrots, cockatoos
Trematodes	Praziquantel	Indirect life cycle. Rare except in imported birds	Wild-caught Grey Parrots, cockatoos

15.18 Frequently identified endoparasites and their treatment. [a] = common; [b] = preferred

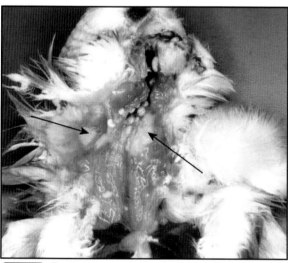

15.19 Post-mortem sample of a Budgerigar with trichomoniasis. Note the changes to the crop mucosa (arrowed). (Photograph courtesy of James Gill.)

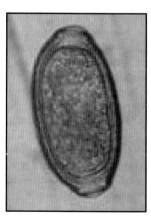

15.20 *Capillaria* egg, faecal flotation, original magnification 400x. (Photograph courtesy of Robert Doneley.)

Ascaridiasis

Ascaridiasis is common in aviary birds on dirt flooring, particularly Australian parakeets. Heavy infestations can lead to intestinal impaction. Birds typically present with weight loss or emaciation. Diagnosis is via a faecal smear or flotation. The prepatent period is 3–4 weeks. In severe infections, birds may die during the occult phase. As well as anthelmintic treatment being initiated, the environment should be cleaned to avoid reinfection. This may involve removal and replacement of the top layer of soil in dirt-floored aviaries (e.g. concreting the aviary), or changing husbandry such that the birds no longer have access to their droppings (e.g. suspended aviary).

Bacterial infection

Bacterial gastroenteritis is common in the psittacine patient (Chapter 13). It is often the result of poor hygiene, concurrent illness or long-standing malnutrition, particularly hypovitaminosis A. Gram-negative organisms, including Enterobacteriaceae, are frequently isolated. *Clostridium* species are becoming increasingly recognized.

Clinical presentations range from vomiting and abnormal droppings through to depression, lethargy and death. Diagnostic tests should include crop washes and faecal cytology, including Gram stains. A monomorphic population of multiplying bacteria is suggestive but culture and sensitivity testing should be considered. Bacterial gastroenteritis can be secondary to a number of other conditions, including proventricular dilatation syndrome, internal papillomatosis or viral gastroenteritis. A thorough investigation should be performed if the patient is systemically ill or refractory to treatment.

Commonly used antibiotics are described below. Supportive treatment can include prokinetic drugs, acidification of drinking water and probiotics.

Oral spiral bacteria (*Helicobacter* series)

These motile bacteria are mainly seen in the pharynx of Cockatiels. Some birds are asymptomatic but clinical signs can include pharyngitis (hyperaemia, increased oral mucus, yawning, head shaking, dysphagia), upper respiratory disease (sneezing, periorbital swelling, rhinorrhoea), anorexia and depression. The current treatment of choice is oral doxycycline (Wade *et al.*, 2003).

Clostridiosis

Psittacine clostridiosis (Chapter 13) can cause a variety of syndromes, depending on the degree of bacterial overgrowth, toxin production and systemic involvement.

- *Localized low-grade intestinal or cloacal infection* usually manifests as abnormal and foul-smelling droppings. Birds are not usually depressed. Papillomatosis is a predisposing factor.
- Flock and individual mortalities have been associated with *ulcerative enteritis*, in which birds present with severe diarrhoea and other gastroenteric signs.
- *Endotoxaemia and/or septicaemia* can also occur, causing peracute to acute morbidity and mortality.

Lories and lorikeets are prone to enteric and acute forms of clostridial infection, as foods high in sugar (such as nectar) foster rapid clostridial fermentation. This is exacerbated in warm weather. Collapsed birds require aggressive fluid, antibiotic and supportive therapy. Birds with low-grade chronic infections need to have antibiotic treatment while the predisposing factors are resolved. Penicillins or amoxicillin/clavulanate are recommended.

Yeast infection

Yeasts are part of the normal GI flora but may multiply under certain conditions. Predisposing factors include warm humid weather, GI motility disturbances, use of antibiotics, hypovitaminosis A, poor hygiene, excessive dietary carbohydrates and generalized ill-health. Young birds, especially Budgerigars and Cockatiels, are often affected. *Candida* is frequently isolated.

Clinical signs depend on the portion of GI tract most affected and can include vomiting, diarrhoea, abnormal droppings, delayed crop emptying, crop stasis or generalized ileus. The mucosa of affected areas may have a 'Turkish towel' appearance, with mucoid or stringy exudate.

Microscopic examination should be performed. Budding yeast is indicative of localized mucosal surface infection, while pseudohyphae suggest more aggressive and possibly systemic infection (see Figure 15.4). Yeast may be present in small numbers in the 'normal' bird. Care should be taken not to misinterpret dead yeast derived from food as representative of infection.

Infections with budding yeast may be treated with nystatin; it is not systemically absorbed, so must be given 20 minutes prior to feeding to allow sufficient mucosal contact time. Severe budding yeast infections or those with pseudohyphae should be treated with systemic antifungal agents such as nystatin or azoles.

Preweaned birds on antibiotics should be prophylactically treated; side effects are unlikely with nystatin, due to the lack of systemic absorption. Although not scientifically proven, probiotics may reduce the likelihood of yeast overgrowth during periods of higher risk.

Megabacteriosis

Several psittacine species have been documented with megabacteriosis infections but Budgerigars are the most commonly affected. The most common presentation relates to chronic maldigestion: breeders refer to the disease as 'going light'. Clinical signs include vomiting, progressive weight loss, emaciation and ill-thrift. Some birds demonstrate a peracute syndrome with bloody faeces and acute death. Diagnosis is made via faecal smear (see Figure 15.5). Organisms are rarely seen on crop wash. The organism is shed intermittently and so repeated faecal examinations should be made in suspect patients. In larger birds with negative faecal examination and suspicious signs, demonstration of the organism may require a proventricular wash.

Oral amphotericin B usually gives good clinical response but it does not eliminate the organism from the bird. In some cases where the response to treatment is poor, histology may demonstrate chronic proventriculitis or proventricular scarring. Fluconazole has eliminated infection in some species but caused mortality in Budgerigars at the required dose rate. Therefore, at least in Budgerigars, infected birds must be considered to be life-long carriers.

Hypovitaminosis A

Hypovitaminosis A (see also Chapter 12) affects a number of organ systems and GI signs vary. Salivary gland lesions present as small to large swellings in the oropharynx. Birds may be inappetent. Diarrhoea may result from intestinal mucosal lesions. Blunted choanal papillae may indicate chronic deficiency. Cytology of uninfected lesions will show predominantly squamous cells, while infected lesions may have bacteria and inflammatory cells present as well. Some species, such as Eclectus Parrots, appear particularly susceptible. The pathophysiology behind this observation is unknown.

The early signs of vitamin A toxicosis may resemble those of deficiency and include epithelial changes, pancreatitis, behavioural changes and loss of condition. Given the difficulty of discriminating between deficiency and toxicity in the early stages, analysis of the vitamin A composition of the diet (including supplements) is crucial to allow the appropriate dietary changes to be made.

Treatment is with oral vitamin A supplementation (with current concerns about hypervitaminosis A, parenteral injections have fallen out of favour). Most birds will improve dramatically on supplementation but some changes are permanent (e.g. blunted choanal papillae). Although lancing and debridement are often recommended, these lesions are usually highly vascular and excessive bleeding may be a problem. A preferred treatment plan is to monitor the bird regularly and to lance and debride lesions only if supplementation fails to achieve an adequate clinical response. Antibiosis is recommended if infection is present. Analgesia should be provided for birds that are inappetent but the effect of non-steroidal anti-inflammatory drugs on potentially compromised renal tubular epithelium should be considered.

Lead or zinc toxicity

Vomiting, regurgitation and depression can be signs of lead or zinc toxicity. Wet smears of crop contents and faeces may reveal reduced numbers of bacteria. This may be due to a locally toxic effect of the heavy metal on GI flora. Diagnosis and definitive treatment are discussed in Chapter 20.

Internal papillomatosis

Papillomas may arise at any point along the GI tract, though the cloaca appears most commonly affected (Chapter 13). Macaws and Amazons are affected most often. Clinical signs of cloacal papillomatosis include weight loss, regurgitation, tenesmus, abnormal droppings, a soiled vent or cloacal prolapse. Closer examination may reveal a fleshy tissue mass, involving a variable amount of the cloacal wall, which will turn white upon the application of acetic acid. Biopsy and histology provide a definitive diagnosis.

Electrocautery, cryosurgery, surgical removal and chemical cautery are among attempted treatments but no treatment thus far has proved universally successful. Some papillomas appear to regress spontaneously. Lesions with secondary infections require antibiosis. Lesions are debulked when causing problems (e.g. with defecation) but scarring is a potential complication. Cholangiocarcinoma may be a sequel to internal papillomatosis (Chapter 13).

Cloacal prolapse

The prolapsed tissue must first be identified. It may be uterine prolapse due to egg binding, rectal prolapse due to enteritis or parasitism, or true cloacal prolapse due to cloacitis or papillomatosis. Hypersexual masturbating birds may prolapse the cloaca due to vent laxity. Viable tissue should then be reduced under general anaesthesia and a horizontal mattress suture placed, ensuring that the bird can still defecate. Purse-string sutures are no longer recommended. Devitalized tissue, if present, must be surgically resected, but confers a poor prognosis. The underlying aetiology should be addressed. Chronic recurrent prolapse refractory to medical therapy may require surgical management in the form of cloacopexy or cloacotomy (Chapter 10).

Therapy of GI disease

Symptomatic treatment

Symptomatic treatment (see also Chapter 5) includes:

- Maintenance of hydration
- Maintenance of caloric intake
- Maintenance of warmth
- Reduction in stress
- Maintenance of peristalsis.

Fluid therapy can be given via oral, intravenous, intraosseous or subcutaneous routes. Any bird that is underweight, inappetent or fails to maintain its body weight should be gavage fed. Gavage feeding will supply a proportion of the daily fluid requirements. Birds should be weighed daily at the same time. Maintaining ill birds in a quiet part of the hospital distant from dogs, cats and other predators will reduce stress.

Absence or reduction in peristalsis is usually treated with metoclopramide and/or cisapride. The former is also anti-emetic. Severe gut stasis can be treated with both drugs. Probiotics and acidification of the drinking water are often used as non-specific supportive agents, although there are few studies to prove that these treatments are any more beneficial than conventional treatment in unwell birds. Acetic acid and organic apple cider vinegar have been used as acidifiers. The advocates of the latter claim there is increased benefit using non-homogenized, non-pasteurized solution. Kaolin and sucralfate have been used as gut-coating agents in cases of ulceration or severe gastroenteritis.

Specific treatment

Commonly used antibacterial agents include: amoxicillin/clavulanate; enrofloxacin; trimethoprim/sulphonamide; and metronidazole. Commonly used antifungal agents include: nystatin; ketoconazole; itraconazole; and fluconazole.

The initial selection of antibiotic or antifungal agent may be empirical, based on the results of cytology and clinical signs, but culture and sensitivity tests should be performed in the case of unusual or refractory infections. Enrofloxacin has no activity against anaerobic infections, while amoxicillin/clavulanate often achieves good results in those instances.

Muscle necrosis can occur in the hospitalized psittacine patient treated with parenteral medication. Wherever possible, medications should be given by the oral route, to reduce muscle damage and patient discomfort. Severely ill patients will need parenteral medication, at least in the initial stages.

Drug side effects

A number of drugs have been associated with vomiting. These include enrofloxacin, nystatin, doxycycline, trimethoprim/sulphonamide, ketoconazole, itraconazole, fluconazole, levamisole, amphotericin B and polymixin B. Although these drugs are often used without clinical side effects, the clinician should be aware of their potential to cause problems. Medicating via crop tube or mixing medication with food may reduce the incidence of these side effects.

Grit

The supply of grit as a food supplement has become a controversial topic (Figure 15.21). Unfortunately, there are very few scientific studies examining this issue in either wild or captive psittaciforms.

Advantages	Disadvantages
• Evolutionary trait that has persisted – must be a reason • Grit is present in the gizzard of most wild birds • Birds tend to consume grit whenever offered • Psychological enrichment • Helps smooth sharp foreign bodies, which may protect the ventriculus from damage	• Addition to diet provided no increase in digestibility in canaries (Taylor, 1996) • Grit impactions possible with overconsumption • Pelleted diets more digestible than wild-type diets and may not require grinding • Enhances absorption of heavy metal objects by speeding dissolution

15.21 Summary of opinions regarding grit supplementation.

Grit may be insoluble or soluble (e.g. crushed oyster shell). Soluble grit is not usually thought to persist for any length of time in the ventriculus and may be considered to be a source of additional dietary minerals, rather than a digestive aid. Insoluble grit, on the other hand, is likely to persist longer in the ventriculus (gizzard) but retention time varies according to grit particle size, quantity of grit within the ventriculus and other physiological factors. Birds using grit tend to replenish the 'lost' amounts continually (Gionfriddo and Best, 1995). Insoluble grit is thought to augment ventricular action by providing an increased irregular surface area against which other food items may be ground. Enhancement of food digestibility may vary according to size, quality and quantity of grit and food type (Moore, 1998).

16

Feather and skin disorders

John Chitty

The external appearance of the bird is of great importance to both the owner and the bird itself. There is a high metabolic and time cost in maintaining plumage; hence many conditions may have a cutaneous manifestation (Box 16.1). The anatomy and physiology of skin and feathers are described in Chapter 2.

Diagnostic approach

Disorders of the skin in psittacine birds, as in other species, require a thorough investigation, including examination and evaluation of the whole bird as well as its skin.

General investigation

A full history should be taken prior to examination, as outlined in Chapter 5. This should be extensive, particularly when dealing with a feather plucker or chewer (see later).

A clinical examination should also be undertaken prior to specific examination of the skin (Chapter 5). It will often prove necessary to take blood for haematology and biochemistry as well as whole-body radiographs. Faecal analysis (Gram stain and flotation for parasites) may also be of value. Coeloscopy and other means of imaging may be required to investigate these clinical findings further.

Specific diagnostics

Examination of skin and feathers

It is essential to understand the normal appearance of plumage for each species (e.g. feather structure, skin colour, plumage colours) as well as the normal structure of feather and skin. There may be differences not only between species but also within species (especially with breeding of colour variants), during the breeding season (e.g. loss of head feathers and yellowing of the exposed skin in breeding Vasa Parrots) and with age (e.g. Grey Parrots). Similarly, there may be differences between imported and captive-bred birds. It is recommended that the clinician dealing with a novel species refers to texts showing normal plumage (del Hoyo *et al.*, 1997; Juniper and Parr, 1998).

Figure 16.1 gives a checklist for the examination of the skin and plumage.

Dermatological testing

The following specific dermatological tests may be appropriate.

Skin scrape: A skin scrape should be taken where there are crusts or hyperkeratotic lesions suggestive of parasitism. The procedure is performed as in dogs or cats, with the scraping being taken into 10% potassium hydroxide or liquid paraffin. Unlike in mammals, the cells in birds are often present as 'rafts' or 'sheets'.

Skin or feather disorders are frequently seen as signs of internal disease. This may be due to the high cost of producing feathers at each moult, with effects on protein metabolism or intake/absorption manifested as interruptions in feather growth ('fret' or 'stress' marks) or malformed feathers. Also, a sick bird may be less willing to expend time preening. This may result in a 'tatty' plumage, retention of feather sheaths (Malley, 1996) or a high parasite burden. Hepatopathies may result in pink feathers in the normal grey areas of a Grey Parrot.

As in mammals, skin turnover is of importance, and nutritional or metabolic disease may manifest as a scaling disorder.

Impaction of the uropygial gland may be caused by hypovitaminosis A. Similarly, underlying disease or nutritional deficiency may act as additional stressors in the plucking bird, while many parrots start plucking or chewing a focal area over a source of pain or discomfort, such as gut pain or colic, arthritis, air sacculitis or abscess. Krautwald (1990) described 'septicaemic alopecia' in Grey Parrots where plucking starts due to rubbing the beak over an area of chronic intracoelomic or hepatic pain: an important differential in these cases is chlamydophilosis.

Endoparasites (especially *Giardia*) have also been implicated as sources of pain, thus triggering feather plucking. However, in these cases the areas affected are generally not related to the abdomen. These cases may represent hypersensitivity to the gut parasite.

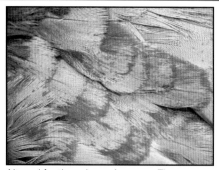

Altered feathers in an Amazon. The blackening is due to poor feather formation allowing yeast colonization. The underlying cause was hepatic lipidosis.

Box 16.1 Cutaneous manifestations of systemic disease.

Colour	Is it uniform? Is there variation on different parts of the body? Is it normal for that species?
Wounds and tears	Is there evidence of self-trauma?
Erythema	Remember that avian skin is extremely thin; apparent 'erythema' may simply be the colour of underlying tissues
Folliculitis	Present?
Lesions	If present, note distribution and type
Masses	Present?
Scale	Lots or none? (Scale should be distinguished from feather dust; see Figure 16.15.)

16.1a Examination of the skin.

State of plumage	'Tatty' or normal?
	Birds rely on perfect plumage to perform roles in flight, insulation, display, etc. Poor quality plumage with tatty 'rough' edges may reflect:
	   • Old feathers needing to be moulted
	   • Lack of or inappropriate preening
	   • Poor nutrition
	   • Internal illness resulting in poor feathering or reduced preening
	   • Damage to feathers in small cage or where perches are too close to bars, in which case only older longer feathers will be damaged

Powder down	Present? In excess?
In moult	Many 'club' or 'blood' feathers Where there are gaps in flight or tail feathers, is there a new feather growing through? If not in moult, when was the last one?
Dystrophy	Are the feathers a normal shape for that part of the body? Note especially: curled feathers; stress/fret marks; incomplete feathers
Colour	Is plumage colour normal? Overall colour changes, or changes in individual feathers?
Damage	Is there loss of structure within the vane? Do barbules interlock? Do areas appear to be 'eaten away'? Is there discoloration of the calamus?
Blood feathers	Do these appear normal? In Grey Parrot, black 'distended' pin feathers on body may show evidence of pulpitis (Box 16.2) on cytology
Feather loss	Feathers normally grow in tracts with featherless areas between (apteria); Cockatiels and cockatoos normally have a featherless area behind the crest May be normal loss of feathers in breeding season ('brood patches') Note distribution of feather loss (e.g. on head will not be self-plucking) Record distribution of feather loss or damage
Follicle loss	Individual follicles are identifiable even without feather where bird has been plucking for only a short period; in long-term pluckers, skin may become quiescent, with few or no identifiable follicles, and owner should be advised feather regrowth in these regions is extremely unlikely
Parasites	Check for feather lice and mites as well as their eggs Feather parasites are rare in psittacine birds (see later) Note that *Dermanyssus* (red mite, rare condition) spends most time off bird; environmental investigation more appropriate than on-bird

16.1b Examination of the feathers.

Feather pulpitis is often found in plucking birds. Affected blood feathers may appear darkened and distended (typically thick black pin feathers on the pectoral area/ventral neck of Grey Parrots) (Figure 16.2) but they may also be grossly normal. Usually there is little reaction in the surrounding skin and follicle, though this may be seen occasionally. Cytology reveals large numbers of inflammatory cells (Figure 16.3) and sometimes bacteria (a normal pulp preparation being relatively acellular). Histopathology shows evidence of necrosis.

The significance of this is not clear. In some cases it appears to be a primary or perpetuating factor and these respond well to antibiotic therapy (e.g. marbofloxacin). Some, however, appear secondary to the plucking and these respond poorly to antibiosis. Some cases show recurrent pulpitis and these may respond to antibiotic therapy on each occasion. By drawing parallels from other species, this may have a possible link to an underlying allergy, though these recurrences may not be seasonal.

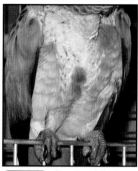

16.2 Swollen black pin feathers, as in this plucking Grey Parrot, are often indicative of pulpitis.

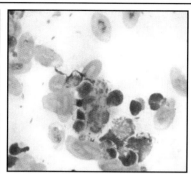

16.3 Pulpitis in a Lovebird: note the numerous heterophils. (Diff-Quik; original magnification 1000x oil immersion)

Box 16.2 Feather pulpitis.

Feather digest: This is useful where there is evidence of feather damage but no parasites are found on gross examination, and also where changes in the calamus (colour or increased opacity) indicate possible quill mite infestation. An erupting or damaged feather is digested in warmed 10% potassium hydroxide before centrifugation and microscopic examination.

Pulp cytology: Two techniques are described for different types of feather (Chitty, 2002). Where birds are chewing large wing feathers (remiges) or tail feathers (retrices) and blood feathers are present:

1. Pull blood feather from the area being chewed. Ideally choose one damaged and one undamaged feather.
2. Clean the calamus, using surgical spirit.
3. Incise along the calamus.
4. Gently squeeze. Small 'pearls' of clear fluid will be seen along the cut. These can be sampled using standard impression smear techniques. Discard blood-tinged fluid.
5. Stain with a standard trichrome stain (e.g. Diff-Quik).
6. If required, a small sterile swab may be inserted into the pulp and/or the whole feather can be preserved in formol saline and submitted for histopathology. The incision in the calamus allows for good penetration by the fixative

When birds are plucking body feathers and blood feathers are present:

1. Using forceps, grasp and remove blood feather.
2. Gently squeeze the distal end, forcing fluid from the proximal end.
3. The first (blood-tinged) drop should be discarded. Subsequent clear fluid can then be collected on a microscope slide and stained using a trichrome stain. A bacteriological swab may be inserted into the collected fluid.

Skin acetate: This is indicated where there is excessive scale, the skin appears 'dry' or there are exudative, crusting or hyperkeratotic lesions (Chitty, 2002b). A piece of acetate tape is laid on the area of scale (Figure 16.4). It is then stuck on a microscope slide with one drop of Giemsa stain prior to examination.

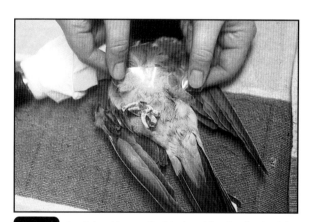

16.4 Acetate strip applied to the skin of a Cockatiel.

Bacteriology: In addition to sampling feather pulp (described above), wetted swabs may be used to sample the skin surface. It should be noted that the normal avian skin (in the UK) supports little bacterial growth and most of those found are Gram-positive. Where bacteria were cultured from abnormal skin, these were often Gram-negative species (N. Harcourt-Brown, personal communication).

Histopathology: Skin biopsy is indicated in any case where there are unusual lesions, where the condition is not responding to logical therapy or in a plucking bird where further information is required. It is worth noting that in the latter case biopsy is often unrewarding and any changes noted may be non-specific or secondary to the plucking. However, it may prove valuable on occasion. The technique is essentially similar to that used in mammals, though the following should be noted.

- Some areas do not lend themselves to biopsy, as it may be impossible to close the wound or the damage inflicted may cause persistent problems (e.g. biopsy of a flight feather follicle).
- The skin should not be aseptically prepared, as this would remove surface cells.
- Avian skin contains a mesh of muscles linking feather follicles (Lucas and Stettenheim, 1972). The consequence of this is that the muscles contract on removal of a section of skin, resulting in a tiny curled biopsy sample and a very large hole (especially if excisional biopsy is used). To reduce this problem, a piece of adhesive tape may be placed over the skin and a sample taken through the tape, using a biopsy punch. This should be done with care to avoid damaging underlying tissues. The sample, with tape attached, is placed in formol saline and submitted for histopathology (Nett *et al.*, 2003).
- A feather follicle should always be included. Where histopathology of the feather is required (e.g. where pulpitis is suspected), feathers should be included separately and a specific request to section these should be made.
- The author recommends 2 metric (3/0) polyglactin for suturing wounds. The owner should be advised that birds (especially self-pluckers) frequently remove the sutures and so the wounds may need to heal by second intention.

Intradermal testing: Although this has been advocated in the diagnosis of allergic disease in parrots and a protocol has been established in the Hispaniolan Amazon, using codeine phosphate as a positive control with allergens injected into the featherless skin on either side of the keel (Colombini *et al.*, 2000), the technique is hindered by the extreme difficulty in achieving a true intradermal injection in such a thin layer and the effects of test site on reaction size (Nett and Tully, 2003). It is now felt that this technique needs further evaluation before its use can be recommended.

Skin disease

Birds, like mammals, present with lesions rather than aetiologies. It is therefore worth considering these skin diseases in terms of their lesional appearance. This applies whether the bird is presented for the lesion, or as a feather plucker or chewer, or whether these are findings on a health check. Useful reviews can be found in Cooper and Harrison (1994), Bauck (1997), Romagnano and Heard (2000), Gill (2001) and Koski (2002).

Wounds

Surgical management of skin wounds is discussed in Chapter 10. Some wounds may not be amenable to immediate surgical intervention, either due to infection, or because there is not enough tissue to close the wound after debridement (e.g. on distal limb), or in chronic wounds where granulation is already progressing. In these cases medical management is essential, either to prepare the wound prior to surgical closure or to allow healing by second intention.

Principles of wound healing and methods available are similar to those in mammals except that the rate of healing in avian patients is much faster and that psittacine birds are generally very unwilling to tolerate dressings. A collar may be used to allow dressings to be applied but it is important to remember that birds often find collars very stressful and that they will still be able to reach extremities (wing tips or feet) whichever collar is used.

When managing this type of wound it is vital to debride any infected or damaged tissue. Bacteriological swabs should be taken and antibiotic therapy should be based on these results. Typically *Staphylococcus* spp. or environmental Gram-negative rods (e.g. *Escherichia coli*) will be found. Amoxicillin/clavulanate is a useful first-choice antibiotic. Antibiosis should be maintained until the wound has completely healed.

The wound can then be managed using dressings such as OpSite or Collamend. The dressings should be changed regularly. Where there are large defects, VetBioSIST is extremely useful in either granular or sheet form.

If the bird will not tolerate a dressing, or if it is desirable to manage the wound in open fashion, daily bathing using povidone–iodine or chlorhexidine followed by application of Intra-Site gel appears to work well. The wound can be further protected by an application of OpSite spray or, if it is in an area likely to be heavily contaminated, the gel can be mixed with a little silver sulphadiazine cream. Surgical closure is indicated as soon as the wound has healed sufficiently.

Crusts and hyperkeratosis

These are typically linked to bacterial and fungal infections or parasitism.

Bacterial and fungal infection

In these cases the crust may consist of 'pus' and so may be classified as a pyoderma. Folliculitis may occasionally present as a crusting lesion. Typically these lesions will be centred on a feather follicle. Similarly, dermatophytosis may be a rare differential diagnosis.

Investigation of the lesion should include skin scraping and cytology, both of the crust and of the underlying skin as the crust is removed. A swab of tissues underlying the crust may be submitted for bacteriology and sensitivity testing. If there is a suspicion of dermatophytosis, a portion of the crust should be submitted for fungal culture. Should lesions fail to respond to logical therapy or should a diagnosis not be apparent after sampling, skin biopsy should be considered.

Therapy of bacterial infections should be based on culture and sensitivity results but marbofloxacin/enrofloxacin or amoxicillin/clavulanate make good first choices.

In fungal infections terbinafine or itraconazole are useful systemic drugs but the latter should be used with extreme caution in Grey Parrots (see Appendix 3).

Topical therapy of bacterial and fungal lesions is useful and the author favours a 1:250 dilution of F10. This can be applied directly to focal lesions or administered by spray or nebulizer for more diffuse lesions.

Skin parasites

It should be noted that, other than cnemidocoptic mange in small species, ectoparasite infections are rare in psittacine birds.

- *Cnemidocoptes pilae* is a cause of 'scaly face' in small psittacine birds (Figures 16.5 and 16.6). It presents as hyperkeratotic lesion of the beak and cere. Often tracts of the burrowing mites may be seen along the beak. In extreme cases deformity of the beak will result.
- Epidermoptid mites are the cause of a relatively unusual condition known as 'depluming itch'. They cause a pruritic, hyperkeratotic lesion on feathered parts of the body. Feather loss is also seen. There are many species which are host-specific. *Myialges* and *Psittaphagoides* spp. have been found in parrots.
- Harpyrhynchid and cheylettielid mites may also be seen in parrots, though disease is rare and is most likely to be seen in recently imported birds or close-contacts. The former cause hyperkeratotic epidermal cysts; the latter cause hyperkeratotic lesions similar to those seen in depluming itch.

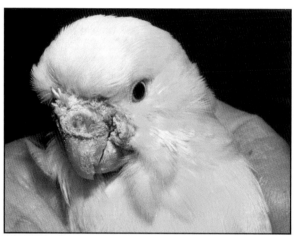

16.5 *Cnemidocoptes* infestation in a Budgerigar. Note the scaling proliferative lesions on the face and mite 'tracks' in the keratin of the beak. Note also the blocking of a nostril by hyperplastic tissue. (Courtesy of John Baxter)

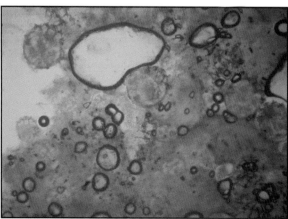

16.6 Scrapings of the lesions in Figure 16.5 reveal many *Cnemidocoptes* mites.

Diagnosis of these skin mites is by recognition of typical lesions, skin scraping, biopsy and response to therapy. Therapy consists of ivermectin given orally or percutaneously. All in-contact birds should also be treated. Often one dose suffices but it may be repeated after a month.

Other mites may be seen on the skin, including both *Dermanyssus* (red mite) and *Ornithonyssus* (northern fowl mite). These do not cause skin lesions but will cause irritation and, in extreme cases, anaemia, as they are blood-feeders.

- *Dermanyssus* is found on birds only when the mite is active at night. It spends the day in the environment and diagnosis usually involves finding the mite there, either by placing a white sheet on the ground at night or by running a piece of white card along cracks in the walls. Therapy centres on removing the source of mites but this usually necessitates destruction of the environment. However, permethrin/pyriproxyfen sprays may be of use. Fipronil spray (on-bird) or ivermectin may also be useful, especially if given prior to moving the bird.
- *Ornithonyssus* spends the whole time on the host, thus causing more acute problems. Diagnosis is by finding the mite on the bird, and therapy consists of fipronil or ivermectin.

Self-trauma and mutilation of the skin

Considering the frequency with which birds are seen plucking feathers and traumatizing their plumage, it is surprising how rare it is to see birds traumatizing or mutilating their skin. Where they do, it is vital to rule out medical causes of ulcerative disease (see below), pruritus (Box 16.3) and, where lesions are focal, disease in the underlying tissues, such as arthritis in a bird chewing over a joint. It is also important to rule out underlying causes such as aspergilloma beneath the lesion. Radiography and haematology/biochemistry

---

When is a bird pruritic? Certainly suspicion should be aroused in the following situations:

- Plucking is continuous or cannot be related to particular times or activities
- Other behaviours are interrupted so that the bird can pluck or chew
- No underlying cause or focus of pain or disease can be identified.

Where pruritus is suspected, investigation of the problem can be focused on dermatological disorders and allergy.

In some cases it may be desirable to use anti-pruritic drugs. Essential fatty acids appear safe but have been relatively ineffective in the author's experience. Similarly antihistamines may have a role and appear to be successful in some cases. Clomipramine appears to be safe and useful but it should be noted that its effects may be due to its action as a tricyclic antidepressant rather than its antihistamine properties. Glucocorticoids can be very effective in some cases but adverse side effects may be common and severe and it is essential to rule out underlying infectious disease (especially chlamydophilosis and aspergillosis) before starting glucocorticoid therapy, as marked immunosuppression may be seen.

Box 16.3 Pruritus.

are essential, as is the taking of a bacteriology swab from the lesion, since secondary infections are often a complicating factor. Biopsy of underlying muscle and/or bone may also be useful.

In severe cases birds may chew through the skin and start to damage underlying tissues and viscera. The prognosis is extremely poor and owners should be advised accordingly. Small macaws (especially Hahn's and Severe) and cockatoos (especially Umbrella and Moluccan) appear most prone to this syndrome. The aetiology often includes diseases of behavioural origin (Chapter 17).

The most common syndrome seen in this category is that of 'split keel'. This is most often seen in Grey Parrots and Umbrella, Greater Sulphur-crested and Moluccan Cockatoos. In Grey Parrots it is generally caused by a poor wing clip resulting in the bird crashing on to its sternum. The resulting bruising causes skin necrosis over the keel and the bird then chews at the lesion as it is so painful. In the cockatoos, injury may be an initiating cause but often it appears to be a mutilation syndrome with a behavioural aetiology. The prognosis in these birds can be poor, as this is an extremely hard condition to control.

It is essential that the bird is stopped from further damaging the tissues and this is one of the few times where a collar may be indicated (see below). Where collars are not practicable, psychotropic drugs may be used but they may not be as effective (Chapter 17).

The wound may be surgically closed or managed as a granulating wound (see above). The author has found VetBioSIST to be of assistance in split keel. It is also useful to apply a padded dressing to protect the wound. Alternatively, the semipermeable hydrophilic dressing Granuflex (Duoderm) may be used to cover and protect wounds, especially in cockatoos, where it blends into the plumage. Healing will typically take weeks to months.

Where the injury has been caused by a poor wing clip, imping of feathers to restore flight may be valuable (Chapter 6).

Collars

While Elizabethan or 'inverted' Elizabethan-style collars may be used, the Stultiens type of collar appears to be better tolerated. These are available commercially but they can also be fashioned from pipe-insulating foam. The tube should be cut to a length equal to the straight length of the neck. It should then be taped round the neck such that there is enough space for food to pass but not enough for the bird to remove the tube (the little finger should be able to pass between collar and skin). In some cases it may be necessary to use a combination collar, where an Elizabethan collar is fitted around the Stultiens collar. After a collar is fitted, the bird should be hospitalized for several days while it gets used to the collar. Food and water bowls should be positioned so that the bird can still reach them. It is important to monitor droppings to check the bird is eating.

Masses and swellings

Cutaneous masses are seen from time to time. First of all, it is important to differentiate normal from abnormal tissue; for example, the pipping muscle on the dorsal neck of the chick may be mistaken for a clinical lesion. Diagnosis may be obvious in some cases (e.g. feather cyst) but in general diagnosis should be made by biopsy (fine-needle aspirate, impression smear or excisional, part or whole) as many of these lesions can appear very similar. Masses may be considered as infectious (Figure 16.7) or non-infectious (Figure 16.8). Swellings of the uropygial gland are considered later in this chapter.

Cause	Appearance	Predilection sites and species (if any)	Clinical approach
Papillomavirus	Proliferative lesions	Grey Parrot: facial skin Amazon: cloaca Macaw: oral cavity	Excision if possible. Otherwise supportive care as many will resolve spontaneously. Autogenous vaccines may help. Where lesions are causing welfare problems (e.g. failure to feed) or in a collection, euthanasia may be considered
Avipoxvirus	Multiple (rarely single) nodules or papules. May appear as vesicles or crusts	All species affected though viral strains may be species or genus specific	Surgical excision of single lesions. Infection is self-limiting but will cause scarring, which may be a problem (e.g. of eyelids). Supportive care (control of secondary infection; assist-feeding, etc) is essential. Euthanasia of debilitated birds or of birds in a collection may be considered. In the latter situation attention should be paid to controlling mosquito vectors and all clinical cases should be maintained in strict quarantine. Use of vaccines designed for pigeons or poultry has not been properly evaluated
Herpesvirus	Dry proliferative lesions on the feet and legs	Cockatoos	Self-limiting
Polyomavirus	Subcutaneous haemorrhage	Especially older Budgerigars	An unusual presentation of this viral syndrome (Chapter13). The lesions may be extensive
Abscess	Subcutaneous (rarely intradermal) mass. Skin may be ulcerated		Typically bacterial; rarely yeast, *Aspergillus* or mycobacteria. Abscess contents should therefore be submitted for cytology and culture/sensitivity. Avian pus is solid, so surgical removal or curettage is the only treatment option

16.7 Infectious causes of skin masses and swellings. (continues) ▶

Cause	Appearance	Predilection sites and species (if any)	Clinical approach
Tick reactions	Huge necrotic haemorrhagic lesions. Tick may have already dropped off	Almost invariably on head and face	Birds may be found dead. Otherwise, fluids (oral/systemic), broad-spectrum antibiotics and short-acting corticosteroids should be given as soon as possible. Exact aetiology of these reactions unknown, but care should be taken not to introduce deer ticks into aviary. Prevention may consist of using permethrin/ pyriproxifen spray in aviary (remember to spray branches or perches as well as ground and nestboxes) and regular on-bird applications of fipronil

16.7 (continued) Infectious causes of skin masses and swellings.

Cause	Description	Therapy
Feather cyst	Failure of developing feather to exit follicle (especially following damage to orifice) results in development of cyst filled with keratinaceous debris. Relatively common in Budgerigars. May be associated with folliculoma	Excision (Chapter 10). Care must be taken not to damage surrounding follicles
Haematoma	Discrete haematomas may form following trauma. Need to distinguish from subcutaneous haemorrhage in polyomavirus infection. If repeated problems or extensive, investigate possible coagulopathy (especially hepatopathy) and/or causes of incoordination (e.g. hypocalcaemia in Grey Parrots)	Generally self-resolving. Non-steroidal anti-inflammatory drugs may be indicated if extensive and/or painful
Constricted toe	Seen in chicks. One or more toes appear swollen distal to tight fibrous band. Distinguish from fibre entanglement. Possible aetiologies include low environmental humidity, egg-related strictures and ergot-like intoxication (Koski, 2002)	Mild cases respond to application of ophthalmic antibiotic preparations which moisten lesion. Severe cases require surgical intervention (Chapter 18). If distal toe appears necrotic, amputation required (Chapter 11)
Neoplasia (Chapter 20)	Many neoplasms described, including: 1 Lipoma 2 Liposarcoma 3 Fibrosarcoma 4 Squamous cell carcinoma 5 Lymphosarcoma 6 Myelolipoma 7 Haemangioma 8 Folliculoma Many types described. Discrete masses should be excised and submitted for histopathology *in toto* and more extensive masses should be sampled for biopsy and submitted for histopathology so treatment plan can be drawn up	1 Benign. Remove if possible or if causing discomfort. Especially common in Budgerigars and may be diet related. Changing to lower-fat diet may result in resolution or shrinkage to point where surgery not required 2 Excise 3 Malignant. If on wing, consider amputation 4 Locally very invasive and can be ulcerative. Very frequently occur secondarily to skin trauma, e.g. burns or dermatitis. Consider if previously improving lesion starts to worsen. Excise if possible but chemotherapy has been described (Koski, 2002) 5 Often around head or neck. Require full systemic work-up. 6 Often on wing-tip or thigh. Very vascular 7 Appear as 'melanoma'. Often involve feather follicle 8 May be linked to feather cysts of flight feathers in Budgerigars
Xanthoma	Dermal masses of cholesterol and lipid-laden macrophages. Skin featherless, thickened and yellow-orange. May be single or multiple, diffuse or discrete. Can be found anywhere on body, especially in Budgerigars and Cockatiels. *Not neoplastic* but may be found overlying other lesions, e.g. lipoma, hernia, chronic inflammation	If suspected (clinical appearance characteristic) evaluate bird thoroughly for systemic disease. Surgical excision if possible, though wound healing poor (Chapter 10). Dietary modification may be useful. Often best left alone

16.8 Non-infectious causes of masses and swellings.

Dermatitis, ulcers, erosions and other inflammatory disorders

As explained earlier, these lesions (Figures 16.9 to 16.12) can be a cause of, or progression from, self-trauma and mutilation. They may also represent underlying disease where the bird self-traumatizes over an area of internal discomfort (Figure 16.13). Similarly they may progress to, or be seen with, crusts and hyperkeratosis.

Cause	Description	Clinical approach
Split keel		See earlier in chapter
Wing web dermatitis (Figure 16.10)	Principally seen in Cockatiels and lovebirds. Presents as area of feather loss with areas of haemorrhage. Skin often thickened. Usually over patagium but lesions may also be seen in 'axillary' area. May progress to squamous cell carcinoma. Many causes proposed, including giardiasis, poxvirus, polyomavirus, circovirus, polyfolliculosis and bacterial infections	Cytology of acetates or impression smears useful. Evaluation of whole bird including faecal tests for endoparasites. Where multiple cases, testing for polyomavirus should be performed. Antibiosis essential, ideally based on culture/sensitivity but marbofloxacin is good first-line drug. Topical therapy useful; author favours daily application of either 1:250 dilution of F10 (Health & Hygiene Pty) or aloe vera gel. Where heavy bacterial contamination, silver sulphadiazine cream used
Polyfolliculosis (Figure 16.11)	Unusual condition seen in lovebirds where multiple feathers erupt from single follicles. Appears to be intensely pruritic (see Box 16.3) and often presents as dermatitis (typically ventral neck or dorsum) often before 'multiple feathers' apparent. In some cases appears to be infectious and polyomavirus has been proposed as cause but many cases test negative for this virus. Changes may also be secondary to self-trauma	Polyomavirus testing if multiple cases. Removal of 'multiple feathers' appears to give some relief from pruritus. May grow back as normal feathers. Antibiosis useful. Topical therapy 1:250 dilution of F10 or aloe vera gel applied daily. Few cases resolve entirely but many improve significantly. May require long-term topical therapy. Where pruritus can't be controlled or where there are concerns about spread of infection then euthanasia should be considered
Folliculitis	Dermatitis centred on feather follicles. Usually related to feather picking and unusual to see gross lesions	Antibiosis based on culture and sensitivity testing
Insect hypersensitivity	Dermatitis on bare areas of face	Control of biting flies. Fipronil spray applied to facial skin. Fusidic acid gel may be applied to lesions
Pododermatitis (Figure 16.12)	Pressure sores on soles of the feet and/or ventral tarsometatarsal area. Often secondarily infected and may become abscessed. In some cases infection may track into deeper structures. Predisposing causes include poor perching, nutritional problems (especially hypovitaminosis A), obesity, lack of activity	Early cases: correction of diet and weight loss (if necessary). Provision of better perching. Some of these can be padded (cotton wool bound on with lint bandage) and disinfectant solutions applied to these each day (e.g. 1:250 dilution of F10 or dilute chlorhexidine). Antibiosis (marbofloxacin, enrofloxacin or amoxicillin/clavulanate). Echinacea cream applied daily to lesions may also be of use. Advanced cases: carry guarded prognosis. Radiography of feet should be performed. Evidence of involvement of deeper structures carries poor prognosis. Full evaluation of bird's health status should be performed to determine causes of inactivity. Antibiosis essential and topical therapies include F10 ointment or silver sulfadiazine cream. If possible abscessed areas should be surgically debrided and closed (if possible) or managed as an open wound
Amazon foot necrosis	Typically involves self-mutilation of feet, legs and/or wings. Lesions consist of necrotic ulcerated areas. Mutilation appears to start after appearance of initial lesion. Underlying causes not known.	Full evaluation of the health status of the bird. Antibiosis and management of infected open wounds. Use of psychotropic drugs and collars may be considered. Poor prognosis

16.9 Dermatitis, ulcers, erosions and inflammatory lesions.

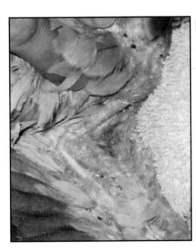

16.10 An unusual case of dermatitis of the propatagium of a Grey Parrot. Bacterial dermatitis was diagnosed and the lesion responded to systemic antibiosis and topical disinfection.

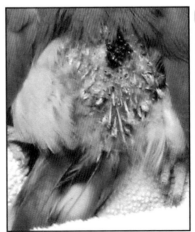

16.11 Polyfolliculosis in a lovebird. Note there are numerous follicles with more than one feather erupting. There is also an accompanying dermatitis.

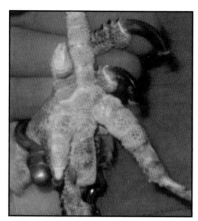

16.12
Pododermatitis in a Blue and Gold Macaw with liver disease. The claws are overgrown, as was the beak.

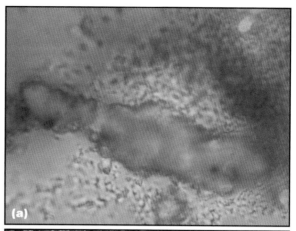

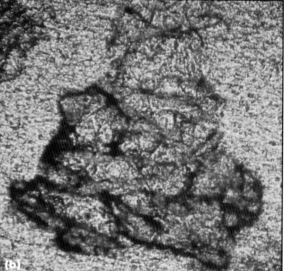

16.15 (a) Powder down (feather dust). (b) Skin scale. Note that skin scale appears as larger, flatter particles than powder down, with scale appearing as flattened squames and feather dust as irregular 'three-dimensional' acellular solid particles. Owners may occasionally be worried by the appearance of large flat pieces of feather sheath (from emerging feathers) that the bird is removing. These pieces are typically much larger and thicker than either scale or feather dust and are of no great concern.

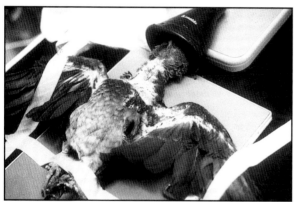

16.13 Grey Parrot with proventricular dilatation disease (PDD). A bacterial dermatitis was present which was initiated by the bird chewing over the ventral body, presumably due to abdominal discomfort. As infection became established, lesions extended over the ventrum. The author has seen this lesion pattern in several Grey Parrots, all of which were later confirmed with PDD.

Scaling and powder down disorders

It is important to consider the differences in scale, which arises from the skin (Figure 16.14), and powder down, which arises from the feathers (Figure 16.15). It should also be remembered that certain birds normally produce a lot of powder down (e.g. Grey Parrots and cockatoos).

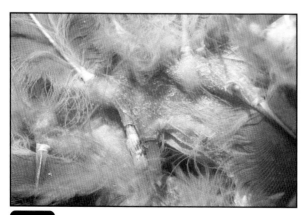

16.14 Normal skin scale on a Blue and Gold Macaw.

- *Reduced powder down.* This may be an early feature of circovirus infections in cockatoos and Grey Parrots, as the powder down feathers are affected. A black shiny beak in these species is a characteristic sign (Figure 13.4).
- *Increased scale.* A dry scaly skin may be associated with pruritus and feather plucking. The most common reason is drying of the skin due to central heating and a lack of water spraying. Other underlying causes include hypovitaminosis A. Secondary infections involving bacteria or fungi (including *Candida* spp. or, rarely, *Aspergillus* spp.) may be involved. Primary infections are rare but this may be seen with epidermoptid mite infestations or dermatophytosis.

Cytology of the skin surface, investigation of husbandry and underlying conditions, and skin fungal culture and biopsy are helpful in unresponsive cases. Therapy generally consists of improving skin hydration by daily spraying. Plain warm water should be used but disinfectants (1:250 dilution of F10 or chlorhexidine) may be used where there are secondary infections. Systemic antimicrobial therapy is rarely needed unless infection is primary or extensive. Evening primrose oil supplements may also be of use.

Feather disease

Feather damage

- *Chewed* by self (see later) or others.
- *Broken blood feather.* Damage to growing feathers may result in extensive bleeding. If not treated correctly (Chapter 6) further blood loss may occur and the damaged feather may be infected or deformed, as may subsequent feathers from this follicle (especially in primaries at end of wing).
- *Malnutrition and systemic disease* may result in malformed feathers or 'stress' marks (Figure 16.16). The latter are horizontal bars or weaknesses across the feather. They occur when feather growth is interrupted. Feathers may easily fracture at these points.
- *Ectoparasites.* Various mite and louse species may be found occasionally on psittacids. Both are highly host and site specific and are *rarely* associated with disease. Finding large numbers generally reflects debility of the host and the bird should be examined thoroughly. Fipronil spray is effective against both. Quill mites may rarely be found within the calamus; the damage may manifest as opacity of the shaft and loss of young feathers 'pinched off' at the tip. Ivermectin may be effective.
- *Damage to distal remiges and rectrices* if the bird is in a restricted cage or is weak and unable to perch.

Distribution of damage and microscopy of the damaged feathers will assist in determining diagnosis. The presence of 'split ends' distinguishes chewed feathers from those cut or broken off at stress marks. Feather digests may assist in finding ectoparasites.

Abnormal feathers

Causes of feather dystrophy are described in Figure 16.17.

Cause/condition	Description	Clinical approach
Circovirus (psittacine beak and feather disease, PBFD) (Figure 16.18) (Chapter 13)	Chronic form of the disease. May present with abnormally shaped feathers, colour change, or loss of powder down. Abnormal shapes include curling, pinching off, stress marks and retained feather sheaths. May progress to beak lesions	Diagnosis by suspicious clinical signs and DNA probe on blood and feather pulp of deformed feathers. Maintain in strict isolation from other birds or euthanase
Polyomavirus (Chapter 13)	Older Budgerigars that survive infection may develop dystrophies similar to those seen in PBFD; may also fail to develop contour feathers	DNA probe of faeces. Euthanasia advised unless birds can be maintained in isolation
French moult	Condition of Budgerigars (also called 'creepers' or 'crawlers') where they have deformed or no flight feathers. Caused by polyomavirus or PBFD. Some PBFD birds also have loss of body feathers	Diagnosis as above or by typical signs. Persistent infection so do not maintain bird in collections
Feather duster disease	Lethal genetic disorder of Budgerigars. Birds show long filamentous feathers	Diagnosis by clinical signs
Polyfolliculosis	See Figure 16.9	See Figure 16.9

16.17 Causes of feather dystrophy.

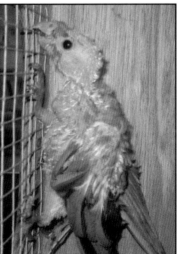

16.18

Psittacine beak and feather disease (PBFD) in a parakeet.

16.16 Fret marks often appear as lines or 'pinches' along feathers. In this young Green-winged Macaw a series of red or yellow (reduced pigment) marks appeared on all growing contour feathers after a stressful event (crop burn). Note also the diffraction pattern on the 'normal' parts of the feathers.

- *Colour changes* (Figure 16.19) may occur due to circovirus infection, hepatic disease, malnutrition, genetic disorders, folliculitis or chronic damage (e.g. plucking). An unusual presentation is that of blackening of body feathers. This occurs after emergence of the feathers, which may also appear damaged. Causes include hepatic disease, malnutrition, yeast infections and contamination with aerosolized particles or grease.
- *Retained feather sheaths* may occur due to circovirus infection, malnutrition or an inability to preen normally.

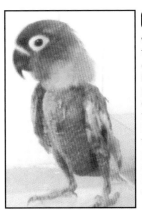

16.20 Plucking lovebird. Contrast this bird with that in Figure 16.18. In this case the feather loss is due to self-removal, as the head feathers are intact and in perfect condition. A positive circovirus test in a case like this is likely to indicate incidental infection, rather than the cause of the plucking. The body feathers are extremely unlikely to grow back, as the follicles appear completely atrophied.

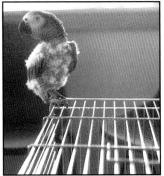

16.21 Typical plucking in a Grey Parrot. Note the white 'fluffy' feathers that result from chewing the feathers as they emerge, thus removing the main part of the contour feather.

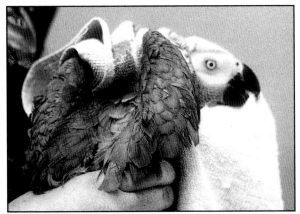

16.19 Red feathers in a Grey Parrot. Circovirus testing was negative and liver function appeared normal. In this case the red feathers had always been present and were presumed to be due to line breeding. In the trade these birds are known as 'King' Grey Parrots.

Feather loss: investigation of plucking and chewing

Where birds are housed together, it is vital to differentiate whether the feather loss is caused by self-plucking or is being done by others. The affected bird should be separated from the others for several weeks to see if feather regrowth occurs before investigating further.

Feather plucking or chewing may be seen in many of the psittacine species (Figure 16.20) but Grey Parrots (Figure 16.21) and Hahn's Macaws may be over-represented. Many medical causes or factors contributing to feather plucking have been documented (Figure 16.22 and Boxes 16.1 to 16.5) in addition to those of behavioural or social origin (Chapter 17). Often cases of plucking will be due to a combination of causes and the clinician needs to identify as many of these as possible in order to resolve the problem. Each factor may not be enough to trigger plucking on its own but each may contribute to the bird's 'stress', eventually resulting in abnormal or stereotypic behaviour such as plucking or chewing.

Each case needs to be thoroughly investigated. This can be very time consuming and requires a thorough knowledge of the bird's husbandry and biological and social needs as well as medicine. If necessary, referral should be considered.

The initial investigation (Figure 16.23) concentrates on treating or ruling out medical causes and obvious husbandry problems, before considering behaviour-related disease (Chapter 17).

Medical causes

Allergy (inhaled; contact; food) (Box 16.4)
Endoparasites
Ectoparasites [a]
Skin irritation
Skin desiccation
Hypothyroidism (Box 16.5)
Pain
Reproductive disease
Systemic illness; especially liver disease
Hypocalcaemia (Grey Parrots)
Proventricular dilatation disease
'Colic'
Chlamydophilosis
Air sacculitis
Heavy metal toxicosis
Folliculitis; bacterial/fungal
Genetic; feather deformities
Malnutrition
Neoplasia

Social causes

Poor socialization
Failure to learn preening behaviours
'Overtiredness' and inappropriate daily routine
Iatrogenic; especially following poor wing trim
Reproduction-related [b]

16.22 Medical and social causes of feather plucking and chewing. [a] Ectoparasites are probably the most frequently blamed cause of feather plucking or chewing. They are, in fact, one of the rarest causes, especially in caged pet birds. This author has never seen a case of plucking caused by ectoparasites. [b] Timing of plucking around times and seasons of reproductive activity may guide the clinician towards this diagnosis. Similarly, the association of plucking with reproductive behaviours (e.g. nest-building) may aid in diagnosis. See Chapter 18 for details of management.

Allergy has frequently been described as a cause of feather picking and chewing. It may be suspected where there is one or more of the following:

• Pruritus
• Skin lesions/appropriate cellular changes on skin histopathology
• Seasonality
• Recurrent pyoderma/superficial infections
• Positive responses on intradermal skin tests
• Recovery after removal of suspected allergen and relapse on re-exposure

The role of allergy is controversial and the means of allergic response uncertain, as birds lack IgE. However, avian IgY may carry out some of the roles performed by IgE in mammals, and mast cells have been demonstrated in avian skin. A useful review is found in Fraser (2002).

Box 16.4 Allergy.

This is commonly cited as a cause of feather plucking but there are few documented cases, possibly because it is a rare cause or due to difficulties in diagnosis, as avian total thyroxine (TT4) levels are normally quite low. Commercial tests may therefore not be evaluated at these low levels (Greenacre and Behrend, 1999). There are also species differences in 'normal' levels and marked seasonality in TT4 levels (Wilson, 1997). Single measurements of TT4, therefore, are rarely adequate for diagnosis of hypothyroidism, especially as many birds may be 'euthyroid sick'.

Thyroid hormones may act as non-specific inducers of moult (depending on photoperiod and season). However, the subsequent feather regrowth may be abnormal, with dystrophic feathers (Van Wettere and Redig, 2001). Supplementation is not recommended unless a diagnosis of hypothyroidism has been made.

The recommended protocol is to use a TSH stimulation test using 1.0 IU TSH i.m. TT4 levels should double in 4 hours.

Interestingly, in experimental models of hypothyroidism birds do not show plucking behaviour but do show dystrophic feathers and abnormal or delayed moult (Voitkevic, 1966).

Box 16.5 Hypothyroidism.

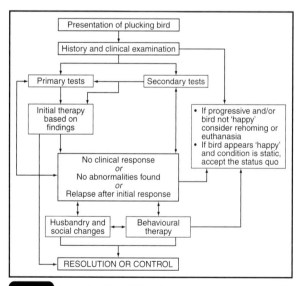

16.23 Investigation of the plucking or chewing parrot.

History

A thorough history should be taken. In addition to the general medical history (Chapter 5), the questions in Figure 16.24 should be considered.

Plucking or chewing history: The timing and manner of plucking or chewing may give clues as to cause. For example, is it related to: separation anxiety; attention seeking; pruritus (see Box 16.3); seasonal factors; reproduction; or allergy (see Box 16.4)?

• Is this the first incidence?
• If not, when did it happen before? For how long? Which feathers were affected? Did the bird re-feather completely before starting again? Details of therapies, etc. Did the problem resolve without therapy?
• When did the bird start plucking? For how long has it been plucking?
• Which feathers were affected first? Has the area affected changed?
• How does the bird pluck or chew? Does it nibble? Aggressive chewing? Does it chew its claws?
• Does the bird rub or scratch itself on the cage or perches?
• When does the bird pluck or chew? Are the owners present or not? If present, what is their response?
• Does it interrupt other behaviours to pluck or chew?

Observation

While observing the bird during the history-taking, what was noted?

• Did the bird appear well? Fluffed? 'Oval-eyed'?
• Did it appear bright?
• Was it quiet/introverted? Or extrovert?
• How did the owner and bird interact with each other?
• Did it pluck or chew? If so, was this an extension of normal preening behaviour? Or did it break off another activity to do this? In the latter case, the chewing or plucking may be a displacement activity while anxious or may show that the bird is pruritic.

Examination and diagnostic testing

After history taking and observation, the bird should receive a full clinical examination (Chapter 5) and dermatological examination (see earlier). Diagnostic tests will invariably be required (Figure 16.25) and may be done at the same time, or in sequence. Coeloscopy, crop biopsy, circovirus tests etc. may be used to follow up specific findings or suspicions.

Therapy

Initial therapy should be based on specific clinical findings and on correcting specific concerns with husbandry. If there are no specific findings, or if there is no response to rational therapy, behavioural aetiologies should be considered (Chapter 17). If a clinical response is seen but not sustained, or if there is relapse, the case should be fully re-evaluated.

The ideal outcome in these cases is a 'happy' normally feathered bird. However, this is not always possible. If all underlying causes have been investigated and treated, the bird appears to be 'happy' and the condition is non-progressive, then it is perfectly acceptable to keep a 'happy' bald bird.

Area of interest	Questions	Notes
Environment (including details of cage, perches and toys)	Are the toys given in rotation? Do the owners smoke? Or do they use air fresheners or sprays near the bird? Is the bird near cooking fumes or open fires? Is there central heating?	Particulate matter may irritate the skin or feathers. Sources of this should be removed, or the bird moved away. Central heating may desiccate the skin
Daily regime	How much time does the bird spend in and out of the cage? Does the bird go outside? If not, is ultraviolet light provided, and how long for? When does the bird 'go to bed'? For how long is the owner with the bird? If the bird is alone, is the radio or television left on? Are there other birds? If so, which species? Details of interactions between the birds and their disease history?	Ultraviolet light is essential in calcium metabolism and is important in controlling activity and seasonal/reproductive cycles. Normally birds will 'roost' as light levels drop. Keeping birds in the living room means that they keep the same hours as the owner (even if the bird is covered). They can become overtired and fractious and start to pluck feathers. It is advised that a 'bedtime' is instigated, with the bird being roosted in the early to mid-evening in a separate darkened room. Parrots tend to live in family groups or pairs within a flock. Being left alone during the day may induce anxiety, especially if hand-reared and imprinted to associate humans as flock members. In these cases it is vital to ensure adequate companionship and to break any 'pair bonding' between owner and bird (Chapter 17)
Spraying	Is the bird sprayed or a bath provided each day? If so, are products added to the water?	This may be a factor in skin desiccation Certain aromatic chemicals sold to be added to spray water may be irritant to some birds
Rearing history	Is the bird hand-reared or parent-reared? If hand-reared, do the owners know when it was taken from the parents? Was it reared alone or with others?	Birds imprinted on people require human company. Rearing young birds in isolation may be a factor in the development of anxiety-related disorders. It may also result in a lack of opportunity to learn certain behaviours (e.g. preening). In the author's opinion this is especially a problem with young feather-chewing cockatoos: the need to preen is innate but the method is learnt and they therefore respond with another innate behaviour – chewing. In some cases these birds may learn correct preening methods if housed with or near another bird so they can observe normal preening behaviour and copy it
Relationship with owners	Is there a favourite owner? Is that favourite male or female? Does the bird feed the owner, or make sexual displays to them? How does the owner handle and stroke the bird? Is the favourite owner away a lot? Has there been any strife or change within the family?	Again, if a pair bond occurs with an owner who is frequently away, anxiety may result. In general, pair bonds with owners should not be encouraged
Reproductive history	Eggs laid? When?	Some plucking cases may be related to reproductive activity (Chapter 18)
Moulting history	When did the bird moult? How long for?	Moulting may be a trigger for plucking, especially in younger birds. Delayed or slow moult may indicate problems in feather production, e.g. nutritional disease
Wing clipping	Is the bird clipped? Has it ever been clipped?	Poor wing clips have been associated with feather chewing. A poor clip may cause direct pain or it may leave split feather ends protruding beyond the covert feathers. These may encourage chewing behaviour. Chapter 6 describes proper clipping techniques

16.24 History taking for cases of plucking.

Primary tests

- Haematology/biochemistry: total protein, albumin, globulin (or serum protein electrophoresis), AST, CK, uric acid, ionized calcium
- Zinc
- Sexing (unless already known)
- Faecal Gram stain
- Skin and feather pulp cytology

Secondary tests

- Radiography: whole body or of a focal area where there is featherloss
- *Chlamydophila* testing
- Faecal parasitology
  Skin biopsy

16.25 Diagnostic testing for plucking and chewing.

Uropygial gland

This holocrine gland is found dorsally at the tail base and is drained via a papilla (with tuft of feathers) on the dorsocaudal surface. The gland is present in most parrots (Chapter 2). Two major conditions are seen:

- *Impaction* (Figure 16.26). May be related to hypovitaminosis A. Gland function is assessed at examination by wiping a finger across the tip; an oily secretion should be present. If not, blockage is likely that may lead to impaction and abscessation. The impacted gland may be squeezed gently to push out contents via the papilla. Some cases may require surgical excision (Chapter 10).
- *Neoplasia*. Adenomas and carcinomas have been reported. Surgical excision is required.

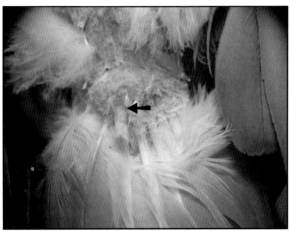

16.26 Grey Parrot with an impacted uropygial gland. Note the dryness of the papilla (arrowed).

Medical conditions of the beak

Trauma, deformities and surgical correction of the beak are discussed in Chapter 11 and beak clipping is discussed in Chapter 6. When presented with a bird with an overgrown beak, it is important to find out why it is so. Beak overgrowth in adult birds may occur due to the following:

- Earlier uncorrected malformation
- Trauma, resulting in malpositioning or loss of part of the beak
- Earlier poor beak clip
- Problems with keratin synthesis and beak growth.

The latter is extremely common and may be due to low-protein, high-fat diets or hepatic disease, especially fatty liver in small psittacids. It is vital to investigate the problem and correct the diet, ideally by giving the bird a commercial pelleted ration or, where the bird will not accept this, by supplementing seed diet with a good quality vitamin and essential amino acid supplement (Chapter 12). Beak overgrowth occurs because the softer poorly formed beak material is unable to keep itself worn down (see Figure 2.3).

Sometimes brown streaks will be seen in the keratin of the beak, especially in Budgerigars. These represent bleeding due to a coagulopathy, generally due to liver disease.

Hyperkeratosis of the beak may be due to infestation with *Cnemidocoptes* mites (see earlier) or due to poor protein synthesis for the reasons mentioned above.

17

Behaviour and behavioural disorders

Kenneth R. Welle

Introduction

Although people have been sharing their homes and lives with pet parrots for the past 2000 years, only recently have most pet bird owners started to realize the potential of these amazing creatures. Originally, the bright plumage and capacity for imitating human speech were the primary appeal. Today, parrots are increasingly recognized as complex, intelligent and highly social animals. Like any other animal, parrots are susceptible to a number of behavioural and psychological disorders. Understanding the bird's perspective can help bird owners to provide their pets with a more appropriate environment and social setting.

A relatively small number of species represent a high percentage of pet birds. Several species (Budgerigar, Cockatiel, Peach-faced Lovebird, Ringneck Parakeet, some Australian grass parakeets) have essentially become domesticated. Among the remaining psittacine birds, most captive individuals are only one or two generations from the wild state. These birds retain many of the wild tendencies but lack the stimuli and training required for full social development.

The life of a wild parrot usually starts in a dark cavity. They are still very embryonic at hatching; their eyes are closed, their ears may be closed, they have no feathers, and know nothing except how to beg for food. They feel physical contact with their warm clutch mates and parents. They are fed frequent small meals throughout the day. Physically, they grow and mature rapidly, achieving adult size in a matter of weeks. Behaviourally and intellectually, however, larger species may continue to learn from their parents for several months to years before they are completely independent. In this time they learn to interact with other birds, establish their social status, learn what to eat, how to find it, how to eat, how to recognize and avoid predators, how to maintain their feathers, and many other important survival skills. Some fly long distances from roosting areas to foraging areas, and (depending on food availability) may spend between 1 and 8 hours finding and consuming food. Some are observed to engage in physical activities purely for fun and exercise. When they reach sexual maturity, they choose a mate, form a pair bond, defend their nest and reproduce, and the cycle starts again (Collar, 1997).

Contrast this with the life of hand-reared parrots. They are still usually hatched in a dark cavity, but then they are moved into a relatively bright brooder, sometimes alone for long stretches of time. They are taken out briefly, fed enormous amounts of liquid food, and returned to the brooder. When they are older, they are not challenged in their social interactions, often rising to the top of the pecking order as adolescents. They have unlimited supplies of calorie-rich food placed in bowls in front of them. They have no foraging challenges and can obtain their calorie needs in a short period of time. They have minimal physical exertion, they have no survival tasks to learn, and they are alone more than they are with their flock. When they become sexually mature, they choose a person as a mate, but that person has another mate. They fight for the mate but, even though they appear to have won, the mate is angry and confines them. It is not surprising that parrots sometimes develop behaviour problems.

Some of the problems start with the selection of the pet bird. The first decision to make is whether a person has an appropriate home for a parrot. Prospective bird owners should be advised to research heavily and decide slowly the type of bird they wish to have, and indeed whether they should have a bird at all (Chapter 3). A couple working 10–12 hours a day should not buy or adopt a cockatoo unless they can safely bring the bird to work, or perhaps find a bird-sitter. Different psittacine species have somewhat different personalities, different needs and different problems. Some desire a tremendous amount of physical contact from the owner. Others are satisfied with visual and verbal interactions. Some species are more inclined to be aggressive, while others may be very fearful. There is tremendous variation within each species, but people should also be made aware of the common problems of a species.

Many people have no idea what to expect from a parrot. In general, most people expect too little and underestimate the potential for their pet. Countless Budgerigars sit unattended in small cages without any social interactions or exercise. They are looked upon as noisy, messy decorations that are replaced every 3–4 years when they die. Their owners have no idea that these little creatures are intelligent and social. As a result the bird becomes a vicious biter, panics when a hand comes near and is, in general, miserable. At the other end of the spectrum are owners who expect their parrot to behave like a person or like a domesticated animal. The birds are given too many liberties, are given no limitations and no guidance, and learn to rule the roost. It is only when people realize that parrots are intelligent, social, wild animals that they can begin to handle them appropriately.

Preventing behaviour problems

Veterinary surgeons have an opportunity to help to prevent many of these behavioural problems. Often, simply discussing some of the social and environmental needs of the bird with a new bird owner will help to prevent some of the more common problems. It should be emphasized that environmental and social enrichment are very important. The availability of a complex environment containing novel circumstances and simple challenges will speed neurological and behavioural development (Neville, 1997). The use of behaviour classes for birds and owners has been very successful in the author's practice (Welle, 1997).

Minimizing fear and stress in the examination room and hospital

Along with the opportunity to help comes the possibility of damaging the human–avian bond. Of course the axiom 'first, do no harm' applies to the behavioural development of parrots as well. One of the benefits of learning more about avian behaviour is that the information can be brought into the examination room. With good handling techniques, the restraint and examination process can be much easier and less stressful to the bird. Aviculture birds that are infrequently handled should be caught and restrained directly from the carrier (Chapter 4). Tame birds (those accustomed to handling) are often taken out of the carrier by the owner prior to the arrival of the veterinarian. If a little time is spent developing rapport with the bird, placement of a towel over them (Figure 17.1) will be much less traumatic. Clients should be advised to play 'peek-a-boo' with their bird, using a towel, from an early age. These birds generally will allow a towel to be laid upon them with little or no stress at all.

When restraining birds, they should be held more vertically (Davis, 1997). Lying on the back is a very frightening and vulnerable position for birds and they will often fight more vigorously in that position. Talking to the bird during the examination will be calming, especially if the owner regularly talks to the bird. The restraint should be kept to as short a period as possible by having everything prepared prior to restraint. For birds that are difficult to catch, as much as possible should be done in one restraint. For others, it is best to use short restraint periods (3 minutes at a time) with rests in between.

When hospitalizing birds, they should be placed in an upper cage bank. When placed in lower cages, birds have to look up at everyone and feel very threatened. More confident birds can be kept at waist height but very frightened birds should be kept higher. Birds should always be kept where they do not see predatory creatures. If possible, they should be kept away from barking dogs.

Socialization

A common misconception is that social behaviour evolved because of a need for companionship. In reality the congregation of groups of animals within a species serves a much more utilitarian purpose. The flock is a protective unit, and affiliation with others is essential to the survival of each individual. The need for social interaction is secondary to the instinct for survival (Davis, 1997b). The presence of conspecifics makes it much more difficult for a predator to stalk and kill a given prey species successfully and the presence of other potential prey items in the vicinity makes it mathematically less likely for an individual to be preyed upon. Behaviours necessary for conflict-free interaction between individuals of a group evolved as a secondary requirement. This makes social interaction even more critical. Not only is an isolated bird lonely; it also feels vulnerable to attack. A close analogy would be a person walking at night: generally people feel more secure and safe when with a group of people than when walking alone.

Most parrots pair-bond. Keas are polygamous. Asiatic parakeets and Eclectus Parrots bond only for the breeding season. Most parrots leave the flock as pairs during breeding, but some, such as Quaker Parakeets, Brown-throated Conures and Patagonian Conures, are colony nesters. Outside the breeding season, parrots live in small to very large flocks.

In order for any animal society to function, communication and conflict-resolution mechanisms must be developed (Collar, 1997). For most social animals a form of hierarchy develops to prevent true combat situations. According to some, most parrot flocks function according to a hierarchical arrangement (Davis, 1997). Young parrots learn to submit to the leader. If they try to share resources, they are bitten and chased away (Harrison, 1994). Others argue that, between

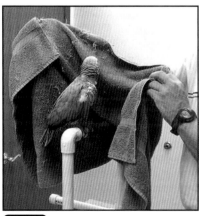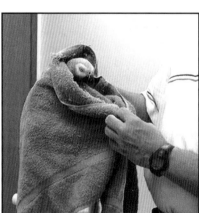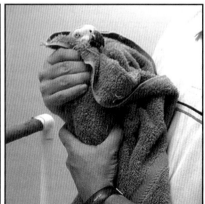

17.1 Gentle towel restraint. Gentle handling can reduce the stress involved with veterinary examinations.

individuals, there appears to be a dominant/submissive relationship; in flock situations no dominance has been described (Luescher, 2004). Because of their intelligence, parrots' social structure may not be a linear dominance hierarchy. There may be a matter of creating alliances more than of dominance. Also, dominance in one situation may not apply in another (Smith, 1999). Pairs may cooperate in agonistic interactions with other birds (Collar, 1997).

Whether there is a true dominance hierarchy system or not, it certainly appears that parrots avoid violent conflict by ritualized posturing and positioning. The responses of one bird to another are likely to be learned or conditioned. Conditioning refers to the process by which behaviour is modified by the outcome of past occurrences of that behaviour. If during one encounter, or repeated encounters, an aggressive bluff gains an advantage for a bird, it is likely that the same behaviour will be used again. If the other bird in this encounter avoids being bitten by deferring to the aggressor, but is bitten when standing his ground, the 'submissive' behaviour is reinforced.

Likewise, parrots learn how best to interact with humans to achieve their goals. In human/parrot interactions it appears that problems do not occur as a result of a failure to 'dominate' a bird, but they commonly occur when a bird is allowed to intimidate or 'dominate' its handler. It is natural for a parrot to be somewhat reluctant to do certain things, such as allow handling by a new person, or go into the cage, or come out of the cage. Even nestlings and fledglings will threaten with an open beak, or lunge at a hand. If the person jerks the hand away, or is otherwise hesitant, the bird learns what a powerful tool aggression can be. Most of the time a threat, or mild nip, is all that is required to achieve the objective. If the handler fails to respond appropriately (in the eyes of the bird), more intensified aggression may occur. Is this dominance aggression? Whether or not these observations describe true dominance behaviour will remain an academic argument for some time. However, it shares enough characteristics with the dominance aggression described in dogs by Overall (1997) that the terms dominance and dominance aggression will be used in the remainder of this chapter (see Figure 17.5).

Vertical placement or height is frequently referred to in avian behaviour literature. It has been said that the dominance order can often be determined by seeing dominant individuals in higher positions (Davis, 1997). Some claim that the apparent relationship of height to dominance may be related to the high spot being the most desirable perch, rather than the height itself (Smith, 1999). Others maintain that the notion of a flock leader and dominant birds sitting higher than submissive birds is a myth (Luescher, 2004). It is unlikely that there is a direct height-to-rank relationship, but clinical observations by the author show that parrots frequently use an inaccessible (i.e. very high) location to avoid human handling. In addition, most parrots dislike being in a very low position, and they are much more likely to step on to a person's hand from a very low vantage point. Following restraint and medical examination, nervous parrots in the author's practice are frequently released from the towel on to the floor. This prevents them from thrashing to the floor and injuring themselves, but, almost without exception, these birds will step on to the hand of the clinician and forgive the examination. Therefore, while the reasoning for some of the traditional advice may not be entirely accurate, it still seems wise to work with most birds at easily accessible heights, i.e. waist level to shoulder level. With particularly difficult birds, working from the floor can facilitate conditioning them to stepping on to a hand.

Most parrots are noisy and communicate vocally. They learn a flock dialect. They also communicate visually with body language and colour (Luescher, 2004). Different vocalizations are used by parrots to signal danger, or food, or to greet another bird (Harrison, 1994; Rach, 1998). Vocalization is critical for keeping flocks together, especially in dense rainforest habitats. Calls are used to bring the flock together at the end of the day. Grey Parrots have been observed exhibiting their remarkable mimicry in the wild as well. The sounds of 10 species (nine avian species and one bat species) have been recorded from wild Greys, but there is no known explanation for why they do this (Cruickshank *et al.*, 1993).

Pairs engage in social grooming and mutual feeding to maintain their bonds. Likewise, parent birds preen and feed immature birds. These interactions are uncommon between other members of the flock (Figure 17.2).

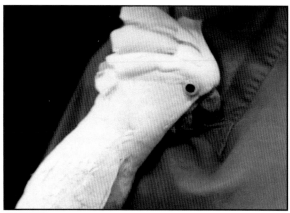

17.2 Excessive physical interaction between owner and parrot may lead to behavioural problems. In the natural state such interactions only occur in a pair or between parent and offspring; the owner–parrot relationship can never adequately fulfil these roles, which will inevitably lead to frustration.

Various behaviours are used by different species for communication with less intimate flock mates (Rach, 1998):

* *Beak clicking*: greeting or warning
* *Beak grinding*: contentment
* *Eye pinning* (dilation/constriction of the pupils): excitement, either good or bad
* *Facial feather twitching*: startled or intrigued
* *Fluffing*: prelude to preening or tension releaser
* *Foot tapping*: territorial defence
* *Tail fanning*: courtship or aggressive display.

Development and learning

For many altricial species (hatched with eyes closed and dependent on parents), including most of the psittacine family, many behaviours tend to be learned. This is true whether the bird is in the wild or in captivity (Welty, 1982) and explains the difficulty in releasing hand-reared orphan birds into the wild. Birds learn various skills more efficiently at certain stages of development, known as sensitive periods or critical periods. One such behaviour is imprinting, which may be either filial (forming social attachments) or sexual (forming an image of a desirable mate) (Smith, 1999). This can lead to conflict when birds are raised by humans, resulting in these birds imprinting upon humans (Harrison, 1994). Such species confusion is compounded when the human caretaker fails to continue the bird's education to include necessary skills for coping with the artificial environment.

Once the bird fledges, it becomes versed in the 'flock experience'. Early learning can be critical for the long-term development of the bird. Any synapses that are not stimulated by early sensory experiences may be 'pruned' by the brain and eliminated (Friedman and Brinker, 2000). Play is used frequently to learn the environment and reaffirm flock position (Rach, 1998). When normal play behaviours of White-fronted Amazons were studied, they included play solicitation, play biting or play fighting, or behaviours associated with pair bonding, such as allopreening and bill nibbling (Harrison, 1994).

Playing with a pet bird can provide effective means of teaching it some necessary skills. Structured training or play sessions can allow owner and pet to interact in an entertaining but structured manner (Horwitz, 1999). The objectives are to teach behaviours required for companionability and behaviours that assure comfort, health and happiness (Friedman and Brinker, 2000). Play should focus on behaviours that the animal enjoys and encourage those that are desirable.

Developing a healthy social environment for pet birds

A healthy human–avian bond requires each side to behave in a manner that promotes this bond. Necessary components of a well adjusted and well behaved pet bird include: respect and trust of the owner and other humans; independence; and a platonic bond. For hand-reared parrots, the first part of the process is providing them with appropriate socialization in the brooder. Keeping clutches together rather than isolating individuals is preferable. Provision of an appropriate amount of physical contact at this stage can be important as well. Inadequate neonatal socialization may result in self-damaging behaviours at a later time. Psittacine feather plucking behaviours bear remarkable resemblance to self-injurious behaviour in primates, which occurs much more frequently in monkeys raised by humans than in those raised by their parents (Orosz and Johnson-Delaney, 2003). Ultimately, the task of taming a parent-reared chick may prove minor compared with the challenge of treating the potential behavioural disorders resulting from inadequate early socialization.

As wild animals, parrots have no concept of the human–animal bond and can only interact with human companions as flock members (Davis, 1997). Initially this may be the role of a parent bird (Athan, 1997). This relationship is relatively easy to accomplish. It is important to set rules for an authority-based relationship, in which the bird understands that the humans are in control (Athan, 1993) – in control of themselves as well as in control of the bird. A lack of confidence by the handler is one of the most certain ways to teach a bird to bite. This is one of the most difficult concepts to convey to parrot owners. Handling should be neither overbearing nor timid. When a hand is offered for a bird to step on to, it should be in a very matter-of-fact manner, with an assumption that the bird will step on. When this confident approach is employed, birds rarely hesitate to step up. Once the parrot has stepped up on to the hand, verbal praise ('Good bird!'), a food treat or other reinforcement can be used to encourage continued performance of the desired behaviour.

Training can begin once the bird has developed adult body conformation and reasonable coordination. The exact age depends on the species. For small species, this may be 6–8 weeks; for larger parrots, 12–14 weeks of age is generally sufficient. While training sessions should be more frequent in young birds, they should continue throughout life to maintain good behaviour.

One of the rules pertains to position. The bird should be positioned to maximize the chances for successful repetitions during training. Whether because of dominance, site-related aggression or other unknown reasons, birds are often more aggressive and hesitant to perform basic tasks when placed in high positions, in close proximity to their cage or other inaccessible retreats (Davis, 1997). Initial training sessions should take place in a room out of sight of the cage, and with few distractions, hiding places or extra people. The bird should be kept below the eye level and in front of the handler. Shoulders are particularly bad locations because they prevent the handler from keeping eye contact and from placing hands properly, and because bites from this position can be particularly dangerous.

The next aspect of maintaining the authority-based relationship is to teach some basic commands and use them frequently. The step-up drill is one that every pet bird should know. In this drill the command 'step up' is given and the bird is coaxed to step up on to the hand (Figure 17.3). Each time this exercise is performed, respect and trust are built. It is not enough that the bird knows what the command means. Practice must be maintained to maintain that mutual trust and respect. Once trust and respect are established, other skills can be taught. Important social skills can include interaction with other birds, playing with water, exploring foods, meeting strangers, and many others (Friedman and Brinker, 2000). These behaviours are learned through imitation. In the home, parrots imitate their companions, whether avian or mammal. If they cannot copy behaviours, they improvise. If the improvised behaviours are reinforced,

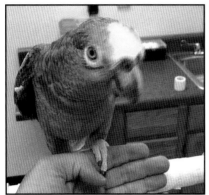

The step-up command is one that should be taught to all birds.

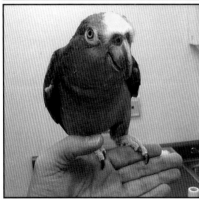

the behaviour can become a pattern. Likewise, desirable behaviours can be encouraged by modelling those behaviours in front of the bird. The motivation to copy behaviours can be enhanced by providing a competitive situation in which the bird learns. This method is known as the model-rival technique and has been pioneered in birds by Dr Irene Pepperberg (Pepperberg, 1999).

Independence and confidence

Contrary to popular opinion, behavioural disorders are not always a result of inadequate interaction with a pet bird. Very often, the interactions are excessive or inappropriate and the bird never develops the ability to be comfortable by itself. Birds that have not been taught independence are much more likely to develop stress-related behaviours.

Most of the strategies a parrot uses to get along in life are learned. Communication, eating, play and what to fear must all be learned for the bird to develop independence. While many types of parrots are independent by nature, others must learn this from carers (Athan and Deter, 2000). When they meet a new situation they look for cues as to how to react: if the carer is happy, the bird will not be afraid. Parrots must be taught to be adventurous. Owners should 'model' playing with the toys or add another bird or person to play, providing a model-rival. These skills are critical for the development of independent behaviour in pet birds.

Many pet bird owners fear spoiling a bird by responding to cries. With juvenile birds displaying baby behaviours such as crying, responding to the bird will not 'spoil' the bird but make it more secure (Athan and Deter, 2000). Particularly in very young birds, withholding food, attention or other necessities can make them doubt the safety of their situation. The common advice of ignoring a vocalizing bird can contribute to a nuisance-screaming problem. A bird that is ignored will continue to scream until something happens. Acknowledging the bird and maintaining some auditory contact can minimize the begging and vocalizations. Vocal cues can be used to calm birds. The key is to plan ahead and consistently use particular words and expressions in the same situations. In this way the association between the word and the situation is clearly patterned. These words can then be used in a threatening situation to give a sense of security (Blanchard, 2000).

Vocal and other games can also promote independence. The games suggested in Figure 17.4 are recommended to owners in the author's practice. These were devised from many suggestions and sources and are not necessarily original. They are written in the same way that they are presented in client education materials. The games should be used daily to weekly (more often early on and less so as the bird matures and adjusts).

Game	Theory	How to play
House Tour	In the wild, fledgling birds follow parents and flock mates around their environment. By seeing the response of the adult birds to various stimuli, they learn what to eat, what to fear, what to avoid, etc. This game is intended to do the same thing.	The bird must be tame and must know the basic 'step-up' command. Carry the bird on the hand and walk around the house. Point out everything you see and say its name. Most importantly, be very calm. By seeing that you are not upset, the bird learns not to be. Introduce all of the human and animal household members. Also, do not neglect sounds. Take the bird near the source of some sounds and do the same exercise. The bonus of this game is that talking birds often learn how to identify people and things in the house.
Colour Game	Parrots are very visually oriented and intelligent creatures. This game helps to stimulate their curiosity.	Take pieces of coloured paper. Say the colour to the bird. Repeat for all of the other colours. Keep in mind that the bird sees colours slightly differently than you do, but can still distinguish them well. In more advanced sessions, ask the bird what colour you are holding. For even better results, do this game with another person in front of the bird. When the parrot gets the answer correct it is lavishly praised.

17.4 Games for building confidence. (continues) ▶

Game	Theory	How to play
Whistle While You Work	In the wild, parrots vocalize to maintain contact with members of their flock. Being alone puts birds at greatly increased risk of predation. Survival depends on maintaining contact. If they cannot hear the response of the group, they think they have lost contact and so they call louder. It is often advised never to respond to a bird's vocalization. Imagine the following scenario. You are at home alone and you hear someone come in the door. You think it is your spouse so you call out his/her name but you get no response. You call again and still no response. At this point you start to panic and get ready to call the police! This is what we are doing to the bird when we ignore their calls.	In order to take the flock contact initiative away from the bird, announce where you are as you move about the house. This is especially true if you are out of sight. Try whistling, humming, singing, or talking as you go.
Trick Training	Parrots are highly intelligent birds. Mental challenges can occupy some of the time they may otherwise use for self-destructive behaviours. Trick training also provides ammunition for counterconditioning. Tricks can and should be relatively natural behaviours that the bird learns to do on request.	Watch your bird for certain behaviours that are interesting. Then start to give a cue, try to get the bird to do the behaviour, and reward even mild attempts at performing. As time goes on, require a little better performance to receive a reward. Rewards can be verbal or food treats. Ideas that may be useful include waving the foot, somersault on the perch or table, holding up wings, holding up objects with the foot, or tearing up a toy.

17.4 (continued) Games for building confidence.

The environment can be critical to the bird's ability to be independent. Birds may perceive many things as dangerous that a large predatory species such as a human would not. While it may seem a good idea to let a parrot look out into the garden to see the bird feeder, it may give more stress than pleasure if the pet sees a hawk coming by and snatching up birds regularly. Location in the home should take this fact into account. Birds should be able to see approaching people and pets from a distance rather than having them appear from nowhere. Placing a cage on a wall right next to a door may be more stressful for a nervous bird.

Parrots may even be sensitive to the emotional 'energies' of those around them and can suffer from this increased stress (Clark, 2000). Such things as marital difficulties, spousal abuse, child abuse or loss of a loved one (even one the bird does not know) may indirectly affect some birds. These can be difficult subjects to approach with clients and must be handled delicately. Some of these factors may be revealed by the owners, others will be more cryptic. Veterinary surgeons are generally not qualified to handle these situations and the appropriate professionals should be consulted when necessary.

The lack of time-occupying activities can contribute to some of the behaviour problems in pet parrots. Without a healthy outlet for its nervous energy, a bird can develop numerous vices. A study in Orange-winged Amazons showed that foraging enrichments reduced feather plucking. These enrichments included requiring the bird to chew through barriers, sort through inedible items, or manipulate food through holes to get food. These foraging enrichments were more effective than other types of enrichment (Meehan *et al.*, 2003).

Bonding

The whole point of having a pet is to bond with it in some fashion. While the role of most birds in a household is simply as companions, occasionally they are kept as surrogates for children, spouses or parents. Sometimes parrots, especially as they are long-lived, can serve as a last link to a loved one who has passed away (Harris, 1997). When the behaviour of a parrot causes this bond to be severed, the results can be devastating to the owner. Unfortunately, placement of these birds into these surrogate roles can lead to an unhealthy social environment. Ideally birds and owners interact as flock members but not as mates. The author often advises owners to behave as a preschool or kindergarten teacher toward their parrot. This helps them to grasp the type of interactions that will challenge and teach parrots without inappropriate pair-bonding behaviours. Social activities for birds may include foraging, playing, flying as a group, and other relatively dynamic activities. Allopreening and cuddling are done primarily with the mate. These interactions should be reserved for evenings and naptimes or when the bird is confronted with unfamiliar things (Athan and Deter, 2000; Clark, 2000).

Many birds will beg for attention and the behaviours they use include shaking toys, sneezing, soft vocalization, displays, crouching and wing quivering, staring, and screaming (Rach, 1998). Interactive dynamic attention given to a begging bird might teach more appropriate behaviour. As opposed to just petting, cuddling or other sedentary social interactions, interactive dynamic attention includes toy play, trick training, word games or exercise. Healthy social environments include social feeding (eating with the owners), which can allow more socialization in a more casual atmosphere. It also gives an opportunity to demonstrate independent eating by eating in front of the bird and offering to share food (Athan and Deter, 2000).

Most psittacine birds remain paired year round and spend a large amount of time together. When the pair is separated by the brooding of eggs, the male will often come repeatedly to the nest to feed the mate. There are few times when there is no contact (Collar, 1997; Rowley, 1997). According to Harrison (1994), 'For such intensely social birds, life in an enclosure with no companionship must be the ultimate "psychological torture".' Realistically, no one can provide 24-hour interaction with the bird. It is therefore best to avoid having the bird develop a pair bond with one person. In addition, birds that develop pair bonds with an owner will tend to be more aggressive.

It is a myth that some species are 'one-person birds'. Interaction with only one person in captivity is contradictory to the psittacid's social nature (Wilson, 2000). Birds should be encouraged to be accepting of multiple people. If a bird is reluctant, 'out-of-territory' interactions such as step-ups, 'rescues' or 'outings' are recommended (Athan and Deter, 2000). 'Rescues' involve such things as a person who is not normally the bird's favourite bringing the bird for a veterinary visit or grooming. Following the procedure, and in this 'hostile' environment, the person that the bird does not like starts to seem very safe and comfortable to the bird. 'Outings' are similar but involve simply taking the bird for a trip out of the home to an unfamiliar area. Again, the person becomes the most familiar thing to the bird. People disliked by a bird should practise step-up exercises in an area unfamiliar to the bird. This 'home field advantage' will often result in a bird that behaves much better towards a person they would normally bite.

Behavioural consultation

Taking a history for behaviour problems

While taking a good history is stressed for nearly every aspect of veterinary medicine, in behaviour medicine it is really the only diagnostic option. It is therefore critical that the history be accurate and thorough. No tests will catch the omissions of the history. The history should be done in a way that is consistent. Each question should be asked every time. It is important that the questions are neither leading nor accusing. If clients feel guilty, or if they perceive that a certain response is desired, they may alter their story.

Some important facts to establish include the bird's source, environment, diet, social interactions and of course the behaviour problems, and what the owners are doing in response to them. It is useful to give clients a survey form to fill out prior to the consultation. An example is provided at the end of this chapter. The standardized form can be augmented by interviewing the owners during the behaviour consultation.

Clinical signs of behavioural problems

The difference between behavioural and 'organic' disease is indistinct. The clinical sign of depression can be caused by many physical conditions, but may also be a behavioural disease. Most other behaviours commonly discussed as behavioural disorders can also have a multitude of physical aetiologies. All behaviours are neurochemically mediated as well. When behaviour problems of birds are discussed, however, certain clinical signs are always included. Aggression or, more specifically, biting, excessive vocalization, feather plucking and excessively fearful responses to stimuli are the most commonly presented behavioural clinical signs. Since veterinary patients cannot be interviewed to determine what this problem is, it can be difficult. Veterinary behaviour specialists have begun to name and categorize some common behavioural problems in dogs and cats. Some of these may have similarities with the avian behaviour diagnoses listed in Figure 17.5 (Overall, 1997).

Diagnosis	Necessary criteria	Sufficient criteria	Avian equivalent
Attention seeking	Animal uses vocal or physical behaviours to obtain attention from people when they are otherwise occupied	Whenever a person is not engaged in activity with animal, animal uses behaviours to direct attention to itself and will interrupt human activity to do so	Same
Compulsive grooming	Grooming in excess of that required for grooming or exploring	Licking in excess of that required for grooming or exploring. Interferes with normal behaviour. Not aborted by interruption	Feather plucking
Depression	Prolonged endogenous or reactive withdrawal from social stimuli, changes in appetite, and changes in sleep/wake cycles not incidental or attributable solely to lethargy	Necessary criteria, accompanied by decreased motor activity and actual physical removal from normal social and environmental stimuli in the absence of any underlying neurological or physiological condition	Same
Dominance aggression	Abnormal, inappropriate, out-of-context aggression consistently exhibited under any circumstance involving passive or active control of the animal's behaviour or access to the behaviour	Intensification of any aggressive response from the animal with any passive or active correction or interruption of the behaviour	Same
Excessive grooming	Grooming by means of licking, scratching or rubbing that is unrelated to hygiene or maintenance and that is more frequent or intensive than previously exhibited	Interruptible (as opposed to compulsive grooming)	Feather plucking

17.5 Behavioural diagnoses in dogs and cats, and the avian equivalents (Overall, 1997). 'Necessary' criteria are those that must be present for the diagnosis to be made. 'Sufficient' criteria are those needed to distinguish a problem from all other conditions. (continues) ▶

Diagnosis	Necessary criteria	Sufficient criteria	Avian equivalent
Failure to groom	From a reduction to a lack of normal grooming behaviours	As for necessary criteria, without concomitant signs of depression	Failure to preen
Fear aggression	Aggression that consistently occurs with signs of fear as identified by withdrawal, passive and avoidance behaviours associated with sympathetic autonomic system	Aggression accompanied by urination/defecation or when aggression is only active or interactive when recipient disengages from behaviour	Same
Fear	Behaviour that occurs with withdrawal, passive and avoidance behaviours/sympathetic autonomic response without aggression	Behaviour that occurs with withdrawal, passive and avoidance behaviours/sympathetic autonomic response without aggression	Same
Generalized anxiety	Consistent exhibition of increased autonomic hyperreactivity, increased motor activity and increased vigilance and scanning that interfere with a normal range of behaviours	Necessary criteria in the absolute absence of provocational stimuli	Same
Neophobia	Consistent, sustained and extreme non-graded response to unfamiliar objects and circumstances; manifests as intense, active avoidance, escape or anxiety behaviours associated with sympathetic autonomic activity	Same; repeated exposure does not vary response	Same
Obsessive–compulsive disorder	Repetitive, stereotypic motor, locomotor, grooming, ingestive or hallucinogenic behaviours that occur out of context to their normal occurrence or in a frequency or duration that is in excess of that required to achieve a goal	As for necessary criteria, and interferes with the animal's ability otherwise to function normally in its social environment	Feather plucking
Possessive aggression	Aggression that is consistently directed toward another individual who approaches an object the aggressor wishes to control	Necessary criteria, but aggression does not occur in absence of object	Same
Protective aggression	Aggression that is consistently directed to a third party in the presence of a certain individual. Occurs in the absence of actual threat	Intensifies with proximity or signs of threat, despite correction or reassurance by person protected	Same
Psychogenic polydipsia	Water consumption in excess of physiological needs of animal	Excessive water consumption is altering time budget and interfering with normal activity	Same
Satyriasis	Excessive solicitation, mounting, thrusting, etc.	Necessary criteria, regardless of degree of provocation, directed interspecifically at animate or inanimate objects	Same
Self-mutilation	Removal of coat with abrasion, petechiation or ulceration to part of the body	Necessary criteria, in the absence of any physiological or dermatological conditions	Same
Separation anxiety	Presence of physical or behavioural signs of distress only in absence of owner	Presence of physical or behavioural signs of distress only in absence of owner	Same
Trichotillo-mania	Pulling out hair	Pulling out hair without injury to skin	Feather chewing
Territorial aggression	Aggression that occurs in a circumscribed area (car, home, cage)	Intensifies as recipient approaches, continues despite correction or attempts to interact	Same

17.5 (continued) Behavioural diagnoses in dogs and cats, and the avian equivalents (Overall, 1997). 'Necessary' criteria are those that must be present for the diagnosis to be made. 'Sufficient' criteria are those needed to distinguish a problem from all other conditions.

Behaviour modification

Behavioural modification requires commitment from the veterinary surgeon and the owner. As behavioural problems rarely stop suddenly, it is helpful to track results by asking owners to log the incidence of problem behaviour. A reduction in the frequency or severity can demonstrate that therapy is having an effect. Some general strategies used by the author for treating common behavioural disorders are given below.

Aggressive behaviour in pet birds

Psittacine aggression is one of the more serious behavioural problems. The strong jaws and hooked bill of a parrot can inflict serious pain and do substantial damage to the owner. Aggression in parrots takes the form of biting or lunging at the object of their aggression. Aggressive behaviour aetiologies in pet birds include: fear; dominance; territorial behaviour; and possessive behaviour (Welle, 1998). Diagnosis of any behavioural disorder is based on the behavioural history. Specifically, the signalment, a description of the environment and social interactions, and a description of the aggression, the circumstances in which it occurs and the owner's reaction to the behaviour are critical to the assessment of a biting bird (Welle, 1999). This should be augmented with observation of the interactions between bird and owner.

Fear biting

Fear is one of the most common motivators for biting. A bird that is frightened by people is simply trying to defend itself. There does not appear to be any age or sex predilection. Certain species are more likely to develop fear of people, despite the fact that they have been raised around them. Grey Parrots are well known for this problem.

Usually, these birds only bite when cornered or caught. They will not normally attack or chase someone. They may learn to attack rather than retreat when the cage door is opened, but they will generally try to get past the handler rather than defend the cage. They will usually not allow handling by anyone, but occasionally a bird will be fearful of a particular person, gender or physical characteristic.

The biting behaviour in this situation is a normal response. What is abnormal is the situation and this is what should be addressed. Treatment of this problem requires a lot of patience. Punishing a fear biter is counterproductive. Affected birds should be gradually desensitized to the presence of people. Desensitization is the process of reducing fear of a given object (or person) by controlled but increasing exposure to this object. Once the bird accepts human presence, careful taming and handling can begin. In extreme cases, drugs such as tricyclic antidepressants can be used to facilitate the early stages of treatment. It is important in these cases to consider the effect of the process of administering the treatments, however. Capturing a bird twice daily to administer medication can overshadow the benefit.

Dominance aggression

Dominance aggression is a controversial classification: the terms 'learned aggression' or 'conditioned aggression' could be used instead. The diagnosis should be applied to the owner–bird pair rather than just to the bird. Over time, the results of interactions between a bird and a handler will influence the behaviour of the bird during future interactions. Individuals will develop behaviour patterns with one another to avoid physical violence. Pet bird owners who have shown a lack of confidence in handling have given their bird an impression that threats and aggression will achieve their goal. Overt aggression will occur when the owner does not behave as expected by the bird.

Dominance aggression may occur in any species but is particularly common in Amazons and macaws. It occurs more often in mature birds than in juveniles. Male birds may be affected more commonly (but the gender of many birds is undetermined). Larger birds are more commonly affected, probably because they more easily evoke fearful responses in the handler. It seems to occur more commonly with birds belonging to people who have weak handling skills, or who have little experience with birds. Biting may occur whenever the bird feels that its authority is being challenged, such as when the owner tries to remove the bird from their shoulder, or put the bird in a cage, or remove the bird from the perch. Affected birds have often learned to manipulate the owner to their wishes. The owner's behaviour may be as useful for a diagnosis as the bird's behaviour. People will often make excuses for the bird's behaviour, take extraordinary measures to prevent upsetting the bird, or otherwise defer to the tantrums of the bird. These birds almost invariably have been removed from the carrier and are sitting on the shoulder of the owner when the clinician enters the room.

Dominant aggressive birds have been patterned to use aggressive behaviour to control the behaviour of their owners, who have been patterned to comply. Both owner and bird may be resistant to changing the situation. After years of being bitten, the owner will be hesitant to be assertive with the biting bird. The bird will initially be confused and will try to re-establish control. Aggression may get worse before it gets better. This type of aggression is similar in some ways to canine dominance aggression, as the bird uses aggressive behaviour to control its interactions with the handler. A major difference, however, is that the aggression in parrots may be severe towards one person and absent towards others. It is the relationship that is abnormal, not the parrot. In some cases, the bird will benefit from placement in a home with a more confident handler.

The wings should be clipped to give the bird one less weapon for controlling situations. The bird should be put in a cage low enough for ease of handling. Macaws sometimes present a problem because their cages are often very tall. Clients of small stature may have difficulty reaching the bird, making the problem more difficult. All handling should take place in neutral territory. If there are any household members who can safely handle the bird, they should bring the bird to the neutral area. If no one can safely handle the bird, the diagnosis should be re-evaluated. Once in a neutral site, out of sight of the cage, step-up exercises should be practised. If the owner cannot keep their hand in front of the bird without withdrawing from its beak, a perch should be used.

The shoulders should be considered off-limits. This can be challenging in its own right if the bird is accustomed to riding on the owner's shoulders. Hand position should be higher than the elbow so the bird does not just climb up on to the shoulder (Figure 17.6). If the

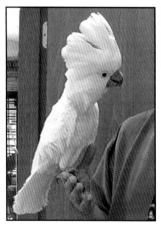

17.6 The position of the hand should be higher than the elbow, to prevent the bird from climbing up the arm.

bird jumps to the shoulder, its feet should be restrained by holding its toes with the thumb. Placing a towel or other object on the shoulder may discourage the bird from jumping on to the shoulder.

When bites occur, the bird should be repetitively stepped up from hand to hand – a process known as 'laddering' (Wilson, 1999). This both provides a reprimand and establishes control. Verbal praise should be given once the bird is stepping willingly. The beak should not be grabbed or struck, as this can escalate the aggression. Birds should never be hit. Shouting or other types of drama can actually be entertaining for some birds, so the victim should always remain calm. The very effectiveness of the bite is what reinforces the behaviour. A slight jerk of the support hand to induce a minor loss of balance, a technique known as an 'earthquake', can be used if the bird is on the hand when the bite occurs.

Drug therapy is not generally required for the treatment of dominance aggression. Prognosis is fair for the bird but guarded for the relationship between the owner and bird.

Territorial aggression

Territorial aggression is particularly common in certain species. Quaker Parakeets are well known for this trait. Conures, dwarf macaws, Grey Parrots and Amazons are also prone to develop this problem. Breeding birds of all species tend to be territorial about their nest area and cage, and this behaviour is considered desirable in these birds. Guarding of the nest territory is an important breeding cue. While the sex of many avian patients is unknown, it appears that territorial aggression is somewhat more common in males than in females.

Diagnostic criteria for territorial aggression are very simple. A necessary criterion is that the aggressive behaviour must occur when the bird is in or on its cage, playpen or other living area (Overall, 1997). If this is not the case, the aggression cannot be territorial aggression. Sufficient criteria are that the aggressive behaviour must be limited to these areas. If the bird exhibits aggression in other circumstances, a definite diagnosis cannot be determined.

Behaviour modification for territorial aggression is multifaceted. In order to achieve the specific goals, general training is essential. The step-up command is an important training tool and obeying it should be automatic for the bird. To avoid injury to the owner, the bird should be removed while servicing the cage. Owners should be schooled on atraumatic but secure towel restraint of the bird if necessary (see Figure 17.1 and Chapter 4). Birds that will not leave the cage without biting should be caught and carried to a separate area. Some birds can be safely handled following voluntary exit from the cage. This will facilitate the other training measures.

Corrections can be given when bites occur but many of the appropriate reprimands will not be applicable. Repeated step-ups can be used, but only if the bird can be brought out of the cage within a few seconds of the bite. Towel restraint can be a useful method of gaining control, especially with smaller birds. Verbal

reprimands can be effective as long as they are stern but calm. Dramatic responses like shouting can be entertaining to birds and should be avoided. Striking the bird and beak grabbing are unacceptable corrections. They further excite the bird, induce fear, and can potentially injure the bird.

An attempt should be made to make the bird less dependent on the cage. This helps in both the prevention and the treatment of territorial aggression. Birds that spend most or all of their time in one cage can become viciously aggressive about defending it (Athan, 1993). In the wild, birds roost in the same area each night. During the day, they travel to other locations to forage, usually with their flock. A two-cage housing set-up helps provide a more natural system. A large, well furnished cage or playpen should be used during the daytime to encourage activity. The cage should be rearranged frequently to promote adaptability in the bird. During the night, a smaller roosting cage with rather sparse accommodation should be used. Each morning the bird can be transported to the larger cage and each evening to the roosting cage. If further measures are needed, the bird can be fed twice daily in another location.

The bird should be integrated into the family social unit. Portable perching stations allow the bird to sit close to the activity of the family. This, combined with consistent handling and training, provides the bird with the social skills needed to be a well adjusted pet. Regularly scheduled handling and training sessions are important for maintaining this socialization. The two-cage housing system described above forces owners to handle birds at least twice daily to transport them.

Psychotropic drugs are not generally indicated in the treatment of territorial aggression in birds. The prognosis for treatment of territorial aggression with behavioural modification alone is favourable.

Possessive aggression

Parrots are prone to developing unhealthy pair bonds with one of their owners. While a bird may bond to more than one person, only one is chosen for a 'mate'. However, if the chosen 'mate' is the only one who ever handles the bird, the aggressive tendencies will be much worse. Also, aggression will be worse if the bird does not respect this person. Possessive aggression occurs most commonly in hand-reared birds of larger parrot species. Amazons, macaws, cockatoos and Quaker Parakeets are all commonly affected. Male birds are most often affected. The behaviour often begins, or becomes more serious, at sexual maturity or during the breeding season.

The aggression will occur in situations where the bird's favourite person is approached by someone else, especially a spouse. The aggression may be directed toward the rival or, paradoxically, displaced toward the favourite person. Occasionally, the aggression may be triggered by an inanimate object such as a telephone. Unlike most other types of aggression, possessive birds will often attack or chase their victims. They are often exceptionally cuddly at other times, at least toward the favourite person.

To help to minimize possessive aggression, the bird should be socialized appropriately. The person to whom the bird has pair-bonded should work to develop a more platonic bond. Interactions should be more active and dynamic, avoiding cuddling and petting. The bird should not be allowed on the shoulder, as this position encourages pair-bonding. All members of the household should take the bird to novel unfamiliar places so that they can be seen by the bird as the familiar comforting figure.

These attacks often involve the face of the victim. The attacking bird should be gently captured in a towel and placed in the cage or other controlled area. Owners should be taught to towel-restrain these birds safely and effectively (see Figure 17.1). While restrained, the bird can be verbally reprimanded in a stern but calm voice. Minor bites on the hand can be dealt with by 'laddering' the bird.

In some cases, the aggressive behaviour can be reduced with hormonal therapy. Leuprolide acetate can reduce the sexual hormones and thereby reduce the intensity of the aggression during the initial phases of behaviour modification. Orchidectomy can reduce aggression in some cases (Bennett, 2002) (Chapter 10).

Nuisance vocalization

Screaming, or excessive vocalization, is another common complaint from parrot owners. It may be responsible for more parrots losing their home than any other problem. Normal vocalizations of some parrots can be quite loud and annoying, but these are not truly a behaviour problem. Attempting to suppress normal vocalizations can be harmful to a bird's psyche.

A normal bird does not constantly squawk. There is usually some 'singing' in the morning and evening and occasionally during the day. Most birds do not vocalize after dark. The most common causes of problem vocalization are attention seeking and flock-cohesion. Parrots quickly learn that making noise will cause owners to yell at them, feed them, squirt them, throw shoes at their cage and so on. If the bird is bored or lonely, these responses are better than nothing. Birds that are seeking attention will vocalize whenever they detect people around and they are not getting attention. This will occur even when the owner is within visual range of the bird. Common advice given for this type of vocalization is to ignore the bird, thereby removing any reinforcement. This process of eliminating a behaviour by removing reinforcement is known as extinction, but it requires prolonged periods of time to accomplish. The vocalizations will become increasingly frantic until some form of reinforcement arrives. Since reinforcement may occur coincidentally at times, the process is very difficult.

Counterconditioning may be a more effective means of controlling this behaviour. A behaviour that is incompatible with loud vocalization, such as whispering, is taught to the bird. Whenever the parrot begins to vocalize loudly, the owner should start whispering without paying particular attention to the bird. When the bird quietens down to hear the owner, the owner turns to pay attention to the bird and encourage whispering. Once the bird makes a low, quiet sound, lavish praise is given. The parrot thus learns a more effective way to get the attention that it craves.

Wild parrots vocalize to maintain flock cohesion. It is important to know where other members of the flock are, for safety reasons. The bird may be reassured if the owner calls softly to the bird if they are out of sight, or carries the bird with them on a portable perch as they move around the house. Many 'attention seekers' may simply be checking on the whereabouts of family members. These birds generally will vocalize when the owners are out of sight. Owners of these birds can take the initiative by 'calling' to the bird by whistling, humming, singing or talking as they move about the house. Even better would be for multiple stations to be placed about the house, allowing the bird to maintain visual contact.

Exaggerated fear

It is natural for animals to fear new and strange things. This is especially true for pet birds, which are naturally a prey species. Fear and panic are usually easily recognized. A fearful bird will generally recoil from the source of its fear. It is often hanging on the back of the cage. If uncaged, the bird may fly, glide or run away. Mild mistrust may be exhibited by the bird constantly watching people. A fearful bird may bite, but generally only if cornered. It generally prefers to flee.

As with any other problem, prevention is far more effective than treatment. Young birds that are exposed to as many things as possible learn how to accept change. Birds that never go anywhere or never see anything new become very suspicious when they do (Voith and Borchelt, 1985). Those that are more 'worldly' accept new things more readily. While prevention is easier, an established fear can be alleviated by slowly and gradually exposing the bird to the source of its fear in a non-threatening setting. Increasing tolerance of the feared item, person or place will eventually be noticeable. This process, known as habituation, can sometimes be facilitated by the use of anxiolytic drugs (Overall, 1997).

The cage of an excessively fearful bird can be elevated so that the bird is above head level. This imparts a feeling of security to the bird. This technique is commonly used in aviculture, where the security and confidence of the birds is critical.

Feather plucking

Feather plucking is one of the most common presenting complaints in avian practice. It is a highly complex clinical sign and has many potential aetiologies. Often the problem is multifactorial, with both medical and behavioural components. It can frustrate both the owner and the clinician. A systematic approach to the diagnosis and treatment of this complex of disorders provides the best hope of resolution (Hillyer *et al.*, 1989; Oppenheimer, 1991). While many cases will still not resolve, a full assessment at least ensures that the feather-plucking bird is healthy and in an appropriate physical and social environment.

Diagnosis

There must be two phases of diagnosis. The first is to determine whether feather plucking is indeed occurring. While this is often obvious, occasionally owners are unfamiliar with the extensive amount of time spent on preening in normal birds and may think that the bird is plucking. Sometimes owners will see the normal apteria when the bird is wet and mistake them for abnormal featherless areas. The most common body sites for feather plucking are the chest, under the wings and on the rump. The least common are the flight feathers. Feather plucking should be suspected in birds with lesion distributions that exclude the head. The head feathers are spared unless the bird (especially a Budgerigar) has learned to rub the head on the cage or other object. The lost feathers will usually exhibit some damage from the beak. Some birds will pluck feathers out; others will chew the feathers in half or chew the barbs off of the shaft.

The next phase of diagnosis involves the determination of the aetiology or aetiologies of the feather plucking. This is the most difficult part. There are many causes of feather plucking. It may be caused by medical problems and a thorough medical workup is indicated (Chapter 16). Figure 17.7 lists some possible behavioural causes of feather plucking.

Behavioural or psychological feather plucking is not a single disease state but a complex of several conditions leading to the same clinical signs. This may explain why most treatment protocols have a low rate of success. Some birds may have overlapping behavioural disorders. If these birds could be accurately diagnosed and treated in a more specific manner, success rates would be higher. Currently no methods of psychological testing in birds are available, leaving the clinician with detailed histories and trial and error as methods of determining how a patient will respond. There are certain tendencies among species. For instance, Grey Parrots appear to have a high incidence of stress-associated feather plucking, cockatoos often have problems associated with inappropriate sexual imprinting, and some macaws appear to have true pruritus. Clients should be warned that many birds will never stop feather plucking. Several treatments may be given in succession until an effective solution is found.

Features	Likely diagnoses	Contributing factors	Recommendations	Drug therapy
Occurs when owner not present	Separation anxiety Boredom	Endorphins Habit	Before leaving: bathing; exercise; meal feed; special toy; encourage independent play	Clomipramine (but drugs not always effective on their own)
Occurs when owner present but not paying attention	Attention-seeking behaviour	Owner's behaviour (drama, attention) Endorphins Habit	Leave room when picking is seen Encourage independent play Reward good behaviour with attention	None
Bird interrupts other behaviour to pluck, not easily distracted from plucking	Obsessive–compulsive disorder True pruritus	Endorphins Owner's behaviour (drama, attention) Habit	Medical work-up Improve social setting Remove feared objects Habituate Encourage independent play Leave room when picking is seen	Tricyclic antidepressants Haloperidol Naltrexone
Bird exhibits signs of excess fear or stress Systemic illness Major change in household	Stress-associated problem	Poor health Endorphins Owner's behaviour (Avoidance) Habit	Medical work-up Remove feared objects Habituate to source of fear Raise the cage Behaviour classes for owner/bird	Tricyclic antidepressants Haloperidol Butorphanol Naltrexone
Problem starts at an extremely young age; hand-fed bird	Genetic Improper preening Poor early socialization	Endorphins Owner's behaviour (drama, attention) Habit	Improve social setting Behaviour classes for owner/bird Leave room when picking is seen	Haloperidol Naltrexone
Involves primarily remiges and retrices Feathers frayed and splintered	Iatrogenic Improper wing trim Feather trauma	Endorphins Owner's behaviour (drama, attention) Habit	Change environment to minimize trauma Feather imping Remove damaged feathers under anaesthesia	Butorphanol NSAIDs
Overly bonded, sexually mature bird Sexual behaviours occur out of context	Reproductive related	Owner's behaviour (drama, attention) Habit Endorphins	Avoid sexually stimulating Limit day length Remove nest-type structures Limit high-calorie and high-moisture foods	Leuprolide acetate, HCG Progestins

17.7 Behavioural causes of feather plucking.

Treatment

Behavioural modification, aimed at removing the initiating cause and redirecting the bird's attention towards more appropriate behaviour, is often the first treatment attempted. Behavioural supportive care should first be provided by improving the physical and social environment of the bird. The cage, its location, the availability of appropriate toys, proper stimuli and cleanliness are all critical to the physical environment. It is important that the bird is socialized well but not overstimulated with a lot of physical contact. Appropriate beak activity such as shredding toys should be encouraged so that it can be used in counterconditioning to an alternative beak activity. Foraging activities especially should be encouraged (Meehan *et al.*, 2003). Foraging behaviours include mixing non-edible materials with the food to force the bird to sort particles, feeding in deep particulate litters (there may be some hygiene concerns here) or the use of simple puzzle toys with food rewards. Bathing should be increased, to encourage normal preening. Several weeks should be given for these changes to be effective. Restraint collars can be used to prevent feather plucking but are only a temporary solution and are usually reserved for those birds that are mutilating skin or muscle. When necessary, pharmaceutical treatments may be added.

Prognosis

With such a complex multifactorial disorder, sudden resolution is uncommon. When success is achieved, it becomes apparent in gradual attenuation of the plucking, followed by the gradual replacement of damaged or lost feathers. As such, owners and clinicians may not note the improvement without good record keeping. Each treatment plan should be followed for a minimum of 8 weeks. Owner observations on the frequency of plucking and visual changes in the plumage should be recorded. Preferably, photographs should be taken regularly so that regrowth can be assessed objectively.

Self-mutilation

Self-mutilation is a more exaggerated problem than feather plucking. In this instance, the bird actually damages the skin itself. The approach to this problem is similar to the approach to feather plucking with a few exceptions:

- A higher percentage of these birds will show physical disease, either as a causative factor or as a secondary consequence. More attention should be paid to assessing the integument (Chapter 16)
- This condition is more painful and has more serious health consequences. Pain management, antimicrobial therapy and wound management should all be included in the treatment plan
- These birds usually require restraint collars or bandages to prevent further trauma.

Behavioural pharmacology

In some cases, behaviour modification can be facilitated by the use of behavioural drugs. There are many drugs that exert an effect upon the behaviour of a patient. Some are used primarily for other purposes; some have been developed exclusively for their behavioural effects. Behavioural drugs exert their effect by enhancing or inhibiting the effects of certain neurotransmitters. Neurotransmitters affected by behavioural drugs include acetylcholine, catecholamines, serotonin, dopamine, gamma-aminobutyric acid (GABA), excitatory amino acids and androgens. Catecholamines, dopamine, androgens and certain amino acids tend to be excitatory, while serotonin and GABA are more inhibitory. This is, of course, an oversimplification, as each neurotransmitter can have different effects depending on the synapse involved. However, it makes it easier to understand the activity of these drugs. Some drugs are non-specific in their effects on these neurotransmitters, others are very specific. More specific drugs require that a more specific diagnosis be made. Efficacy of the drug can then lend credence to the diagnosis.

There are several classes of drugs used for behaviour therapy. Most work by enhancing serotonin or GABA activity, or inhibiting dopamine activity. Tranquillizers are used for a variety of behavioural disorders but they are not recommended for long-term use.

- *Benzodiazepines* such as diazepam function as dopamine inhibitors and GABA potentiators. They have some central sedative effects. They have a muscle-relaxing action and can cause some motor impairment. They have been successfully used for inter-cat aggression, spraying and noise phobias. These drugs can interfere with learning ability, making training less effective (Overall, 1997).
- *Butyrophenones* include the drug haloperidol. Drugs in this class inhibit dopamine. While not generally used for canine and feline behaviour problems, haloperidol has been used in birds for both self-mutilation and feather plucking (Lennox and Van Der Heyden, 1993); the study was very small but therapy was effective in most cases of self-mutilation, though less effective for feather plucking. Success was best for feather plucking in cockatoos, suggesting differing aetiologies in various species. Side effects included depression, decreased appetite, agitation and excitability.
- *Antihistamines* such as diphenhydramine and hydroxyzine act by inhibition of histamine receptors. The side effect of mild sedation may account for any behavioural benefit (Overall, 1997). Diphenhydramine is sometimes recommended for use in feather pickers but clinically appears to have very limited success (Johnson-Delaney, 1992).
- *Anticonvulsants* such as phenobarbital potentiate GABA. They are rarely effective for behavioural disorders, though the author had one feather-plucking Red-lored Amazon that also began to have seizures: when phenobarbital was started, both the seizures and the feather plucking ceased.

- *Progestogens* (including medroxyprogesterone acetate) potentiate GABA, have a non-specific calming effect and have some anti-inflammatory properties. Medroxyprogesterone acetate has proven effective, in both injectable and silicone implant forms, for the treatment of feather plucking in birds (Harrison, 1989; Hillyer *et al.*, 1989). The side effects, including obesity, liver degeneration and diabetes mellitus, are frequent enough that long-term usage of this drug is not recommended. Leuprolide acetate, a GnRH agonist, has been used to inhibit reproductive hormones and behaviour as well. While it appears clinically effective in many cases, dosing and frequency are currently determined empirically.
- *Tricyclic antidepressants* (TCAs) have the major effects of sedation, anticholinergic activity, and potentiating serotonin by inhibiting re-uptake. The net effect is the alleviation of anxiety and depression. These drugs are also potent antihistamines, making them potentially useful for pruritic disorders. Amitriptyline, doxepin and clomipramine are all examples of this group. Both doxepin and clomipramine have been discussed for use in feather plucking in birds (Johnson, 1987; Ramsay and Grindlinger, 1992). Although they were effective in only a small proportion of cases, no differentiation between behavioural aetiologies was made. The combination of these drugs with behavioural modification may improve efficacy. Side effects of tricyclic antidepressants are the result of anticholinergic responses. They include dry mouth, constipation, urinary retention and potentially arrhythmias. Patients should receive a baseline ECG prior to treatment and periodically during treatment to assess for arrhythmias.
- *Serotonin-specific re-uptake inhibitors* such as fluoxetine have the serotonergic effects without the anticholinergic or antihistaminic activity. Fluoxetine has been used clinically for feather plucking with mixed results (Bauck, 1997).
- *Narcotic agonists and antagonists* act at the opiate receptors in the brain. They can block endorphine responses that may reinforce self-injurious behaviours. Naltrexone was effective in deterring feather plucking in 26 of 41 cases in one study (Turner, 1993). Collars were used in this study, making it impossible to assess the efficacy of the drug critically.

In order to maximize success, the same principles apply as in treatment of other medical disorders. A treatment plan is proposed, including any behavioural modification or drugs indicated by the problem. If the initial treatment plan does not resolve the problem, an alternative plan is formulated and tried. Each treatment plan should be given 6–8 weeks to work. Figure 17.8 lists some drugs that have been used to treat behavioural disorders in birds.

Drug	Oral dosage	Primary effect	Indications	Side effects
Clomipramine	0.5–1.0 mg/kg q24h or q8h	Serotonergic Antidepressant Anxiolytic Antihistamine	Feather plucking Anxiety Fear Phobia	Regurgigation Transient ataxia Drowsiness Arrhythmias
Diazepam	0.5 mg/kg q12h or q8h	Tranquillizer Anticonvulsant	Excessive fear or phobia	Sedation Long-term liver damage
Diphenhydramine	2–4 mg/kg q12h	Antihistamine Sedation	Pruritus Irritation	Drowsiness
Doxepin	0.5–1.0 mg/kg q12h	Serotonergic Antidepressant Anxiolytic Antihistamine	Feather plucking Anxiety Fear Phobia	Regurgitation Drowsiness Arrhythmias
Fluoxetine	1 mg/kg q24h	Serotonergic	Feather plucking	None reported
Haloperidol	0.15–0.2 mg/kg q12h	Tranquillizer	Self-mutilation	Anorexia Depression Excitability Agitation
Leuprolide acetate	0.25–0.75 mg/kg monthly	Suppresses reproductive hormones	Feather plucking Aggression	None reported
Medroxyprogesterone acetate	5–25 mg/kg every 4–6 weeks	Suppresses sexual activity Calming Anti-inflammatory	Feather plucking Aggression Egg laying	Obesity Diabetes mellitus Liver damage
Naltrexone	1.5 mg/kg q12h	Narcotic antagonist	Feather plucking Self-mutilation	None reported
Phenobarbital	3.5–7 mg/kg q12h	Anticonvulsant	Feather plucking associated with seizures	Sedation Long-term liver damage

17.8 Drugs used for behavioural problems.

Addendum: Example of a history-taking form, as used by the author.

Owner		Bird's name	
Address		Species	
Phone		Age	
Work		Sex	
FAX		Determined	
Email		Color	

Please check which of the options below that you would prefer.

	I would like to proceed with the behavior consultation and I agree to the fee of _____.
	I do not wish to proceed with the consultation but retain this for my bird's medical record.

Medical and Grooming Information

My bird: *has*		*has not*		been examined by my veterinarian in the past 6 months.
My bird: *has*		*has not*		been examined by my veterinarian for this problem.

Have your veterinarian send a copy of your bird's medical record if he/she is not one of our patients.

My bird's wings are: *fully flighted*		*clipped*		

First wing trim was done: *before weaned*		*after weaned*		*when mature*

Wing trim style:

Wing trim is:		*one side*		*both sides*

Bird Source

I got my bird from : *a pet store*		*a breeder*		*a show*		*shipped*
My bird was: *wild caught*		*domestic parent raised*		*hand raised*		

When I took my bird home, he/she was:

still being hand fed		*just weaned*	
weaned a while but sexually immature		*sexually mature*	

If you hand fed this bird, did you:

allow to wean on his/her own		*force weaning*	
continue hand feeding beyond 6 months of age			

Other than the breeder or pet store, my bird has had:	*0*		*1*		*2*		*several*		previous owners.

Prior to bringing my bird home I: *never*		*occasionally*		*frequently*		visited him/her.

Environment

Describe the bird's cage. Give brand name, size, etc. _____

List all furnishings and contents of the cage _____

How many hours per day does your bird spend in the cage? _____

Describe other areas where your bird spends time. _____

How much time is spent here? _____

List toys your bird has access to. _____

Draw a map of your house and put in the bird's cage, play area, as well as areas where family members spend time.

Sit or stand at bird height in the location of the cage. Describe everything you see and hear in all directions, including up and down. If you can photograph or video record this, much more information can be determined. _____

_____

How many hours per day is your bird alone? _____

What sights, sounds, and other stimuli are available to your bird while you are gone? _____

_____

When are the lights in the bird's area turned off at night? _____

When does light first come in the morning? _____

Would you consider the light intensity: *bright* ☐   *dim* ☐   or *moderate* ☐

What types of lights are used in the area where the bird is kept? _____

Describe your bird's diet in detail. Give brands of pellets. Describe your bird's preferences. _____

_____

What is your bird's feeding schedule? _____

_____

What are your bird's favorite treats? _____

_____

Are there any smokers in the household? _____

Do they smoke around the bird? _____

Are there any other sources of odors or fumes in the household? _____

_____

How often and in what way is your bird bathed? _____

_____

Do you dry the bird following a bath? How? _____

_____

Your Bird's Flock

List all human members of the household. _____

_____

List all of the animal members of the household. _____

_____

List the ages of children within the household _____

_____

Who does the primary maintenance of the bird? _____

Who spends the most time with the bird? _____

Who does the bird appear to prefer? _____

Who does the bird appear to dislike? _____

Bird's Behavior

Would you say that your bird steps on your hand: *easily* ☐   *hesitantly* ☐   *rarely* ☐

Is your bird allowed on your shoulder: *often* ☐   *occasionally* ☐   *rarely* ☐   *never* ☐

How does your bird greet you when you come home? _____

_____

How does your bird greet other family members? _____

_____

Describe your bird's play behavior. _____

_____

Does your bird talk?   *Yes* ☐   *No* ☐

Vocabulary: *<10 words* ☐   *10-30 words* ☐   *>30 words* ☐

Does your bird use words appropriately?   *Yes* ☐   *No* ☐

Does your bird like to be petted: *on the head* ☐   *on the back* ☐   *over the tail* ☐   *under wings* ☐   *other* ☐

When out of the cage, is your bird in physical contact with someone:

constantly ☐   *intermittently* ☐   *rarely* ☐   *never* ☐

How well does your bird tolerate restraint?

doesn't mind at all ☐   *doesn't like it but tolerates it* ☐   *gets very stressed* ☐

How does your bird respond to the following situations:

	anxiety	fear	calm	happy	excited	aggressive	can't tell
Favorite approaching:							
Other approaching:							
Stranger approaching:							
Favorite opens cage:							
Other opens cage:							
Stranger opens cage:							
Favorite hand in cage:							
Other hand in cage:							
Stranger hand in cage:							
Favorite step-up:							
Other step-up:							
Stranger step-up:							
Favorite petting/touching:							
Other petting/touching:							
Stranger petting/touching:							
Favorite hands food:							
Other hands food:							
Stranger hands food:							
Other approaching favorite:							
Favorite approaching other:							
Stranger approaching favorite:							
Favorite approaching stranger:							
Stranger approaching other:							
Other approaching stranger:							
Favorite to other transfer:							
Other to favorite transfer:							
Favorite to stranger transfer:							
Stranger to favorite transfer:							
Other animal approaches:							
Favorite out of vision:							
Other out of vision:							
Loud noises:							
New objects out of cage:							
New object in cage:							
Strange places:							

Which behavior problems does your bird exhibit? Check all that apply.

Biting		Screaming		Feather plucking/ chewing		Self mutilation		Irrational fears	
Other		Describe							

Specifically describe the situations in which these behaviors occur. _____

Describe what you do when these behaviors occur. _____

For feather plucking, chewing, or self mutilation, answer these questions.

What parts of the body are affected? _____

Are feathers pulled or damaged: (Check all that apply)

when they first appear? ☐ *when they start to open up?* ☐ *when they are mature?* ☐

when you're not home? ☐ *when you're not paying attention?* ☐ *when you're paying attention?* ☐

Does behavior interrupt:

playing? ☐ *eating?* ☐ *other activities?* ☐

This behavior can be interrupted by:

attention? ☐ *reprimand?* ☐ *food?* ☐

When this behavior occurs:

bird acts like it hurts? ☐ *bird acts like it itches?* ☐ *bird acts like it doesn't bother him/her?* ☐

18

Reproduction and paediatrics

April Romagnano

Sex determination

Psittacine birds are predominantly sexually monomorphic. This means that to humans the male and female are visually indistinguishable from each other. Although a few general characteristics may help a guess at the bird's sex, these are only indicators that are often incapable of accurate gender determination. They include the size of the head and beak, overall size of the bird, iris colour, feather colour and aggressive behaviour.

Since the first requirement for successful captive breeding is heterosexual or true pairs, gender determination is important. Accurate sex differentiation is also important because 'sexing' is a veterinary service, and the avian practitioner is making a diagnosis. Various options are available; the practitioner can choose the method most suitable to the patient, the client, and the veterinary surgeon (Figure 18.1).

Cytogenetics can be used to evaluate the complete karyotype of a bird. As well as gender, cytogenetics can identify chromosomal defects. Cytogenetic defects of parrots include chromosomal inversions, chromosome translocations, triploidy and ZZ ZW chimaerism; these reduce fertility significantly.

Method	Comments	Advantages	Disadvantages
Visual	Only suitable for a few adult dimorphic species (Figures 18.2 and 18.3). May become more useful when technology allows viewing in ultraviolet range where many more species are dimorphic	Easy	Limited application
Physical characteristics	E.g. vent sexing in Vasa Parrots and (possibly) lovebird species. Width between pubic bones in smaller psittacine species	Non-invasive	Requires experience, applicable to a limited number of species, some results questionable
Surgical	Endoscopic sexing via left lateral approach (Chapter 9) developed in 1970s	Instant results so enables ringing and certification. Provides information about other body organs as well as physical characteristics of gonads, i.e. may give more information on possible infertility problems as well as gender determination. Applicable to all species, immature and mature	Anaesthetic risks. Invasive; risk of damage and infection, though these should be minimal with experience and good sterile technique. Newly weaned birds of some species (e.g. macaws) may have undifferentiated gonads. Expensive equipment and requires some degree of experience
DNA (feather)	Modern DNA sexing relies on identification of products from W chromosome of heterozygous female, i.e. birds sexed as 'female' and 'non-female' (i.e. male)	Easy. Non-invasive. Can be done from an early age	Need to collect sufficient DNA; test is done on cells attached to freshly plucked feather, *not* feather itself, therefore not appropriate to use moulted feathers and several should be sent. Inappropriate to issue sexing certificate unless bird is closed ringed and feather personally collected. Contamination: not appropriate technique if birds housed together as scale from female birds may alter result of male bird; seen in about 4% of samples; reverse not seen due to the testing method. Results take over a week. No information re fertility
DNA (blood)	Relies on identifying female chromosome	Relatively non-invasive, requires whole blood. Can be done from hatching by clipping a toenail or from a blood vessel inside the eggshell	Human error main source of inaccuracy. Identifying individuals can be difficult if birds too young to ring or Indentichip

18.1 Methods of sex determination.

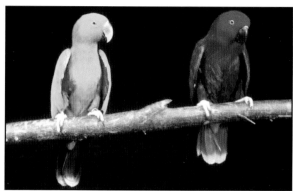

18.2 Eclectus Parrot. The male (left) is green; the female (right) is vibrant red and purple.

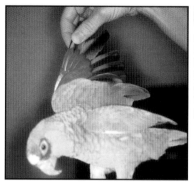

18.3 White-fronted Amazon. The male has red feathers on upper wing coverts, edge of the carpus and alula. In females these are green.

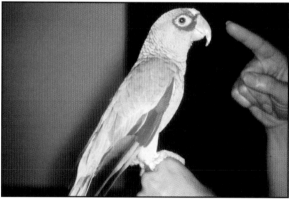

Reproductive disease

Females

Obstetrical problems have many causes, and prognosis varies according to cause. The avian clinician must obtain a thorough general and reproductive history and perform a physical examination. The decision on whether to proceed with diagnostic tests, or to commence emergency supportive treatment immediately, is made on a case-by-case basis.

A blood sample (complete blood count, electrophoresis and biochemistries), cloacal culture, radiography, endoscopy and ultrasonography are important diagnostic tools.

Egg binding and dystocia

- Egg binding is the failure of an egg to pass through the oviduct at a normal rate (delayed oviposition). The typical laying interval is 48 hours.

- Dystocia is the mechanical obstruction of an egg in the caudal reproductive tract. It can occur at the level of the caudal oviduct/uterus, the vagina, or the vaginal–cloacal junction. Obstruction can result in cloacal impaction and/or prolapse.

Causes of egg binding include: hypocalcaemia and other nutritional deficiencies; dysfunction of oviduct, uterus or vaginal muscle; excessive egg production; large, misshapen or soft-shelled egg(s); age of hen; obesity; oviduct tumour; oviduct infection; lack of exercise; hyper- or hypothermia; breeding out of season; first-time layer; hen afflicted with persistent cystic right oviduct; lipoma; abdominal wall herniation; genetics; or hen not given an appropriate nesting place.

Life-threatening circulatory disorders, shock and nerve paralysis can occur during dystocia. These occur secondary to compression of pelvic and renal vasculature and nerves. Cessation of normal defecation and urination can lead to severe metabolic disturbances, including gastrointestinal ileus and obstructive renal disease. Pressure necrosis of the oviduct results in oviduct rupture.

Clinical signs: The clinical signs of dystocia and egg binding vary with size. Smaller species such as Budgerigars, Cockatiels and lovebirds are more commonly affected by dystocia. Limited reserves, high-energy requirements and compact anatomy warrant more aggressive therapy in small versus large species. Usually the egg-bound bird is depressed, lethargic, quiet and tachypnoeic. It has a wide non-perching stance and may have uni- or bilateral paresis/paralysis. The abdomen and cloaca are usually 'doughy' and swollen; an egg may be palpable. Tail wagging, straining, decreased defecation frequency, increased defecation volume or dyspnoea, as well as nesting behaviour, may be seen. In cases of severe dystocia, the bird's feet may become 'blue-white', indicating vascular compromise and warranting immediate intervention.

Stabilization: Following physical examination, patient stabilization is critical. Ideally fluids (saline or lactated Ringer's solution) should be given subcutaneously (Chapter 6), but initially supplementation with an intravenous bolus may be needed. Placement of a jugular or metatarsal vein intravenous catheter, or an intraosseous catheter, should be reserved for cases of severe dehydration (Chapter 6). Subcutaneous 10% calcium borogluconate should be given in all situations (Figure 18.4). The patient should be placed in a warm, humid and steam-filled oxygenated incubator. The incubator should be covered and the bird should be kept quiet.

Diagnosis: Depending on the condition of the patient, a radiograph, complete blood count (CBC) and biochemistry may be warranted. Hypocalcaemia, a frequent cause of egg binding, occurs secondary to either low-calcium diets (especially those high in fat) or aberrant calcium metabolism (Figure 18.4). A cloacal culture and sensitivity should be performed and parenteral antibiotics initiated. If present, prolapsed tissues should be cleaned with warm sterile saline and coated with sterile lubricant. If no tissues are prolapsed and abdominal palpation does not reveal an egg, radiography and or ultrasonography should be performed. Radiography should show medullary bone in most long bones (Chapter 2) (Figure 18.4). Well developed medullary bone suggests adequate calcium reserves for egg production. Ultrasonography is useful for the diagnosis of impacted soft-shelled eggs, ectopic soft-shelled or shell-less eggs, and salpingitis, as well as to differentiate oviduct masses from other caudal abdominal masses.

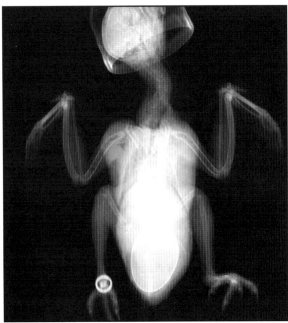

18.4 Radiograph of an unwell egg-bound conure showing a normal-sized egg surrounded by shell. The medullary bone has been used from the long bones (compare with Figure 2.8) to produce the shell, making hypocalcaemia the most likely aetiology. Note also the displacement of the bird's viscera, reducing the size of its air sacs. The bird was given calcium supplementation and the egg was laid within half an hour. The egg had a thinner shell than normal and lacked a cuticle.

Therapy: The author's preferred treatment is to use the supportive care described above and minimal surgical intervention described below. However, the following hormonal treatments are available.

Prostaglandin E_2 and E_1 (PGE$_2$ and PGE$_1$) are known to relax the uterovaginal sphincter and increase uterine contraction. PGE$_2$ gel (0.1 cc/100 g body weight) and PGE$_1$ liquid are recommended topically, applied to the uterovaginal sphincter. If the uterus is intact and free of disease or neoplasia, and the egg is not adhered to the oviduct, then the contractions produced by PGE$_2$ gel are forceful enough to expel an egg safely within 15 minutes of application. Prostaglandin $F_{2\alpha}$ is dangerous when compared with PGE$_2$. It is not the prostaglandin of choice in birds as it elicits generalized smooth muscle contractions and does not specifically relax the uterovaginal sphincter.

Oxytocin has been recommended to stimulate the oviduct but it is not produced in birds and, when given parenterally, it produces profound cardiovascular effects in addition to generalized, very painful but ineffective, smooth muscle contractions.

If oviposition has not occurred within 2–14 hours of treatment, one of two non-surgical techniques should be tried. With the bird under anaesthesia, the cloaca is lubricated with intracloacal sterile KY Jelly and the vagina is gently dilated with a fine pair of haemostats. The egg is palpated through the abdominal wall, fingers are placed above the egg (between it and the caudoventral keel) and constant pressure is applied, encouraging the egg to be expelled from the oviduct. Care and firm pressure are needed to avoid breaking the egg, causing a prolapse or damaging the kidneys. This manipulation is contraindicated in cases of uterine constriction, torsion, rupture or ectopic eggs.

Ovocentesis – the aspiration of the egg contents with a large-bore needle (21 or 23 G) – is warranted if oviposition does not occur with digital pressure. If the tip of the egg can be seen through the cloaca, transcloacal ovocentesis is safest. Sometimes it is necessary to aspirate with a needle placed through the abdominal wall. It is useful with soft-shelled eggs that are easily passed after being collapsed. Following aspiration, firmer eggshells may need to be collapsed gently before removal. All shell pieces need to be removed carefully, as sharp pieces can cause uterine damage and retained pieces can serve as a nidus for infection.

Surgical removal is warranted if the egg is lodged in the caudal oviduct or urodeum. An episiotomy should be attempted in these cases. A ventral laparotomy and possibly a hysterectomy are indicated if: the egg is severely adherent to the oviduct wall; the uterus is ruptured; a soft-shelled egg is located cranial to the oviduct; or the egg is ectopic.

Prolapsed oviduct

Prolapse of the oviduct, uterus, vagina and/or cloaca can occur secondary to dystocia, normal egg laying, physiological hyperplasia, various disease states affecting these tissues, general debilitation and malnutrition. The uterus is the most commonly prolapsed tissue, but any part of the oviduct (Figure 18.5) or intestine is possible. Exposed tissues are susceptible to infection and devitalization; they should be kept moist and clean

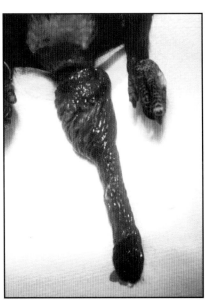

18.5

Prolapsed oviduct in Eclectus Parrot (see also Chapter 10).

with warm sterile saline flushes. Immediately before flushing, samples should be taken for cloacal culture and sensitivity testing, CBC and chemistry. Parenteral antibiotics and fluids should be administered. Next, sterile lubricant mixed (1:1) with sterile 50% dextrose can be applied to the prolapsed tissue to help to decrease oedema. Moistened shrunken tissues are gently replaced with a lubricated swab. Recurrence is common and re-replacement should be attempted. If necessary, one stay cruciate suture can be placed laterally on either side of the vent to help prevent recurrence. This allows the tissues to regress in size naturally, but also leaves an aperture while maintaining an exit for urine, urates and faeces. If the cloaca repeatedly prolapses, a cloacopexy is warranted. If the uterus repeatedly prolapses, a hysterectomy is warranted or, if the bird is a breeder, the dorsal or ventral uterine ligaments should be repaired.

If treated promptly, the prognosis for prolapsed tissues is good. Chronic prolapses have a poor prognosis for survival of the prolapsed tissue and of the patient. Surgical debridement, or possibly a hysterectomy may be required once the patient is stabilized (Chapter 10).

Egg-related peritonitis
Septic egg yolk peritonitis is a term used to describe a frequently fatal condition associated with the presence of infection and egg yolk material in the coelomic cavity. Prognosis is better in cases caught early and treated before they become infected. Hence, non-septic yolk peritonitis has a better prognosis, since the yolk itself only causes a mild histiocytic response and is gradually reabsorbed. A group of syndromes may contribute to egg yolk peritonitis and include ectopic ovulation secondary to reverse peristalsis, salpingitis, metritis, neoplasia, cystic hyperplasia, ruptured oviducts, and stress or physical restraint of the egg-laying hen.

Acute signs of egg yolk peritonitis include decreased or ceased egg production, depression, anorexia, mild weight loss, and a history of broodiness or recent egg laying. Diagnosis and immediate treatment improves prognosis. Abdominal swelling and ascites are common chronic clinical signs, especially in smaller psittacines.

Acute septic egg yolk peritonitis causes a severe inflammatory response, paralleled by that seen in chlamydophilosis, aspergillosis and osteomyelitis, hence white blood cell (WBC) counts may be > 30,000/μl but can also be normal. Radiography, abdominocentesis, endoscopy and laparotomy are helpful diagnostic aids. Egg yolk peritonitis is most frequently described in Cockatiels, Budgerigars, lovebirds and macaws, especially Scarlet Macaws. Other syndromes associated with egg yolk peritonitis include egg-related pancreatitis (which may lead to temporary diabetes mellitus) and yolk emboli (which can result in a stroke-like syndrome, especially in Cockatiels).

Therapy: Treatment depends on the severity of the clinical signs. Traditional medical management of chronic cases includes long-term parenteral antibiotics based on culture and sensitivity, and supportive care as needed, including abdominocentesis to reduce abdominal pressure and relieve dyspnoea. The aetiological agent of egg-related peritonitis is often a coliform

(usually *Escherichia coli*) but *Yersinia pseudotuberculosis* and staphylococci have also been associated with this condition, and anaerobes and *Chlamydophila* have been implicated. Endoscopy should be performed in the stabilized patient to assess the severity of the internal pathology. If an excessive amount of yolk, an inspissated egg or adhesions exist, then surgery, consisting of a laparotomy with abdominal flushing, is indicated in the stabilized patient (Chapter 10). Prognosis is dependent on prompt detection and early treatment. Traditionally, most cases resolve with medical therapy alone when detected early, but chronic egg yolk peritonitis remains the most common fatal obstetric condition in avian species.

Chronic egg laying
Chronic or excessive egg laying occurs when a hen has repeat clutches, regardless of the presence of a natural mate or the proper breeding season, or when she lays larger than normal clutch sizes. This phenomenon occurs commonly in Cockatiels, Budgerigars and lovebirds, and infrequently in hand-raised psittacine hens that are imprinted on humans.

Excessive or chronic egg laying leads to calcium deficiency, and eventually egg binding, osteoporosis and severe malnutrition. Sexual stimulation induced by toys, nest boxes, human beings, inappropriate mates or natural mates should be eliminated. Decreasing the photoperiod to 8 hours of light per day interrupts the hormonal balance, stopping egg production. The eggs of an excessive or chronic egg layer should be left in the nest, or replaced with artificial ones, as an empty nest stimulates the hen to lay again, exacerbating the problem.

Clinical signs: In addition to excess egg production, clinical signs attributable to end-stage chronic egg laying include: weight loss and dehydration secondary to chronic regurgitation; feather loss and dermatitis around the vent secondary to masturbation; and abnormal egg production, oviduct inertia, muscular weakness and pathological fractures secondary to chronic calcium depletion. Unfortunately, these late signs are typically the first ones noted. Acute or early clinical signs include repetitive or increased frequency of egg laying, increase in numbers of eggs laid and excessive broodiness. These signs are particularly noticeable in determinate layers (i.e. Budgerigars), who will normally only lay a set number of eggs per clutch regardless of removal or destruction. The majority of parrots are thought to be indeterminate layers, who will continue to lay after egg removal or destruction until they recognize the correct number of eggs in their clutch. Studies in Cockatiels indicate that reproductive behaviour is associated with photostimulation, nest box presentation and access to a 'mate', which in hand-reared birds is usually the owner. Levels of luteinizing hormone (LH) were indeed elevated in Cockatiels.

Therapy: Treatment of chronic or excessive egg laying includes addressing malnutrition, beginning medical or pharmacological treatment, and potentially salpingo-hysterectomy. Nutritional and/or vitamin supplementation should be addressed in all cases.

Pharmacological medical management of chronic egg layers is controversial and varied. Medroxyprogesterone injections or implants have been used to interrupt the laying/ovulatory cycle. Side effects include obesity, lethargy, polyuria, polydipsia and hepatic lipidosis. This treatment is contraindicated because medroxyprogesterone is likely to precipitate a fatal gluconeogenic catastrophe in a bird that may already have fatty liver.

Long-acting leuprolide acetate, a very expensive superactive gonadotrophin-releasing hormone, has been safely used to prevent egg laying in Cockatiels and many other psittacine birds. Leuprolide acetate can be safely divided into Cockatiel-size doses after reconstitution and frozen for future use. When thawed it is still active if used immediately. Psittacine birds injected every 2–3 weeks with leuprolide acetate, a minimum of three times, may cease chronic egg laying. Some Cockatiels may respond to leuprolide acetate by ceasing egg production for from one to several years, while others may continue to lay indiscriminately despite injections. Experimental studies on Cockatiels have shown that some birds need up to seven injections in order to shut down egg production. Refractory cases are candidates for salpingohysterectomy (Chapter 10).

It has been suggested by some authors that the LH activity of human chorionic gonadotrophin (HCG) given at the appropriate stage of follicular development may cause follicular atresia and therefore may be used as a means to control ovulation. However, its reported efficacy and safety are questionable and its use is not recommended. Synthetic LH supplements are very safe and can be effective.

Ultimately only a salpingohysterectomy will stop a chronic egg layer. This intricate surgery is generally considered safe in most medium to large psittacine birds. It requires a very skilled surgeon for Cockatiels, lovebirds and Budgerigars. If left untreated, chronic or excessive egg laying can lead to egg binding, osteoporosis and severe malnutrition; thus preventive medicine and client education are very important in the treatment of this condition.

Neoplasia

Ovarian neoplasia is more common than oviduct neoplasia in psittacine birds. Cloacal carcinomas are less frequent.

Ovarian tumours can enlarge to one-third of the bird's body weight, causing massive organ displacement. Herniation, ascites and cysts are frequent sequelae to neoplasia of the ovary and oviduct. The most significant clinical sign secondary to abdominal enlargement is dyspnoea, but cere colour changes from pink or blue to golden brown are also seen in the Budgerigar, as is unilateral or bilateral paresis or paralysis. Diagnostic testing includes palpation, radiography and ultrasonography, but definitive diagnosis is based on biopsy and histopathology. Commonly reported ovarian tumours include adenocarcinomas, adenomas, granulosa cell tumours, lipomas, fibrosarcomas and carcinomatosis. Due to the active and invasive nature of most ovarian tumours, they are usually inoperable.

Tumours of the oviduct include adenomatous hyperplasia, adenocarcinomas, adenomas and carcinomatosis.

Males

Infertility of the male may be due to age, obesity, inbreeding or infection. After a clinical examination, infertility in male birds should be investigated by examination of the vent and cloaca (bacteriology, cytology, histology), taking and examining a semen sample, and endoscopic examination of the testes and vasa deferentia with testicular biopsy if appropriate (Chapter 11).

Orchitis

Infection of the testes can originate from cloacitis or renal obstruction or, in the Vasa Parrot with its protruding cloaca, prolapse or ulceration can cause a retrograde infection. The most commonly found bacteria in orchitis are *Escherichia coli*, *Salmonella* spp. and *Pasteurella multocida*. Clinical signs are similar to those expected for any generalized infection. Treatment is best achieved with antibiotics based on culture and sensitivity of cloacal, semen and testicular cultures.

Neoplasia

Testicular neoplasia can involve one or both testes and is regularly seen in Budgerigars. Clinical signs include unilateral paresis, progressive weight loss and abdominal enlargement. Affected males may become more feminine in nature as secondary sexual characteristics are reduced. Metastasis from testicular tumours usually affects the liver. Seminomas are the most common testicular tumour diagnosed in birds, and behavioural changes, such as aggressiveness, have been associated with this tumour. Sertoli and interstitial cell tumours have also been described. Lymphoma can cause infertility by infiltrating the testis.

Incubation

Successful incubation and hatching require intensive husbandry. Similarly, altricial psittacine chicks require intensive care from day 1. Neonates hatch with eyes closed and with little or no down; they are unable to thermoregulate and need to be hand fed on a scheduled basis. Thus, in addition to preventive and triage medicine, the veterinary surgeon can help the aviculturist by evaluating the following processes: incubation, hatching, hand feeding, neonatal development and weaning.

Natural incubation

Natural incubation by captive psittacine birds is affected by many factors, including the demonstration of normal breeding behaviours by both parents, their health, diet, species, origin (wild caught or hand reared), experience, environment and design of nest box. Perhaps the most important of these is the demonstration of normal breeding behaviours. The female should act broody and prepare for and care for her nest of eggs. The nest should be built with the help of her mate and be kept clean and well protected. The male should take on the role of provider and feed the female constantly and consistently throughout the pre-laying and the post-laying period. He should become even more attentive to her nutritional needs once the eggs hatch and the mother and he are feeding the offspring

Broken eggs commonly result when birds are startled, especially cockatoos, Grey Parrots and macaws; poor quality eggshell should always be suspected and the diet should be checked. Cracked eggs are susceptible to bacterial infections and should be repaired topically with nail polish and incubated artificially.

Reduced breeding success has been reported with some domestic hand-reared and inexperienced psittacine breeding pairs when compared with wild-caught parents or domestic parents raised with experienced birds. However, this has not been this author's experience and these reports may be disproved as the numbers of domestically raised pairs increase. Nest box parameters (e.g. cleanliness, shape, depth, width, height and degree of openness) and the amount of lighting are important for breeding success.

Artificial incubation

Hatchability of artificially incubated eggs pulled (removed from the parents) at day 1 is lower than that of those naturally incubated for the first 7–14 days. Further, large psittacine eggs seem to be more tolerant of incubation from day 1 than the eggs of smaller psittacine birds. Smaller eggs are most difficult at the start of incubation. Their natural required temperature gradient is difficult to mimic in an incubator. In general, they should be incubated a few degrees higher than normal at the start of incubation. Nevertheless, the larger avicultural collections typically incubate eggs from day 1 to increase production. This dichotomy occurs because pulling the eggs at day 1 encourages the hen to lay again, thus increasing the number of eggs laid per clutch, as well as the number of clutches laid per year. Eggs need to be carefully identified; a soft lead pencil is safest.

Successful artificial incubation depends on several parameters, including temperature, humidity, airflow in the incubator or hatcher, vibration and egg rotation. Egg rotation (turning) is very important in artificial incubation. It is required to prevent embryo adhesion to the shell membranes. In natural incubation, parents will rotate their eggs as often as every 35 minutes. Inadequate turning in artificial incubation results in early dead-in-shell, malposition or late dead-in-shell embryos. Good quality commercial incubators will turn eggs at different rates on various types of timed mechanical rollers with 10 turns per day being the average. A minimum of 5 turns per day is required in machines where automatic turning is not an option.

Artificial incubators and hatchers should be cultured for bacteria and fungi several times a year, and tested by DNA-probe for polyomavirus and psittacine beak and feather virus. Units should also be cleaned and gas-sterilized annually.

Incubation temperature and relative humidity vary for different psittacine species, but range from 37.2 to 37.4°C (98.9 to 99.3°F) and 30% to 45%, respectively. Digital hygrometers work best to monitor humidity.

Temperature in the incubation room is ideally maintained at 22.8–23.9°C (73–75°F) with a humidity of 43–48%. Psittacine embryos are best hatched at 37.5°C (99.5°F) with a hygrometer reading of 65–75%.

Incubation times vary for different psittacine species (Figure 18.6) and range from approximately 18 days in Budgerigars to approximately 30 days in Palm Cockatoos.

Species	Egg number	Incubation (days)	Nestling period (days)
Grey Parrot	2–3 (4)	21–30	80
Senegal Parrot	2–4	25	63
Peach-faced Lovebird	4–6	23	38
Scarlet Macaw	1–4	24–28	100
Blue-fronted Amazon	1–5	23–25	60
Pionus parrots	3–6	26	60
Lesser Sulphur-crested Cockatoo	2–3	27	70
Moluccan Cockatoo	1–3	28–29	100
Cockatiel	3–7	20	35
Budgerigar	4–6	18	30
Kakarikis	5–9	20	35
Green-cheeked Conure	3–4	22–24	42
Ringneck Parakeet	3–4	22	50

18.6 Incubation periods. Incubation is usually performed by the female alone, except in cockatoos where it is done by both sexes.

Embryo development and candling

Artificially incubated eggs are 'candled' to monitor development. A penlight can be used for candling weekly or bi-weekly. The eggs should be moved to the bottom of the incubator, and no longer turned, once drawdown (creation of the air space) has been noted, as this is when internal pipping begins (see below).

Psittacine eggs are less tolerant of handling than poultry eggs but candling (a necessary form of handling) is important in determining embryo fertility and viability. The critical periods of development for psittacine embryos are the first few days of incubation and the time from internal pip until hatching. During these times the embryo is most susceptible to adverse handling and improper incubation parameters. An egg monitor can be used to assess heart rate at this stage.

The first signs of fertility are blood vessels radiating uniformly from the embryo in a branching pattern from days 3 to 5 (Figure 18.7). Eggs with clear yolks showing no signs of blood vessels or development by day 7 are either infertile or early 'dead-in-shell', and should be removed from the incubator (or nest). Mortality during the first 7 days of natural incubation is usually due to poor incubation by the parents or the artificial incubator, but can be due to egg-borne infection or contamination, or genetic abnormalities. Some causes of early embryonic death during artificial incubation include

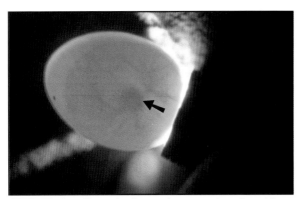

18.7 Candling a fertile egg between days 3 and 5 reveals a small early embryo (arrowed) with blood vessels radiating from it. Over the next few days the embryo and its associated vasculature grows and by mid incubation the egg is opaque.

improper handling, excessive or insufficient temperature or humidity, excessive vibrations, improper egg turning or poor ventilation resulting in the build-up of carbon dioxide.

A healthy developing psittacine egg should lose between 11 and 16% (average 13%) of its water weight by diffusion during incubation (day 1 to external pip). The air cell forms at the rounded end of the egg during this period of weight loss. If the humidity is too high, the air cell will be small; if it is too low, the air cell will be larger. (Dirt on eggs should be removed when dry. Washing parrot eggs is not recommended.)

The normal psittacine embryo develops with its head below the air cell. Psittacine embryos have shorter and thicker necks than chicken embryos and do not normally have their heads under their right wing. Instead, they barely tuck their head and typically lay it close to the right wing tip.

Hatching

Hatching is the time of greatest embryo mortality. It occurs in stages: drawdown; internal pip; external pip; and emergence from the egg.

1. *Drawdown* is defined as the creation of the air cell space (see Figure 2.14). About 24–48 hours prior to internal pip, the air cell expands and extends (draws) down one side of the egg, occupying 20–30% of its volume.
2. The gaseous exchange needs of the embryo are no longer met by the allantoic circulation, and carbon dioxide levels rise, causing the hatching muscle in the neck to twitch and move the head, forcing the egg tooth through the chorioallantoic membrane into the air cell (*internal pip*). The embryo is now a chick, as it breathes air within the air cell.
3. As the lungs begin to function, the right-to-left ventricular shunt in the heart closes, and in certain species a peeping sound may be heard from the egg. The egg no longer needs turning and is placed on the bottom of the incubator. Twitching of the abdominal muscles, which occurs secondary to breathing, causes the yolk sac to be drawn into the chick's abdomen. With subsequent breaths,

the level of CO_2 within the air cell rises to 10% and the hatching muscle again begins to twitch, causing the egg tooth to penetrate the shell (*external pip*). At this time the eggs are moved out of the incubator and into the hatcher. The time between internal and external pipping is typically 24–48 hours (range 3–72 hours).

Embryo and chick mortality

In artificial incubation, malposition and inadequate moisture loss are the most common causes of embryonic mortality prior to hatching. Malpositioning commonly occurs secondary to hyperthermia or elevated temperatures, which also cause premature pipping. The commonest malpositions are when the head is located at the small end of the egg or when the beak is rotated away from the air cell. Eggs incubated below optimum temperatures develop more slowly and typically have increased problems with hatching. High humidity prevents adequate water loss and the oedematous 'wet chicks' drown at pipping, due to excessive albumin. Low humidity and too much water loss cause the shell membrane to adhere to the chick, preventing normal pipping.

All dead eggs should be necropsied. During the gross necropsy the embryo's general condition and position are assessed. Abnormal tissues and fluids are cultured or sent off for histopathology. The shell is examined for colour, texture, shape and the presence or absence of stress lines. Thickness of the shell is assessed by differences in texture, as well as transparency and the degree of porosity.

Care of chicks

Once hatched, chicks should be housed in incubators.

Hand feeding

All chicks should be started on a dilute commercial formula (e.g. Kaytee Macaw Exact) for their first 3 days of life. The macaw formulas are higher in fat and calcium and lower in vitamin D, all of which are important to the developing embryo and subsequent chick. The diluted formula (35 cc bottled water and 1 tablespoon Kaytee Macaw Exact) is given every 2 hours of the first and second day, except during the night, when crops are allowed to empty. On day 2, chicks should be given a probiotic formula (0.1 cc) at their first feed. Feedings on day 3 are every 3 hours.

By day 4, chicks should be started on an undiluted formula mixture. The schedule of formula feedings after day 3 goes from five times a day for the smallest of birds, to four times a day, to three times, to twice, to once, to weaning for birds of conure size and up. The rate at which the number of feeds is reduced is related to species and individual size (slowest for larger species). The amounts fed are based on body weight (BW) early on, and later by species (see below). For example:

- On day 4, Kaytee Regular Exact is fed to all the white and pink or salmon-coloured cockatoos. They are fed at 10% BW until reaching the three times a day feeding, when they are switched to 8% to prevent hepatic lipidosis.

- Birds that require more fat, such as the black or grey cockatoos, Thick-billed Parrots, Hyacinth Macaws, Green-winged Macaws, Queen of Bavaria's Conures and Slender-billed Cockatoos, must be fed a special diet based on a macaw hand-feeding formula with added fat and fibre. The Hyacinth Macaw is fed such a formula at 12% BW and the Green-winged Macaw at 11%; all the other birds in this group are fed at 10% BW.
- The rest of the macaw species, Grey Parrots, caiques, Sun Conures, Eclectus Parrots, and Hawk-headed Parrots do best on the Macaw Exact hand-feeding formula. All these birds are fed at 10% BW, except for the Buffon's Macaw, which is fed at 12% BW.
- Once the birds reach their twice-a-day feeding, they are gradually changed to a once-a-day predetermined maximum for their species. For example, the maximum daily volume for a Cockatiel is 5 cc, Sun Conure 25 cc, Grey Parrot 50 cc and Hyacinth Macaw 140 cc.

Weaning

At two feedings a day juvenile birds should be offered solid foods such as pellets, fruits and vegetables, and treat items such as pine nuts and almonds. Water bowls should be introduced when the birds are on one feed a day. Once birds are drinking and eating on their own, they can be moved into flight or larger cages, where available. There they can be trained to use an automated drinking device before their water bowls are removed.

Birds should always be weighed and monitored closely during the weaning process. They should never be forced; instead, each should be treated as an individual and weaned at its own pace.

Paediatrics

History taking

- Note the parent's health and breeding history, the condition of the siblings, and any problems the chick may have had during incubation and hatching.
- Evaluate diet, its preparation, and the amount and frequency of feeding.
- Determine whether the bird's crop is empty for each feed, especially the first feed of the day.
- Assess environment, housing and substrate for cleanliness, safety and warmth.
- Enquire as to the behaviour of the chick, its feeding response, and the colour, consistency and volume of its faeces, urine and urates.

Physical examination

Physical examination of the chick entails evaluating available weight charts for daily gain and assessing overall appearance, proportions and behaviour. In neonates, this examination should be performed in a warm room with pre-warmed hands. Knowledge of growth rates, development and behavioural characteristics of different species is helpful.

Newly hatched chicks (with down feathers)

Psittacine chicks are altricial: nourishment, warmth (34–36°C), food and a safe place must be provided.

- Most abdominal organs can be seen through the neonate's skin: normally visible are a liver, duodenal loop, yolk sac, ventriculus and occasionally lung.
- The lungs and heart should be auscultated.
- Body mass should be assessed by palpation of elbows, toes and hips, as keel muscle mass is not a reliable indicator of body mass in the very young.
- The crop should be examined visually for size and colour and carefully palpated for thickness, tone, burns, punctures or the presence of foreign bodies. The crop should also be transilluminated to attempt to evaluate and describe their contents.
- Skin should be evaluated for colour, texture, hydration and the presence of subcutaneous fat. Normally, psittacine chicks should have beige-pink, warm and supple skin. Dehydration causes a chick's skin to become dry, hyperaemic and tacky.

Older chicks (with growing contour feathers)

The chick's requirements for extra warmth decrease as its feathers grow. Chicks are able to move around actively before they are skeletally mature, but this should be discouraged.

- Feathers should be examined for stress marks, colour bars or shade changes, haemorrhage, or deformities of shafts and emerging feathers.
- The musculoskeletal system should be palpated and assessed for skeletal defects or trauma in chicks of all ages. Until weaning, cockatoo chicks sit back on their hocks and are balanced forward on their large abdomens, whereas macaws prefer to lie down. Chicks normally have prominent abdomens, due to a food-filled crop, proventriculus, ventriculus and small intestine.
- Beaks should be examined for malformations when the bird's mouth is closed. Pump pads (the soft fleshy part of the baby bird's beak at its commissures) should be examined for wounds and the feeding response elicited. Generally, a healthy baby bird should exhibit a vigorous feeding response when stimulated at the beak's lateral commissures.
- The eyes and the periocular region should be examined for any abnormalities, including lid defects, swelling, discharge, crusting or blepharospasm. Normally a clear discharge is noted in the eyes when they are first opening, which typically occurs unilaterally. Eyes begin to open on days 14 to 28 for macaws, 10 to 21 for cockatoos, and 14 to 21 for Amazons.
- Nares and ears should be examined for discharge and aperture size or absence.
- The oral cavity should be examined for plaque, inflammation, or injuries.

Diagnostic tests

Clinical pathology
Haematology and clinical chemistry should be performed on blood from the right jugular vein. As with adults, blood samples drawn should be < 1% of the bird's body weight. Toenail clips should be reserved for blood sexing only. Young chicks have lower PCVs and lower total proteins than do adults. Their albumin and uric acid values are lower and their alkaline phosphatase and creatine kinase values are higher.

Microbiology
Cloacal cultures, crop cultures, faecal cytology and Gram staining should be performed during routine examination. Normally, cloacal and crop flora are Gram positive and consist of *Lactobacillus, Corynebacterium, Staphlylococcus* and non-haemolytic *Streptococcus* spp. Most Gram-negative and anaerobic bacteria are considered pathogenic, as are yeasts. Choanal cultures should be taken if upper respiratory tract disease is suspected or if choanal papillae are abnormally blunted.

Radiography
The crop, proventriculus and ventriculus are normally enlarged in neonatal and juvenile birds before weaning, and the latter two take up much of the abdominal cavity on radiographs. Furthermore, muscle mass is reduced.

Endoscopy
Endoscopy and surgery in general are best performed on the fasted paediatric patient, since the proventriculus, ventriculus and intestines are normally enlarged in unweaned birds. If the birds are kept warm and stable, anaesthesia and endoscopy are quick. It is safest to 'scope only after weaning, but the author has safely 'scoped much younger birds, three times daily feeds being the 'cut-off' point. Hypothermia, hypoglycaemia and hypocalcaemia are easily avoidable if feeding occurs soon after recovery. Endoscopy is useful for foreign body retrieval, syrinx examination, surgical sexing and laparoscopy.

Treatments

Antimicrobials
Antibiotic treatment should be based on culture and sensitivity for 7 days. The author feels strongly that all paediatric patients on antibiotics should be given the antifungal nystatin. *Lactobacillus* supplementation is also highly recommended after antimicrobial treatment and at the beginning of life, 2 days after hatch. Mild yeast infections can be treated with nystatin alone for 14 days. Intractable yeast infections should be treated with the systemic antifungal ketoconazole in combination with nystatin for a minimum of 21 days. Refractory yeast infections should also be treated with an acetic acid crop gavage at the end of the antifungal treatment, followed by *Lactobacillus*.

Fluids
In paediatrics, patient stabilization centres on temperature and rehydration, which means that oral, subcutaneous and intravenous fluids should be warmed up and given as needed. Subcutaneous fluids are the most frequently used. In the severely dehydrated neonate, a jugular catheter is the preferred rehydration route.

Common paediatric problems
Birds that are being reared by their parents tend to be more resistant to disease and much less likely to be affected by physical problems than birds that are being hand reared. However, poor quality diets will produce deformity and illness in any growing bird.

Unretracted yolk sac
The yolk sac provides the chick with nourishment and maternal antibodies. It should be retracted into the body in the last stages of incubation and is then completely absorbed. Sometimes the yolk sac does not retract before hatching, usually due to incubation hyperthermia but sometimes due to infection. Healthy chicks with unretracted yolk sacs should be placed on clean towels in the hatcher or the incubator, and the umbilicus swabbed with chlorhexidine scrub. Crop and cloacal cultures should be performed, as well as yolk sac cultures if the sac is leaking, and the chicks should be placed on appropriate antibiotics and oral antifungal treatment. Chicks should also be treated with fluids. If the yolk sac fails to become internalized, surgery is necessary: it should be borne in mind that the yolk sac enters the body and connects to the small intestine; its blood vessels run to the liver. Retention of the yolk sac within the abdomen commonly occurs secondary to *Escherichia coli* omphalitis.

Stunting
Stunting, commonly caused by malnutrition, is most pronounced in the first 30 days of life. Affected birds have poor growth rates, low weight, an enlarged head relative to their body size, and abnormal feather growth, including delayed emergence (on the body), misdirection (top of head) and feather stress or colour bar lines.

Leg and toe deformities
Splay leg, a common deformity, usually occurs as a result of malnutrition, especially calcium and vitamin D deficiency exacerbated by too much exercise, obesity or a congenital defect. Usually one leg is affected, but both can be. Chicks can be packed in paper towels or hobbled (Chapter 11). Juveniles that splay on pellets or other slippery substrates may straighten up on towels or packed towels. Treatment options also include hobbling and possibly surgery. Crooked, crossed or forwardly directed toes can be corrected by splinting if caught early on, otherwise surgery may be indicated (Chapter 11).

Constricted toes
Constricted toe syndrome occurs most commonly in Eclectus Parrots, macaws (Figure 18.8) and Grey Parrots. The lesion consists of an annular ring constriction usually on the last phalanx and most frequently affecting the inner toes.

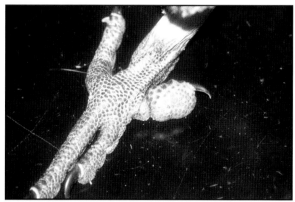

18.8 Constricted toe syndrome. This half-grown Green-winged Macaw was being hand reared after poor parenting. Digit I was very swollen and there is a constriction (on the other foot, digit I had been the same and the portion of toe distal to the constriction dried up and dropped off). The constriction was relieved surgically and the toe returned to normal over 3 weeks.

1. Under isoflurane anaesthesia and magnification, rule out cloth or other fibres as a cause.
2. Debride the circumferential fibrous annular band with fine forceps.
3. Put two full-thickness longitudinal incisions, medially and laterally, through the constriction band, express accumulated serum, bandage, and monitor for swelling.
4. Soak in warm dilute chlorhexidine solution and massage daily, then re-bandage.

Chicks should have cloaca and crop samples cultured, and be given parenteral antibiotics and oral antifungal treatment. Frequently the toe becomes dead distal to the constriction and requires amputation. The aetiology remains unproven but it has been suggested that a dry atmosphere may be a cause.

Beak malformations
The three most common beak malformations are: lateral deviations of the maxilla (scissor beak); compression deformities of the mandible; and prognathism (pug beak). Lateral deviation is thought to be congenital or induced by poor hand-feeding technique; mandibular compression is thought to be induced by rough hand-feeding technique; and prognathism is thought to be congenital. The first two are most common in macaws, while the third is most common in cockatoos. When the chicks are young and the beaks are most pliable, physical therapy and trimming are indicated. After calcification, frequent trimming, acrylic implants or extensions are often needed to correct the malformations (Chapter 11).

Regurgitation
During weaning, the crop normally shrinks in size. Hence, regurgitation of small amounts of food after feeding signals the need to reduce feeding frequency and to begin introducing solid foods such as pellets, fruits and vegetables. Typically, as a bird grows, feeding volumes are increased and the frequency is decreased. Younger birds will regurgitate if overfed and this can lead to aspiration pneumonia. Repeated regurgitation in a chick that is too young to wean or regurgitation of large volumes may indicate disease or mechanical blockage. Foreign bodies, crop or lower gastrointestinal fungal or bacterial infection, gout and proventricular dilatation disease (PDD) should be ruled out. Drugs such as trimethoprim/sulphonamides, doxycycline and nystatin can cause regurgitation, especially in macaw chicks. Chicks should be worked up and started on antibiotics and antifungal treatment as needed. Note that, in cases of regurgitation, antibiotics should be given parentally.

Oesophageal or pharyngeal punctures
Oesophageal or pharyngeal punctures occur secondary to syringe or tube feeding. They are most common in vigorously pumping birds, such as macaws. Oesophageal punctures usually occur midway between the pharynx and the thoracic inlet in the cranial-most aspect of the crop. Pharyngeal punctures usually occur in the caudal aspect of the pharynx, slightly caudal to the right of the glottis. Emergency surgery is needed to remove subcutaneously deposited food, create a drain, and begin flushing of the wound. The bird must be tube fed so that food does not come into contact with the wound during healing. The crop, cloaca and choana should be cultured, CBC and blood chemistry should be performed, and the bird should be started on antibiotics and antifungal treatment.

Crop stasis
Crop stasis is very common in neonatal and juvenile birds. Primary causes of crop stasis include infection, crop foreign bodies (such as feeding tube or syringe tips), atony, burns, dehydration of food in the crop, hypothermia, cold or hot food and environment. The most common primary cause of crop stasis is yeast or candidiasis. Secondary causes include distal gut stasis due to ileus, intestinal intussusception, bacterial or fungal infection, sepsis, dilation, PDD, polyomavirus, gastrointestinal (GI) foreign bodies, renal failure or hepatic failure. Medical and mechanical management are typically needed for the treatment of crop stasis. Diagnostics as described above are very important, especially culture, crop and faecal cytology, and blood work. Further diagnostics, such as radiography, crop biopsy and/or reduction, should be performed as needed without hesitation (Chapter 10).

Fluids are vital for the treatment of both crop and other GI stasis cases. Oral fluids rehydrate inspissated crop material and hasten its passage. Subcutaneous fluids are the treatment of choice for systemic rehydration. Intravenous fluids are best in the severely dehydrated patient. In these cases, placement of a right jugular intravenous catheter is preferred; such catheters are safely maintained for days. If the crop is severely impacted, repeated flushing with warm saline may be needed to empty it. A 'crop bra' (Figure 18.9) is a simple form of mechanical management for the overstretched crop. In a severely overstretched crop, reduction surgery may be necessary to facilitate emptying. Hypoproteinaemia may occur secondary to severe chronic crop stasis. In these cases, whole-blood transfusions and metoclopramide or cisapride may be indicated, as long as GI obstruction has been ruled out.

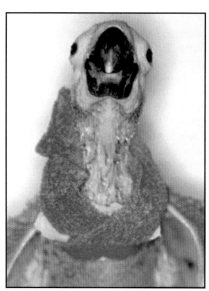

18.9

Crop 'bra' designed to support an overstretched crop.

Chronic non-responsive crop stasis may involve mural candidiasis. These cases are best diagnosed with biopsy and require long-term systemic antifungal and antibiotic treatment and acetic acid gavage. Acetic acid acidifies the crop's contents and discourages yeast and bacterial growth. The most common clinical signs of crop stasis are a visibly oversized static crop and regurgitation. Although a manageable problem, crop stasis can be a fatal condition due to dehydration and sepsis and it therefore demands immediate intervention. Crop stasis, the most common paediatric problem, causes dehydration. Sepsis typically follows dehydration, and together these conditions are the most common killers in birds during hand rearing.

Crop burns
Crop burns of the mucosa and skin occur secondary to feeding excessively hot food (> 43°C). The burn must fistulate through before surgery is indicated and this may take several days to weeks (Chapter 10).

Foreign body ingestion or impaction
Neonates and juveniles are curious and will ingest foreign bodies. If these are large and in the crop, they can be removed by digital manipulation; forceps may be needed. Small pieces, such as wood shavings, may pass through the crop, causing lower GI impactions. Emergency surgery is often indicated (Chapter 10).

Less common paediatric problems

Rectal prolapse
Secondary to hypermotility or infection, rectal prolapse has been reported in macaws. If the prolapsed tissues are fresh, the bird may be saved. Emergency surgery is indicated (Chapter 10).

Intestinal intussusception
Intestinal intussusception has been seen in juvenile Amazons but could occur in any species. Although the birds require fluids, antibiotics and antifungal treatment, emergency surgery is necessary. The prognosis in baby parrots is poor and euthanasia should be considered (Chapter 10).

Hepatic haematomas
These are suspected to be secondary to rough handling/trauma or possibly dietary deficiencies. Most reports have been in macaws, where the aetiology is unknown. Blood work and cultures should be taken; chicks should be given vitamin K_1 and blood transfusions if necessary.

Hepatic lipidosis
Hepatic lipidosis occurs secondary to overfeeding or individual susceptibility, primarily in handfed Umbrella Cockatoos, Moluccan Cockatoos and Blue and Gold Macaws, but it can occur in other birds. Affected chicks have severely enlarged livers (see Figure 7.32d) visible through the skin, and enlarged abdomens, and may be pale and dyspnoeic. These birds need to have their volume of food reduced but number of feeds increased, which immediately helps to improve their dyspnoea. The dietary fat content should be reduced. A blood sample and faecal culture are useful. The birds should be given milk thistle and lactulose.

Gout
Gout, a clinical sign, occurs secondary to severe renal disease and severe dehydration. In juvenile macaws, gout is thought to occur secondary to excess vitamin D_3 and calcium in the diet. A genetic predisposition is suspected in Blue and Gold Macaws, Red-fronted Macaws, Cockatiels and Palm Cockatoos.

Wine-coloured urine
Red-stained urine normally occurs in juvenile Grey Parrots, Amazons and Pionus parrots. It may occur secondary to certain hand-feeding formulas, and is most obvious on white or light towels.

Infectious diseases in the nursery
Infectious diseases (Chapter 13) are uncommon if a breeder keeps a closed flock and does not visit bird shows, auctions and other collections. At the other end of the spectrum, some breeders will raise chicks with unknown disease problems for other breeders; this is a high-risk procedure.

Polyomavirus
This is the most common viral disease encountered in psittacine nurseries. It is highly contagious, has an estimated incubation period of 2 weeks and is typically widespread before detection. Most affected birds die within 24–48 hours. Macaws, conures, Eclectus Parrots and Ringneck Parakeets between 2 and 14 weeks old are most commonly affected. If clinical signs appear at all, they consist of weakness, pallor, subcutaneous haemorrhage, anorexia, dehydration, crop stasis, regurgitation, vomiting and depression (see Figure 7.18). Haemorrhage is noted at injection sites, plucked feathers bleed excessively, and petechial and ecchymotic haemorrhages appear on the skin. Survivors exhibit poor weight gain, polyuria, gut stasis, and abnormal feathering similar to that caused by circovirus (PBFD). Asymptomatic infection keeps this virus in the psittacine population. A polyomavirus PCR test is available to identify actively shedding birds. A vaccine is available in the USA. Strict nursery husbandry and a closed nursery policy should be practised.

Proventricular dilatation disease (PDD)

PDD is also an important viral disease of the paediatric patient. Affected birds are 10 weeks and older; the disease is ultimately fatal. In the nursery, chicks may exhibit regurgitation, crop stasis, voluminous faeces, weight loss, weakness and neurological signs, including head tremors. Biopsy of the ventriculus, the proventriculus or the crop may be diagnostic if lymphocytic plasmacytic infiltrates of myenteric plexi are noted. A 'closed' nursery and impeccable husbandry are the best tools available to control the virus.

Psittacine beak and feather disease (PBFD)

PBFD is highly contagious and easily spread by powder down. This viral disease is characterized by abnormal feather growth and is most often noted in fully feathered chicks. Feathers can be clubbed, have circumferential constrictions, sheaths and blood feathers may be retained, and so on. A PBFD PCR test is available. Positive birds should be isolated and retested for 90 days, as some may clear the virus. The disease course may be acute or chronic, depending on the age and immuncompetence of the individual. Strict nursery husbandry and quarantine should be practised. All chicks should be tested before leaving the nursery. If baby birds are being sold to pet shops there is a significant risk that they can contract circovirus infection in the pet shop from infected powder down – many Budgerigars are symptom-free carriers. Young birds should be exposed to this risk only when they have a fully developed immune system.

Avipoxvirus

In the USA, this virus is a problem in neotropical parrots where chicks remain in the nest for any length of time or where juveniles are housed outdoors. In Europe the situation is different (Chapter 13).

Microbial infections

Microbial alimentary infections are among the most common problems in psittacine chicks. They are typically diagnosed by cloacal and crop cultures and Gram stains. Gram-negative bacteria or yeast infections are abnormal in psittacine chicks. Some strains of *Escherichia coli*, *Klebsiella* spp. and *Enterobacter* spp. are thought to vary in pathogenicity and can be isolated from completely normal chicks. Birds should be treated only if they exhibit clinical signs or if Gram-negative bacteria or yeast are identified in large numbers. Further, they should only be treated based on culture and sensitivity testing. As mentioned above, all paediatric patients given antibiotics must also receive the antifungal nystatin. In cases of regurgitation or stasis, antibiotics should be given subcutaneously until crop emptying or stasis improves. Microbial disease organisms of importance in the nursery include *Escherichia coli*, *Klebsiella* spp., *Enterobacter* spp., *Pseudomonas* spp., *Salmonella* spp. and *Candida* spp.

Chlamydophila should be looked for in all cases of nursery mortality, especially if the collection contains Budgerigars or Cockatiels (Chapter 13).

19

Neurology and ophthalmology

Thomas N. Tully, Jr

Neurology

Neurological diseases can be primary or secondary and affect the central or peripheral nervous system. Signs associated with central nervous system disease include convulsions (seizures), depression, ataxia, paresis, paralysis, tremors, circling, head tilt, nystagmus, torticollis, visual defects and/or behavioural abnormalities.

Brain and brainstem

The avian brain consists of the proencephalon (telencephalon and diencephalon) and the caudal brain (medulla, pons and mesencephalon). The cranial nerves are similar to those of mammals (Figure 19.1). Birds are highly visual creatures of mainly reflex behaviour.

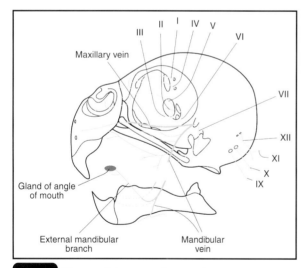

19.1 The cranial nerves of a parrot.

Spinal cord

The spinal cord is the same length as the vertebral column and the spinal cord segment is at the same point as the vertebral column segment (King and McClelland, 1984). The internal vertebral venous plexus serves as a conduit for infectious agents or neoplasia as it anastomoses with the drainage of the kidney.

Nerves found in the thoracic and pelvic limb originate from the brachial plexus (thoracic limb) (Figure 19.2; see also Figure 2.6) and the lumbosacral plexus (pelvic limb) (Figure 19.3; see also Figure 2.7).

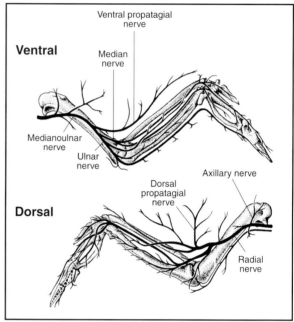

19.2 Peripheral nerves of avian wing.

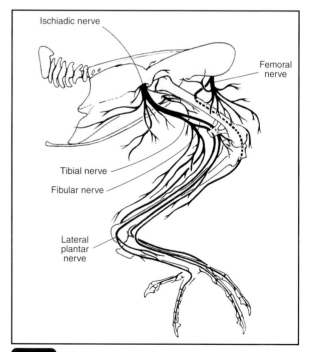

19.3 Peripheral nerves of avian leg.

The long ascending and long descending pathways of avian species have not been studied to the extent of those in mammals but there is enough evidence (King and McClelland, 1984; Orosz, 1996) to correlate the pathways with their mammalian counterparts and to speculate on, if not to verify, their action in birds (Figure 19.4).

Pathway	Action
Long ascending pathways	
Dorsal column	Information from body wall. Touch, pressure, kinaesthesia. Proprioception of the joints
Dorsolateral ascending bundle	Unconscious proprioception of wing
Ventrolateral ascending bundle	Unconscious proprioception of body
Dorsolateral fasciculus	Transmit tactile information
Spinoreticular tract	Delivery of pain information
Propriospinal system	Sense of non-localized pain
Long descending pathways	
Lateral reticulospinal tract	Visceral motor function
Rubrospinal tract	Enhance flexor tone of muscles
Cerebrospinal tract	Provides upper motor neuron input to motor neurons in ventral horn of cervical region
Vestibulospinal tract	Flight and ability to move freely in three-dimensional space
Reticulospinal tract	Altering somatic and visceral motor tone
Tectospinal tract	Coordination of reflex movements between eyes and upper body, primarily cervical area

19.4 Long ascending and long descending pathways.

Neurological disease diagnosis

Clinical signs associated with neurological disease in avian species are often generalized, making it difficult for many veterinary surgeons to obtain a diagnosis, much less establish a viable differential diagnosis list. Understanding neuroanatomy and physiology will aid in isolating the anatomical region or cause of the neurological signs. It is extremely important to obtain a thorough history and perform a clinical examination.

The first observational criterion to be evaluated is the mental status of the patient. A good baseline determination is the owner's opinion of the bird's mental status. In the clinic, the bird will behave differently but should still be assessed. Is it bright, alert and responsive, or depressed? Is the patient exhibiting neurological signs such as ataxia, torticollis, paralysis, opisthotonus (Figure 13.3) or convulsions (seizure activity)? Convulsions in birds are similar to those in mammals: a pre-seizure phase (aura); the seizure phase (ictal), consisting of tonic clonic convulsions; and the post-seizure phase, generally with lethargy and depression (Jones and Orosz, 1996).

A postural reaction test can evaluate a bird's ability to perform complex actions that require integration of the proprioceptive sensory systems for initiation and the motor systems for response (Jones and Orosz, 1996). Parrots can have these reflexes tested by making them step up on to a perch and by extending and releasing the wings, checking for normal placement upon release.

It is difficult to localize a neurological lesion through sensory examination (e.g. temperature changes and light touch) and so most veterinary surgeons concentrate on the pain pathways. Spinal reflex evaluation is best performed using a haemostat to pinch the distal wing tip and/or toe – the bird should pull its limb away, look at the haemostat and maybe preen or bite it. A haemostat pinch to the cloacal or vent epithelium should cause constriction of the vent and reaction from the bird. Decreased muscle tone is often associated with lower motor neuron disease but can be found in upper motor neuron disease. Upper motor neuron disease often causes increased muscle tone with increased muscle irritation and facilitation (Jones and Orosz, 1996).

The poorest prognosis for return to function is loss of deep pain, because deep pain is the last sensory level to be lost after a serious injury. The order of neurological deficits after a compressive injury to the spinal cord is loss of: (i) consciousness; (ii) unconscious proprioception; (iii) motor function; (iv) superficial pain; and (v) deep pain (Oliver and Lorenz, 1993).

Cranial nerve evaluation

To determine whether the central nervous system (CNS) is involved, a thorough examination of the cranial nerves needs to be performed. If a single cranial nerve is involved, the lesion is usually localized; multiple nerve involvement is observed as extensive damage (Bennett, 1994). Patients with CNS lesions often present with clinical signs affecting proprioception, pain localization and upper motor neuron abnormalities but the mental status of the bird is not altered (Figure 19.5) (Oliver and Lorenz, 1993; Jones and Orosz, 1996).

Cranial nerve (CN)	Signs of dysfunction
CN I (olfactory nerve)	Impaired smell
CN II (optic nerve)	Impaired sight
CN III (oculomotor)	(Motor) ventrolateral deviation; (Motor) drooped upper eyelid; (Parasympathetic) dilated pupil
CN IV (trochlear)	Dorsolateral deviation
CN V (trigeminal nerve) – facial sensation (sensory supply to the face, cornea, and eyelids; partial supply to the jaw)	Facial hypoaesthesia; wide palpebral fissure; unable to close jaw
CN VI (abducens)	Medial deviation; third eyelid immobility
CN VII (facial)	Asymmetry of face; poor taste; decreased secretions of most glands of head
CN VIII (vestibulocochlear)	Impaired hearing; nystagmus; head tilt
CN IX (glossopharyngeal)	Poor taste and feel; dysphagia; voice loss
CN X (vagus)	Regurgitation; voice change; increased heart rate; no crop mobility
CN XI (accessory)	Poor neck movement
CN XII (hypoglossal)	Tongue deviation

19.5 Clinical signs of dysfunction of the cranial nerves in birds (Clippinger *et al.*, 1996).

Diagnostic testing

To increase the chances of localizing a lesion that confirms a neurological diagnosis, it is recommended that all available information be used. The neurological examination should be followed by diagnostic tests, including a CBC, plasma chemistry panel, radiography, cytology, faecal Gram staining and parasite evaluation. Lead and other toxins should be considered (Chapter 20).

Although not available to most veterinary surgeons, electrodiagnostic testing (e.g. electroencephalography, electromyography, electroretinography) can be used to detect cerebral disease, myopathies/neuropathies and retinal health, respectively (Sims, 1996). Scans such as magnetic resonance imaging (MRI) and computed tomography (CT) are useful.

Because birds do not have a cauda equina, lumbar myelograms are difficult to perform and the vertebral venous plexus makes the cisterna approach unreliable. It is difficult to obtain a cerebrospinal fluid (CSF) sample due to location of the collection site, the viscous nature of the CSF and lack of technical experience. There are no recorded normal values for CSF in parrots.

Neurological diseases and conditions

Metabolic diseases

Hypocalcaemia: Hypocalcaemia may be the most common metabolic disease diagnosed in psittacine birds. Clinical signs often associated with hypocalcaemia include convulsions (seizures), tremors, weakness and long bone defects in chicks. Unfortunately it is often difficult to diagnose early-onset hypocalcaemia, because serum/plasma calcium levels are often within normal range. Affected birds may have total blood calcium levels < 2.0 mmol/l. Total calcium measurements are imprecise; they vary not only with the amount of calcium in the bird but also with the albumin levels, as most of the calcium is protein bound.

Ionized calcium is the best measurement to determine the true level of physiologically active calcium (Michael Stanford, personal communication). The normal range of ionized calcium levels in Grey Parrots has been established at 0.96–1.22 mmol/l and any measurement below 0.75 mmol/l is considered suspicious. Birds exhibiting clinical signs of hypocalcaemic tetany have ionized calcium levels of < 0.6 mmol/l and low vitamin D_3 levels. If a Grey Parrot has ionized calcium in the normal range but is clinically ill, an explanation may be due to an alkalosis shifting the calcium level.

Causes of hypocalcaemia in psittacine species include inability to maintain serum calcium levels (e.g. Grey Parrot), which is usually due to a diet lacking in calcium and vitamin D_3 coupled with a lack of sunlight or a phosphorus:calcium imbalance (Chapter 12). A viral infection has been speculated as a cause of parathyroid pathology resulting in an inability of the Grey Parrot to mobilize skeletal calcium, but no viral organism has been identified (Lumeij, 1994b). Kidney or parathyroid abnormalities and infectious disease affecting those organs may reduce the bird's ability to maintain calcium levels. Oral tetracyclines can be chelated with cations such as calcium and magnesium and cause deficiency (Flammer, 1994).

Treatment varies, based on the underlying cause of the hypocalcaemic condition, but calcium and vitamin D_3 supplementation (Chapter 12) should be administered as well as removing the cause of calcium loss.

Hepatic encephalopathy: Convulsions (seizures), ataxia, paresis, depression, anorexia, stupor, coma and proprioceptive deficits are signs described in patients diagnosed with hepatic encephalopathy (Bennett, 1994; Lumeij, 1994a). The clinical signs are associated with portosystemic shunts or hepatic disease resulting in disturbances in brain and brainstem function (Tyler, 1990a,b). Pathophysiological theories for hepatic encephalopathy include:

- Increased levels of neurotoxins, including ammonia
- Alteration of monoamine neurotransmitters as a result of perturbed aromatic amino acid metabolism
- Alteration in amino acid neurotransmitters, gamma-amino butyric acid–glutamate
- Increased cerebral concentrations of endogenous benzodiazepine-like substances (Jones and Orosz, 1996; Tyler, 1990a,b).

Dietary management, treatment of liver disease and treatment with lactulose may help to reduce the neurological signs associated with hepatic encephalopathy (Chapter 20).

Renal disease: Renal disease that may result in renal failure will cause neurological signs similar to those described for other metabolic diseases above: convulsions, stupor, coma, anorexia, vomiting and depression (Lumeij, 1994b). Unfortunately the clinical signs are not present until end-stage renal failure. The pathophysiology of renal-based neuropathy is believed to be uricaemic/uraemic toxins or impaired excretion of other substances (e.g. parathyroid hormone, gastrin) (Lumeij, 1994b).

Hypoglycaemia: Malnutrition, hepatic disease, endocrine disorders, septicaemia, renal diseases, malabsorption and neoplasia are causes of hypoglycaemia in parrots, especially young birds (Forbes, 1996; Jones and Orosz, 1996). Depression, ataxia and seizures are most often noted with birds suffering from hypoglycaemia. Initial treatment should involve glucose supplementation with prolonged therapy concentrated on the disease process that may be involved with the cause of the hypoglycaemic condition.

Toxic diseases

Toxic diseases are discussed in more detail in Chapter 20.

- Lead and zinc are considered the most common causes of metal toxicosis in pet birds, but lead is the primary source that causes neurological signs. Ataxia, convulsions (seizures), paralysis, torticollis, blindness and head tremors are clinical signs associated with lead toxicosis in parrots. Rarely will an owner offer information that will aid in the diagnosis of lead toxicity.

- Chocolate has been identified as a cause of hyperexcitability, seizures and death. Other foods and substances may cause abnormal behaviour.
- Pesticides can cause many neurological signs, usually paralysis of the legs and/or wings.
- Iatrogenic toxicosis through the treatment of protozoal parasites with dimetridazole and metronidazole may cause convulsions, wing beating and opisthotonus; these are reversible by stopping treatment and giving supportive care.
- Although rare, plants or seeds that are ingested may be toxic to parrots (Chapter 20). A good history, which is often provided by the owner, along with some of the plant material will aid in a rapid diagnosis. Until the specifics of the toxin are identified, supportive treatment (including fluid therapy and oral activated charcoal) is recommended, to reduce the absorption of the toxin in the gastrointestinal tract and dilute the toxin's effects within vital organs. Non-specific neurological signs are often associated with cases initiated by plant toxins.

Nutritional diseases

Adverse neurological signs may also be seen with nutritional deficiencies and toxicoses in parrot species. Many birds are fed nutritionally deficient diets (Chapter 12). Most of the neurological disorders associated with nutrition are associated with dietary deficiencies. These nutritional deficiencies will be the focus of this section.

Vitamin E and selenium deficiencies result in encephalomalacia, where a patient will often present with non-specific nervous signs accompanied by muscular dystrophy or exudative diathesis. The nervous signs noted by veterinary surgeons include ataxia, weakness, straddle legs, torticollis, opisthotonus, head tilt and tremors. Diagnosis is made through history, clinical signs, blood testing (blood levels of selenium and/or vitamin E), response to therapy or post-mortem examination of gross lesions and histopathological evaluation of brain/muscle tissues. Gross lesions in a bird suffering from vitamin E and selenium deficiencies are characterized by extensive haemorrhage and oedema in the brain, with necrosis and degeneration of neurons; petechial haemorrhage and oedema are often noted when examining the cerebellum (Klein *et al.*, 1994).

Young birds (7–20 days old) presenting with curled toes, paralysis and weakness fit the parameters for vitamin B_2 (riboflavin) deficiency. Treatment for riboflavin deficiency is vitamin B-complex injections, which are also recommended for the uncommon nutritional deficiency of vitamin B_6 (pyridoxine) in which a bird presents with convulsions, flapping wings and/or a nervous jerky walk. Although vitamin B_1 (thiamine) deficiency is uncommon in pet birds, thiamine may be given to all birds presenting with nervous signs (Forbes, 1996). Common clinical signs observed in parrots that have a thiamine deficiency are opisthotonus, ataxia and/or paresis. Supplementation with thiamine will often cause birds with vitamin B_1 deficiency to have a rapid positive clinical response.

Trauma

Injuries are often the cause when a parrot presents with non-specific neurological signs such as paralysis, paresis, ataxia, torticollis and/or tremors. Owners will readily provide historical accounts of the bird flying into objects such as ceiling fans, sliding glass doors or walls. An important consideration for the veterinary surgeon is the possibility of a neurological cause of the bird flying into that solid object. It should not be assumed that the neurological presentation is only associated with the flight collision trauma. Peripheral neurological deficits may be the result of collateral neurological damage caused by fractured bone fragments, brachial/pelvic nerve avulsion or egg pressure on the ischiadic nerve.

Traumatic CNS injuries require fluid and anti-inflammatory therapy and, if necessary, mannitol and furosemide. In egg-bound hens, the patient should be assessed and treatment should be initiated (Chapter 18). Limb fractures should be stabilized as soon as possible to prevent secondary vascular and nerve damage to the affected extremity.

Neoplasia

Occasionally neoplasia can affect the central or peripheral nervous systems. It is often difficult to diagnose tumours in birds that only present with neurological clinical signs. Often the clinician must carefully rule out other disease diagnoses before listing neoplasia at the top of the differential diagnosis list. Diagnosing tumours, especially CNS neoplasia, is made more difficult because of the expense of CT and MRI as diagnostic aids.

If diagnosis is confirmed, there is little hope for treatment and resolution. Peripheral neuropathies associated with tumour growth may be treated with surgery or chemotherapy. As with any cancer treatment, the bird's owner must be informed of the tumour type, prognosis and quality of life anticipated after treatment.

Budgerigars are the psittacine species most commonly affected by tumours of the nervous system. Tumour types that have been identified with the CNS include astrocytomas, glioblastomas, oligodendrogliomas, choroid plexus papillomas, neuroblastomas, ganglioneuromas, haemangiosarcomas, teratomas, lymphosarcomas and meningiomas and pituitary adenomas (Moulton, 1990; Jones and Orosz, 1996).

Budgerigars are often affected by unilateral leg lameness. Usually trauma must be included as a differential diagnosis but, in Budgerigars, trauma is less likely a cause of unilateral leg lameness than a peripheral neuropathy due to compression of the ischiadic and/or pudendal nerve from an adrenal, gonadal or renal neoplasia (Jones and Orosz, 1996). The most common tumour types that cause ischiadic and/or pudendal nerve compression are renal adenocarcinomas, ovarian or testicular tumours, adrenal tumours and embryonal nephromas. Schwannomas and malignant schwannomas have also been identified as tumour types that cause peripheral neuropathies in parrots.

Abscess

The joints between notarium and synsacrum can be a site of septic arthritis. This forms an abscess that causes spinal cord compression, giving progressive hindlimb paralysis and loss of sensation. The abscess can usually be seen on radiography and, like most septic arthritis, is unresponsive to treatment. There is usually a history of trauma within the last 6 weeks. It is wise to give a course of antibiotic (marbofloxacin is useful) to any bird that is presented after it has flown into a window etc.

Infectious diseases

Infectious diseases are covered in more detail in Chapter 13 but some cause neurological signs.

Viral diseases: There are many viral diseases that cause neurological signs in psittacine species. In some of the viral infections, clinical signs alone will be enough for the veterinary surgeon to make a diagnosis, while others can only be diagnosed by using serological testing or pathology examinations of affected tissue (Chapter 13).

Paramyxoviruses (PMV), containing at least nine known serotypes, are the cause of some of the most well known diseases that produce neurological signs in parrots (Alexander, 1987). Newcastle disease, a paramyxovirus (PMV-1), can cause sudden death, depression, ataxia, torticollis, head tremors, leg/wing paresis and opisthotonus (Forbes, 1996) and is a notifiable disease. Other paramyxovirus serotypes that have been identified in psittacine species are PMV-2, PMV-3 and PMV-5 (Alexander, 1987) (Chapter 13). If the bird survives the acute infection, chronic neurological signs may persist for months (Jones and Orosz, 1986).

Polyomavirus can cause generalized body tremors and ataxia. Other clinical signs include structural feather abnormalities and subcutaneous haemorrhages.

Psittacine proventricular dilatation disease (PDD), while primarily identified with the gastrointestinal tract, has been reported to involve both the central and peripheral nervous systems (Ritchie, 1995). Young birds (< 1 year of age), especially cockatoos, are often the most common group to exhibit neurological signs. Although no specific viral entity has been identified as the aetiological agent for this disease, histopathological evidence points to a virus as the cause.

The togavirus family includes eastern, western and Venezuelan equine encephalitis virus, Highland J virus and avian viral serositis virus (AVSV). Within this group, AVSV has been identified with psittacine species most often; it can result in focal cerebral meningitis, necrotizing encephalitis and non-suppurative encephalitis (Jones and Orosz, 1996). Eastern equine encephalitis has been connected to disease in Eclectus Parrots and Palm Cockatoos. Cross-protection of eastern equine encephalitis has been obtained in psittacine species by using the equine vaccine.

Ataxia and torticollis are the common clinical signs identified in parrots infected with influenza A virus (Ritchie, 1995), another notifiable disease. Although not a common infection in parrots, it has been identified and will cause clinical signs associated with a diseased CNS.

Reovirus is another rare viral infection diagnosed in parrots; Grey and Senegal Parrots and cockatoo species seem to be the most commonly affected. Clinical signs are ataxia, depression and anorexia. Paresis may occur secondary to vascular thrombosis of extremities, resulting in peripheral neuropathies (Forbes, 1996). Diagnosis of reovirus infection is based on histological examination of affected tissues and/or viral isolation.

Bacterial diseases: *Listeria monocytogenes* and *Mycobacterium* spp. can cause granulomas or abscessation in the brain and/or pre-auditory infraorbital sinus that results in CNS neurological signs, including ataxia, depression, torticollis and lateral recumbency. *Staphylococcus aureus*, *Enterococcus* spp., *Salmonella typhimurium*, *Escherichia coli*, *Pasteurella* spp. and *Klebsiella* spp. are other bacteria that may cause neurological signs consistent with an encephalitis (Jones and Orosz, 1996). Lethargy, tremors, seizures and opisthotonus have been noted in parrots infected with *Chlamydophila psittaci*, especially birds that are chronically infected (e.g. Cockatiels) (Gerlach, 1994).

Fungal diseases: Fungal diseases are uncommonly identified as the causative agent of central neurological signs in pet birds. Aspergillosis can develop into secondary cerebral infection and toxin-induced peripheral neuropathies (Greenacre *et al.*, 1992; Forbes, 1996). Mycotoxins in contaminated food can cause generalized neurological signs prior to death and are very difficult to diagnose (Chapter 20). Paralysis or paresis of the legs can be caused by *Aspergillus* invading the kidneys and invading or compressing the lumbosacral plexus; weakness of the wing(s) can be caused by *Aspergillus* in the clavicular air sac invading or compressing the brachial plexus.

Parasites: CNS clinical signs have been caused by *Sarcocystis* spp. and *Filaroides* spp. Although uncommon, the effect of the parasitic infection will often lead to debilitating neurological conditions (e.g. torticollis, wing and leg paresis and/or paralysis, ataxia, circling and muscle tremors). Prevention is the best treatment. Anti-parasitic medications often cannot resolve the initial trauma by eliminating the parasite. Therefore the prognosis is guarded. Another parasite, *Baylisascaris procyonis*, has been identified in North America as a cause of cerebrospinal nematodiasis in psittaciforms (Jones and Orosz, 1996).

Miscellaneous conditions

Other conditions and diseases have been associated with neurological signs in psittacine species. The conditions in this section are rare but should be considered when evaluating a neurological case. Congenital defects, although uncommon, may increase in the future due to reduced genetic diversity as well as artificial incubation. Hyperthermia is a powerful teratogen in embryos.

Idiopathic epilepsy, cerebral vascular complications, stroke, fat embolism during egg laying and atherosclerosis of carotid arteries of Amazons are some of the more obscure disease diagnoses that may be the aetiology behind parrots presenting with neurological clinical signs.

Emergency therapy

As with all cases that present with neurological clinical signs (e.g. seizure, ataxia, paralysis), thorough history taking is recommended and a physical examination to isolate the cause of the condition. If convulsions (seizures) are occurring upon presentation, diazepam (0.3–1.0 mg/kg, i.v. or i.m.) can be given (Forbes, 1996). However, many parrots will require a general anaesthetic, which controls the convulsions, followed by radiography (to look for lead etc.) and a blood sample for glucose and ionized calcium. If the results are not available immediately, the bird should be injected with calcium borogluconate, glucose and edetate calcium disodium (CaEDTA). Anti-inflammatory agents, fluid therapy and antibiotics should also be considered.

Whilst hypocalcaemia, hypoglycaemia and lead poisoning are the commonest causes of convulsions in captive parrots, there are many others (Figure 19.6). If the bird is still convulsant after initial medication, diagnostic testing must be initiated and appropriate treatment given until there is evidence to discontinue.

Neuropathy	Clinical disease
Metabolic	Hypocalcaemia Hepatic encephalopathy Hypoglycaemia
Toxic	Lead Zinc Pesticides Drug reactions Plant
Nutritional	Vitamin E and selenium Thiamine, vitamin B_1 Hypocalcaemia
Trauma	Central nervous system Spinal Peripheral nervous system Neoplasia
Infection	Bacterial Fungal Viral Parasitic
Miscellaneous	Congenital Idiopathic epilepsy

19.6 Differential diagnoses for the convulsant/ neurological case.

Ophthalmology

Parrots have laterally placed eyes and a visual field of about 300 degrees. Their eye is able to discern all the colours that humans can see plus ultraviolet reflected colours. In both companions and aviary birds the ocular anatomy, along with the fact that parrots are prey species, may contribute to owners not being aware of an eye problem in their birds. Avian patients with unilateral ocular disease often face the owner and examiner with their 'good' eye, making assessment of

the affected eye difficult. Understanding parrot ocular anatomy (Chapter 2) will aid the veterinary clinician in examination, diagnosis and prognosis of ophthalmological disease.

Examination

A clinical history should be obtained and a full clinical examination performed as well as an ocular examination. Often primary systemic diseases, both infectious and non-infectious, can lead to secondary clinical signs involving the eye and surrounding structures.

The ophthalmic examination should include menace and palpebral reflexes, Schirmer tear testing, intraocular pressure, fluorescein staining and nasolacrimal function as well as examination of the globe, orbit, lids, conjunctiva, nictitating membrane, cornea, anterior chamber, iris, pupil and lens, vitreous and fundus (Figure 19.7).

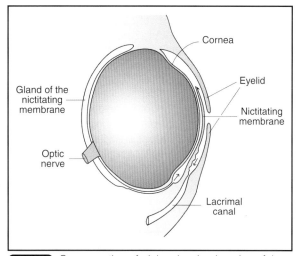

19.7 Cross-section of globe showing location of the gland of the nictitating membrane in relation to the nictitating membrane (third eyelid) and lacrimal canal (see also Figure 2.18).

To examine a parrot's eye, the bird must be restrained in a manner that will allow minimal head and body movement while at the same time inducing little stress and restriction of breathing. With larger parrots, one person may need to hold the body and another to hold the head. Small parrots can be held by one person. General anaesthesia may be required to allow ophthalmological evaluation. The eyes should be examined grossly with a good light such as a pen torch or a Finhoff transilluminator. Magnification is often needed.

- Eyelids should be examined for mobility and abnormal appearance or function. A cotton bud or finger tip should be used to touch around the medial and lateral canthus. The upper eyelid is less mobile than the lower lid, which may aid one's ability to culture the underlying conjunctiva but reduces the exposure of the underlying globe.
- The nictitating membrane (see Figure 2.18) should be clear to translucent and very mobile and can be induced to cover the eye by trying to touch the cornea with a cotton bud or finger.

- The nictitating membrane may trap a foreign body (e.g. sand, dirt) so should be examined on its ocular surface by extension with atraumatic forceps, which will require anaesthesia.
- To test corneal sensation, the cornea should be touched with cotton teased from the tip of a cotton bud.
- To test that the eyes can move within their orbit, the head should be held and the bird allowed to follow a finger or cotton bud using its eyes only.
- Interpretation of the pupillary light reflex is complicated by voluntary constriction and dilation of the pupil. The optic nerves of the parrot decussate completely and so there is no neuronal consensual light reflex (Levine, 1955).

Tear production test

Evaluation of tear production by the Schirmer tear test (STT) (Figure 19.8) is imprecise in parrot species. The published data regarding STT normal values in parrot species are 8 ± 1.5 mm (mean ± SD) for larger psittaciformes and 4 ± 1 mm (mean ± SD) for smaller species (Korbel, 1993). To aid insertion of 6 mm STT strips into the small avian lid margin, the strips should be cut to approximately 4 mm. Tear production should always be measured prior to the administration of anaesthetic eye drops or ophthalmic medication.

Tear production in parrots could be measured using the phenol red thread tear test, a very sensitive method using a fine cotton thread that rapidly absorbs tears and changes colour as the tears soak into it, but there are no reported normal values for psittacine species.

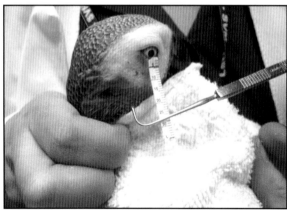

19.8 Schirmer tear test being performed on a Grey Parrot. A blunt-tipped 90 degree probe is used to place testing paper under the ventral lid.

Ocular pressure

Both increased and decreased intraocular pressure can also be measured with slight pressure applied to the anaesthetized cornea using a moist cotton swab. Indentation in the normal eye is approximately 1–2 mm while a hypotonic eye will indent to a greater degree. To desensitize the cornea, a topical anaesthetic agent should be applied to the cornea 15–20 seconds prior to measuring the intraocular pressure. The Schiøtz tonometer and Tonopen (Mentor O&O, Norwell, Maine, USA) produce accurate values (Figure 19.9). The most reliable results are obtained from eyes with corneal

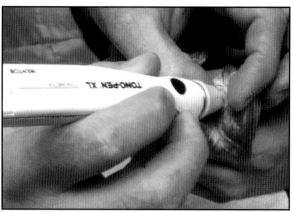

19.9 Tonopen being used to read intraocular pressure in an avian patient.

diameter of 9 mm or larger (e.g. large parrot); they are more imprecise for eyes with corneal diameters of 5–9 mm (e.g. Cockatiels) and unreliable in Budgerigars (Korbel, 1993). In a study using non-psittacine avian species, physiological values of intraocular pressure measured with the Tonopen were 9.2–16.3 mm Hg.

Culture samples

Bacterial and fungal eye infections require culture and sensitivity. Samples should be taken from the conjunctival area under the upper lid prior to the administration of any topical agents. Corneal samples should be taken from the centre and edge of the affected area. Small swabs should be used. The common bacteria from eyes of a clinically normal group of captive parrots were *Staphylococcus* spp. and *Corynebacterium* spp. (Wolf *et al.*,1983).

Anterior and posterior segment evaluation

Anterior segment evaluation should be performed using good light and magnification and, preferably, a slit beam. Normal corneal appearance is clear, smooth and moist. Fluorescein dye should be applied to check for ulceration. The fluid within the anterior chamber should be clear and free of defects. Iris colour varies between species and even in individuals; the normal appearance is uniform, smooth and similar to the other eye. The lens should also be smooth and clear.

To examine the posterior segment, the pupil must be dilated. For a conscious parrot, the drug of choice is vecuronium: one drop applied topically, followed by one drop 2 minutes later, of an 0.8 mg/ml solution in 0.9% NaCl without a surface-acting penetrating agent. If vecuronium is not available, darkening the room may be effective in producing sufficient dilation of the pupil for the posterior chamber and retina to be observed, or the bird can be examined under general anaesthesia, which abolishes the blink and third-eyelid reflex and passively dilates the pupil by relaxing the muscles in the iris. Normal vitreous is clear and intact, while the retina of parrots is grey with a red undertone from the choroid layer. The pecten sits on the optic nerve head. Direct and indirect ophthalmoscopy are both useful. Indirect ophthalmoscopy requires a 30D lens for large parrots; smaller parrots (pupil size > 5mm) require 78D; and Budgerigars require 90D.

Other diagnostic tests

- For cytology, conjunctival cells are obtained from the dorsal inner lid margin. A sterile platinum spatula or a small sterile brush can be used on the conjunctiva and/or cornea.
- Radiography is a useful tool when examining for bony abnormalities within the globe (e.g. scleral ossicles), retrobulbar abscesses, neoplasia or orbital fractures (Paul-Murphy *et al.*, 1990).
- Ultrasonography requires a transducer size of 10–15 MHz.
- Electroretinography can evaluate retinal photoreceptor degeneration and has been evaluated in avian species other than psittaciforms; there may be species differences (Roze, 1990).

Ocular problems

Avian ophthalmic disease categories are similar to those in other animals treated in veterinary clinics, such as trauma and infectious, non-infectious, congenital and nutritional diseases.

Conjunctivitis

Conjunctivitis can be caused by trauma but is often associated with upper respiratory tract infections (Figure 19.10), because discharges and bacteria track back up the tear duct. If there is an abscess associated with the conjunctival inflammation, this should be removed and the area cultured. Although topical antimicrobial treatment will aid in treating conjunctival infections, veterinary surgeons recognize and treat more generalized disease processes in order to prevent recurrence.

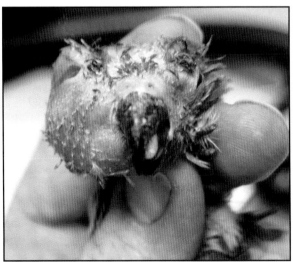

19.10 Sinusitis in a Rainbow Lorikeet. Note the swelling is around the eye. Many cases of sinusitis are presented as ocular problems.

Corneal ulceration

Birds with a corneal ulcer have blepharospasm and photophobia. Causes are foreign bodies, trauma, infection and dry eye. Fluorescein dye is useful. Treatment is usually with a topical antibiotic. Some ulcers worsen rapidly and should be treated with an appropriate antibiotic plus *N*-acetylcysteine or serum (whole blood is taken from the bird and allowed to clot; serum is separated and one drop applied four to six times daily). Both these treatments negate the effects of matrix metalloproteinases. If the corneal ulcer is severe, a third eyelid flap or conjunctival graft may be indicated (see ruptured globe, below).

Dry eye

Keratoconjunctivitis sicca has been identified in parrots suffering from hypovitaminosis A due to a poor and unsupplemented diet (Chapter 12). As well as vitamin A, the bird should receive artificial tears until it has improved.

Enophthalmos

Sunken eye syndrome, or enophthalmos, is often the sequel to a severe upper respiratory infection where periorbital tissues swell (Figure 19.10), or atrophy of the supporting fat pads of the globe or dehydration, in which case the eye sinks into the orbit.

Iris colour

Iris colour is determined by the individual, species, age and gender. It may be modified by disease, injury and dietary deficiency. Most captive parrots have a dark iris that lightens over their first year and becomes lighter until they are geriatric. In older macaws the iris actually changes back to a darker colour from the lighter adult phase (Clubb and Karpinski, 1993). In white cockatoos the male has a darker iris while the female has a red to reddish-orange iris. If the cockatoo's irises that are being examined are not easy to classify as red or black, other means of sexing the bird are required (Chapters 9 and 18). Uveitis will cause the iris to change colour.

Uveitis and vitreal haemorrhage

Uveitis can be due to trauma but may be a sign of systemic disease or autoimmune conditions. The iris will darken with inflammation and there is often an aqueous flare. Treatment is with antibiotic and anti-inflammatory (NSAID or corticosteroid) topically and parenterally. If possible, the pupil should be dilated with an intracameral injection of a mydriatic such as D-tubocurarine (Verschueren and Lumeij, 1991). Usually, topical corticosteroid agents are administered only when no corneal ulceration is present. Idiopathic chronic recurrent uveitis has been described in macaw species. No specific aetiology for this recurrent uveitis was identified but the condition responded to topical corticosteroid treatment and atropine for a short period of time (Lawton, 1993). Primary ophthalmic complications from untreated or recurrent uveitis cases are cataracts and posterior synechiae.

Vitreal haemorrhage may occur after a head injury. The pecten (Chapter 2) is often injured where it attaches to the vitreous. Resolution of the haemorrhage may take months. Detachment of the retina due to clot, scar and adhesion formation is a possible consequence. This can be limited by prolonged anti-inflammatory treatment and mydriasis.

Trauma
Companion parrot species injure their eyes by flying into windows or glass doors or into moving objects such as fans. Eyes can also be injured by other birds in the house or cagemates, or by foreign bodies.

- Eyelid lacerations can be repaired using 0.3–0.5 metric (7-0 to 9-0) polydioxanone. Avoid placing the suture as a full thickness bite through the lid or it may irritate the corneal surface.
- Foreign bodies can become trapped under the eyelid or nictitating membrane. Under local or general anaesthesia, lift the lids and examine carefully, using magnification. Liberal flushing with ophthalmic solution helps to remove the foreign body.

Trauma to the globe often results in ocular presentations of lens luxation, lens capsule rupture, skeletal damage to the orbit and scleral ossicles, iris prolapse, corneal perforation, uveitis and hyphaema; these injuries can result in glaucoma. Anti-inflammatory drugs and mydriasis help to prevent glaucoma. Intraocular pressure should be measured in companion birds as a part of their eye examination.

Ruptured globe
Ruptured globes are an uncommon presentation for psittacine species. If the cornea cannot be repaired, enucleation should be performed (see below). If the cornea can be repaired, a conjunctival graft or a third eyelid flap will support the repair. The flap should be left for 2 weeks; a graft can be left for longer. Both require general anaesthesia. To anchor the third eyelid it is pulled, using atraumatic forceps, from its position in the superior medial fornix of the conjunctiva and sutured to the inferolateral bulbar conjunctiva with two small 0.7 metric (6/0) polydioxanone mattress sutures. This is useful in small birds such as Cockatiels. In large birds the third eyelid's muscle is very strong and sutures usually pull out. In these birds a tarsorrhaphy or even a conjunctival graft may be needed.

A conjunctival graft can be made from the dorsolateral conjunctiva and sutured to the cornea and sclera using 0.7 metric (6/0) polydioxanone on a spatulate cutting needle. The conjunctiva is not as voluminous and the cornea of the bird is thinner than in the dog or cat but the technique is similar to that in dogs and is very useful. It is also possible to suture a collagen graft over a corneal defect.

Retinal degeneration
Retinal degeneration is rarely diagnosed. There is only one report of retinal degeneration in a psittacine species: a 3-year-old Budgerigar. Cataracts were suspected of initiating the degeneration (Tudor and Yard, 1978). As parrots live longer and cataract formation coincides with longevity, this may lead to an increased incidence of retinal degeneration.

Nutritional deficiencies
Although hypovitaminosis A is often associated with respiratory mucosal breakdown, it also affects the epithelium of the eyelids and conjunctiva. Hyperkeratosis leads to swollen eyelids and occluded nasolacrimal ducts. The eyes and respiratory tract become more susceptible to infectious disease, in particular fungi and bacteria. Vitamin supplementation and dietary correction are required, as well as appropriate medical treatment.

Neoplasia
Neoplasia of the eyelids, nictitating membrane, conjunctiva, intraocular tissues and brain have all been recorded. Most ocular tumours do not tend to metastasize but a few have been considered secondary to a distant primary tumour. Tumours associated with the psittacine eye include melanoma, lipogranuloma, basal cell carcinoma, squamous cell carcinoma, xanthoma, cystadenoma, pituitary adenoma, medulloepithelioma and lymphoreticular neoplasm. A fine-needle aspirate followed by excisional biopsy is usually diagnostic. Radiography, ultrasonography and biopsy of underlying tissue are also useful.

Exophthalmos is one of the most common clinical signs associated with a retrobulbar mass. Although abscesses within the infraorbital sinus are common, some cases have an underlying tumour. It is important to find the primary diagnosis so that the owner can be informed about disease assessment, prognosis and possibility for treatment success.

Corneal degeneration and cataracts
Corneal degeneration has been reported in psittacine species but no definitive cause has been identified. Punctate keratitis, possibly caused by an unidentified viral infection and the stress of capture and shipping, was noted as small focal scars on the corneas of quarantined Orange-winged Amazons in the USA at the height of bird importation.

Cataracts have been identified in a number of psittacine species, primarily older birds. The degree of opacity and the stage of progression are used to determine the stage of maturation; cataracts are also classified as congenital and juvenile to senile, depending on the age of onset (Brooks, 1997). Cataract formation has also been associated with skeletal malformations, genetic disorders, nutritional deficiencies, infection, trauma, senescence, toxic effects, uveitis and retinal degeneration. Many large parrots show signs of old age by 30–40 years. Lens opacities are part of the ageing process and microsurgical extracapsular extraction of the lens can help to restore partial sight. An experienced veterinary ophthalmologist should be consulted for any of the surgical procedures mentioned in this chapter.

Infectious diseases

Viral infections: Pet parrots are sometimes affected by ocular viral infections (Chapter 13). Avipoxvirus, a papilloma-like virus, papovavirus and adenovirus-like inclusions have all been associated with ocular disease in parrots, but mostly in imported wild birds. While poxvirus lesions can present as raised nodules on and around the external ocular anatomy (e.g. lids, conjunctiva) most of the viral presentations are non-specific blepharitis and conjunctivitis. Hygiene measures and treatment of secondary fungal and bacterial infections allow most birds to recover from avipoxvirus infections.

Bacterial and fungal infections: Bacterial infections are very common in pet parrots. *Chlamydophila psittaci*, *Mycoplasma gallisepticum*, *Haemophilus* spp., *Nocardia asteroides*, *Pseudomonas aeruginosa*, *Aeromonas hydrophila* and *Staphylococcus* spp. are just a few of the bacterial species that have caused eye disease, and therefore culture and sensitivity are very important.

Mycotic eye infections are rare in parrots but can occur. *Candida albicans*, *Cryptococcus* and *Aspergillus* will cause conjunctival, corneal and intraocular disease. As with bacterial ocular infections, proper antimicrobial therapy is essential to the success of treatment. It is often more difficult to treat mycotic ocular infections, because they tend to invade the mucosa and epithelium. The side effects of parenteral treatment must be considered and the therapeutic regime reassessed if any complications are observed.

Parasites: *Cnemidocoptes pilae*, the scaly face/leg mite, is the most common external parasite infestation in companion avian species. It usually affects Budgerigars and may be passed from parents to the young in the nest. The mite only becomes a clinical problem when the host is immunocompromised, usually through stressful conditions. The scaly face mite causes hyperkeratosis of the featherless areas around the face, including the lids. Diagnosis is made through a skin scraping of affected tissue and observing the mites on a microscope slide under low power. Treatment includes topical mineral oil (to debride the hyperkeratotic tissue and moisten the thickened dry skin) and ivermectin given at 200 µg/kg s.c. or orally. Oral administration requires the water-soluble formulation of ivermectin rather than the propylene glycol product.

Thelazia spp. and *Oxyspirura* spp. are two nematodes that have been identified in the periocular tissues of companion psittacine species. Ivermectin is the drug of choice to treat nematodes in parrots. Nematode infections are rare in companion avian species unless there is contact with imported birds.

Congenital abnormalities: Ocular congenital or developmental abnormalities are rarely reported. Cryptophthalmos, a condition where the skin is continuous over the orbit with no evidence of a ciliary margin, and ankyloblepharon, where the ciliary margins are formed but remain fused, have been reported in four Cockatiels (Buyukmihci *et al.*, 1990). Attempts at surgical correction by reconstructing the palpebral fissures were unsuccessful; the lid margins returned to their preoperative state within 2–3 months of the surgery. A personal attempt to correct a case of an Amazon with a partial ankyloblepharon was successful in separating the fused ciliary margins. The attempt to form a functional ciliary margin in ankyloblepharon cases would appear to have a greater chance for success, since the margins are formed rather than fused as in cryptophthalmos. A congenital symblepharon of the third and upper eyelids was diagnosed in a 6-month-old cockatoo that presented with lagophthalmos and exposure keratitis. The keratitis was resolved by performing a permanent partial lateral canthorrhaphy (Kern *et al.*, 1996).

Choanal atresia (the incomplete development of the choanal openings into the oral cavity) is associated with chronic ocular and nasal discharge. This condition is evident as soon as the chick is first observed in the nest. Nest material is often adhered to the nares and around the eyes. Surgical correction of the choanal atresia (Chapter 11) alleviates the ocular discharge problem.

Ocular surgery

General anaesthesia is required for avian ophthalmic surgery. The bird should be intubated and placed on a mechanical ventilator or have manual positive pressure ventilation administered during surgery. Air sac perfusion anaesthesia may be a reasonable alternative to endotracheal anaesthesia when performing surgery on the head of an avian patient. Air sac perfusion through an air sac cannula does require a higher percentage of anaesthetic gas and volume of oxygen to maintain a surgical plane of anaesthesia than does perfusion through an endotracheal tube. Pulse oximetry or capnography is also recommended. Monitoring of the heart rate is important during eye surgery because of the oculocardiac (trigeminal–vagal) reflex that occurs with the manipulation of the globe; if the rate slows, atropine should be injected.

Proper ophthalmic instrumentation is required for ocular surgery, including magnification (×3 to ×10). Radiosurgery is recommended for surgical techniques where blood loss is a concern; it is an excellent choice for incision, mass removal and vascular haemostasis. Cellulose sponge wedges, cotton-tipped applicators and haemostatic foam will also aid in removal of blood from the surgical field and haemostasis. Haemostatic foam is especially useful when placed in the orbit of a patient that has just had its globe removed. The foam product can be left in the orbit upon closure. The use of 0.7 metric (6/0) or smaller suture material is usually required for eye surgery procedures, and basic surgery techniques used on other small animals are applied to the avian patient.

Enucleation

Severe trauma, ocular tumours, abscesses and panophthalmitis are presentations that may indicate the need for globe removal or evisceration of a parrot eye. Two methods that may be used are a transaural approach and a globe-collapsing procedure. In both techniques a lateral canthotomy is performed prior to a 360 degree subconjunctival dissection. The subconjunctival dissection undermines the conjunctiva, membrana nictitans and periorbital fascia. Surgeons should be aware of two major vessels when performing the subconjunctival dissection: one at the dorsal medial canthus area and the other at the ventrolateral canthus area. Preparation for haemostasis for these vessels will aid in preventing blood loss.

In the transaural approach blunt/blunt tenotomy scissors are used to dissect the globe from the orbit.

Once lifted, haemostats may be used on the vascular attachment prior to separating the globe from the orbit. Gauze sponges and pressure should be used to administer haemostasis to the exposed orbit. Gelatin foam sponge is then placed in the orbit for continued haemostasis and the lid margins are closed with simple interrupted sutures after approximately 2 mm of the ventral and dorsal lid margins are removed along with the conjunctiva and nictitating membrane.

With the globe-collapsing technique, Mayo scissors are used to sever the sclera and its associated ossicles once after subconjunctival dissection. Forceps are then used to access the posterior part of the globe, at which time it is removed similar to the technique described for the transaural approach.

Evisceration of the ocular contents is a procedure that may be considered as an alternative to enucleation. The evisceration technique has been used on companion avian species to preserve the natural symmetry of the head, though there will be collapse of the lid margins closed over the orbit. The cornea, third eyelid and conjunctiva should be removed prior to performing the tarsorrhaphy.

Cataract surgery

The lens of birds is very soft and easily aspirated and their eyes are relatively resistant to postoperative inflammation. Birds seem to be able to focus their eyes after cataract removal: parrots that have had bilateral cataract surgery can fly and alight on a perch. Cataract surgery is relatively easy and rewarding.

Phacoemulsification, using ultrasonic waves emitted through a single needle tip that also includes irrigation and aspiration lines, has been used successfully in avian species to remove cataracts. Because of the size of instrument needed for phacoemulsification, smaller psittacine eyes are not large enough for the widespread use of this technique for the removal of cataracts.

Phacoaspiration using a 26 G needle on a 1 cc syringe is feasible:

1. Place the needle into the lens by insertion through the cornea at the 5 o'clock position, close to the sclera. Avoid touching the iris (it bleeds easily) and enter the lens.
2. Aspirate and infuse the lens' contents to remove the cataract. Aspiration and infusion should be continued until all the lens material is removed.
3. Close the cornea at the site of the needle entry with one 0.5 metric (7/0) absorbable suture.

Postoperative care for phacoaspiration and phacoemulsification includes artificial tears, a topical and parenteral non-steroidal anti-inflammatory medication (carprofen or meloxicam) and topical antibiotic therapy for approximately 10 days.

20

Systemic non-infectious disease

Alistair Lawrie

Hepatic disease

Hepatic disease is commonly encountered in the pet psittacine bird but the identification of liver disorders and differentiating them from other conditions can be difficult for the clinician. The liver can be affected by a variety of conditions that may show no clinical or biochemical evidence of their existence whilst part of the organ is functioning normally. Liver disease is most commonly diagnosed in Amazons, Cockatiels, Budgerigars and cockatoos.

Liver disease may be divided into acute or chronic conditions, many of the acute conditions being infectious (Chapter 13) or toxic. Non-infectious conditions include hepatic lipidosis (fatty liver), fibrosis, haemochromatosis, toxicoses, amyloidosis, neoplasia and hepatic congestion.

Clinical signs

Clinical signs can be very non-specific and are often the classical 'sick bird' signs of anorexia, fluffed-up feathers, depression, polydipsia and polyuria. Poor feather quality, condition and 'darkening' of feather colour may be seen. Beak and claw overgrowth and flaking can occur.

Biliverdinuria is the most obvious sign of extensive hepatic pathology, with affected birds passing green or yellow urates. Visible icterus (hyperbilirubinaemia) of the skin and sclera is not a common feature of hepatic dysfunction in birds, since little bilirubin is produced by erythrocyte degradation. Vomiting, coelomic swelling and dehydration may be observed. Coelomic swelling due to hepatic enlargement may cause tachypnoea or dyspnoea by pressure on the lungs and air sacs.

In cases of 'fatty liver syndrome' there may also be tachycardia and tachypnoea associated with the high viscosity and lipid content of the blood. Weight loss despite polyphagia can be a feature of chronic disease.

If hepatic encephalopathy is present, there may be neurological signs too. These can include tremors and seizures and may be due not solely to raised blood ammonia levels but to the presence of other metabolic products as well (from protein degradation). A vast variation in the blood ammonia levels in healthy parrots is documented and thus signs cannot be correlated with ammonia levels.

Palpation of the caudal border of the enlarged liver is possible in some birds just beyond the caudal edge of the sternum. The 'abdomen' of the normal parrot is small and convex, and distension by organ enlargement or ascitic fluid should be easily detected. Hepatic enlargement can alter the position of the gizzard and make it more easily palpable. In the smaller, thinner patient the liver edge may be visualized by applying surgical spirit to the skin surface.

Diagnosis

Careful history taking is needed, together with observation of the clinical signs and a thorough clinical examination. Blood sampling and a full haematological and plasma biochemical analysis followed by radiography to estimate the size of the liver silhouette (which can be enlarged or smaller than normal) should then be performed. Ultrasonography is better for examining the hepatic architecture (more useful than radiography if the bird is ascitic) and it may be possible to visualize abscesses, cysts or evidence of metastatic disease. A definitive diagnosis is often only possible after laparoscopic examination and liver biopsy (see Figures 9.20 and 9.21).

Haematology

Estimation of the packed cell volume, haemoglobin and leucocyte counts should give some indication of the degree of dehydration, anaemia and the possibility of an infectious cause.

Plasma biochemistry

Plasma biochemical parameters are rarely specific for liver disease in birds (Chapter 7). Elevated aspartate aminotransferase (AST) alone does not establish liver disease, as levels are also raised following muscle cell damage. To differentiate liver from muscle damage, bile acids and creatine kinase (elevated in muscle damage but *not* in liver damage) should also be measured. AST is not necessarily increased in chronic liver conditions and levels may be normal in birds with relatively severe liver pathology.

Moderate to severe elevations in bile acids (250–700 µmol/l) indicate a marked loss of hepatic function and poor prognosis (e.g. severe hepatic fibrosis, bile duct hyperplasia, infections). Minimally elevated levels (50–150 µmol/l) suggest discrete liver lesions with some normally functioning liver remaining (e.g. advanced liver neoplasia such as lymphoma or bile duct carcinoma). Variable elevations in bile acids are seen in fibrosis, lipidosis, hepatic vacuolation and cholangitis. It should be noted that haemolysis and lipaemia may falsely elevate results.

Imaging

An enlarged hepatic silhouette will often be seen (Figure 20.1) but this does not indicate the underlying pathology. It must not be confused with proventricular enlargement (Chapter 9), and barium contrast studies may be needed to differentiate between them (see Figure 21.7). The shadow of a normal liver will fall within a line drawn between the shoulder and the hip joints on the ventrodorsal view. An assessment of cardiac and hepatic shapes and their relationship should be made, since enlargement of both may be from cardiac failure, pericardial effusion, etc. Microhepatica, a feature in some macaws and cockatoos, is of undetermined significance.

Ultrasonography can be useful for differentiating some of the above.

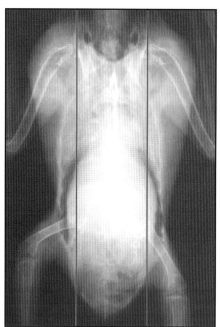

20.1 Hepatic enlargement in an Amazon. The liver silhouette extends beyond (imaginary) lines drawn from shoulder to hip.

Biopsy

Liver biopsy is needed for the definitive diagnosis of hepatic disease. Although it is relatively easy to perform (Chapter 10) the procedure does carry a risk, since blood clotting ability may be compromised in birds with liver disorders. Birds that have prolonged bleeding times after venipuncture or have evidence of thrombocytopenia are not good candidates for liver biopsy.

Indications for liver biopsy are in patients where there is obvious gross pathology or in those that have persistently elevated bile acid values despite therapy (usually for infectious disease) (Chapter 13).

Examination of ascitic fluid

Ascitic fluid should be collected (midline below sternum) and examined. The colour, consistency, pH and specific gravity should be estimated. Liver-related ascitic fluid will normally be a clear transudate or modified transudate. Ascitic fluid may also be present because of reproductive tract, cardiac, peritonitic or other infection-related pathology. Cytology of the fluid is essential (Chapter 7).

Treatment

For some liver diseases there will be very limited or even no therapy. A specific diagnosis may in some cases indicate euthanasia. Treatment in most cases of non-infectious hepatic disease will be supportive or symptomatic.

- Heat and fluids together with feeding by crop tube three or four times a day may be needed.
- Fluid therapy may lead to oedema formation in the hypoalbuminaemic bird and colloids may be needed.
- The administration of lactulose syrup may decrease enteric ammonia production and reduce the pH in the intestines, and giving milk thistle extract is believed to aid liver cell function.
- Vitamin supplementation is definitely worthwhile, as is diet modification, especially in cases with lipidosis. There must be adequate amounts of biotin, choline and methionine.
- Specific antibiotic therapy is indicated if the causative organisms are identified.

Liver diseases

Figure 20.2 summarizes different types of hepatopathy.

Metabolic conditions
Gout (visceral)
Fatty change (e.g. poor diet, diabetes mellitus, hypothyroidism, corticosteroid use, starvation, toxicoses, inherited metabolic problems, amyloidosis)

Neoplastic conditions
Bile duct carcinoma or adenoma; lymphoid leucosis; fibrosarcoma; haemangiosarcoma

Toxic conditions
Aflatoxicosis; corticosteroids; haemochromatosis

Infection-related conditions
Viral: Herpesvirus (Pacheco's disease); polyomavirus; adenovirus; leucosis/sarcoma virus
Bacterial: *Mycobacterium avium*; *Pasteurella multocida*; *Salmonella*; *Yersinia pseudotuberculosis*; *Escherichia coli*; *Chlamydophila psittaci*
Fungal: *Aspergillus fumigatus*
Parasitic: *Plasmodium;* trematodes

20.2 Examples of different types of liver disease.

Hepatic lipidosis

Hepatic lipidosis is a syndrome where there is excessive fat storage and deposition in the liver. The aetiology may involve nutritional (e.g. high dietary fat content, amino acid deficiencies, vitamin deficiencies; Chapter 12), hereditary or toxic factors (lead, arsenic, phosphorus, aflatoxin). There is a high incidence of lipidosis in Amazons and Cockatiels. It may be exacerbated in the egg-laying bird by vitellinogenesis in the hepatic cells (medullary bone may be visible radiographically). Inactivity and being unable to exercise may also be contributing factors.

Clinical signs: These may be variable but include depression, anorexia, polyuria and diarrhoea, biliverdin-uria, poor feather condition, dyspnoea, abdominal enlargement and obesity. Signs of hepatic encephalopathy (ataxia, convulsions and muscle tremors) may also be observed if the liver function is seriously impaired.

Diagnosis: Diagnosis is based upon a complete physical examination and analysis of plasma biochemistry. Plasma enzyme values can be invalidated by the severe lipaemia that is often present, resulting in the blood resembling a strawberry milk shake (Figure 20.3). Bile acid, AST and cholesterol levels may be raised; total protein and albumin levels may be decreased. Radiography will often reveal hepatomegaly but definitive diagnosis requires a liver biopsy.

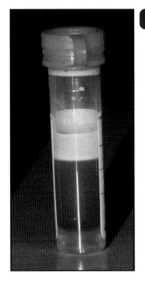

20.3 Lipaemic blood from a macaw.

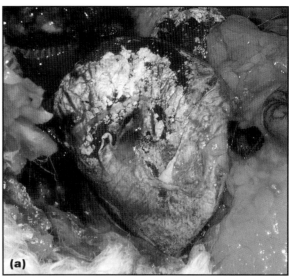

(a)

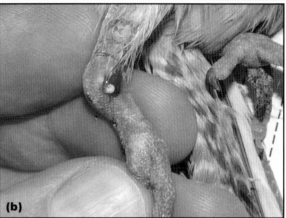

(b)

20.4 (a) Pericardial gout. (b) Articular gout; the diagnosis has been made by nicking the skin covering an affected area (using a 23 G needle), allowing the subcutaneous paste-like uric acid to ooze out.

Treatment: A low-fat diet should be supplied but the bird must not be 'starved' into eating it. Suitable diets are complete formulated pellet diets (Chapter 12) together with fruit and vegetables. Many of the affected birds will be 'addicted' to high-fat seeds and dietary change may be difficult. Intensive care including fluids, heat and nutrition via crop tube may be needed in some patients. They can be critically ill when presented and may still die despite therapy.

Giving additional liver function support by the administration of milk thistle extract has been advocated and also administering lactulose to decrease blood ammonia levels and acidify intestinal contents. L-Carnitine supplementation has been shown to lower blood triglyceride and fatty acid levels in lipomatous Budgerigars (De Voe *et al.*, 2003).

Gout

Visceral gout occurs when uric acid crystals (as white flecks) are deposited on the serosal surface of the liver and other organs (e.g. kidneys and pericardium; Figure 20.4a). It is a serious disease with a poor prognosis. Articular gout is often subcutaneous or periarticular (Figure 20.4b) and together with visceral gout can be as a result of renal disease, high dietary protein and calcium levels and D$_3$ hypervitaminosis.

Clinical signs: These are non-specific and may include weight loss, anorexia and emaciation. Sudden death is not uncommon and may relate to cardiac embarrassment from the pericardial and epicardial urates.

Diagnosis: Plasma uric acid levels are usually elevated but these are not diagnostic, since other conditions can elevate uric acid levels. In a suspected case, laparoscopy is the single most useful investigative procedure. Many cases will only be diagnosed on post-mortem examination (PME) (see Figure 7.34).

Treatment: In the acutely ill bird intensive supportive therapy (especially fluid therapy) is needed with vitamin A administration and an improved diet. Allopurinol administration helps to reduce the plasma levels of uric acid but has no effect on the previously deposited urates.

Haemochromatosis

Haemochromatosis occurs where there is excessive accumulation of iron, causing pathological changes in the liver (and in other organs). It is diagnosed most commonly in toucans and mynah birds but does occur in psittacine birds (particularly lories). The condition seems to arise from an altered intestinal absorption of iron, possibly from an inherited defect, and also from a high dietary iron content.

- Foods high in iron content include: dark green vegetables; grapes; raisins; egg yolk.
- Foods low in iron content include: apples; bananas; pears; plums; pineapples; figs; melons; maize.

Clinical signs: These relate to the physical changes in the liver, namely hepatic enlargement, ascites and swollen abdomen. Fluid accumulation can lead to weakness and respiratory signs (e.g. coughing). Sudden death without previous signs is not uncommon.

Diagnosis: Plasma biochemistry may show an increase in AST levels and a decreased level of plasma proteins, while radiography may reveal hepatomegaly, ascites and sometimes cardiomegaly. Examination of ascitic fluid will show a yellowish transudate. Liver biopsy is required for definitive diagnosis (Prussian blue stain for iron) and monitoring (serial biopsies).

Treatment: Ascitic fluid drainage is imperative if the bird is dyspnoeic. Thereafter, daily removal of 1–2% of the bird's blood volume should be performed until either there is a clinical improvement or the haematocrit reaches the lower end of the range for the species involved. Weekly phlebotomy may need to be carried out to remove blood volumes of about 1% of body weight. Serum albumin should be monitored to ensure that the patient does not become hypoalbuminaemic.

A (pelleted) diet should be fed that is low in iron (below 100 ppm and possibly as low as 25 ppm for frugivorous birds) together with a low vitamin C content (citrus foods, strawberries, kiwi fruit and tomatoes enhance iron uptake). Deferoxamine can be given to reduce the level of iron in body tissues and tea can be given instead of drinking water (tannins decrease iron uptake). The normal level of serum iron is 200 µg/dl.

Even with intensive therapy, the prognosis is not good. Death can be due to myocardial necrosis.

Amyloidosis
Rarely reported in psittacine birds, this disease is usually secondary to chronic infectious or inflammatory conditions. It is diagnosed by biopsy and is progressive and often fatal. Colchicine and ascorbic acid may be useful therapeutically (Chapter 7).

Neoplasia
Metastatic or primary neoplasia can occur. The most common hepatic tumour is the bile duct carcinoma, which is seen most often in Amazons and Green-winged Macaws. Birds affected by cloacal papillomas can develop cholangiocarcinoma and pancreatic neoplasia later. Primary lymphomas, haemangiomas and adenomas may also occur (Chapter 7).

Hepatotoxins
Hepatotoxins can cause necrosis of the parenchymal cells. This results in replacement with fibrosis or lipidosis and can be a progressive situation (chronic active hepatitis) even in the absence of the initial toxin. Widespread fibrosis will result in cirrhosis.

Renal disease

Renal disease is generally greatly under-diagnosed in the avian patient, since signs are mild or non-specific until the advanced stage of the disease is reached. The owner's description of 'diarrhoea' is often polyuria.

Anatomy and physiology
The avian kidney differs significantly from the mammalian kidney in both anatomy and physiology (Chapter 2).

The main nitrogenous waste product of the bird is uric acid, most of which has been synthesized by the liver. Some is filtered through the glomeruli but in a normal healthy psittacine bird over 90% is secreted by the cells of the proximal convoluted tubule. Once in the urine, it combines with proteinaceous mucus to become the familiar white colloidal condensate.

Uric acid secretion is barely affected by the glomerular filtration rate until very low levels of urine flow result in the precipitated materials being unable to flow through the tubules. Blood uric acid levels do not tend to rise in the dehydrated psittacid until dehydration is severe, so that elevated uric acid concentrations indicate either severe dehydration or extensive proximal tubular damage (renal function is below 30% of normal function before uric acid levels are elevated).

Uric acid concentrations above 600 µmol/l may result in tophi (uric acid crystals) being deposited in and around joints (articular gout) or internal organs (visceral gout).

Some birds with extensive renal damage can have normal uric acid concentrations because: (i) some uric acid is eliminated by filtration even though there is secretory tubular damage; (ii) renal failure cases will often be polydipsic/polyuric and thus will have an increased filtration rate; and (iii) uric acid production may be decreased by compromised liver function or anorexia.

Regulation of sodium and water excretion is by the aldosterone–vasotocin–renin–angiotensin system. In the face of water deprivation, birds (unlike mammals) are also able to increase their plasma osmolarity gradually. Again unlike in mammals, plasma potassium and phosphorus levels do not tend to rise significantly nor plasma calcium levels decrease in cases of renal failure.

Urine
Most healthy parrots will produce a moderate amount of urine containing white urates (Appendix 2). They may become coloured for a number of reasons (Figure 20.5). If urates are not examined when recently voided, other colours may leach into them (e.g. from the faecal component or from newsprint).

Because of the close association with urates and faeces, analysis of urine alone can be difficult, but examination of the urinary sediment is worthwhile.

- The normal sample may reveal the presence of casts (very few), some cells (possibly from the cloacal epithelium), small numbers of Gram-positive bacteria (from the faeces/cloaca) and some erythrocytes and leucocytes (not normally >3 per high power field). The presence of many casts indicates renal pathology.

Colour	Possible causes
White	Normal
Green	Biliverdinuria – severe hepatic disease (e.g. chlamydophilosis, herpes hepatitis, fatty liver syndrome)
Brownish/yellow or golden yellow	Hepatic disease Vitamin administration Herpes hepatitis
Red/brown/chocolate	Lead poisoning/other toxins Nephritis Haemolysis Polyomavirus Warfarin-type poisons

20.5 Avian urates. (See Appendix 2.)

- The urine has a lower specific gravity (1.005–1.020 g/ml) than that of mammals.
- The pH values range from 6.5 to 8.0 and a trace of protein may be present.
- Urobilinogen is not present in urine.
- Occasionally a trace of glucose may be detected. This may be stress-associated, or evidence of proximal tubular damage.
- High levels of glycosuria may be seen in diabetic patients or after parenteral dextrose administration.
- Dehydration is probably the commonest of the non-urogenital causes of oliguria.
- Polyuria is not necessarily a sign of renal disease and may have many causes, including stress (Figure 20.6).

Type of disease	Examples
Dietary	Excessive fruit ingestion or pelleted diet; vitamin A deficiency; hypervitaminosis D_3; excess salt or fluid
Psychogenic and stress	Recently weaned; fear; excitement
Hypocalcaemia	
Diabetes mellitus	Glycosuria
Pituitary tumours	Especially Budgerigars; diabetes insipidus; Cushing's syndrome
Systemic infectious diseases and peritonitis	Polyomavirus
Hepatitis	Herpes; chlamydophilosis; tumours; other bacterial infections
Renal disease	Nephritis; neoplasia; gout
Toxins	Lead; zinc; salt; mycotoxins
Chronic disease	Aspergillosis
Iatrogenic	Antibiotics (aminoglycosides); steroids; diuretics
Physiological	Egg-laying female

20.6 Causes of polyuria.

Clinical signs

In most cases, there will only be mild symptoms and renal disease may not even be suspected. In birds, most urinary tract diseases are part of systemic diseases affecting many organs, but there are some diseases that affect only the urinary tract.

- Abnormal urinary output can be polyuria, anuria or oliguria.
- Polydipsia will often accompany polyuria and there may be depression, dehydration and convulsions.
- Polydipsia can be either the *cause* of polyuria (behavioural) or the *result* of polyuria (renal, endocrine). It is a non-specific sign and needs investigation.
- Some renal cases have no change in urinary output.
- 'Normal' urinary output varies with age, species and physiological state and these factors must also be taken into account in the suspected 'renal patient'.

Lameness is a feature of some cases of renal disease and is caused by pressure on the ischiadic nerve by the swollen kidney (Chapter 19).

Aetiology

Infectious agents

These are covered in more detail in Chapter 13 but include the following.

Bacterial infections: Bacterial infections are most commonly acquired from the haematogenous route, resulting in both interstitial nephritis and glomerulonephritis.

Ascending infections appear to be rare in psittaciformes, but tend to be acute and rapidly fatal when they occur. Increased numbers of urinary leucocytes, bacteria and casts might be expected. Culture of urine is indicated but interpretation of blood cultures may be made difficult, since healthy birds can be bacteraemic. Septicaemic birds would usually show signs associated with generalized disease.

Polyuria is often seen in bacterial infections without there being demonstrable renal pathology. A bile pigment nephrosis has been demonstrated in birds with biliverdinuria from hepatitis.

Viral infections: A number of viruses can affect the kidney, including herpesvirus, adenovirus, paramxyovirus and avipoxvirus, as part of a generalized infection process. Polyomavirus infection can induce an immune-complex glomerulonephrosis in nestling psittacids but these birds generally die from other manifestations of the infection and therefore the renal pathology itself is not clinically important.

Fungal infections: Kidney infection by fungal agents is usually as a result of direct spread from air sac granulomas, usually from respiratory mycosis commonly

249

caused by *Aspergillus* spp. Because the infection is localized, specific renal signs are unlikely to be seen, though there may be polyuria or other symptoms of a severe systemic disorder. Thrombotic hyphae in the kidney are sometimes seen as an end-stage lesion in terminal mycotic disease, but this will be a pathological rather than a clinical diagnosis.

Protozoal infections: Microsporidia have been found in association with nephritis in lovebirds. They can be identified in the urine but have not always been associated with histological evidence of inflammation.

Toxicities
Heavy metal toxicity in Amazons is often associated with haematuria and polyuria. Nephrosis may occur in conjunction with liver disease and biliverdinuria. Myoglobin and haemoglobin are known to cause renal conditions in mammals and have been implicated in crush injuries in birds. Poisonous plants, aminoglycosides and other drugs are all potential nephrotoxins in birds and may affect the tubular epithelium directly without inducing an inflammatory response. Polyuria is seen in toxaemias, mycotoxicoses and with excess salt in the diet.

Renal dysfunction
Excessive vitamin D intake (> 100 IU/kg of feed) can cause metastatic mineralization of the kidney and other soft tissues. Polyuria, polydipsia and an inability to concentrate urine may be seen, followed by uricaemia and gout. Metabolic conditions such as gout, haemochromatosis and amyloidosis have all been recorded as causes of renal dysfunction.

Ureteral obstruction (Figure 20.7) can occur as a result of severe dehydration and, it has been postulated, as a result of hypovitaminosis A where there is squamous metaplasia of the ureteral epithelium resulting in obstruction of the ureter. Cloacoliths, tumours and pressure from egg binding are other possible causes of obstruction. Elevated uric acid levels may be seen in these cases.

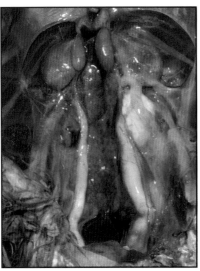

20.7

Nephritis, ureteral blockage, distension and rupture in an Amazon.

Diagnosis
The clinical signs and history may suggest renal problems or the signs may be non-specific (e.g. polyuria). A thorough physical examination is always indicated. To diagnose renal disease accurately, a thorough clinical investigation (including kidney biopsy) is needed.

- Urinalysis is performed by collecting droppings on cellophane or greaseproof paper under the bird's perch and then obtaining as uncontaminated a urine sample as possible by using a syringe or capillary tube to draw it off.
- Routine haematology and complete blood biochemical analysis are needed to differentiate diseases of other organ systems causing renal signs.
- Radiography is essential and ultrasonography useful for visualizing kidney size and density. The renal density and size will vary with dehydration (smaller and more dense), renal gout and nephritis (possibly swollen). Lateral projections are the best radiographic views for size interpretation.
- The colour (normally an evenly coloured dark red/brown), size and shape of the kidney can easily be observed by endoscopy, and biopsy can be performed without causing significant renal compromise. Cysts, neoplasia, renal or visceral gout, aspergillosis, renomegaly and even the absence of a kidney can all be identified.
- By virtue of the lobulated arrangement of nephrons in the avian kidney, it is easier to obtain a representative sample than from a mammal. Usually the cranial and middle lobes are biopsied via a lateral approach through the caudal thoracic air sac (Chapter 9). If a coagulopathy is suspected, a biopsy may be inadvisable.

Other tests include the following:

- Plasma uric acid, total protein and albumin levels are useful parameters to measure and the packed cell volume can be used to assess dehydration.
- Filtration must decrease by 70–80% before plasma uric acid is elevated. The bird can have renal disease but still have normal uric acid levels, since a large number of tubules need to be damaged before the levels rise.
- Hyperphosphataemia is not a significant finding in birds with renal failure but will be seen if there is any degree of sample haemolysis, muscle necrosis or metabolic bone disorder. Similarly, haemolysis (plasma should be separated immediately, or a patient-side test performed) and muscle necrosis are common causes of false hyperkalaemia.

Treatment
It is most important to provide symptomatic therapy until a diagnosis is reached and then identify and treat the underlying cause. Heat, nutritional support and

especially fluids via crop tube should be given to all psittacids with suspected renal disease. Parenteral fluid therapy via intravenous or intraossoeus routes will be required in the most severe cases (Chapter 6).

In debilitated birds, response to treatment will be seen as an increase in appetite, weight gain and improvement in general demeanour. Blood uric acid levels may also decrease in the recovering patient.

Anuria and oliguria

If the patient is anuric or oliguric, the fluid given should be restricted to 20 ml/kg/day to equate with daily fluid loss. Body weight must be accurately monitored daily for signs of over- or under-hydration. Furosemide should be given to increase diuresis. A good quality low-protein diet or a high-calorie diet with little or no protein, sodium or potassium should be fed.

Polyuria

To prevent dehydration, hyponatraemia and hypokalaemia, the hydration and electrolyte status of polyuric birds in acute renal failure must be monitored. Lactated Ringer's solution (Hartmann's) should be administered. Antibiotics are indicated in all cases, since there is a higher susceptibility to renal invasion by portal vein-carried enteric organisms.

It is imperative that non-nephrotoxic antibiotics are administered and that due regard is given to the use of any other potentially toxic drugs in the psittacine bird that is renally compromised.

Vitamin A should be given to birds on poor diets or to those with elevated uric acid levels, many of which will have renal tubular changes. Administering vitamin E and the vitamin B complex will also be of value, especially since many of these birds will have other systemic problems, including anaemia, hepatic disease and anorexia.

Theoretically, uric acid levels are lowered by oral allopurinol. However, it must be borne in mind that long-term use may result in renal damage. In severe cases concurrent use of colchicine may be of some value.

Endocrine diseases

Reproductive hormones are discussed in Chapter 18.

Diabetes mellitus

Diabetes mellitus occurs most commonly in Budgerigars and Cockatiels but has also been reported in Amazons, macaws, Grey Parrots and others. The cause would appear to be related to glucagon excess (plasma glucagon levels 10–50 times those in mammals) rather than hypoinsulinaemia.

The importance of insulin is not well understood in birds and it is released in response to a wide range of stimuli, not just to glucose. It would appear that adrenocorticotrophic hormones and prolactin have a greater effect on blood sugar than insulin has. Many of the diabetic cases seen may, in fact, be Cushingoid. Mitotane therapy could therefore be expected to be successful. Pituitary tumours are common in Budgerigars (Schlumberger, 1954). Glucagon release is normally inhibited by glucose, insulin and somatostatin. Normal avian blood glucose levels are higher than those in mammals and a persistently elevated blood glucose level above 20 mmol/l is needed before a diagnosis of diabetes can be made. It should be noted that glycosuria alone does not indicate diabetes mellitus: it may instead indicate uric acid contamination or the mixing of faeces with urine in the cloaca, as well as renal disease.

Clinical signs: Polydipsia, polyuria, polyphagia, dullness and depression are common. There may be weight loss despite the polyphagia.

Diagnosis: Diagnosis is made on the evidence of persistently high blood glucose levels and response to a glucose tolerance test (2 g glucose/kg is administered orally to the fasting bird and the blood glucose is measured at 10 minutes and 90 minutes after administration).

Treatment: Treatment is not always easy or successful. Many of these birds are relatively small; a highly variable insulin dose is needed for individual birds; and there can be problems of owner compliance with administration of insulin. Insulin resistance can occur and there may also be concomitant pancreatic insufficiency and atrophy.

The dosage of insulin can vary from 0.067 to 3.3 IU/kg q12–24h, but the starting point for most birds will be between 0.1 and 0.2 IU/kg. A glucose curve should be obtained, from which the dose and frequency of administration can be calculated. It can vary from twice daily up to once every few days.

Simply giving a low-carbohydrate diet, such as one of the complete pelleted diets, will often improve many cases. Supplemental vitamins and liver support may also be useful, since some of the birds will be obese and have hepatic lipidosis.

Obviously hypoglycaemia should be avoided and injectable dextrose should be given if this occurs. Some birds will improve clinically yet still have glycosuria and hyperglycaemia. ACTH levels and anti-glucocorticoid therapy should be considered.

Thyroid disease

Hypothyroidism and thyroid hyperplasia (goitre) are more commonly encountered in the smaller psittaciforms (Chapter 21). Hypothyroidism is often suspected in psittacine birds but documentation of the condition is poor (Chapter 16). Many may have low iodine intakes.

Clinical signs: These can include poor feathering (including abnormal colour and defective structure), obesity, stunting, absence of moulting and lipoma formation. As in mammals, thyroxine (T_4) levels can be low due to many factors (e.g. systemic illness, stress, drug therapy). Birds further complicate the picture by having a distinct diurnal variation in T_3 and T_4 levels that may not be detectable at their lowest normal levels. Rapid degradation of these hormones causes a very short half-life (a few hours).

251

Diagnosis: Definitive diagnosis depends on a thyroid-stimulating hormone (TSH) stimulation test. A baseline T_4 is measured and then is measured again 6 hours after TSH administration (1 IU/kg for psittacine birds). A less than 2–3-fold increase over baseline levels is indicative of hypothyroidism. It can be difficult to find laboratories that can accurately measure the low T_4 levels or to source TSH (bovine or human). Hypothyroidism should not be diagnosed by apparent response to therapy alone.

Treatment: Levothyroxine should be administered once or twice daily. Over-supplementation to undiagnosed or euthyroid birds must be avoided, since polydipsia, polyuria, tachycardia, weight loss, convulsions and death can occur.

Parathyroid disease

Parathormone (PTH) is secreted in response to a decrease in plasma calcium concentration. The primary target tissues are kidney and bone, PTH being of particular importance during egg laying where calcium is moved from medullary bone to the eggshell.

Renal production of vitamin D_3, which is also regulated by PTH, can raise blood calcium and inorganic phosphate levels by increasing intestinal absorption. It is also thought to increase renal absorption of calcium and to increase loss of phosphate (Chapter 12). Oestrogens and prolactin stimulate the renal production of vitamin D_3 and so there is a marked increase in blood calcium levels about 4 days before ovulation (partly due to yolk protein-bound calcium).

Nutritional secondary hyperparathyroidism (Chapter 12) is the most common disease process affecting the parathyroids and relates to dietary deficiency of calcium and vitamin D_3 or inappropriate calcium/phosphorus ratios. The result is 'metabolic bone' disease and varying degrees of muscle weakness, tetany and seizures. It is a particular problem in Grey Parrots, which can have difficulty maintaining their blood calcium levels.

Adrenal disease

There is no distinct cortex or medulla. Corticosteroids, aldosterone, epinephrine and norepinephrine are secreted by the cells. Adrenal disease is found at PME of diseased birds and hypo/hyperadrenocorticism may therefore exist. Clinical signs are probably masked by other disease processes in the sick bird. Adrenal neoplasms are rare.

Cardiovascular disease

Cardiovascular disease has for many years been under-diagnosed in the psittacine patient. An awareness that it even exists is important, and that there are now diagnostic techniques that allow cardiac investigation. Electrocardiograms (ECGs), radiography and ultrasonography have advanced the understanding of cardiovascular disease, but there is still a paucity of information.

Cardiovascular examination can be challenging to the clinician, since the rapid heart rate can make detection of murmurs and arrhythmias difficult and there is often difficulty in peripheral pulse detection.

Clinical signs

Signs of heart disease become more obvious with increased severity of the disease. Some are similar to those in mammals (Figure 20.8). Hepatic congestion, dyspnoea and ascites can be seen but coughing is not usually a feature nor is exercise intolerance observed in the caged bird. Sudden death without premonitory signs can occur. Both dyspnoea and ascites can have many other causes in birds, however.

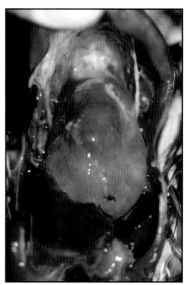

20.8
Grey Parrot with congestive heart failure and pericardial fluid.

Diagnosis

Diagnosis is based upon the history, physical examination (which may have to be brief) and auscultation. A complete haematology and plasma biochemistry analysis together with radiography, ECG and ultrasonography should be performed.

Murmurs can be difficult to classify as systolic or diastolic and there may be cardiac muffling. This can be due to liver enlargement or pericardial effusion. Radiography and ultrasonography should allow an assessment of the cardiac/liver outlines and whether there is cardiomegaly, pericardial effusion, hepatomegaly, ascites or even microcardia. Microcardia is normally associated with hypovolaemia and dehydration.

Electrocardiography

A paper speed of 100 mm/sec and 1 cm = 1 mV is desirable. Recordings are made by placing the patient in dorsal recumbency under anaesthetic and attaching the four leads to the metal part of 25 G needles placed through the skin (propatagium and medial thighs) (Figure 20.9). Alternatively, adhesive pads may be used for ECG lead attachment. Lead II is normally used for monitoring and interpretation.

The amplitude of the waves tends to be low in avian patients and there is little information correlating cardiac pathology and changes in the ECG. It is assumed that the significance of major abnormalities will be similar to that in mammals (e.g. atrial fibrillation, ventricular premature complexes, AV block). ECG abnormalities are described in Figure 20.10.

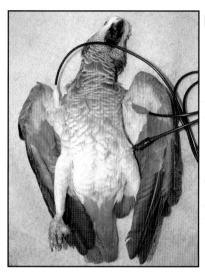

20.9
ECG leads attached to a Grey Parrot. Examination under anaesthetic with the use of ECG, radiography and ultrasonography is probably the most useful way of obtaining a diagnosis for cardiovascular disease.

Abnormality	Possible causes
Atrial premature contractions, fibrillation or flutter	Serious atrial dilatation due to valvular insufficiency
Ventricular premature contractions	Hypokalaemia; thiamine deficiency; vitamin A deficiency; paramyxovirus; avian influenza; myocardial infarction (due to lead toxicity); digoxin toxicity
Ventricular tachycardia, fibrillation and premature contractions	Hypoxic conditions: changes in T wave indicate hypoxia, and more serious abnormalities may follow
Atrioventricular (AV) block	Drug administration (e.g. xylazine); congestive heart failure; atherosclerosis
Small T waves and increasing R waves	Deepening anaesthesia
Arrhythmias	Hypothermia

20.10 Electrocardiographic abnormalities.

Heart diseases

Myocarditis and pericarditis can occur. Pericardial effusion has been recorded together with ascites in cases of congestive cardiac failure. Various infectious agents can also cause pericardial effusion (e.g. *Chlamydophila, Mycobacterium* and other bacteria). Valvular bacterial endocarditis and valvular insufficiencies have also been seen.

Atherosclerotic lesions are common in older parrots and are usually found in the aorta (Figure 20.11), myocardial vessels and brachiocephalic trunk. Many are diagnosed at PME but calcified vessels may be seen on radiographic and ultrasonographic examination.

Treatment

Therapy is based on mammalian treatment regimes:

- Tachycardia and poor contractility can be improved by administering digoxin daily. Digoxin should be used with care and the response monitored with an ECG, since the drug can

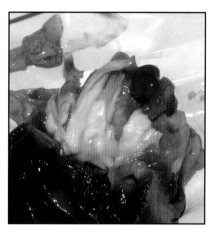

20.11
Atherosclerosis in the aorta of a Grey Parrot.

cause serious side effects such as AV block, bradycardia and atrial fibrillation. Therapy should be discontinued if any arrhythmias develop.
- Diuretics such as furosemide can be given in an attempt to reduce ascites, etc. Monitoring of weight and potassium levels is advised so that hypovolaemia and hypokalaemia can be prevented. This is especially important if furosemide is used together with digoxin.
- Angiotensin-converting enzyme (ACE) inhibitors have been used and may have a place in therapy but there is little information available on their use.

Toxicology

Illness caused by toxins is less common than illness caused by infectious disease. However, the inquisitiveness and chewing behaviour of many members of the Psittaciformes must always make intoxication a possibility (Figure 20.12). In the wild, macaws have the ability to 'neutralize' the effects of eating toxic plants by the ingestion of clay (Gilardi, 1996). Birds in captivity may also be 'programmed' to eat toxic items but do not have access to the necessary dietary antidotes. Their extremely efficient respiratory systems allow inhalant toxicoses to exert a rapid and profound effect. This susceptibility to inhaled toxins has been recognized for a long time.

Route	Examples
Ingestion	Non-food items/foreign bodies Drugs prescribed for people or other pets Toxic food items (chocolate, salt) Infected/spoiled food Storage diseases (mycotoxins) Heavy metals (lead, zinc)
Inhalation	Polytetrafluoroethylene (PTFE) and aerosols
Contact	Nicotine Insecticides Tricothenes
Iatrogenic	Drugs administered by owner or veterinary surgeon (e.g. ivermectin)

20.12 Routes of poisoning.

In the UK, in cases of toxicosis it is worth contacting the Veterinary Poisons Information Service (VPIS), a subscription service that provides advice on all aspects of the treatment of acute toxic exposures. Information received may also help to increase their database. Veterinary practices registered with the VPIS may use either of the following numbers to obtain advice 24 hours a day: (Leeds) 0113 245 0530, (London) 020 7635 9195.

Figure 20.13 outlines a general approach to the treatment of toxicoses.

Prevent further exposure to toxins

Remove bird from source of exposure to toxin
Remove any toxins from feathers, skin or eyes:
* Flush eyes for 30 minutes with saline. Wash feathers with mild, warm detergent
* Thoroughly rinse with water
* Flush acid or caustic alkali with water. (Do not try to neutralize with sodium bicarbonate or vinegar: exothermic reactions cause more damage)
Decrease absorption from GI tract:
* Repeated gavage of crop or proventriculus. Must intubate bird and avoid aspiration. Best carried out within 3 hours of exposure, using activated charcoal or saline
* Surgical removal of solid objects
* Use sodium or magnesium sulphate as cathartics if toxin in lower GI tract (0.5–1 g/kg orally)

Institute supportive therapy

Heat
Warmed oxygen
Fluids – including correcting acid–base balance if needed
Reduce stress

Provide specific antidote if available

20.13 General approach to treatment of toxicoses.

Ingested toxins

Lead poisoning
Lead ingestion is a common cause of poisoning in psittacine birds. There are many source of lead in houses, especially in older houses: lead curtain weights, leaded windows, lead putty, paint, solder, electrical and plumbing clips are fairly obvious examples. Chronic intoxication from car exhaust fumes and licking or chewing lead batteries can also occur.

After ingestion, particulate matter is usually retained by the ventriculus and, because lead is very radiodense, it is easily visible on radiographs. It is important to be aware that the lead particles may have already passed through the bird's enteric tract or that the source of lead may not have been of the particulate variety in the first instance (inhaled or licked).

Lead and its salts are relatively insoluble but the small percentage that is dissolved and absorbed from the gastrointestinal (GI) tract is stored in the bones and soft tissues of the bird. Lead is excreted by the kidneys very slowly (over months).

Clinical signs: Signs of lead poisoning (Figure 20.14) relate to the effect of lead on various body systems and may include blindness, convulsions, tremors, paresis, depression, weakness, vomiting, polydipsia/polyuria, haemoglobinuria (reported in some Amazons and Grey Parrots) and death.

Clinical signs	Reasons for signs
Anorexia, regurgitation, vomiting, diarrhoea ± blood in faeces	Necrosis of GI tract
Anaemia	Damage to erythrocytes and bone marrow depression
Emaciation and polyuria	Hepatic degeneration and necrosis
Seizures, blindness, head tilt, ataxia and paresis of legs and wings	Capillary damage and cerebral oedema
Green/yellow urates	Biliverdinuria from hepatic dysfunction
Pink, red or fawn urates	Haematuria/haemoglobinuria – especially Amazons and Grey Parrots

20.14 Signs of lead poisoning.

The severity of clinical signs varies with the acuteness or chronicity of the intoxication. Speed of onset and severity can also be related to the size of lead particles that have been ingested (small particles having a greater surface area) and also to the amount of abrasive material that is present in the ventriculus.

Diagnosis: A tentative diagnosis can be based on the clinical signs and history. Confirmation is by radiography and finding elevated blood lead levels. Radiography may show extremely radiodense particulate material in the GI tract and sometimes ileus of the upper GI tract (lead shot in muscle does not usually cause symptoms of lead poisoning).

For blood samples, whole blood is collected into lithium heparin tubes (*not* EDTA):

* Levels >0.2 ppm (20 µg/dl, 1.25 µmol/dl)) are suggestive of lead poisoning.
* Levels of 0.5 ppm (50 µg/dl, 2.5 µmol/dl) or above are diagnostic of lead toxicosis.

Treatment: Many of the birds with symptoms of lead toxicosis are extremely unwell and it is imperative that supportive care is instituted before even the full diagnostic work-up is undertaken.

Supportive care: Control of convulsions is the first priority (diazepam), then fluid deficits must be attended to since some individuals will have been vomiting and many will be polyuric. In patients that are vomiting, fluids need to be given by parenteral routes (Chapter 5). General nursing care should include heat, oxygenation, increased humidity and quietness. Low perches should be provided, or consideration given to removing perches if there are central nervous system signs.

Chelation therapy: Intramuscular injections of edetate calcium disodium (CaEDTA) or versenate should be given. Penicillamine can be used, or a combination of both the above therapies.

Chelation therapy is used until signs of toxicosis have resolved (Figure 20.15). It is known that CaEDTA can induce renal damage in mammals; therefore it is generally recommended that therapy is given intramuscularly for 5 days and then stopped for 2 days and repeated as needed, though it has also been given for up to 10 consecutive days or on alternate days for 10–14 days. Oral penicillamine therapy may need to be continued for 36 weeks, although this is unusual.

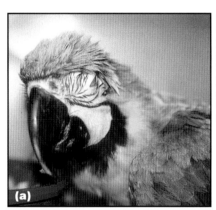
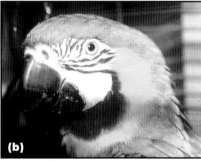

20.15

Lead poisoning in a Blue and Gold Macaw before (a) and after (b) CaEDTA therapy.

Particle removal: Endoscopy or surgery can be postponed as long as the bird is receiving chelation therapy and is improving. Small particles will be passed (confirmed by radiography after 7 days) once intestinal motility has returned and with the aid of bulk diets. Mineral oil, peanut butter, corn oil, sodium sulphate and magnesium sulphate or bulk laxatives can be used to aid the passage of small particles through the GI tract. It may also be necessary to treat the induced diarrhoea.

Surgery: Once the patient's condition is stable, particle removal can be by endoscopic or surgical means. Endoscopic access may be via the oral route or via ingluviotomy, depending upon the size of the patient (Chapter 10).

Gavage: The need for particle removal by gavage is debatable, given the inherent danger of fluid aspiration and the need for the patient to be physiologically stable enough to withstand the procedure. The patient is anaesthetized and intubated with an endotracheal tube of appropriate size. By elevating the rear half of the bird and keeping its head and neck facing downwards, it is possible to flush out the contents of the ventriculus with saline at body temperature (beware of the risk of both hyper- and hypothermia). The flushed-out contents are collected for lead particle examination, or radiography is performed to confirm particle removal.

Zinc poisoning

Genuine zinc poisoning in psittacine birds may occur more frequently than is diagnosed. Conversely, it may be 'over-diagnosed' as a cause of feather chewing. One of the most common sources is newly galvanized wire, which should be treated by brushing with a wire brush and mild acetic acid solution to remove powder and particulate matter before being used in aviaries. Galvanized dishes, coins, car keys, wire, staples, 'Monopoly' game-pieces and even leg rings (some containing up to 17% zinc rather than being pure aluminium) are all sources of zinc, as are some fertilizers.

Unlike the situation with lead toxicity, the ingestion of zinc particulate matter is not as common and therefore radiography is not so helpful diagnostically. Zinc storage is mainly in soft tissues rather than in bones and so, theoretically, removal of the source of zinc should result in reduction of zinc levels in the body.

Clinical signs: These include weakness, polydipsia, polyuria, GI disturbances, weight loss, anaemia, hyperglycaemia and convulsions. Lethargy, weight loss, dysphagia and depression may be more common in chronic cases, and ataxia, recumbency, convulsions and diarrhoea in acute cases. The clinical signs relate to storage in and damage to soft tissue structures, namely pancreatic necrosis and damage to the kidneys, liver and GI system. Elevated blood zinc levels have also been found in some birds that are feather picking or chewing (Chapter 16).

Diagnosis: Zinc toxicosis can exist without radiographic signs or there may be metallic densities in the ventriculus. The measurement of serum zinc concentrations is necessary for confirmation of a suspected diagnosis. Care must be taken with the sampling technique and blood samples must be taken with all-plastic syringes and put into containers of glass or plastic without contact with rubber (e.g. rubber stoppers or syringe plungers). Serum zinc levels > 2 ppm (200 µg/l, 32 µmol/l) are suggestive of zinc toxicosis. The pancreas is the best tissue for post-mortem determination of zinc levels.

Treatment: Treatment for zinc toxicosis is the same as that for lead toxicosis.

Other metal toxicoses

Other metals, such as copper and mercury, may be implicated in cases of metal toxicosis, either by themselves or together with lead or zinc. Penicillamine is the treatment of choice for copper toxicosis.

Chocolate poisoning

Consumption of even small quantities of chocolate can be fatal for psittacine birds. The toxic effects are due to total cocoa solids, theobromine and caffeine content. Bitter (dark) chocolate is generally even more toxic than milk chocolate. Sudden death can occur but more commonly signs of vomiting, diarrhoea and passing dark-coloured faeces are seen. There may also be seizures, cardiac arrhythmias, hyperactivity and ultimately death. Treatment is by administering gastroenteric protectants, cathartics and the provision of general supportive and symptomatic care. Activated charcoal will significantly decrease the half-life of theobromine.

Salt poisoning

If salt is ingested in excessive quantities, signs of salt poisoning may be seen. These are related to the induced cerebral oedema and haemorrhage. Signs are of polydipsia and polyuria, together with neurological disturbances (tremors, opisthotonus, ataxia and convulsions) that can result in death. Diuretics (furosemide) and low sodium fluids may be administered.

Avocado poisoning

Any part of the avocado fruit (*Persea* spp.) may be toxic (stone and flesh – toxin unidentified) for psittacine birds. The toxicity may vary between different varieties of avocado but none of them should be fed to birds. Deaths have been seen as quickly as 10 minutes after eating avocado but more commonly 10–15 hours later. Signs are of anorexia, fluffed feathers, increased respiratory rate, outstretched wings and then death. Subcutaneous oedema has been reported in some birds and pulmonary congestion is seen at PME. Treatment is non-specific and is supportive and symptomatic, such as warmth, fluids and oxygen. Diuretics and activated charcoal can be given.

Household plant toxicities

Many household plants may be poisonous to birds (Figure 20.16) but cases of toxicity may be less common than expected, because the birds will often tear and chew houseplant leaves rather than ingesting them. Toxicity may also be minimized by their fast gut-transit time. In the wild, studies have shown that the deliberate ingestion of clay by some of the psittaciforms helps to adsorb toxins of plants that would otherwise cause poisoning. Treatment is symptomatic.

Mycotoxins

Mycotoxins are chemical metabolites produced by some fungi; for a particular fungus, the conditions for the production of a mycotoxin may be very specific. There are many mycotoxins but the clinically significant ones for the psittacine bird are aflatoxin, ochratoxin, deoxynivalenol (vomitoxin) and tricothenes (contact dermatitis is a possibility with the tricothenes).

Mycotoxins are undetectable by sight, smell or taste and may be present with no visible signs of mould (fungus) growth (e.g. aflatoxin in peanuts). The amount of toxin produced may vary and is also variable within different parts of a batch of food. If birds are fed soaked or sprouted seeds, thorough and regular rinsing is needed to prevent bacterial and fungal growth.

Clinical signs: These relate to hepatotoxicity and there may be prolonged clotting times, kidney dysfunction and depressed immune system function. Depression, haemorrhages, anorexia, polyuria, erosive lesions of the oral mucosa, constriction of digits, immunosuppression and neurological disorders can all be seen.

Diagnosis: This is difficult in the live bird since signs are non-specific and vague or mimic other diseases. Diagnosis is based on the finding of mycotoxins in the food or the GI tract. Unfortunately, the food may not be available for testing since it may all have been ingested or consumed some time previously. Culturing the fungi and identifying mycotoxins can be a lengthy process.

Common name	Species	Common name	Species
Aloe	*Aloeaceae* spp.	Kalanchoe	*Kalanchoe* spp.
Asparagus fern	*Asparagus plumosus*	Lily-of-the-valley	*Convallaria* spp.
Autumn crocus	*Colchicum autumnale*	Lupin	*Lupinus* spp.
Avocado	*Persea americana*	Mistletoe	*Viscum album*
Azalea	*Rhododendron* spp.	Mother-in-law's tongue	*Sansevieria trifasciata*
Castor bean	*Ricinus communis*	Narcissus	*Narcissus* spp.
Christmas rose	*Helleborus* spp.	Oleander	*Nerium oleander*
Clematis	*Clematis* spp.	Onion	*Allium* spp.
Cyclamen	*Cyclamen persicum*	Philodendron	*Philodendron bipinnatifidum*
Daffodil	*Narcissus* spp.	Poinsettia	*Euphorbia pulcherrima*
Deadly nightshade	*Atropa belladonna*	Rhododendron	*Rhododendron* spp.
English ivy	*Hedera helix*	Swiss cheese plant	*Monstera deliciosa*
Foxglove	*Digitalis* spp.	Tiger lily	*Lilium lancifolium*
Gladiolus	*Gladiolus* spp.	Tomato plant	*Lycopersicon esculentum*
Holly	*Ilex* spp.	Tulip	*Tulipa* spp.
Hyacinth	*Hyacinthus* spp.	Virginia creeper	*Parthenocissus quinquefolia*
Hydrangea	*Hydrangea* spp.	Yew	*Taxus* spp.
Iris	*Iris* spp.		

20.16 Some plants toxic to psittacine species.

Post-mortem examination:

- Aflatoxin (*Aspergillus* spp.) is hepatotoxic and causes hepatic cell degeneration and bile duct necrosis. An enlarged pale liver and enlargement of the spleen and pancreas are seen on PME. GI haemorrhage from altered clotting ability is common. Often it is peanut-associated.
- Tricothenes (*Fusarium* spp.) cause necrotic lesions from ulceration of the oropharynx and GI tract.
- Ochratoxin (*Penicillium* and *Aspergillus* spp.) signs are non-specific, and often secondary infections are present due to immune system depression (e.g. air sacculitis). It is also both hepatotoxic and nephrotoxic.

Pesticides

Pesticide intoxication can arise from the direct application of pesticides to the bird, indirect contact (e.g. impregnated insect repellent strips), or by contact with household pesticides. The risk from residual pesticides applied to foodstuffs is unknown. Accidental ingestion of insecticide is also possible (e.g. naphthalene and para-dichlorobenzene, found in mothballs).

Pyrethrins (often combined with piperonyl butoxide) have the lowest toxicity for birds when applied topically. However, they can be toxic if applied at high concentrations or following inhalation.

Clinical signs: Signs of toxicity are weakness, anorexia, central nervous system signs, dyspnoea and death. With organophosphate exposure, delayed toxicosis can occur 7–10 days later. These signs are due to an induced neuropathy rather than inhibition of acetylcholine activity.

Diagnosis: Diagnosis is made on the history of possible exposure to pesticide and on the clinical signs. A plasma cholinesterase assay (to measure depression of cholinesterase) may confirm organophosphate and carbamate toxicity. Post-mortem diagnosis from GI contents or tissues is possible.

Treatment: Atropine and pralidoxime chloride (2-PAM) are administered for acute organophosphate toxicosis, and atropine alone for carbamate poisoning. Supportive care and treatment of lung oedema may be needed.

Inhaled toxins

Polytetrafluoroethylene (PTFE) poisoning

PTFE is a gas released by heating 'non-stick' coatings such as Teflon, which is found on the surface of irons, ironing-board covers and non-stick pans (Chapter 14). Heating to 260°C (530°F) causes pyrolysis and release of the PTFE gas (hydrogen fluoride, carbonyl fluoride, perfluoroisobutylene plus irritating particles) which is odourless and invisible. The avian lungs are the primary target area of the toxin.

Clinical signs: Sudden death or collapse are the commonest manifestations of toxicity. If the bird is still alive, clinical signs are those associated with haemorrhage and congestion of the lungs: wheezing, dyspnoea, rales, ataxia and terminal convulsions.

Treatment: Death usually occurs too rapidly for treatment to be given. If the patient is still alive, intensive therapy is indicated. The bird should be placed in an oxygen chamber and systemic and nebulized prednisolone and/or heparin administered. Warmth, fluids and broad-spectrum antibiotics may help, together with diuretics (furosemide) to treat the pulmonary oedema.

Confirmation: Haemorrhage and congestion of the lungs are found on PME and occasionally PTFE particles may be found histologically.

Nicotine poisoning

Passive inhalation occurs in psittacine birds that reside in households with heavy smokers. Toxicity can also occur through ingestion of tobacco from cigarettes or from the bird's feathers. Cotinine, a nicotine metabolite, has been found in birds at almost the same levels as in human smokers in the same household (Chapter 7).

Clinical signs: Signs may be of a respiratory or ocular problem. There can be sneezing, coughing, sinusitis and conjunctivitis due to chronic respiratory tract irritation. Nicotine exposure can be part of feather chewing or plucking syndromes or other contact dermatoses, including facial dermatosis (Grey Parrots or macaws with non-feathered skin) or pedal dermatosis (Chapter 16). Contact with nicotine-contaminated fingers can be enough to cause signs. Self-mutilation can occur and there may also be excitability, vomiting, diarrhoea and seizures. The amount of smoking/nicotine-related disease in birds (e.g. cardiac, cancer and allergies) is unknown at present. The ingestion of nicotine, even in small quantities, can cause death.

Treatment: Treatment is supportive, with activated charcoal, mineral oil and fluids, and symptomatic therapy as in cases of ingested toxicosis. In respiratory syndrome cases, the bird must be removed from sources of nicotine.

Household toxins

Most household aerosols will cause direct irritation of the pet psittacine bird's respiratory system, through either the fluorocarbon content or the particulate matter within the aerosol. Care must be exercised when using deodorant sprays, perfumes and other household aerosols.

Any household gas leak or carbon monoxide build-up can result in sudden death of birds in the house. Carbon monoxide combines with haemoglobin to form carboxyhaemoglobin and reduces the ability of oxygen to dissociate from haemoglobin. Cases occur more commonly in late autumn, when heating systems are switched on. Signs of dyspnoea and sleepiness may be seen, and death results from hypoxia. The tissues and blood may appear bright pink on PME. Treatment is by providing a quiet, oxygen-enriched environment (but oxygen toxicosis can occur if birds are given 100% oxygen for long periods).

Overheating of cooking oils releases toxic acroleins and will also cause smoke inhalation problems. Smoke causes hypoxaemia by displacement of oxygen from the air and thermal burns to the respiratory system. If a humidified, oxygenated and stress-free environment is provided and supportive treatment for lung oedema and bronchospasm are given, pulmonary failure as a result of irritant gases may be delayed. Treatment and monitoring may be needed for up to 3 weeks after exposure.

Iatrogenic toxicoses

For vitamin overdosage and supplementation, see Chapter 12.

Ivermectin

Fatalities have occurred after ivermectin injection. They can be due to overdosage of the ivermectin but may also be from possible propylene glycol toxicity in the smaller psittaciforms (e.g Budgerigars). Blindness, seizures and death can occur. Intensive nursing and fluids may save some patients. Administering dexamethasone has helped some cases of toxicity.

Dimetridazole/metronidazole

Toxic signs are tremors, convulsions and extensor rigidity. Deaths have been seen in Budgerigars and Cockatiels following administration in drinking water. An increased consumption of water by breeding female birds and whilst rearing young will increase the risk of toxic problems. Nestlings in this situation will also be at risk. Toxicity is usually reversible if fluids are administered. Multiple haemorrhages and pale, enlarged livers and kidneys are seen on PME.

Antibiotics

Nephrotoxicity may be seen with aminoglycoside administration and where there is impaired renal perfusion. Cephalosporins, tetracyclines and parenteral amphotericin B may also be nephrotoxic.

Drugs

Although not classed as toxicoses, some drugs will cause GI tract disturbances in certain birds. Macaws are particularly sensitive to the administration of trimethoprim/sulphonamide and doxycycline suspensions and also to ketoconazole. Reddening of the facial skin, vomiting and depression can occur.

The vomiting bird

Vomiting in birds is a diagnostic challenge and often necessitates a full diagnostic investigation before a specific diagnosis can be made. Some birds vomit because of GI problems (Chapter 15) but many cases are not GI-related (Figure 20.17).

Vomiting must be distinguished from regurgitation:

- *Regurgitation* is expulsion of ingesta from the crop and is physiologically normal (e.g. courtship/ feeding behaviour to a mate, owner or mirror)
- *Vomiting* is expulsion of ingesta from the proventriculus or crop and is associated with illness and, commonly, depression and dehydration. It may occur alone or in conjunction with other GI signs.

Infectious agents (Chapter 13)

Viruses
Bacteria: Gram-negatives; *Chlamydophila; Mycobacterium*
Fungi: *Candida albicans; Mucor;* 'megabacterium'
Parasites

Metabolic dysfunction

Liver: infection; metabolic change (fatty liver, haemochromatosis); toxicity; neoplasia
Kidney: gout; nephritis; infection
Endocrine: thyroid hyperplasia; pancreatitis?
Reproductive: egg binding; egg peritonitis

Toxicity

Pesticides: organophosphates; carbamates; organochlorines
Household: bleach; detergents; disinfectants; matches; PTFE (Teflon); houseplants
Heavy metals: lead; zinc; mercury; copper
Food: mycotoxins; chocolate; alcohol; avocados; salt
Drugs: levamisole; enrofloxacin; doxycycline; trimethoprim; azoles

Miscellaneous

Behavioural: fear; excitement; motion sickness; courtship
Physiological: over-feeding
Nutritional: food allergy; vitamin A and E deficiencies
Crop stasis: bacterial or yeast infections; hand-rearing food at incorrect temperature; impactions; pendulous crop
Foreign bodies: ingluvioliths
Neoplasia
Goitre
Intussusception
Ileus
Callus formation after coracoid fracture

20.17   Causes of vomiting.

Signs

Food or mucus may be found on the floor of the cage, feathers, face (often on crown), perches and walls. Observation of the demeanour of the patient and for evidence of polydipsia/polyuria are important.

Some conditions may be commoner in certain species, such as *Trichomonas* infection in Budgerigars, hepatitis and Gram-negative infections in Amazons, megabacteria and thyroid hyperplasia (goitre) in Budgerigars, and haemochromatosis in lories.

History

If numerous birds are affected, infectious or toxic agents are more likely. Single birds in isolation are more likely to be affected by toxic, foreign body, reproductive, nutritional or neoplastic conditions.

The life stage may be important (for example, being hand fed increases the likelihood of candidiasis and crop burns), as is the dietary history (e.g. the type of food, freshness, high iron content or the overeating of grit).

Physical examination

A complete physical examination is essential:

- Check for oral lesions such as ulcers, plaques, papillomas, granulomas or pox lesions
- Palpate the crop and look for impaction, distension, foreign body, excess grit or burns
- There may be weight loss, with or without abdominal distension and GI signs; for example, tenesmus or abnormal droppings might be observed
- Respiratory signs can occur either as part of systemic disease or due to liver enlargement and air sac restriction. Egg binding must also be considered.

Vomiting with neurological signs can occur in viral diseases, such as Pacheco's disease, polyomavirus infection or proventricular dilatation disease (Chapter 13), or with liver disease or lead or zinc toxicosis.

Investigation

A diagnostic plan is essential. It is important that the condition of the severely ill bird is stabilized before stressful investigations are performed. Tests are selected based on history, signalment, physical examination and evaluation of droppings.

- Make impression smears of oral lesions (Chapter 7) and then perform a crop aspirate (both a wet mount and Gram's stain), with or without culture and sensitivity and fungal culture.
- Faecal examination should include gross examination, flotation for parasites and Gram staining for bacteria and avian gastric yeasts. The colour and form of droppings (Appendix 2) and the presence of undigested seeds are important. These tests are simple, cheap and relatively stress-free and should always be carried out.

- Perform a complete haematological and blood biochemistry examination, looking for infectious, inflammatory, metabolic or toxic causes (aspartate aminotransferase (AST), urea, creatine kinase (CK), total protein, amylase, lipase and bile acids if liver involvement suspected).
- Radiography is important to identify lead and zinc particles, grit, ingluvioliths, enteritis, foreign bodies, trauma and liver and proventriculus size and to evaluate the respiratory tract and abdominal organs (for eggs too). Be aware that lead and zinc toxicity can occur without radiographic signs.

The following tests, although useful, may be limited by financial constraints or lack of expertise and equipment in general practice:

- Fluoroscopy/barium studies can assess proventricular activity and dilatation; and biopsy samples and endoscopy can be peformed as indicated.
- PCR testing can be used for specific organisms, e.g. *Chlamydophila,* polyomavirus.

Treatment

Therapy obviously depends upon the cause of the vomiting and therefore a *specific* diagnosis is needed (Figure 20.18).

- Treat the underlying cause and provide supportive care while treating that cause (e.g. fluids).
- Withhold food until the vomiting has stopped.
- Metoclopramide has been used intramuscularly twice daily but be aware of potential side effects (sedation and extrapyramidal effects).

Disease	Therapy
Oral lesions	Poxvirus, vitamin A therapy, bacterial infections: symptomatic treatment
Crop lesions	Surgery – for burns and foreign bodies, crop flushing; support 'bra' for pendulous crops (see Figure 18.9); proventricular tube placement; correct dehydration by giving liquid food; iodine if goitre
Candidiasis	Nystatin, fluconazole or ketoconazole
Trichomoniasis	Metronidazole, dimetridazole or carnidazole
Proventricular lesions	Megabacteriosis: amphotericin B plus cider apple vinegar in drinking water
Proventricular dilatation disease	See Chapters 13 and 15
Gizzard worms	Fenbendazole or ivermectin
Enteric bacterial disease	Treat according to culture and sensitivity testing
Hepatic disease	Supportive: antibiotics, B vitamins, choline, lactulose syrup, milk thistle extract; low-protein, high-carbohydrate diet; metronidazole or neomycin to reduce colonic bacterial numbers
Poisoning	See Toxicology
Reproduction-related	See Chapter 18 – treat the cause

20.18 Therapy for vomiting.

Abdominal/coelomic distension

The 'abdomen' of the normal, healthy psittacine bird is relatively small and externally is concave from the pelvis to the sternum. The body wall is composed of skin, muscle and peritoneal lining and is usually a fairly thin structure. Any gross alterations in the size of the abdominal organs or accumulations of fluid are thus easily detectable, but swelling may not be noticed by the bird's owner until relatively late in the disease process.

Early signs may be faecal material sticking to the cloacal area as the abdomen distends and pushes the cloaca dorsally. The swelling may progress to feather loss over the area, difficulty in perching and trauma to the skin. Pathological changes in the muscle or skin (e.g. xanthomatosis) may lead to weakness and hernia formation (Figure 20.19).

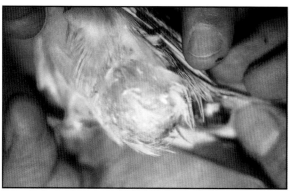

20.19 Coelomic distension and hernia in a Budgerigar.

The absence of a diaphragm in the coelomic cavity of the bird means that any increase in intracoelomic pressure can result in a variety of symptoms due to the effects on various organ systems. The air sacs will be restricted and can result in quite serious 'respiratory' symptoms (Chapter 14). Similarly, there may be vomiting, anorexia, signs of intestinal obstruction or difficulty in passing droppings.

Abdominal distension is a normal feature of the neonatal psittacid, with the liver appearing enlarged and the viscera being visible.

Distension caused by organ enlargement

The normal liver is not palpable as it does not extend beyond the ventral border of the sternum. It may increase in size because of infection (Chapters 13 and 15), congestion (cardiac failure), neoplasia, or other liver pathology, such as cirrhosis or haemochromatosis, lipidosis or hepatoma (see Figure 7.32). Visualization of the posterior border of the enlarged liver is often possible in the thin bird by application of surgical spirit to the skin. *Chlamydophila* infection must always be considered as an important cause of hepatic enlargement. Radiography will indicate whether there is hepatic enlargement.

Splenic enlargement will often be concurrent with hepatic enlargement as part of a systemic infection. Splenic tumours and lymphoid infiltration must also be considered. The spleen may easily be visualized by radiography (Chapter 9).

Minor swelling of the kidneys may not be detectable as a cause of coelomic distension, but may cause other signs (e.g. lameness). Greater enlargement will cause obvious coelomic distension and often displacement of other organs (e.g. ventriculus). This may be palpated or seen radiographically to be in an abnormal position. A fairly common syndrome in Budgerigars is that of renal neoplasia associated with leucosis/sarcoma virus, often manifested as unilateral lameness with coelomic distension.

Pathological conditions of the GI tract may cause abdominal distension, either by neoplastic infiltration or by distension of various parts of the GI tract. Proventricular dilatation may produce an obvious distension and may have a number of causes (Chapter 15). Radiography (plain and contrast studies) and fluoroscopy are particularly useful in these cases.

In the smaller, thinner psittacine bird, intestinal lumen distension from heavy parasite (ascarid) infestations may result in a palpable coelomic distension and signs of intestinal obstruction (Chapters 15 and 21). Faecal examination should aid diagnosis.

Reproductive tract disorders are fairly common causes of coelomic distension and the sex of the patient needs to be known. Physiological enlargement of the testicle (although occasionally quite massive) when males are in breeding condition does not usually result in abdominal distension; neither does orchitis. Testicular tumours, however, can grow to a considerable size and will often result in abdominal distension together with a variety of other signs. These may include feminization, vomiting, weight loss and lameness. Seminomas and Sertoli cell tumours both occur (Chapter 18), as can retrovirus-induced neoplasms (leucosis/sarcoma virus).

Disorders of the female reproductive tract (Chapter 18) are commonly associated with coelomic distension. They may vary from simple cases of 'egg binding' to more chronic salpingitis and oviductal enlargement or oviductal tumours. Ovarian cysts and tumours may also occur. Older hens may have abdominal hernias concurrently with reproductive tract problems. Egg peritonitis may result in the accumulation of coelomic fluid. Ova are ovulated directly into the coelomic cavity or are ejected from the oviduct by reverse peristalsis. Diagnosis is aided by paracentesis, cytological examination of the fluid and detection of 'egg yolk' in blood samples (Chapter 7).

Fluid may also be present as a result of sepsis (e.g. intestinal perforation) or as an effusion from neoplasia. Intracoelomic haemorrhage can also occur. Abdominal fluid that is present as the result of congestive heart failure or hepatic failure is genuinely 'ascitic' fluid. Other clinical signs and fluid analysis should help the diagnosis.

Air sac distension may cause coelomic enlargement if the bird is unable to expel air from the caudal thoracic and abdominal air sacs because of anterior airway obstruction (e.g. aspergillosis). Parrots that are excessively fat or that have internal lipomas can also have abdominal distension.

Investigation

The patient with abdominal swelling should be observed, inspected and then gently palpated. There is a distinct risk of organ or fluid rupture into the air sacs and death by drowning. Palpation of the gizzard and identifying its position may give some indication of the location of an abdominal mass. Abdominocentesis must be done with care so that there is no leakage of fluid into the air sacs. Good restraint, asepsis and accurate mid-line needle puncture below the sternum are needed.

With radiography and ultrasonography, extreme care must be taken if the bird is to be placed in dorsal recumbency, as respiratory function can be compromised. Standing survey radiographs taken with the patient in a cardboard box are much safer (see Figure 9.7). The presence of medullary bone in the femur and humerus will point to ovulatory activity in the female bird.

Ultimately organ biopsy or exploratory laparotomy may be needed (Chapter 10) for diagnosis or treatment. Treatment depends on the cause and may be medical or surgical.

The thin bird

As the normal weight of many species of parrot has a wide range (e.g. Grey Parrots 385–585 g), an assessment is made of the bulk of pectoral muscle mass and the amount of subcutaneous fat present. 'Thinness' can be the end result of many conditions. Psittacine birds will become thin as a result of starvation, anorexia or cachexia associated with disease processes.

A diagnosis of malnutrition requires some knowledge of the patient's nutritional history and the absence of any clinical signs of disease. The type and quality of food offered must be known, as must also the amounts given and, more importantly, the amount consumed.

It will be necessary to assess whether the bird is actually able to eat (e.g. problems in the oral cavity, damaged beak) and whether it recognizes the substances offered as 'food' (e.g. changing from seeds to pellets) (Figure 20.20). Some birds may want to eat but have been kept away from food containers by more dominant companions; others may be thin because of normal physiological conditions, such as after feeding consecutive nests of young.

Birds that have suffered some weight loss and then become dehydrated will appear to be even thinner. An assessment of their hydration state and their weight at initial examination is therefore needed. Dehydration may be the end result of inadequate fluid intake but is more likely to be because the patient is experiencing excessive fluid loss from either vomiting or diarrhoea.

Many thin birds will, of course, be eating normally, or even excessively, depending on what the underlying pathological condition is (Figure 20.21).

A full diagnostic investigation is needed to find the cause of thinness (Chapters 6, 7 and 9). This must include full haematology, biochemistry, diagnostic cytology of crop and faeces and radiography. Investigations (Appendix 1) are necessary for diagnosis of the causes of wasting. Severely ill or debilitated birds should be stabilized before intensive or invasive investigations begin.

Type of disease	Examples
General systemic illness	Hepatitis/splenitis/air sacculitis Respiratory problems where patient is either dyspnoeic or tachypnoeic and has difficulty eating Sinusitis and ocular inflammation can also greatly reduce bird's appetite
Conditions of the GI tract	Oral cavity – injuries to beak, hypovitaminosis A and associated tongue lesions, papillomatosis Crop problems – impactions, infections, obstructions (e.g. thyroid gland enlargement), ingluvioliths Proventricular dilatation disease, Megabacteria (?pain from proventricular ulceration) Intestinal obstruction (e.g. parasites) Coelomic masses – tumours, air sac masses, eggs, fluid accumulation Toxicoses – ingested heavy metals (e.g. lead, zinc)
Terminal illness	Too ill to eat
Painful limb joints	Some birds that use their feet to eat (e.g. cockatoos) may have difficulty eating if they have painful limbs

20.20 Causes of not eating.

Type of disease	Examples
GI conditions	Parasitic infections: ascarid worms or protozoal infections (e.g. *Giardia, Trichomonas*); tapeworm infections Enteritis: chronic inflammation from bacterial infections Fungal infections: 'megabacteriosis' results in alteration of pH and digestive function of proventriculus; candidiasis can cause weight loss or lack of weight gain, especially in young bird Insidious blood loss from ulceration may also contribute to general debility Tumours: anywhere within GI tract or associated organs, e.g. pancreas and bile duct (especially in older macaws and Amazons that have had cloacal papillomas) Chronic hepatic disease: chronic hepatitis or other pathological changes in liver Chronic or mild forms of proventricular dilatation disease
Renal diseases	Nephritis: under-diagnosed in all birds. Some have obvious clinical signs of polyuria, haematuria, etc., most diagnosed by complete diagnostic work-up, possibly including kidney biopsy (Chapter 10)
Chronic infections (Chapter 13)	*Mycobacterium avium, Aspergillus* spp. and *Chlamydophila* infections (severe hepatic damage can lead to thin bird) Chronic peritonitis – especially in egg-laying females
Musculoskeletal problems	Trauma to wings, e.g. badly healed fractures or ankylosed joints and unable to fly will have atrophy of pectoral muscle masses. Thin but otherwise healthy. Birds that have had severe wing clips at early stage in lives often never develop pectoral muscle mass properly

20.21 Causes of weight loss in the presence of normal or excessive appetite.

Proventricular dilatation

Proventricular dilatation can occur as a specific neurological disease (PDD) (Chapter 13) or as a result of non-specific factors (proventricular dilatation syndrome) (Figure 20.22).

Type of disease	Examples
Neurogenic	Proventricular dilatation disease (PDD) (Chapter 15) Ingestion of lead or other heavy metal that results in generalized ileus
Non-neurogenic causes	Foreign body ingestion, intussusceptions or impaction Distension due to extraluminal masses or pressure Neoplastic changes, e.g. viral papillomas causing obstruction and subsequent dilatation
Inflammatory disease or infection	Disease of mucosa may affect motility

20.22 Causes of proventricular dilatation syndrome.

Clinical signs

These may be associated with acute obstruction or more chronic GI hypomotility, or be related to other signs from ingested toxins. In obstructive cases there may be no or scanty faeces.

Diagnosis

Diagnosis depends on a combination of history, physical examination, full blood biochemistry and haematology, and radiology. Specific sampling for blood lead and zinc levels is indicated (see Toxicology). Radiographic investigation may reveal impaction of the crop and distension of the proventriculus.

Barium contrast studies are often useful for differentiating hepatic enlargements from proventricular distension. Administering barium to the conscious bird, putting it on a perch in a cardboard box and performing radiography or fluoroscopy can give a rapid assessment of proventricular function. In cases of PDD, there may be segmental dysfunction of the GI tract.

Lead or zinc particles may be visualized radiographically but their absence does not rule out toxicosis.

If PDD is suspected, a biopsy of the crop (or proventriculus) (to include a blood vessel – and thus a nerve too) should be performed. A negative result does not rule out PDD.

Therapy

Treatment depends upon the diagnosis and may be specific therapy (e.g. for metal toxicity) or supportive care and anti-inflammatory drugs for PDD cases (Chapter 13).

Crop feeding with easily digested foods, laxatives and fluids may be needed.

Oncology

Neoplasia accounts for between 3% and 4% of psittacine histopathological submissions. Neoplasms from Budgerigars account for at least two-thirds of these samples, of which lipomas are the most frequently diagnosed conditions (10–40% of Budgerigar neoplasms). Pituitary tumours have been commonly found (Schlumberger, 1954).

Neoplasms can be classified according to their tissue origins (e.g. connective, fibrous, muscle) or by their cellular composition and activity (e.g. benign or malignant). The cause of most tumours is unknown but some are associated with viral infections, such as epithelial papillomas (papillomavirus), cloacal papillomas (herpesvirus) and some Budgerigar renal tumours (leucosis/sarcoma virus). They may present as obvious palpable masses (e.g. some cutaneous tumours) or may occur within major organs (e.g. liver or gonad), where their presence may be more difficult to diagnose at an early stage (Figure 20.23).

Integument	
Papillomas	Occur on skin of face, feet and legs and have been shown to be viral induced (papillomavirus found in Grey and Timneh Parrots)
Squamous cell carcinoma	Malignant tumour that can present as ulcer or proliferative irregular mass. Tends to be locally aggressive, has low metastatic potential and can develop at sites of chronic irritation. Has been diagnosed on various parts of skin but also affecting beak and uropygial gland
Adenomas or adenocarcinomas	Uropygial gland. Histology necessary both for diagnosis and differentiation from gland inflammation (adenitis) or metaplasia (vitamin A deficiency). Common neoplasms in Budgerigars and early surgical excision advised
Basal cell tumours	Occur anywhere on skin as firm broad-based masses, often with central ulcerated area
Malignant melanomas	Have been recorded in Grey Parrot on beak and face
Cutaneous lymphomas	Usually found around face as multifocal diffuse yellow/grey skin thickenings
Lipomas	Benign fatty masses most commonly seen in sternal areas of Budgerigars, Cockatiels and Amazons. Also found over abdomen, internally and over inner thighs. May show rapid tumour growth with increased vascularity and ulceration of overlying skin. Liposarcomas rarely occur and are firmer, more vascular and infiltrative

20.23 Neoplasia. (continues) ▶

Integument *continued*

Malignant fibrosarcoma	Reported more commonly than benign fibroma. Locally invasive, rarely metastasize and frequently ulcerate. Recurrence after excision is potential problem and amputation of wing or leg is often treatment of choice. Also recorded on face, beak and internal organs (Figure 20.24)
Benign haemangiomas	Circumscribed soft red to black masses. Less commonly the malignant haemangiosarcoma. Can resemble melanomas
Osteosarcomas	Under cere or beak may cause swelling or cracking of beak itself. Also on wings
Non-neoplastic skin masses	Feather cysts containing keratin and xanthomas (Chapter 16) may resemble tumours

Gastrointestinal tract

Papillomas of oral cavity	Should be differentiated from cutaneous form. Oral form associated with herpesvirus infection and may occur in choana, throughout GI tract (sometimes causing obstruction) and in cloaca where reddish friable masses can be found. Also linked to subsequent development of bile duct and pancreatic neoplasia. Commonest in Amazons, Hawk-headed Parrots and macaws. Local excision, cryosurgery, cautery and mucosal stripping. Birds with cloacal papillomas should be regarded as being potentially infectious to other individuals and appropriate measures to prevent transmission need to be undertaken
Squamous cell carcinomas	Can resemble cloacal papillomas. Also recorded in beak, oesophagus, oral cavity and proventriculus
Infiltrative adenocarcinomas	At proventricular/ventricular junction can cause clinical signs of regurgitation and chronic wasting. May be thickening of wall with necrosis and haemorrhage. Contrast radiography or endoscopic biopsy needed for diagnosis
Leiomyomas and leiomyosarcomas	Tumours of smooth muscle of intestine occasionally seen in wall of tract; rarely metastasize
Melanomas	Beak region of Grey Parrots. Infiltrative and metastatic
Lymphoma	Recorded on beak

Liver and pancreas

Liver tumours	Primary (arising from bile ducts, hepatocytes or hepatic stromal tissue) or secondary metastatic lesions. Metastases have few distinguishing features, often multiple foci throughout liver parenchyma. Histopathology needed for identification and diagnosis. Care needed with liver biopsies – excessive haemorrhage may be sequel. Vitamin K-dependent coagulation factors may have been compromised by the liver disease. Consider pre-treatment with Vitamin K
Bile duct carcinomas	Commonest neoplasm of liver (cholangiocarcinoma). Association with intestinal papillomas and can be solitary or multiple, firm white masses
Hepatocyte adenomas and carcinomas	Can be solitary, affecting one lobe, or multiple. Grow by infiltration and can be accompanied by tumour necrosis
Lymphosarcoma	Commonest lymphoid neoplasm in psittacine bird. Not all birds with lymphosarcoma are leukaemic and therefore haematological examination may not be particularly helpful for diagnosis
Vascular neoplasms	Can also affect liver
Malignant lymphoma	Hypercalcaemia has been reported in two Amazons. May be multisystemic or single organ that is grossly involved
Pancreas tumours	Adenomas, adenocarcinomas or carcinomas – usually firm greyish white masses. Possible relationship with previous cloacal/intestinal papilloma infection (Figure 20.25)

Urogenital system

Renal adenocarcinomas and adenomas	Most often seen in Budgerigar where presenting signs may be lameness or abdominal swelling. Lameness usually unilateral and caused by pressure on ischiadic nerve beneath swollen kidney In Budgerigars, association with leucosis/sarcoma virus infection. Surgical treatment usually impossible
Testicular tumours	Seminomas, Sertoli cell tumours or interstitial cell tumours. Budgerigar has highest incidence of testicular tumours. Radiographically, abdominal mass may be seen and in the case of Sertoli cell tumour, polyostotic endosteal hyperostosis may be seen (increased oestrogen levels). Surgical treatment sometimes possible
Ovarian tumours	Adenocarcinomas, carcinomas, cystadenomas and granulosa cell tumours. Cockatiel and Budgerigar commonly affected. Signs of weight loss or abdominal swelling and ascites (cytological examination useful). Paralysis of left leg recorded in a bird with a cystadenocarcinoma. Ovarian carcinomas can metastasize widely
Oviductal carcinomas and adenomas	Some, if discrete, can be successfully treated by salpingectomy; others spread directly to abdominal cavity and may be inoperable

20.23 (continued) Neoplasia. (continues) ▶

Musculoskeletal system	
Osteosarcomas and osteomas	Both have been identified in long bones of legs and wings. Firm tumours that cannot be easily cut. New bone proliferation and lysis may be seen on radiography. Diagnosis relies on histology
Rhabdomyosarcoma	Metastasizing case reported in Budgerigar. Muscle tumours have been infrequently seen
Fibrosarcomas	On wings and limbs. Amputation may be necessary
Respiratory tract	
Upper respiratory tract	Variety of neoplasms have been identified. Include choanal papillomas, squamous cell carcinomas, melanomas and lymphoma of nasal sinuses and oral cavity. Present as red infiltrative masses that can cause distortion of facial bones
Lower respiratory tract	Neoplastic disease rare. Adenocarcinomas and fibrosarcomas reported and also metastatic spread of neoplasia from other organs. Air sac adenocarcinomas can arise in air sacs of long bones and abdominal cavity. Space-occupying lesions may be identified by radiography
Endocrine system	
Thyroid adenomas and adenocarcinomas (less frequently)	Most often reported in Cockatiels and Budgerigars (Chapter 21). Occur in thoracic inlet and can lead to voice changes (pressure on syrinx) or partial crop obstruction. Differentiation needed from more common thyroid hyperplasia which is usually bilateral and can be managed medically by addition of iodine to diet
Pituitary gland adenomas	Reported to be common in Budgerigar. May cause clinical signs related to space-occupying lesion in brain, e.g. incoordination, seizures, blindness and exophthalmos. Polyuria/polydipsia related to antidiuretic hormone decrease, or increase in adrenocorticotrophic hormone and glycosuria from increased ACTH levels

20.23 (continued) Neoplasia.

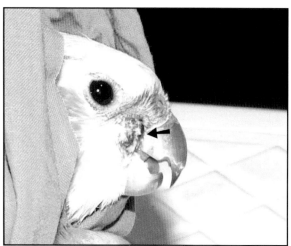

20.24 Fibrosarcoma (arrowed) at the junction of the upper and lower beak in a 12-year-old Cockatiel.

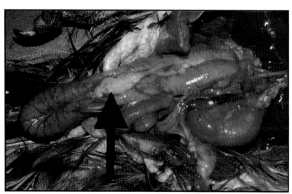

20.25 Pancreatic carcinoma in a Green-winged Macaw. This was related to cloacal papillomatosis. (Compare Figure 15.16.)

Lymphosarcoma

Although birds have aggregates of lymphoid cells around blood vessels and in various locations in the body, they do not have encapsulated lymph nodes and so lymphadenopathy is not a feature of neoplastic disease. Lymphoid leukaemia originates in the bone marrow. Lymphosarcoma usually originates in the primary or secondary lymphoid tissue and can spread to other parts of the body. Multicentric lymphosarcoma does occur, and is the most common lymphoid neoplasm. There may be diffuse or nodular involvement and the liver is the most commonly affected organ, followed by the spleen and kidneys. Other organs that are typically infiltrated include the skin, bone marrow, GI tract, thyroid gland, oviduct, lungs, sinuses, brain, periorbital muscles, pancreas, testes and thymus. There may be isolated whitish or yellow nodular lesions on the skin and these may ulcerate.

No viral cause in psitttacine birds has yet been found (unlike in poultry). Typical histology is of uniform populations of lymphoblasts and mature lymphocytes. Mitotic figures are common.

Diagnosis is usually from biopsied material, since many birds with lymphosarcoma are not leukaemic and therefore haematology is not useful in these cases. The organs involved are generally enlarged and pale and must be differentiated from amyloid, fatty liver, hepatitis, mycobacteria infection and other neoplastic cases.

Definitive diagnosis

A definitive diagnosis is only reached by performing a biopsy and histopathology. The presence of a neoplasm can be suspected by using some or all of the ancillary diagnostic aids. For internal neoplasia, radiography, ultrasonography, clinical chemistry and biopsy may all need to be employed.

Therapy

Therapy may involve simple excision or cryosurgery but other treatment modalities are increasingly being developed and employed, such as chemotherapy and radiotherapy.

Surgery

The treatment of choice for most neoplastic masses is radical excision. This may involve localized surgery, amputation or cloacal mucosal stripping. Many neoplasms are either disseminated or inaccessible and so other treatment regimes are being developed. A combination of treatment methods may be needed, such as surgical de-bulking, chemotherapy, intra-tumour injections and radiation therapy.

Chemotherapy

Figure 20.26 outlines chemotherapeutic agents and regimes.

Radiation therapy

Low-energy X-rays (orthovoltage) have been used in some cases (lymphoreticular neoplasia and squamous cell carcinoma) (Quesenberry, 1997) either alone or in combination with chemotherapy. Doses of 4 Gy have been used at varying intervals and lengths of treatment, e.g. three times weekly for 10-week regimes, or larger doses at weekly intervals. Specialized facilities are needed for radiotherapy. Results have been encouraging and protocols are still being developed for combined chemotherapy/radiotherapy treatments.

Agent	Neoplasm	Patient	Route + dose	Treatment time
Doxorubicin	Osteosarcoma	Amazon	i.v. 60 mg/m^2	Monthly × 4 months
Cisplatin	Fibrosarcoma	Macaw	Intra-tumour	Plus orthovoltage X-ray 3 × weekly for 11 weeks
Chlorambucil	Lymphocytoma	Macaw	20 mg/m^2	Weekly for 6 weeks, repeated after 12 weeks
Vincristine plus chlorambucil	Cutaneous lymphosarcoma	Cockatoo	i.v. 0.1 mg/kg (V) Orally 2 mg/kg (C)	Weekly until patient dies or is cured OR Twice-weekly for 17 weeks
Carboplatin	Squamous cell carcinoma	Amazon	Intra-lesion 5 mg/kg (in sesame seed oil)	Single treatment
Cisplatin	Healthy birds	Sulphur-crested cockatoo	Infusion 1 mg/kg over 1 hour	Gives therapeutic plasma platinum levels

20.26 Chemotherapy: some agents and regimes that have been used.

21

The sick small psittacid

Ron Rees Davies

Introduction

Frustratingly, one of the most common psittacine bird presentations is one of the most difficult to deal with: that of a sick small parrot or parakeet which is presented merely as being 'off colour' or 'fluffed up'. The common pet species in this category are Budgerigars and Cockatiels; other small species include lovebirds and grass parakeets.

Such cases present a number of diagnostic challenges. The size of the bird limits the amount of information that can be gained from physical examination, and may limit the sample sizes available for clinical pathology. The frailty of the birds may limit the degree of invasive diagnostics or therapeutic intervention that can be used. In some cases (though notably not all), there are severe financial constraints over the clinical approach, and even where diagnosis is possible some cases present only in the terminal stages of a chronic unnoticed disease process.

The most difficult aspect of small psittacine bird medicine can be communicating with the distraught owner about where the boundaries of both clinical possibilities and financial limitations lie. In some cases it will be necessary to determine whether euthanasia would actually be better for the bird's welfare than attempted investigations or treatment.

This chapter provides some practical suggestions on approaching all these problems. In doing so it necessarily duplicates some basic information available elsewhere in this book, but omits much of the detail (for which readers should turn to the appropriate chapters).

History taking

The successful small psittacid consultation revolves around a thorough understanding of the ways in which the patient is housed and kept. Clients are usually desperate to impart details about the current illness, but it is essential to step back and start by asking, either verbally or in the form of a questionnaire, a number of important questions about the bird's environment before it became ill. Taking a full history may seem superfluous when a bird is presented with what seems like an obvious problem such as a traumatic injury, but it is important to take a holistic approach to these birds and attempt where possible to correct underlying husbandry deficiencies as a preventive measure.

Source, and time in owner's possession

The range of diseases likely to be encountered will be much greater with a bird recently acquired from a major bird wholesaler than a pet bird that has been in solitary confinement for many years.

Type of husbandry

Not only does the type of husbandry (pet, indoor aviary, outdoor aviary, breeding colony) affect the likelihood of various disease processes, but importantly it will probably affect the required approach to the disease. An owner with 200 breeding Budgerigars is unlikely to want a full work-up on an individual sick bird, whereas a pet owner will probably be unimpressed by a suggestion of culling and post-mortem examination. In particular, birds housed in colonies, especially if in outdoor aviaries, will be more prone to parasitic diseases (e.g. ascaridosis, trichomoniasis, red mite infestation). Some diseases will be solely encountered in one type of husbandry (e.g. tick-associated disease in outdoor aviaries).

Normal enclosure

A number of factors involving the enclosure may be important, including the site (e.g. polytetrafluoroethylene and cooking fumes if in the kitchen; temperature fluctuations if in direct sunlight), construction (e.g. lead or zinc toxicity from consuming fragments of cage materials; pesticides or other treatment present on perches), lighting intensity and photoperiod (a factor in female reproductive diseases).

Exposure to other birds

Although unusual in housebound pets, there are a number of infections to which small psittacine birds are prone. These include psittacosis (chlamydophilosis), trichomoniasis, giardiasis and viruses such as paramyxovirus, polyomavirus, circovirus and reovirus (Box 21.1).

Infection may be more likely if the bird has recently been exposed to others, such as during boarding whilst the owner is on holiday, or at an exhibition, or by the introduction of a new bird. Some diseases can be transmitted by fomites, such as in feather dust on the clothes of an owner that has visited an aviary, bird show or pet shop, or may be harboured asymptomatically for many months or even years before clinical signs develop.

At the time of writing (mid 2004) there was an ongoing epornitic in the UK Exhibition Budgerigar population. Early unconfirmed reports of serious losses in Budgerigar breeding colonies began in early 2002, with confirmed outbreaks being seen in the winter of 2002/3 and spring 2003. There was then a respite, but a further four outbreaks occurred in late 2003 and early 2004. Almost all of the cases could be traced to a single source in South-East England. There had been an estimated total of 30 cases altogether.

Virus isolation at the Central Veterinary Laboratory, Weybridge, yielded a reovirus. Epidemiological work suggested that the virus had an incubation period of about 10 days, with variable mortality of 45–95%, and surviving birds appeared to become viral 'carriers' for at least 6 months. Transmission was thought to be faeco-oral, though oro-oral and feather dust transmissions were also possible.

Affected birds showed non-specific signs of being 'fluffed' and anorectic and were found on the floor of the cage. All had diarrhoea and a proportion had CNS disturbances such as tremors or incoordination. Some birds died suddenly. In an outbreak there may be a lot of deaths over a short period, but typically deaths were of several birds every day for several weeks. Immunosuppressive effects of the virus were suspected, as many birds had concurrent infections such as chlamydophilosis or *Escherichia coli*.

Some control of the disease could be effected by 'fogging' the birdroom with F10, and the use of sanitizing agents in the drinking water.

Box 21.1 The 2002 Budgerigar reovirus outbreak (JR Baker, personal communication, 2004).

Diet

The type of dietary intake is possibly less of a problem with most small psittacine birds than with the larger parrots. Most of the small species are parakeets, which eat predominantly seeds in the wild, and so the standard 'budgie mixes' or 'cockatiel mixes' are at least a reasonable basis for nutrition. However, depending on the source and variability of the seeds presented, a number of nutritional problems can occur (e.g. iodine-responsive goitre in Budgerigars), and the *ad libitum* access to food without adequate exercise provision leads to obesity in some birds.

Owner's ability to handle

A particular problem with many small psittacids is often the owner's complete inability to handle the bird, and thus also to administer medication if required. The bird may well be presented to the veterinary surgeon within a cage that it has not left for many years, and this constrains the choice of medication route and therefore choice of treatment protocol for birds that need therapeutic drugs.

Examination within the cage

Where possible, pet-owning clients should be encouraged to present their bird in the cage in which it normally resides. Much more information about the suitability and maintenance (and indeed legality) of the cage can be determined from a first-hand inspection than from any number of husbandry-oriented questions. It is also often less stressful for the bird to travel in its own cage, provided it is not too cumbersome.

Examination of the cage will allow the veterinary surgeon to begin to make an assessment of the bird's clinical condition by evaluating the state of the droppings (laboratory examination of droppings at this stage may help to direct clinical examination of the bird later), by looking for evidence of regurgitation or vomition and by assessing the number and state of feathers on the floor of the enclosure. Owners should be strongly discouraged from 'spring cleaning' the cage prior to a visit to the surgery, but perhaps encouraged to place a sheet of writing-paper over the cage floor to allow assessment of which droppings are fresh, to facilitate assessment of the physical characteristics of the dropping (Appendix 2) and to allow microscopy without the annoying inclusion of sand grains (which make fresh wet-preparation examination exceedingly difficult).

Presentation of the bird in its own cage, rather than an enclosed cardboard box, also allows the veterinary surgeon to examine the bird at rest during the history taking. This is important, because many birds will efficiently mask the signs of illness when they are in a stressful situation (e.g. travelling; a noisy waiting room) or when they know they are being observed. If a bird is presented within an enclosed box, it can be useful to transfer the bird to a hospital cage during the history taking for such observation.

Signalment

Type

An assessment of the species and type of bird being presented can also be made at this stage. Several of the small psittacids have been bred in captivity for many generations and various 'colour mutations' exist. Some of these, particularly the 'ino' (albino and lutino) varieties, appear to have weaker immune systems than their wild-type counterparts. This effect of selective breeding is perhaps seen at its most extreme in the Budgerigar where, because of a bottleneck in the population in the 1940s and subsequent strongly selective inbreeding for size and feather density, there are now two subpopulations: the 'pet type' bird, which is smaller and sleeker and lives on average for 10–15 years; and the 'exhibition type', which appears larger, has a roughened ('buff') appearance due to its feathering and has a dramatically shortened lifespan (breeders expect stock to live on average only 18 months to 3 years).

Age

Age determination is usually not possible by visual inspection. Some species have pronounced differences between adult and juvenile plumage – particularly Budgerigars, which have a series of fine horizontal lines across the forehead as youngsters ('barheads') that become clear once the bird moults to adult plumage at 12 weeks of age. This appearance is masked in some colour varieties, though with experience feather texture can be used.

Iris colour can also be used, and in many species babies have completely dark irises, which become lighter with age. In the Budgerigar the iris in most varieties begins black, and from 4 months of age passes through a range of grey colours, finally becoming silver or white at 8–10 months old.

Otherwise the age of a bird generally remains unknown unless it has been fitted with a closed ring, which is usually stamped with the year and so at least defines the maximum age the bird could be. Plastic rings and 'split' rings do not carry useful information on the age of a bird.

Sex

Sex determination may be possible at this 'in cage' assessment stage in Budgerigars and Cockatiels, though most of the distinguishing features are not evident until adulthood and are suppressed or absent in certain colour mutations. Sex determination features of various small psittacids are discussed in Figures 21.1 and 21.2. Budgerigars may have altered or even apparently transitional cere coloration if they are ill and in particular if they have gonadal neoplasia.

Species/variety	Male (cock)	Female (hen)
Budgerigar: Immature	Until 3–5 months of age both sexes have a purple or flesh coloured smooth cere (fleshy area over beak).	
Budgerigar: Adult (most varieties)	Blue smooth cere. Brighter and shinier when in 'breeding condition'.	Cere fawn to chocolate brown and roughened in appearance. Deeper, richer brown colour when in 'breeding condition'.
Budgerigar: Some colour mutations (particularly Albino, Lutino, Recessive pied, Lacewing)	No blue colour. Cere remains flesh coloured as for youngster but remains smooth and can develop a bluish sheen.	As for other varieties, often more pronounced brown colour.
Cockatiel: Immature	Up to 6–8 months of age all look similar to adult females, with dull facial patterns (only a few spots of yellow) and marked regular yellow 'spotting' or 'barring' of otherwise dark flight and tail feathers. Crests usually grey.	
Cockatiel: Adult 'Normal Grey' (Grey and Yellow) varieties	Bright yellow face, deep orange cheek patch, no regular pale markings on flight and tail feathers. Crest is yellow with only grey tips to the feathers.	Retain immature plumage appearance – dull face with obvious barring of tail and flight feathers.
Cockatiel: Other Grey varieties	With many other grey-bodied varieties, pattern is same but without yellow on face. Male's crest and face white, female's remains grey and female has tail bars.	
Cockatiel: Lutino	Lutino Cockatiels lack all grey pigment, instead having white to cream background colour. The remaining patterns (brighter cheek patch and yellower crest in males, yellow-on-cream barring in females) may be evident but can be difficult to identify on very pale individuals. Try holding tail or flight feathers up to light to look for regular spots or bars.	
Cockatiel: Lutino whiteface, Pieds	Cannot be reliably sexed by visual inspection.	
Bourke's Parakeet	More blue and pink on the breast, bluer forehead.	Barring under tail when mature.
Splendid Parakeet	Blue head, red chest.	No blue on head or red on chest. Generally duller colours.
Turquoisine Parakeet	Chestnut red on wings.	No chestnut on wings. Generally duller colours.
Red-rumped Parakeet	Red rump patch.	Rump green. Barring under wings when mature.
Scarlet-chested (Splendid) Parakeet	Chest feathering red.	Chest feathering green.
Abyssinian Lovebird	Red patch on forehead and lores.	Red patches absent.
Madagascar (Grey-headed) Lovebird	Grey head, neck and breast.	Green head, neck and breast.
Other lovebird species	Cannot be reliably sexed by visual inspection.	

General notes:

• Behavioural attitude toward another bird or owner of known gender is *not* a reliable method of sex determination.

• Male cockatiels may sing and whistle more than females. This is not a reliable method of sex determination but may be apparent before moulting to adult plumage. Male Budgerigars are generally easier to train to talk than females.

• As some colour mutations are genetically 'sex-linked', breeders may be able to tell the sex of the bird reliably from its parentage, even whilst in the nest.

21.1 Common sex determination features of small psittacids.

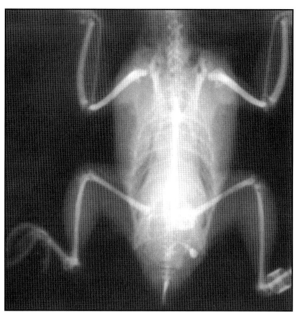

21.2 Medullary bone formation in a female Budgerigar. This alerts the clinician that the bird is female (if not already known) and that she is reproductively active, which may have a bearing on disease syndromes likely to be present.

Clinical examination

Restraint and handling

It is necessary to catch the bird to examine it. Although many veterinary surgeons have reservations and fear that the bird will 'drop dead from fright' at being handled, it is important to recognize that this is an extremely rare occurrence and almost always the result of examining a bird that was moribund in the first place. Nevertheless, the examination within the cage should allow the veterinary surgeon to warn the owner of this risk if the bird does indeed seem to be severely compromised, but to point out that the only chance of saving the bird is to examine it.

A firmly restrained bird will struggle less and have less risk of iatrogenic damage than one that is restrained too lightly. Where possible, handle the bird using a towel (a supply of thin tea towels or handkerchiefs is ideal but paper towels will suffice). The towel helps to restrain the bird by enclosing the wings (Chapter 4) and also helps to avoid perspiration from the veterinary surgeon's hands causing feathers to be pulled out unnecessarily. Some birds, in particular Cockatiels, will readily drop many feathers during even gentle handling.

In many cases, clinical examination needs to be brief to avoid excessive stress to the bird. All materials that may be needed for the examination should be at hand. With birds that seem particularly ill on the 'in cage' examination it may be worth having a selection of appropriate 'shotgun' medications prepared in advance to avoid having to handle the bird a second time.

Clinical examination of small psittacids can seem daunting because of the apparent lack of observable criteria. However, by paying particular attention to the following areas a reasonable reduction in the differential diagnosis list can be obtained.

Scoring body condition

Palpation of the sternum gives a reasonable guide to current nutritional or metabolic status. In a normal bird the sternal keel should be just palpable, with the convex-shaped pectoral muscles almost level with it on either side, though this will vary with the amount of flying the bird is allowed. Shape of the muscle mass can give an idea of chronicity of the disease. Initial loss of muscle mass occurs relatively rapidly, possibly due to depletion of glycogen stores rather than true catabolism, and the convex shape can turn to a marked concave within a few days. Further muscle loss occurs gradually until, with debilitating diseases of weeks to months in duration, the pectoral muscle mass becomes almost completely lost and the shape of the underlying bone can be determined easily.

Obese birds may have a layer of subcutaneous fat on palpation of the sternal area, and it is important to recognize that with subacute diseases it is quite possible for a bird to show marked loss of pectoral muscle mass and yet still be obese. A further complication of this is that in some birds, especially Budgerigars, the sternum is a predilection site for fat distribution and lipoma formation (Figure 21.3).

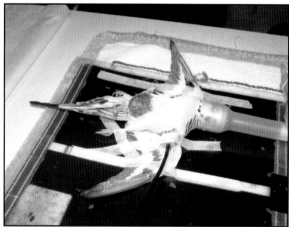

21.3 Lipoma overlying the abdomen of a Budgerigar. The bird has been anaesthetized and prepared for surgery. Note use of a syringe case as an induction mask and the positioning of a Doppler device over the wing to monitor pulse rate and strength. Minimal heat loss is critical in these cases so the bird is positioned on a heat mat and as small an area as possible has been plucked.

Head area

The feathering of the head should be examined. There may be 'pin feathers' (ensheathed growing feathers) present that provide evidence of current moulting. (It is not unusual for a reportedly 'feather plucking' or 'pruritic' small psittacid to be simply moulting, or for these pin feathers to be interpreted as mites or ticks.) If there is genuine feather loss, it should be determined whether this is self-inflicted or done by a cage mate (Figure 21.4). There may also be matting of the feathers around the eyes, around the ear canal or above the nares as evidence of abnormal discharges from these sites. Small psittacids, especially Cockatiels, are prone to a conjunctivitis associated with chlamydophilosis (Figure 21.5).

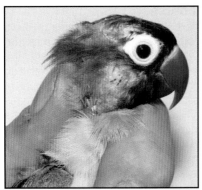

21.4

Another common cause of 'plucking' is barbering by a cage mate.

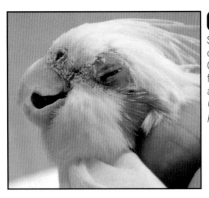

21.5

Sinusitis/ conjunctivitis in a Cockatiel. This is frequently associated with *Chlamydophila psittaci* infection.

There may be evidence of vomition or regurgitation. Some birds, particularly Budgerigars, flick their heads upwards as they vomit, and the vomit tends to cause matting of the feathers in the forehead area, which often have a characteristic odour. Birds showing sexual regurgitation bob their head up and down, but regurgitated seeds (usually not malodorous) are generally either deposited on cage items, cage mates or the owner or are simply allowed to dribble down underneath the mandible.

A number of conditions cause other alterations around the head area.

- Changes of the facial skin include cnemidocoptic mange infestation, which causes scaling or proliferative outgrowth with a characteristic pinpricked or honeycombed appearance of the beak and surrounding areas (mainly in Budgerigars but occasionally on the facial or pedal skin of other small psittacids).
- Hypertrophic changes can occur to the cere, particularly of female Budgerigars where it has been referred to as 'brown hypertrophy'. The excess keratin material can often be simply chipped of with a thumbnail and rarely causes clinical problems, but occasionally it occludes the nares and it can be present secondary to underlying disease.
- Normal birds should never need their beak clipping. Overgrowth or excessive flaking or crumbling of the beak can be due to earlier trauma or be idiopathic, but can also be a form of 'hepatocutaneous syndrome' and ideally liver investigations should be considered. Once a beak starts growing abnormally it will need repeated clipping on a regular basis for the rest of the bird's life.

- Although conjunctivitis does occur, swellings around the eye area are usually related to infection of the underlying paranasal sinuses. Even conjunctival foreign bodies (e.g. canary-seed husks, sand) may be secondary to the bird rubbing at an already inflamed periorbital area. Sinus swelling can also present as an outpouching between the lateral oral commissure and the medial canthus of the eye. Diagnostic samples of nasal or ocular discharges, or sinus flush samples (Figure 21.6), can be taken for cytology, culture or DNA analysis.

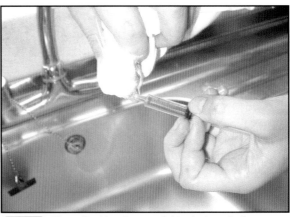

21.6 Sinus flushing is a useful technique in the therapy of sinusitis. The bird is held upside-down over a sink. A syringe of an antimicrobial is held against a nostril and injected into the nasal cavity. Fluid should pass through the sinuses and exit via the opposite nostril, choana and conjunctival sacs. For diagnostic sampling, sterile saline is used and the flush sample collected in a sterile container.

Examination of the mouth can be difficult, but with practice paperclips of assorted sizes can be used as specula. Abscesses and abnormal discharges are occasionally seen but are unusual. Evaluation of mucous membrane colour is generally unreliable, as many birds normally have greyish or pigmented mucosae.

Crop

Palpation of the crop is useful. A normal bird should have a crop with a small to moderate amount of seed with little fluid palpable within the crop. An empty crop may indicate anorexia, or simply withholding of food during a long journey. If the owner reports that the bird has been eating recently yet the crop is empty, the food bowl should be checked for evidence of dehulled seeds (especially the very dark kernels of canary seeds). Anorexic small psittacids (especially Budgerigars with megabacteriosis) will display 'sham-eating' behaviour: they appear to have a normal appetite but drop the dehulled seeds back into the food bowl.

Palpable fluid within the crop can be a sign of gastrointestinal stasis, crop infection (ingluviitis) or polydipsia. Air within the crop area can be a result of fermentation of materials within the crop, or aerophagia due to dyspnoea, or may actually be emphysema around the crop as a result of a punctured or ruptured air sac.

Aspiration of crop contents is a valuable yet inexpensive tool in investigating disease of small psittacids. A metal ball-tipped crop tube (or a Spreull needle) is inserted gently through the mouth down to the crop, where the tube tip can be palpated. Fluid can be aspirated, or if the crop is empty instillation of 0.7 ml warmed saline along with 0.3 ml air followed by brief gentle massage allows retrieval of a diagnostic specimen.

Trichomoniasis (see Figure 7.38) is a common cause of ingluviitis and vomiting in Budgerigars, especially (but not exclusively) those housed in colonies. Bacterial and yeast overgrowths can also be found, though these may be secondary problems as a result of gastrointestinal stasis.

Abdominal area

Palpation of the 'abdominal' area is restricted to probing in the area bordered cranially by the caudal margin of the sternum and laterally by the ribs and pubic bones. Both a 'finger and thumb' lateral approach cranial to the pubic bones and a 'single finger' midline approach between the pubic bones should be used. In the normal bird the only identifiable palpable object in this area is the gizzard, which is a smooth rounded structure (5–10 mm in diameter) in the left craniolateral quadrant and should not be misinterpreted as an egg or a neoplasm, though hepatomegaly or space-occupying masses may displace the gizzard into a more obvious position than usual (Figure 21.7). Otherwise the area should generally have an 'empty' feel.

A 'full' or 'spongy' feel may be an indicator of obesity but could indicate increased soft tissue structures within the abdomen, such as a dilated female reproductive tract (normal during egg laying) or gastrointestinal tract. Eggs and neoplasms are also sometimes palpated, and Cockatiels in particular seem prone to egg-related peritonitis, possibly as a consequence of oviduct torsion. Fluid within the peritoneal cavity causes a generalized distension of the area.

Aspiration can be performed but there is a risk of iatrogenically introducing fluid into the air sac system. The ventral midline is generally the safest approach.

Cloaca and uropygial gland

The cloaca and the surrounding feathering should be examined. Birds with diarrhoea or polyuria will often have matting and staining of these feathers, whilst faecal accumulations ('clagging') can occur in birds that have been unable or unwilling to groom themselves for some time.

The uropygial gland and surrounding area should be examined for signs of ulceration, asymmetry, pain or self-mutilation (particularly a problem in this area in lovebirds). The gland is a predilection site for the formation of squamous cell carcinomas.

Limbs

Both wings should be palpated and extended, looking for injuries, deformities or abnormal masses (the distal wing tip is a site of predilection for the formation of feather cysts and xanthomas; Figure 21.8) but also particularly at the featherless area (apterium) on the

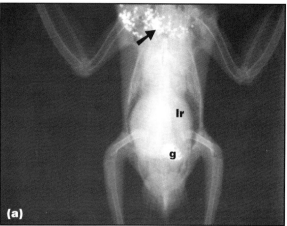

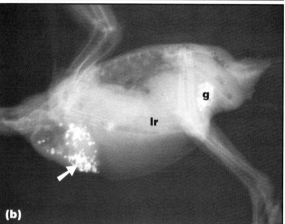

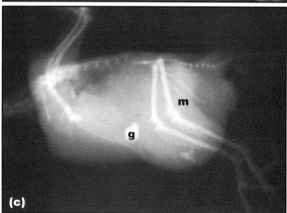

21.7 The gizzard position enables the clinician to determine the nature of masses that are displacing it. Radio-opaque material within it acts as a positive contrast material. (a,b) The gizzard (g) in this Cockatiel is displaced caudally by an enlarged liver (lr). The radio-opaque material in this case (arrowed) is metal, later found to be zinc. The presence of this metal within the crop shows that the intake is current and ongoing. This enables the clinician to locate the source within the bird's immediate environment. (c) The gizzard (g) in this Budgerigar is displaced cranially by a large abdominal mass (m), which was later found to be an ovarian tumour. (Courtesy of John Chitty.)

inner aspect of the elbow, where several veins can be visualized. The appearance of the skin and the veins can give a crude indication of dehydration or anaemia. This area and the axilla can be a site of self-mutilation, particularly in Cockatiels.

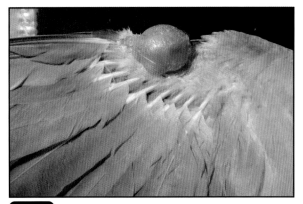

21.8 Xanthoma on the wing of a lovebird.

The legs should be examined, and especially the joints and soles of the feet, which may be abnormal for dietary (vitamin A deficiency), perching (Figure 21.9) or metabolic (gout) reasons. The feet may show different degrees of wear, indicating that the bird has been lame on the less-worn leg for some time.

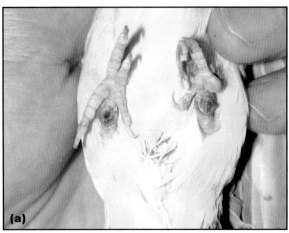

(a)

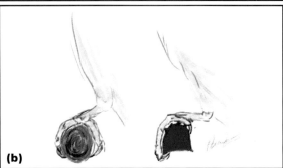

(b)

21.9 (a) Poor perching can cause severe foot lesions. (b) The weight distribution on the perching feet can be seen, where the correct-shaped perch (left) enables even perching, while incorrect shapes result in abnormal pressure on different parts of the feet.

Clinical pathology

Both financial considerations and sample volumes may constrain the amount of laboratory testing that is possible and so it is important to make best use of what samples are available.

Cytology

Much information can be gained from simple cytology, a rapid and inexpensive tool (Chapter 7). Aspirated material from the crop and fresh faeces (or cloacal wash samples) can be examined, initially using direct wet-preparation examination (for motile protozoans, nematodes, cestodes, inflammatory cells). Later the same samples can be dried, fixed and stained with either rapid cytological stains (e.g. Diff-Quik, Rapi-Diff) to evaluate inflammatory and other host-cell populations, or with Gram staining, which allows more reasoned choice of antimicrobial where appropriate and in particular allows examination for the 'megabacterium' yeast (Figure 21.10).

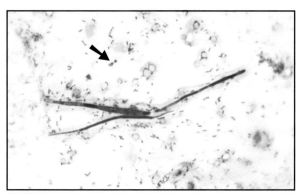

21.10 'Megabacterium'; this yeast has been reclassified as *Macrorhabdus ornithogaster*. Two bacterial cocci are arrowed for comparison. (Gram stain, original magnification 1000x)

Further testing of faeces by an outside laboratory may be indicated where *Chlamydophila* (formerly *Chlamydia*) *psittaci* is suspected, with a range of tests available (including modified acid-fast staining, immunofluorescent staining and DNA techniques). Similarly acid-fast staining may in some circumstances be used as a tool for identifying *Mycobacterium* infection.

The use of urinalysis in birds is limited, but again the sample is freely available without stress to the bird and may be worth evaluating. Dipstick analysis is complicated by the admixture of faecal and urine components within the dropping, so a positive glucose or protein test cannot necessarily be relied upon. However, a negative urine glucose would rule out diabetes mellitus (symptoms similar to which are seen commonly in Cockatiels, especially following use of corticosteroids) in a polydipsic bird. Cytological examination may reveal blood cells or renal casts in cases of pyelonephritis.

Cytological techniques should also be applied routinely for cases with masses and swellings. In particular, swellings of the joints associated with gout will often yield a white pasty material with microscopically characteristic needle-like crystals on aspirated cytology specimens. The identity of the crystals can be confirmed using the 'Murexide' test: mix an aspirated sample with one drop of nitric acid on a slide; evaporate over a Bunsen flame; cool; then add one drop of ammonia. A reddish purple colour develops if urate material is present.

Blood sampling

When considering blood sampling of small psittacids, prioritization is of utmost importance. Sample volumes can be at most 1% of the bird's body weight, which means that at most 0.35 ml will be available even from a typical healthy 35 g Budgerigar. However, modern laboratory techniques allow a surprisingly comprehensive range of tests from such a sample.

Where possible a differential list should be considered before taking a sample, and it should be decided which tests are most appropriate. Some tests are not particularly accurate in birds (protein tests, for example; serum protein electrophoresis would be a better alternative but is not widely available and requires a larger sample volume) or their significance may be doubtful (AST and LDH are the most widely used 'liver' enzymes, but levels are likely to be elevated simply because of the muscle catabolism in an underweight bird). In particular, certain tests (full haematology, bile acids) usually require a larger amount of sample than most biochemistry tests. The laboratory should be consulted regarding suitable samples before the blood is taken. Small-volume heparin tubes are available and should be used rather than a small volume of blood being put into a full-sized tube. Sending two air-dried smears of non-anticoagulated blood will help the pathologist to elicit more information.

In non-specific 'sick small bird' cases where no realistic differential diagnosis can be developed, this author's preferred order of testing would be as follows:

- Total white blood cell count (with differential WBC from whole blood where possible or from the buffy coat of the PCV if necessary)
- Packed cell volume (PCV)
- Uric acid
- Calcium: ionized (Ca^{2+}) if available, with total calcium as well if sample size allows
- Bile acids (if sample size will allow)
- Zinc and lead (if tests available and sample size allows)
- Total protein
- Albumin (and calculated 'globulins')
- Aspartate aminotransferase (AST)
- Creatine kinase (CK)
- Glucose
- Cholesterol
- Electrolytes
- Amylase

- Lactate dehydrogenase (LDH)
- Phosphorus
- Triglyceride
- Gamma-glutaryl transferase (GGT)
- Creatinine

Diagnostic imaging

Radiography can be a useful tool, but it takes some practice to get good quality images from such small subjects. It carries the drawback that either stressful conscious restraint or light isoflurane anaesthesia will be necessary in order to obtain the desired positions. An accurate exposure chart for birds of varied body weights should be developed by analysing previous radiographs or, where necessary, by radiographing carcasses of dead small birds. Even then, it is often useful to 'bracket' the exposure factors – taking exposures of the same patient position using several different exposure factors on the same cassette. By using a Perspex sheet for restraint, such multiple exposures add little to the anaesthetic time but can greatly reduce the need for further exposures.

An additional useful tool is digital imaging of the radiographs. By using a digital camera to photograph the radiograph, the image can be enlarged and the brightness, contrast and colour saturation altered to enhance the imaging of certain structures. The images can be transferred directly to the computer record, and printed out for the client.

In small psittacids, radiography is particularly of use in investigating fractures, ingested foreign metallic materials (Figure 21.7), egg retention in females and, with the aid of barium contrast, gastrointestinal disorders and particularly coelomic extraintestinal masses displacing the intestinal tract from its normal position.

Other diagnostic imaging techniques are either difficult to perform because of the patient's small size (ultrasonography) or underused because of financial constraints (computed tomography, magnetic resonance imaging).

Differential diagnoses

A list of common small psittacid presentations, with some possible differentials and positive and negative indicators for those differentials, is provided in Figure 21.11.

Presentation	Differentials	Suggested tests	Notes
Ill bird with 'fluffed-up' feathers	End-stage chronic disease	Haematology and biochemistry	Clinical examination shows both muscle and fat loss. Many cases will have secondary bacterial, yeast or fungal infections
	Anorexia	History Examination of bird and cage	Check for presence of food in the crop. Look for specific underlying diseases unless simple starvation. Budgerigars in particular show 'sham-eating' behaviour (sit by bowl and dehusk seeds but not swallow them): examine food bowl for dehulled seeds. This is particularly a feature of megabacteriosis ('megabacterium' yeast infection)

21.11 Differential diagnoses for specific presentations. (continues) ▶

Presentation	Differentials	Suggested tests	Notes
Ill bird with 'fluffed-up' feathers *continued*	Systemic infection	Haematology Chlamydophilosis testing	Doxycycline is treatment of choice for chlamydophilosis
	Hepatic lipidosis	Signalment (especially prevalent in Budgerigars and diabetic Cockatiels) Clinical examination Radiographically enlarged liver Biochemistry (AST, bile acid) Biopsy/histopathology	Most small psittacids have evolved to eat almost entirely seed-based (high fat and carbohydrate) diet but to have very high levels of exercise to burn off energy intake (wild Budgerigar colonies fly hundreds of miles especially in search of food). Captive inactivity and overeating (possibly accompanied by thyroid dysfunction due to iodine deficiency in Budgerigars) can lead to lipid overload, which may present as chronic hepatic lipidosis, with hepatocutaneous signs (common reason for overgrown or deformed beaks and nails) or overt lipomas. Chronic lipidosis can present as apparently acute syndrome of hepatic failure with lethargy and anorexia. Acute lipidosis can also be precipitated by corticosteroid therapies. Therapy: both short-term supportive therapy (lactulose, anabolic steroids) and long-term nutritional correction (increased exercise, iodine supplementation and conversion to improved diet)
	Acute organ failure	Haematology and biochemistry	
Regurgitation	Trichomoniasis	Crop wash cytology (see Figure 7.38)	Contact birds likely to be infected also, may be subclinical. Consider wild birds as a source of parasite in naive colonies
	Megabacteriosis ('megabacterium' yeast infection of proventriculus)	Faecal Gram stain (see Figure 21.10)	Usually present with chronic weight loss, often with 'sham-eating' behaviour (see Anorexia). Can be sudden death due to acute haemorrhaging gastric ulcer. Organism can be suppressed using amphotericin-B, but is rarely eliminated so relapses are probable
	Heavy metal toxicity	Radiography Serum metal analysis Haematology (lead) Amylase (zinc)	Chelation with EDTA possible
	Systemic infection, air sac infection	Haematology Biochemistry Chlamydophilosis testing	
	End-stage chronic disease	Haematology and biochemistry	Clinical examination shows both muscle and fat loss. Many cases have secondary bacterial, yeast or fungal infections
	Foreign body in crop; mass at crop or thoracic inlet	Clinical examination Radiography	See also hypothyroid goitre under Dyspnoea
	Acute metabolic failures	Haematology and biochemistry	
	Proventricular dilatation disease (PDD)	Contrast radiography Crop biopsy	Uncommon in small psittacids but possible, especially in Cockatiel
Polyuria/Polydipsia	Hepatic disease	Biochemistry Radiography	
	Renal disease	Lameness Biochemistry	
	Heavy metal toxicity	Radiography Serum metal analysis Haematology (lead) Amylase (Zn)	
	Steroid administration	History	Steroid administration can lead to hepatopathy or to syndromes similar to iatrogenic Cushing's syndrome or diabetes mellitus. Sudden withdrawal of drug can induce a syndrome similar to Addison's disease. Use of steroids should be avoided in small psittacids

21.11 (continued) Differential diagnoses for specific presentations. (continues) ▶

Presentation	Differentials	Suggested tests	Notes
Polyuria/Polydipsia *continued*	Diabetes mellitus	Weight loss Glycosuria Persistent hyperglycaemia Fructosamine	Existence of true diabetes mellitus is debatable. Suggestive clinical signs may be due to hyperadrenocorticism, steroid administration, or glucagonoma
Diarrhoea			Unusual. When taking history and examining cage, need to distinguish true 'diarrhoea' (malformed faecal portion of dropping) from abnormalities of urine and urate fractions, which are more common. Diarrhoea as result of dietary factors possible
	Physiological at egg laying	History Signalment (gender) Clinical examination	Females normally pass voluminous masses of faecal and urate portions of dropping during period around egg laying
	'Clagged vent'	Clinical examination	Accumulation of droppings on feathers around vent Non-specific sign, seen in many 'fluffed' birds due to positional and grooming effects of generalized weakness, also seen as consequence of obesity and of 'buff' feathering in exhibition-type Budgerigars
	Cloacitis/cloacalith	Clinical examination including examination of fresh droppings Abdominal palpation	Cloacitis often presents as 'clagging' Droppings may show mixing of faecal and urate components, possibly with some blood flecks
	Nematodes	Faecal wet-preparation cytology Faecal flotation	Nematodes unusual in pet birds, though possible. More common in colonies of some parakeet species. Can cause weight loss and eventually death due to intestinal obstruction
	Protozoa (*Giardia*)	Faecal wet-preparation cytology (see Figure 7.7)	Widely reported in Cockatiels in USA; uncommon in UK
	Chlamydophilosis	Faecal testing Zoonotic symptoms	Asymptomatic carrier status common in small psittacids Doxycycline is treatment of choice Test or treat all contact birds Warn owner of zoonotic signs
	Proventricular dilatation disease (PDD)	Contrast radiography Crop biopsy	
	Heavy metal toxicity	Radiography Serum metal analysis Haematology (lead) Amylase (zinc)	
	Enteritis	Bacteriology History (multiple cases)	
Lameness	Trauma – muscle/ligament Fracture Dislocation (rare)	History Clinical examination Radiography	
	Pelvic bruising following or during egg laying	History Signalment Radiography	
	Renal or gonadal neoplasia	Abdominal palpation Radiography ± contrast	Budgerigars particularly prone to gonadal and renal neoplasms. Hindlimb innervation lies between kidney/gonad and bony plate of synsacrum. Neoplasms press on nerves, presumably causing 'numbing' of limb
	Spinal disease	Clinical/neurological examination Radiographic abnormalities	
Feather loss, feather plucking and mutilation	Behavioural	Rule out internal and infectious problems	Difficult to diagnose definitively and to treat
	Systemic disease Metabolic disease	Haematology Biochemistry	

21.11 (continued) Differential diagnoses for specific presentations. (continues) ▶

Presentation	Differentials	Suggested tests	Notes
Feather loss, feather plucking and mutilation *continued*	Dermatitis	Clinical examination Cytology of feather pulp Skin biopsy	Various bacterial and fungal dermatoses can occur but can be difficult to differentiate primary inflammatory causes from inflammation secondary to self-trauma, which in turn may be result of internal disease processes
	Circovirus (psittacine beak and feather disease, PBDF) Polyomavirus	DNA-PCR testing of blood and feather pulp (circovirus) or cloacal swab (polyomavirus)	Both can cause 'French moult' in Budgerigar fledglings and typical dermatological and immunosuppression signs in all species (Polyomavirus also causes specific mortality in Budgerigar chicks)
	Pain	Clinical examination Radiographic abnormalities	
	Mites (rare)	Generalized pruritus (± anaemia): examine aviary or cage for *Dermanyssus*	Needs environmental eradication, rather than simple treatment of affected bird(s)
		Localized lesions: clinical examination reveals crusting typical of *Cnemidocoptes* on face and/or legs	Responds readily to avermectins, fipronil or other local antiparasitics
Chronic weight loss	Acute vs chronic	Often difficult to determine. Acute cases often present with moderate loss of pectoral muscle mass and other signs of clinical disease (regurgitation, fluffed etc). Subcutaneous fat may still be present or extensive even in face of marked acute weight loss Chronic cases usually more advanced and little fat present	
	Megabacteriosis ('megabacterium' yeast infection of proventriculus)	Gram-staining of faeces and 'crop wash' specimens	Usually present with chronic weight loss, often with 'sham-eating' behaviour (see Anorexia above) Can be sudden death due to acute haemorrhaging gastric ulcer Organism can be suppressed using amphotericin-B but is rarely eliminated so relapses probable
	Parasitism	Faecal wet-preparation cytology and flotation *Dermanyssus* found in aviary	
	Systemic infection Organ failure	Haematology Biochemistry *Chlamydophila* testing	
	Diabetes mellitus	Glycosuria Persistent hyperglycaemia Fructosamine	See notes under 'Polyuria/Polydipsia'
	Mycobacteriosis	Faecal acid-fast cytology (see Figure 7.22) Lesion biopsy	Mycobacterial (avian TB) infections usually enteric
Dyspnoea	Air sac infections Chlamydophilosis Aspergillosis (unusual)	Radiography Haematology *Chlamydophila* testing Bacteriology Endoscopy	
	Thyroid hyperplasia	Clinical examination Dietary history	Predominantly in Budgerigars on all-seed diets Characteristic click, wheeze, squeak or grunt on expiration Suggested to be independent of functional hypothyroidism, yet many affected birds obese Most respond well to iodine supplementation
	Non-respiratory factors	Haematology Biochemistry Radiography ± contrast	Dyspnoea is commonly result of poor ventilation of air sacs due to space-occupying 'abdominal region' lesions, including eggs, egg-related peritonitis, ascites, hepatomegaly and neoplasia

21.11 (continued) Differential diagnoses for specific presentations. (continues) ▶

Presentation	Differentials	Suggested tests	Notes
Facial swellings or discharges	*Cnemidocoptes*	Clinical examination Cytology	Very characteristic honeycombed crusting around beak, cere and sometimes legs of Budgerigars Unusual in other species May remain asymptomatic for long periods before becoming clinically apparent – consider immunosuppressant trigger factors
	Sinusitis	Clinical examination Cytology of nasal discharge or sinus flush sample *Chlamydophila* testing Bacteriology	Many cases of apparent 'ophthalmic' disease in small psittacids are actually sinus infections
	Rhinitis/rhinolith	Clinical examination	Likely to be associated with sinusitis (see above)
	Conjunctival sac foreign body	Clinical ophthalmological examination	May be secondary to underlying sinusitis and subsequent rubbing
	Otitis	Periauricular swelling or discharge	Uncommon
	Neoplasms	Cytology Biopsy	
	Mycobacteriosis	Faecal acid-fast cytology or histopathology	May appear to be localized neoplasms Dermal mycobacteriosis in birds may be associated with human (*Mycobacterium tuberculosis*) rather than avian (*M. avium-intracellulare* complex) as former, being respiratory pathogens, able to grow at lower temperatures

21.11 (continued) Differential diagnoses for specific presentations.

Therapeutics

The ideal therapeutic approach can only be designed once an accurate and specific diagnosis has been made and so this should always be the aim. However, for many reasons it is often not possible to reach this point and so some generalizations must be made, bearing in mind the findings of the investigations detailed above.

One of the problems particularly encountered in small psittacid therapeutics is that of how to deliver medications. Many owners find it difficult or impossible to handle their birds. Some birds are so ill that repeated handling needs to be avoided and so there may be benefits to longer-lasting injections, but a small proportion of birds will have adverse reactions to the injection procedure, especially with larger volumes. Nebulization therapy can be considered as a short-term method of delivering humidified air (which may even provide some rehydration) and of providing therapy for respiratory infections without having to handle the bird at all. For the longer term, in most cases medications will need to be given either by repeated injections, which will probably necessitate hospitalization of the bird, or by the oral route. In-food medication is possible (if the bird will eat it, a 'soft food' or mashed fruit with medication added can be prepared) but will result in unreliable intake of the drug. Similarly, in-water medication should generally be reserved as the last option, as the desert-dwelling parakeet species (especially Budgerigars) have evolved to be able to reduce their water intake dramatically at times when palatable water is unavailable. Both in-food and in-water intake will also be dramatically altered by the disease process itself – birds may be anorectic and may be adipsic or polydipsic.

The most reliable method of administration of medications is direct oral administration, either by using a crop tube for larger volumes or, for most medications, by simple administration of a few drops (up to 0.1 ml) directly into the bird's mouth. Palatability can again be a problem and the bird may accept the medication better if it is flavoured with a fruit juice or cordial, or mixed with jam, peanut butter or honey. Some medications, particularly avermectins, are absorbed readily through the skin and can be applied topically.

For a detailed discussion of appropriate therapeutic agents in psittacids see the Formulary (Appendix 3) at the back of this book. Figure 21.12 provides a ready reference for medications of frequent use in small psittacids, including a discussion of treatments that may have some merit as part of a 'shotgun' or 'coverall' approach to cases where any one of a number of clinically indistinguishable differentials could be causing the bird's disease.

Drug	Dosage (with practical 'rough dose' guide for common UK preparations in square brackets assuming 30–45 g Budgerigar and 90–120 g Cockatiel)	Indications / advantages	Disadvantages / contraindications
Amoxicillin	150 mg/kg i.m. q24h (long-acting preparation) [Duphamox LA injection 150 mg/ml (Fort Dodge): 0.05 ml per Budgerigar; 0.1 ml per Cockatiel] 150 mg/kg orally q12h [Duphamox palatable drops 50 mg/ml (Fort Dodge): 0.1 ml per Budgerigar; 0.3 ml per Cockatiel]	Bacterial infections Can be used as once daily 'LA' (long-acting) injection (do not substitute penicillin LA) Good choice to accompany enrofloxacin where serious bacterial infection suspected, as covers Gram-positive and anaerobes	Possible by oral route but requires 2 or 3 times a day administration In-water possible but only available as large-scale poultry/pigeon measures
Doxycycline	25–50 mg/kg orally q24h 520 mg/l water [UK licensed: Ornicure (Alpharma)] 100 mg/kg i.m. q7 days [Vibravenos injection 100 mg/5 ml (Pfizer): 0.2 ml per Budgerigar; 0.5 ml per Cockatiel]	Broad-spectrum antibiotic cover, including activity against Chlamydophila psittaci and mycoplasmas	No convenient suspension for oral dosing, use dispersible tablets In-water use licensed but for individual birds water intake very variable and doxycycline may make water less palatable Avoid calcium-containing supplements including grit and cuttlefish during oral therapy due to chelation effects Injection useful for birds that cannot be handled for dosing but only available under terms of 'Special Treatment Authorization' in UK
Edetate calcium disodium (EDTA)	35 mg/kg i.m. q12–24h 100 mg/kg i.m. once	Indicated as therapy for confirmed or suspected heavy metal toxicity	Potentially nephrotoxic Some prefer to dilute concentrated injection 1:5 with saline before administration.
Enrofloxacin (UK licensed)	10–15 mg/kg i.m., orally q12h [Baytril 2.5% (Bayer): 0.05 ml = 1 drop per Budgerigar; 0.1 ml = 2 drops per Cockatiel]	Bacterial infections. Broad-spectrum cover against many avian bacterial pathogens including some effect vs Chlamydophila and Mycoplasma Oral administration possible in drinking water	Not fully reliable in drinking water May decrease appetite (+ water intake if in-water) Not effective against anaerobes and some Gram-positives
Fluid therapy	15–20 ml/kg orally, s.c., i.v., intra-osseous q6–24h [1 ml per Budgerigar; 2 ml per Cockatiel]	Indicated for many sick small psittacids by oral, subcutaneous or in extreme cases intravenous or intraosseous routes	Avoid intraperitoneal route due to the risk of penetrating air sacs
Iodine	'Lugols' or 'Aqueous Iodine' [Make stock solution of 0.5 ml in 7.5 ml water. Store in dark bottle. Add 3 drops to every 100 ml drinking water.]	Thyroid goitre and possibly obesity in Budgerigars	
Metronidazole	40 mg/kg orally q24h 25 mg/kg orally q12h [Flagyl suspension 40 mg/ml (Hawgreen): 1 drop per Budgerigar; 0.1 ml per Cockatiel]	Main uses against trichomoniasis in Budgerigars, and giardiasis Also anaerobe antibiosis – useful adjunct to enrofloxacin or doxycycline where septic conditions suspected	
Multivitamin supplementation	Various forms available See notes on specific product labels Do not use more than one supplement concurrently	Deficiencies, particularly vitamin A	In-water medication unreliable On-seed medication unreliable Best route is powder on to fresh food or in 'soft food' if bird will consume Hypervitaminosis A possible, especially if multiple products used or manufacturer's guidelines exceeded

21.12 Therapeutic medications for use in small psittacine birds. (continues) ▶

Drug	Dosage (with practical 'rough dose' guide for common UK preparations in square brackets assuming 30–45 g Budgerigar and 90–120 g Cockatiel)	Indications / advantages	Disadvantages / contraindications
Non-steroidal anti-inflammatory drugs (NSAIDs)	Meloxicam: 0.2 mg/kg orally/i.m. q24h [Metacam oral solution 0.05 mg per drop (Boehringer Ingelheim): 'a quarter of a drop' per Budgerigar; 'half a drop' per Cockatiel] Can be diluted with honey immediately prior to administration where appropriate Carprofen: 4 mg/kg i.m. q24h [Rimadyl 50 mg/ml injection (Pfizer): 0.001 ml per bird]	Pain, inflammation Meloxicam available as palatable formulation in UK	Potential GI ulceration and renal disease Side effects rare in psittacine species
Nystatin Amphotericin B	Nystatin: 300,000 IU/kg orally q12h [Generic nystatin suspension 100,000 IU/ml: 0.1 ml per Budgerigar; 0.3 ml per Cockatiel] Amphotericin B: 100–300 mg/kg orally q12h [Fungilin oral suspension 100 mg/ml (Bristol-Myers Squibb): 1–2 drops per Budgerigar]	Oral or crop yeast infections Not systemically absorbed – works by contact Amphotericin B effective at suppressing 'megabacterium'	Must be delivered to site of infection – crop tube administration misses oral and proximal oesophageal lesions Nystatin not effective against 'megabacterium'
Potentiated sulphonamide	100 mg/kg orally q12h [Septrin Paediatric Suspension 240 mg/5 ml (GlaxoSmithKline): 0.1 ml per Budgerigar; 0.2 ml per Cockatiel]	Broad-spectrum antibiosis	Available in UK in convenient and palatable banana-flavoured suspension
Probiotics	Various in-water and on-food products available	Alterations to GI flora; stress	
Prokinetics (Cisapride, metoclopramide)	Cisapride: 1 mg/kg orally q8–12h [Prepulsid suspension 1 mg/ml (Janssen-Cilag): 1 drop per Budgerigar; 2 drops per Cockatiel] Metoclopramide: 0.5 mg/kg orally, i.m. q8h [Generic 5 mg/ml injection: 0.005 ml per Budgerigar; 0.1 ml per Cockatiel; 1 mg/ml oral products: 1 drop per bird]	GI motility alterations, particularly regurgitation and crop stasis.	Cisapride appears more effective, but in UK is only available (Prepulsid suspension) under terms of 'Special Treatment Authorization'

Useful combination therapies:
The following mixtures have few data supporting pharmacological stability, but are easy to administer and have been used by the author and editors with apparent success.

Amphotericin B and metronidazole	1 part Fungilin to 4 parts Flagyl [0.1 ml per Budgerigar q12h]	Indicated for vomition or regurgitation of undiagnosed cause in Budgerigars. Combines effects against Candida, 'megabacterium', Trichomonas, Giardia and some other bacterial infections
Enrofloxacin and meloxicam	10 parts Baytril 2.5% oral to 1 part Metacam oral [1 drop per Budgerigar; 2 drops per Cockatiel; q12h]	Useful combination for treatment of inflammation or pain with possible bacterial involvement, e.g. traumatic and surgical wounds

21.12 (continued) Therapeutic medications for use in small psittacine birds.

22

Zoonotic, legal and ethical aspects

Peter Scott

Zoonoses

Many zoonoses are transmissible from psittacine birds (Figure 22.1) and the legal aspects of these diseases are important. The Health and Safety at Work Act (HSWA) 1974 and the Control of Substances Hazard-ous to Health (COSHH) regulations 1988 both apply here. Civil law relating to negligence also has a bearing with regard to clients or indeed veterinary staff who may become infected or injured (Animals Act 1971). It is now necessary to prepare COSHH sheets related to zoonotic diseases.

Disease	Causal organism	Means of spread	Effect on host		Possible control measures	Comments
			Bird	*Human*		
Salmonellosis	*Salmonella* spp.	Usually ingestion, occasionally other routes	Varies from subclinical (non-apparent) to acute systemic disease	Varies. Often gastrointestinal, sometimes fever	Hygiene Routine health checks	Latent infection is common in some species
Chlamydophilosis (psittacosis or ornithosis)	*Chlamydophila psittaci*	Usually inhalation, occasionally other routes	Varies from subclinical to acute systemic disease	Varies from subclinical to severe respiratory; can be fatal	Minimize contact Hygiene Routine health checks Screening of in-patients Safe post-mortem technique	Can also be contracted from other (non-psittacine) species
Yersiniosis (pseudotuberculosis)	*Yersinia pseudotubulosis* and *Y. enterocolitica*	Usually ingestion	Varies from subclinical to acute disease	Alimentary signs	Control rodents Minimize contamination of food by rodents or wild birds Hygiene	Wide range of animal hosts
Tuberculosis (mycobacteriosis)	*Mycobacterium* spp.	Usually ingestion, occasionally other routes	Varies from local lesions to systemic disease: cutaneous lesions commonly *M. tuberculosis*; systemic lesions commonly *M. avium*	Varies from local lesions to extensive involvement of respiratory or urinary tract	Hygiene Routine health checks	Immunosuppressed people are particularly susceptible to mycobacteria, including atypical species
Ectoparasite infestation	Many species, especially *Dermanyssus gallinae*	Contact	Varies from subclinical to pruritus and anaemia	Pruritus and skin lesions	Hygiene Routine health checks	Some birds seem more susceptible than others

22.1 Examples of zoonotic diseases associated with psittacine birds.

Psittacosis (Chlamydophilosis)

Psittacosis is perhaps the most significant zoonosis associated with parrots and it must be noted that people have died after becoming infected by their birds. At the same time it is a popular diagnosis (or misdiagnosis) in humans following disclosure that they have a pet bird.

The **Zoonoses Order 1989** made under the Animal Health Act 1981 designates organisms of the genera *Salmonella* and *Brucella* as zoonoses, enabling powers (including powers relating to the slaughter of poultry) under the Animal Health Act 1981 to be used to reduce any risk to human health of these organisms. Under this Order the term 'poultry' has been extended to include birds of any species. The order provides for the imposition of control measures that include quarantine, movement restrictions, cleansing and disinfection.

The **Psittacosis and Ornithosis Order 1953** provides for the detention and isolation of birds and for other powers to prevent the spread of disease. This order extends the definition of the expression 'disease' for the purposes of the Diseases of Animals Act 1950 to include 'psittacosis' or 'ornithosis'. The order also provides for the detention and isolation of birds affected (or suspected of being affected) with this disease, and for the cleansing and disinfection of premises and utensils for such birds. The order, together with the Diseases of Animals (extension of Definition of Poultry) Order 1953, also enables powers of compulsory slaughter to be used, at the government minister's discretion, in respect of poultry affected with or in any way exposed to psittacosis/ornithosis. This regulation brings 'parrots' within the definition of poultry.

Compulsory slaughter of psittacine birds has never been carried out on the grounds of psittacosis. A number of veterinary surgeons have recommended this as a course of action but it is not required in the UK (and indeed is not necessary in the view of this author) and may lead to claims for compensation. Certain specific situations regarding the health of the owner (immunosuppression) or the level of risk (uncontrollable exposure to the public) may result in a decision to euthanase a bird.

Various treatment regimes for psittacosis have been published (Chapter 13) and the licensed drug for use in the UK is doxycycline (Ornicure) (see Appendix 3). The owner must be advised about the zoonotic risks and about the difficulty and problems in guaranteeing a complete clearance of organisms. Different requirements for dealing with psittacosis may exist in other countries and it would be sensible for veterinary surgeons to check national requirements.

Despite all of this, psittacosis in humans is not currently a notifiable disease in the UK. For a time, for the sake of gathering information, it was made notifiable in three local authority areas (Cambridge City, South Cambridgeshire and East Cambridgeshire). DEFRA (Department for Environment, Food and Rural Affairs) laboratories making the diagnosis in psittacine birds will usually report the incident to the local medical officer of health, who will usually want to know that a veterinary surgeon is dealing with the case and advising the owner about treatment and disinfection.

The **Diseases of Animals (Seizure) Order 1993** lists psittacosis (ornithosis) amongst the diseases to which this order applies and includes the following:

- An inspector or veterinary inspector shall have power to seize anything (other than a live animal), whether animate or inanimate, by or by means of which it appears to him that a disease to which section 35(1) of the Animal Health Act 1981 applies might be carried or transmitted.
- An inspector or veterinary inspector exercising powers under this Order shall dispose of the thing seized by destruction, burial, treatment or such other method of disposal as he thinks expedient to prevent the spread of disease.

This essentially provides for collection of samples, which then allows for the exclusion of Newcastle disease or avian influenza.

Avian influenza and Newcastle disease in Psittaciformes

At present the official view of DEFRA in the UK is that, under the **Diseases of Poultry (England) Order 2003**, both avian influenza and Newcastle disease are notifiable. This means that anyone who suspects either of these diseases in a bird or carcass must inform the local DEFRA Divisional Veterinary Manager (DVM). The same applies to a person who examines or inspects any bird or carcass or who analyses any samples taken from any bird or carcass and suspects these diseases.

The DVM will give telephone advice and arrange to investigate the report. A notice will be served on the occupier or person in charge of the premises (Schedule 1, Part 1 of the Order) where disease is suspected specifying certain restrictions and requirements; for example, that birds are kept in their living quarters or some other place where they can be isolated and that nothing liable to transmit disease is moved from the premises.

If disease is confirmed, the objective of the control is to prevent virus production. The most effective way of doing this at present is by slaughter of affected birds. Contacts would be traced to identify other birds that might have been exposed to disease. Where disease is confirmed in poultry, an infected area would be declared (with a minimum radius of 10 km) and restrictions applied to that area. However, this may not happen if disease is confirmed in captive birds or racing pigeons unless there was a serious risk that the disease could affect poultry.

Under the Animal Health Act 1981, compensation is paid for birds that are slaughtered because of an outbreak of avian influenza or Newcastle disease but which are not diseased.

The Control of Substances Hazardous to Health (COSHH) Regulations

The COSHH Regulations apply to biological agents and there is a Biological Agents Approved Code of Practice (ACOP) in addition to the general COSHH requirements. Biological agents are classified into

Groups 1 to 4, with Group 1 being the least and Group 4 the most dangerous. A suitable and sufficient risk assessment (Figure 22.2) must be carried out for any work activity involving the deliberate use of biological agents (e.g. research, medical care) or any exposure where exposure is incidental to the activity (e.g. veterinary work, farm work). The assessment should cover the agents, their form, effects and hazard groups, the likelihood of exposure and disease, the possibility of substitution by a less hazardous agent, the control measures, monitoring and health surveillance. Detailed guidance is available on appropriate control measures, especially for intentional work with biological agents. The Health and Safety Executive (HSE) must be notified of the use, storage or consignment of biological agents. Protective clothing and equipment should not itself become a means of transmitting agents. Monitoring of exposure should be carried out if a suitable technique is available. Information should be provided to employees in writing, particularly when dealing with highly infective agents.

Other legislation

Other legislation relevant to zoonoses includes:

- **Public Health (Control of Disease) Act 1984** This is regarded as the key piece of legislation covering communicable diseases and gives various powers to the medical authorities.
- **Public Health (Infectious Diseases) Regulations 1988** This is the key legislation listing notifiable diseases in humans and updating controls. It includes rabies, tuberculosis, leptospirosis and anthrax.

Endangered species legislation

CITES

The 'Washington' Convention on International Trade in Endangered Species of Wild Fauna and Flora, more commonly known as CITES, aims to protect certain plants and animals by regulating and monitoring their

A suitable and sufficient risk assessment must:

- Identify all the hazards – that is, those aspects of work that have the potential to cause harm:
    Substances
    Equipment
    Work processes
    Work organization
    Biological agents
- Identify any specific regulations that must be complied with
- Assess all the risks – that is, the likelihood that the harm will occur from the hazards identified
- Be systematic in approach
- Ensure that all aspects of the work activity are considered:
    Waiting room
    Consulting room
    Laboratory
    Operation room/preparation room
    Kennels/hospitalization facilities
- Address what actually happens in the workplace, not what the staff handbook or practice manual says should happen.
- Ensure that everyone who might be affected (employees and others) is considered, e.g.:
    Veterinary staff (vets and nurses, kennel staff)
    Office staff
    Night cleaners
    Maintenance staff
    Visitors
- Identify groups of workers particularly at risk, such as:
    Young workers
    Inexperienced workers
    Lone workers
    Workers with disabilities
    Pregnant workers
- Take account of existing preventive or precautionary measures and whether they are working properly:
    Isolation
    Effects of treatment
    Disinfection
    Air flows

22.2 Risk assessment.

international trade to prevent it reaching unsustainable levels. The Convention came into force in 1975 and the UK became a Party in 1976. There are now over 150 Parties. The CITES Secretariat is administered by the United Nations Environment Programme (UNEP).

The species covered by CITES are listed in three Appendices, according to the degree of protection they need:

- **Appendix I** includes species threatened with extinction. Trade in specimens of these species is permitted only in exceptional circumstances.
- **Appendix II** includes species not necessarily threatened with extinction, but in which trade must be controlled in order to avoid utilization incompatible with their survival.
- **Appendix III** contains species that are protected in at least one country, which has asked other CITES Parties for assistance in controlling the trade.

The psittacine species listed in these Appendices are shown in Figure 22.3.

A specimen of a CITES-listed species may be imported into or exported (or re-exported) from a State that is party to the Convention only if the appropriate certification has been obtained beforehand and presented for clearance at the port of entry or exit. There is some variation in the requirements from one country to another and it is *always* necessary to check on the national laws.

EC Wildlife Trade Regulation
CITES has been implemented in the European Union since 1984 through a number of Regulations.

- **Council Regulation (EC) No. 338/97** deals with the protection of species of wild fauna and flora by regulating the trade in these species.

- **Commission Regulation (EC) No. 1808/2001** (which replaced **Commission Regulation (EC) No. 939/37**) sets out the rules for the import, export and re-export of the species to which they apply. The regulation of trade is based on a system of permits and certificates that may only be issued when certain conditions are met.

Within the EU, the lists are described as A, B and C rather than I, II and III. This may appear confusing but the lists may differ a little; the system allows for tighter controls within Europe than perhaps are operated elsewhere and so, whilst operating CITES as a basis, the EU may upgrade the level of 'supervision' given to a species.

In the European Union the CITES Appendices are replaced by Annexes to EC Regulation 338/97. Current species lists are held by the UNEP World Conservation Monitoring Centre and can be viewed by visiting their web site.

- **Annex A** includes all species listed in **Appendix I** of CITES, plus certain other species included because they look the same, need a similar level of protection, or to secure the effective protection of rare taxa within the same genus.
- **Annex B** includes all the remaining species listed in **Appendix II** of CITES, plus certain other species included on a 'lookalike' basis, or because the level of trade may not be compatible with the survival of the species or local populations, or because they pose an ecological threat to indigenous species.
- **Annex C** includes all the remaining species listed in **Appendix III** of CITES.
- **Annex D** includes those non-CITES species not listed in **Annexes A** and **C** that are imported into the Union in such numbers as to warrant monitoring.

Appendix I

Amazona arausiaca	*Ara couloni*	*Propyrrhura couloni*
Amazona barbadensis	*Ara glaucogularis* (often traded as *Ara caninde*)	*Propyrrhura maracana*
Amazona brasiliensis	*Ara macao*	*Psephotus chrysopterygius*
Amazona guildingii	*Ara militaris*	*Psephotus dissimilis*
Amazona imperialis	*Ara rubrogenys*	*Psephotus pulcherrimus* (possibly extinct)
Amazona leucocephala	*Cacatua goffini*	*Psittacula echo*
Amazona ochrocephala auropalliata	*Cacatua haematuropygia*	*Pyrrhura cruentata*
Amazona o. belizensis	*Cacatua moluccensis*	*Rhynchopsitta* spp.
Amazona o. caribaea	*Cyanopsitta spixii*	*Strigops habroptilus*
Amazona o. oratrix	*Cyanoramphus forbesi*	*Vini ultramarina*
Amazona o. parvipes	*Cyanoramphus novaezelandiae*	
Amazona o. tresmariae	*Cyclopsitta diophthalma coxeni*	
Amazona pretrei	*Eos histrio*	**Appendix III**
Amazona rhodocorytha	*Eunymphicus cornutus*	
Amazona tucumana	*Geopsittacus occidentalis* (possibly extinct)	*Psittacula krameri* (Ghana)
Amazona versicolor	*Guarouba guarouba*	
Amazona vinacea	*Neophema chrysogaster*	**Appendix II**
Amazona viridigenalis	*Ognorhynchus icterotis*	
Amazona vittata	*Pezoporus wallicus*	The rest of the Psittaciformes (e.g. Blue-fronted Amazon, Grey Parrot) but excluding the
Anodorhynchus spp.	*Pionopsitta pileata*	Budgerigar and Cockatiel, which are not included
Ara ambigua	*Probosciger aterrimus*	in the Appendices.

22.3 Parrot species listed in CITES Appendices.

Aside from trading restrictions (see below), CITES also requires that anyone breeding or displaying for commercial gain any species listed on Annex A requires a licence under Article 10, referred to as a 'specimen specific' licence. Sale of a bird requires an Article 10 certificate. The Red-fronted Kakariki (*Cyanoramphus novaezelandiae*) and Hooded Parrot (*Psephotus dissimilus*) are commonly bred in captivity and are exempt from these requirements, under Article 32(a). They can therefore be sold, exchanged or displayed without the need for an Article 10 certificate. However, they must be closed-ringed and there must be documentary evidence that they were bred in captivity. Zoos with many Annex A animals usually apply for Article 30 licences, which are collection specific and act as a blanket licence for all of the animals and plants they hold. All Annex A birds are required to be permanently marked with either a closed ring or a microchip.

Implementation of CITES regulations

The Global Wildlife Division of DEFRA is the UK's CITES Management Authority, responsible for ensuring that the Convention is implemented in the UK. Its role includes enforcement and issuing permits and certificates for the import and export, or commercial use, of CITES specimens. All enquiries regarding Article 10 licensing should therefore be referred to this division. Applications for CITES permits are referred to a designated CITES Scientific Authority for advice on the conservation status of the species concerned.

In the UK, CITES is enforced principally through the **Control of Trade in Endangered Species (Enforcement) Regulations 1997**, known as COTES. It was widely felt by conservation groups that the weak powers of this legislation accounted for the relatively few prosecutions under it, and this concern resulted in harsher penalties being introduced in 2003. There are provisions within COTES for power of entry and provision for offences by corporate bodies. Prosecutions may also involve the Customs and Excise Management Act 1979 for import offences, which has more substantial penalties.

It is advisable to check current lists and requirements on the internet or with DEFRA, as they change fairly frequently.

Global Wildlife Division of DEFRA:
www.defra.gov.uk/wildlife-countryside/gwd/cites/index.htm
UK CITES: www.ukcites.gov.uk
UNEP World Conservation Monitoring Centre: www.unep-wcmc.org

Also see:
Joint Nature Conservation Committee: www.jncc.gov.uk
Red List of Endangered Species: www.redlist.org

Import and export

Importation of psittacine birds into the UK from within the EU is covered by Directive 92/65 EEC (the 'Balai' Directive). This requires an official export health certificate.

Importation from Third Countries (i.e. countries outside the EU) requires general licences with conditions laid down in Commission Decision 2000/666/EC,

which currently allows imports only from countries that are members of the Office International des Epizooties (OIE). The imported birds must have an approved-format health certificate and must be quarantined in approved premises for 30 days. During quarantine they will be kept with sentinel chickens that are then blood tested towards the end of the quarantine to ensure that they are clear of Newcastle disease and avian influenza. Where private owners are importing pet birds it may be possible for birds to be quarantined in the owners' homes. They should be inspected by an official veterinary surgeon within 24 hours of arrival and again 35 days later. All waste materials from the bird must be destroyed during this period and any illness must be reported to the local Divisional Veterinary Manager. Imports must comply with the Importation of Birds, Poultry and Hatching Eggs Order 1979.

Exports are dealt with in a similar fashion. Certification of birds for import/export is complex and requires consultation every time with DEFRA. Export papers often require certification that an area is clear of Newcastle disease but this cannot be certified without the prior confirmation and permission of DEFRA.

Some practical pointers for those involved with importing and exporting birds are given below.

Determine the species. This sounds easier than it may be in practice and it could be crucially important in moving a bird to another country.

For the owner:
• Check with the Global Wildlife division of DEFRA regarding any CITES requirements. If appropriate, obtain certificates and submit to the destination country for their CITES team to approve import. (Failure to do this could lead to confiscation.)
• Submit to DEFRA for CITES approval. They will then issue an import certificate.

For the veterinary surgeon:
• Advise the owner to clarify the situation with the Global Wildlife Division.
• Check with DEFRA Animal Health division.

Commercial importation

This is a complex business involving a number of steps, covering both CITES and internal health controls:

1. Before importing, the importer must provide a prior export permit from the country of origin.
2. This is presented to the UK CITES Office (DEFRA), which checks with the government scientific management adviser, the Joint Nature Conservation Committee (JNCC), which considers the application.
3. If JNCC approves, it advises DEFRA to issue a permit.
4. The birds are then brought in through Heathrow, where they and the certification are checked by the Customs CITES team.
5. The birds are held in quarantine and inspected three times prior to release for sale.

CITES Appendix A species cannot be traded commercially but applications must go through the same procedure.

The practical pointers to be borne in mind concerning import are the following:

- Obtain prior export certificate from country of origin.
- Submit to DEFRA for CITES approval; they then issue import certificate.
- Check with DEFRA Animal Health.

It is necessary to be aware that CITES rules are implemented differently in different parts of the world.

Performing animals cause special problems where they may be imported into a country for a particular job, which may be for a matter of days, or on a contract for several years. If the stay is long term but ownership is not changing, it may be necessary for the animals to travel back to the country of origin simply for renewal of paperwork.

Biological and veterinary diagnostic samples

It is important to note that, currently, CITES rules apply to all tissues from CITES specimens, including samples taken for diagnostic purposes. The Global Wildlife Division of DEFRA should be contacted and appropriate paperwork obtained prior to sending samples outside the EU.

Zoo legislation (UK)

The **Zoo Licensing Act 1981 (Amendment) (England and Wales) Regulations 2002** includes all places where animals not normally domesticated in the UK are displayed to the public for 7 days or more per year, whether a charge is made or not. This could range from a conventional zoo or bird garden to a local council-operated park with aviaries. This Act was primarily concerned with public safety, though animal welfare issues were also covered. The recent Amendments comply with the EC Zoos Directive (1999/22/EC) to provide for good standards of animal care, and set the framework for the participation of zoos in conservation, research and education.

The Secretary of State's Standards for Modern Zoo Practice are the standards to which zoos and public aquaria must operate in the UK. The general standards are based around the 'Five Freedoms', presented as Five Principles:

- *Provision of food and water* – requiring attention to nutritional content, method of presentation and natural behaviour of the animal or bird
- *Provision of a suitable environment* – consistent with species' requirements; spatial requirements are included, as are appropriate three-dimensional environments
- *Provision of animal healthcare* – to protect the animal from injury and disease
- *Provision of an opportunity to express most normal behaviour* – taking into account enrichment and husbandry guidelines
- *Provision of protection from fear and distress* – including group composition, sex ratios and stocking levels.

These principles provide a good structure for assessing any parrot accommodation. The current standards are available via the internet or direct from DEFRA.

Performing animals (UK)

The **Performing Animals (Regulation) Act & Performing Animals Rules 1968** require any person who exhibits or trains any performing (vertebrate) animal to be registered with a local authority. The term 'exhibit' is defined as 'exhibit at any entertainment to which the public are admitted, whether on payment of money or otherwise…'. To 'train' means 'train for the purpose of any such exhibition'.

This applies to circuses and also to other situations (such as cabarets, film making and plays) that involve animal performances, and there is no exemption for zoos. The definitions in the Act also appear to cover some of the training and performance with animals that take place in zoos. However, it might be expected that training that was carried out to assist in the routine management of an animal (and not intended as preparation for a performance) would not involve registration.

Ethical considerations

Psittacine birds have been kept in captivity for a relatively short time and with the exception of very few species (Budgerigar and Cockatiel) they cannot really be considered domesticated.

There are several ethical issues related to the keeping of parrots.

In the past, parrot keeping has been unsatisfactory at various levels. Birds brought under human 'stewardship' or 'ownership' should be given consideration. People make a choice to keep them for their own reasons. The birds have not been changed in any way from the wild bird, other than losing freedom, the very least that can be done is to give them what they need. The Five Freedoms mentioned above have been used in a wide range of animal-related areas to assess welfare and are also applicable here.

Behavioural disorders shown by pet birds can perhaps be legitimately used as evidence that some birds may be relatively unsuited to captivity. The Grey Parrot is the classic example: a flock bird, which in the wild eats predominantly one food item (the fruit of an oil palm), is captured in large numbers, shipped through the supply chain and may end up as a single bird in a small cage. At some stage its diet is changed, ultimately to a poor one consisting mainly of sunflower seed (a seed that Grey Parrots do not see in the wild but which they take to because of its high fat content). These birds very often develop feather plucking problems. It appears that the cause of these behavioural problems may be multifactorial, but many of those factors have a human cause. Captive-bred Grey Parrots will often develop the same sorts of problems.

Bringing into captivity

The majority of species have now been bred in captivity yet some species are still collected from the wild for the pet trade (e.g. Grey Parrot). The concept of sustainable wildlife resources is used to support this practice and, since the concept is one that now has support from some of the wildlife conservation organizations, it cannot be ignored.

The very important captive-breeding work now being carried out with a wide range of parrots (including Spix Macaws) is based on pioneering work by serious aviculturists rather than zoos. The serious zoo contribution is relatively recent. But it is still important to distinguish between a pet keeper and an aviculturist (although aviculturists were probably all pet keepers once).

Basic 'keeping' practices

Cages for pet birds have been extremely unsatisfactory. Many birds have been kept for their captive life in cages too small to spread their wings.

There is provision in Section 8 of the **Wildlife & Countryside Act 1981** which regulates the size of cage in which any bird (excluding poultry) may be kept. The cage or other receptacle must be sufficient in height, length or breadth to permit a bird to stretch its wings freely, unless: the bird is being moved by any means; or it is being shown or exhibited and is not so kept for longer than 72 hours; or it is undergoing treatment or examination by a veterinary surgeon; or it is being trained for exhibition and is not so kept for any longer than 1 hour in any period of 24 hours.

In practice this can make it difficult to find cages suitable for macaws and makes many of the parrot cages currently in use potentially illegal. The aim is laudable but it has resulted in criminalizing many people who should rather have been educated to want better accommodation, and to demand it for their birds. The dealer who sells the bird with an inadequate cage is perhaps the one who should be prosecuted.

Feeding of pet birds especially is often poor. Owners may be lazy or ignorant of the bird's needs ('Birds eat seeds, don't they?'); they may simply feed what the bird selectively chooses (e.g. sunflower seeds: despite these being nutritionally deficient, they taste nice). At this stage little is known by the scientific community of the true dietary needs of parrots, yet there is now a switch to 'complete diets' that fail to provide any of the behavioural rewards such as finding food, husking seeds or squeezing fruit. Birds eat from what they are given and it is the owner's fault if a diet is deficient nutritionally or by behavioural deprivation.

Wing clipping as a practice causes problems. It is a fact that, if a bird is to be kept, controlling its flight by means of training, harnesses or wing trimming does make certain tasks easier to carry out. Over the years even pinioning (in this context widely accepted as an unnecessary mutilation) has been used on these birds.

It can be argued that wing clipping permits the bird greater access and freedom and is therefore good, but in reality it simply makes the owner's life easier and as such is difficult to justify. It is perfectly possible to use harnesses (Figure 22.6) to control flight temporarily when necessary.

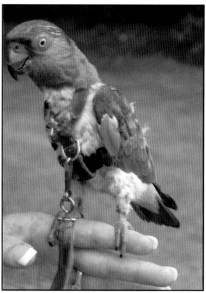

22.6

Senegal Parrot wearing harness and leash. This enables the owner to take the bird outside with them on walks; therefore the bird's wings do not need to be clipped. (Courtesy of John Chitty.)

Setting aside the various techniques that may cause injury due to unbalancing a bird or may trigger feather plucking, the practice of wing clipping inevitably frustrates the bird's ability to fly and causes it to lose a 'gift' that renders birds unique. It is suggested that the removal of flight leaves a bird psychologically 'exposed' to predators and that this may be a cause of stress. When carried out in a young bird that has never flown, the psychological effects may be even worse.

Section 14(1) of the Wildlife & Countryside Act 1981 makes it an offence for a person to release or allow the escape of an animal (including birds) of a kind that is not ordinarily resident in and is not a regular visitor to Great Britain in a wild state; or a species listed in Schedule 9. This affects those people who might wish to free-fly their birds (zoos and private keepers), and if in doubt people wishing to do this should contact DEFRA's wildlife inspectorate for advice.

Supply of medicines

The **Medicines (restrictions on the administration of veterinary medicinal products) regulations 1994 (SI 1994/2987), as amended by SI 1997/12884 (Amelia 8)**, establish in UK law the prescribing cascade, and the requirements for minimum withdrawal periods and for record keeping by veterinary surgeons that were adopted by the European Community in 1990. These requirements were incorporated in the Code of Practice for the Prescribing of Medicinal Products by Veterinary Surgeons introduced by the British Veterinary Association (BVA) in 1991 and, subsequently, in the Guide to Professional Conduct of the Royal College of Veterinary Surgeons.

In summary, when no authorized veterinary medicinal product exists for a condition in a particular species, and in order to avoid causing unacceptable suffering, veterinary surgeons exercising their clinical judgement may prescribe for one or a small number of animals under their care in accordance with the following sequence:

(i) A veterinary medicine authorized for use in another species, or for a different use in the same species ('off-label use')
(ii) A medicine authorized in the UK for human use
(iii) A medicine to be made up at the time on a one-off basis by a veterinary surgeon or a properly authorized person.

There are additional requirements for treating food-producing animals.

The 'small number of animals' limitation and the requirement to follow the three stages of the cascade in strict order do not apply to non-food-producing animals of minor or exotic species. The Veterinary Medicines Directorate suggests that, as a working rule, 'minor and exotic species' is taken to cover all companion, laboratory and zoo animals (other than any whose produce might enter the food chain) other than cats and dogs.

Other UK legislation affecting psittacine birds

The **Protection of Animals Act, 1911 (1912 Scotland)** deals with the subject of unnecessary suffering. It states that:

1.1 If any person –
  a) shall cruelly beat, kick, ill-treat, over-ride, over-drive, over-load, torture, infuriate, or terrify any animal, or shall cause or procure, or, being the owner, permit any animal to be so used, or shall, by wantonly or unreasonably doing or omitting to do any act, or causing or procuring the commission or omission of any act, cause any unnecessary suffering, or, being the owner, permit any unnecessary suffering to be so caused to any animal; or
  b) shall convey or carry, or cause or procure, or, being the owner, permit to be conveyed or carried, any animal in such manner or position as to cause that animal any unnecessary suffering, …
such person shall be guilty of an offence of cruelty within the meaning of this Act, …

Cooper (1987) discussed the implications of this in detail and explained that, to show that an offence under Section 1 has been committed, it is necessary to show that an act both causes suffering and that it was unnecessary. It also needs to be unreasonable and, by case law, 'substantial'. This may change with the new legislation currently being drafted.

Under the **Pet Animals Act, 1951 and Pet Animals Act, 1951 (Amendment) Act 1982**, BVA and local authority consultative groups have Guidelines for Inspections that specify cage dimensions and standards for shops. Considerations during an inspection should include:

- The basic Five Freedoms or Five Principles as outlined
- Suitable food
- The cage size requirements from the Wildlife and Countryside Act
- Isolation/separate accommodation available if necessary
- Signs of behavioural problems (e.g. feather plucking).

One part of this Act is being used to control sale of birds (mainly parrots) at bird shows and auction:

2. If any person carries on a business of selling animals as pets in any part of a street or public place, at a stall or barrow in a market, he will be guilty of an offence.

It would seem likely that the point of putting this in the original Act was to safeguard animals from the milling hordes of people in a market, and to protect them from the influence of the weather, by putting the sale of animals into shops where the public and the conditions could be controlled. Some degree of argument has been used to license some such premises where the 'public' enter for a fee as pet shops, since they are not simply 'open'.

Such sale days and fairs do perform a function in allowing breeders (unlicensed in any other way) to come together and sell surplus birds in a reasonably controlled, inspected environment. This should be viewed as a better alternative than no control at all.

The **Abandonment of Animals Act, 1960** makes it an offence of cruelty under the 1911 Act to abandon an animal without reasonable excuse in circumstances likely to cause it suffering. Prosecutions have been sought in regard to pet Cockatiels released when an owner moved house.

Under the **Animals (Scientific Procedures) Act 1986**, as amended, regulated procedures involving pain, suffering, distress or lasting harm in live vertebrate animals and the octopus must be authorized. Researchers and premises must also be authorized. The Act applies to zoos and fieldwork but it does not apply to procedures that are recognized veterinary, agricultural and animal husbandry practices. Most behavioural observation is not covered by the Act.

The **Animals Act 1971** makes provision with respect to civil liability for damage done by animals. It places liability on the keeper, who at the time may not necessarily be the owner.

Other useful web sites

- Health Protection Agency: www.hpa.org.uk
- Health and Safety Executive: www.hse.gov.uk/pubns/ais2.pdf

Leaflet AIS2, *Common Zoonoses in Agriculture*, can be found at the HSE site. The HSE also publishes *The Occupational Zoonoses*.

References and further reading

References

Aguilar RF and Redig PT (1995) Diagnosis and treatment of avian aspergillosis. In: *Kirk's Current Veterinary Therapy XII*, ed. JD Bonagura, pp. 1294–1299. WB Saunders, Philadelphia

Alexander DJ (1987) Taxonomy and nomenclature of avian paramyxoviruses. *Avian Pathology* **16**, 547–552

Altmann RB, Clubb SL, Dorrestein GM and Quesenberry K (1997) *Avian Medicine and Surgery*. WB Saunders, Philadelphia

André J and Delverdier M (1999) Primary bronchial carcinoma with osseous metastasis in an African grey parrot (*Psittacus erithacus*). *Journal of Avian Medicine and Surgery* **13**, 180–186

Antinoff N (2001) Understanding and treating the infraorbital sinus and respiratory system. *Proceedings of the Annual Conference and Expo of the Association of Avian Veterinarians, Orlando, Florida, August 22–24*, pp. 245–260

Antinoff N, Hoefer HL, Rosenthal KL and Bartick TE (1997) Smooth muscle neoplasia of suspected oviductal origin in the cloaca of a blue fronted Amazon parrot (*Amazona aestiva*). *Journal of Avian Medicine and Surgery* **11**, 268–272

Antinoff N and Hottinger HA (2000) Treatment of a cloacal papilloma by mucosal stripping in an Amazon parrot. In: *Proceedings of the Annual Conference of the Association of Avian Veterinarians, Denver, USA*, pp. 97–100

Bartels KE (ed.) (2002) Lasers in Medicine and Surgery. *Veterinary Clinics of North America* **32**(3)

Bauck L (1995) Nutritional problems in pet birds. *Seminars in Avian and Exotic Pet Medicine* **4**, 3-8.

Bauck L, Hillyer E and Hoefer H (1992) Rhinitis: case reports. *Proceedings of the Annual Conference and Expo of the Association of Avian Veterinarians*, pp. 134–139

Baumgartner R, Hoop RK and Widmar R (1994) Atypical nocardiosis in a red-lored Amazon parrot (*Amazona autumnalis autumnalis*). *Journal of the Association of Avian Veterinarians* **8**, 125–127

Bavellar FJ and Beynen AC (2003) Influence of amount and type of dietary fat on plasma cholesterol concentrations in African Grey Parrots. *Journal of Applied Research in Veterinary Medicine* **1**, 1–7

Bennett RA (2002) Reproductive surgery in birds. *Proceedings, North American Veterinary Conference*

Best R (1996) Breeding problems. In: *Manual of Raptors, Pigeons and Waterfowl*, ed. PH Beynon, NA Forbes and NH Harcourt-Brown, pp. 208–215. BSAVA, Cheltenham

Blanchard S (2000) Teaching your parrot self-soothing techniques. *Pet Bird Report* **9**(6), 52–53

Bowles HL and Zantop DW (2002) A novel surgical technique for luxation repair of the femorotibial joint in the Monk parakeet (*Myiopsitta monachus*). *Journal of Avian Medicine and Surgery* **16**, 34–38

Brooks DE (1997) Avian cataracts. *Seminars in Avian and Exotic Pet Medicine* **6**, 131–137

Brown RE, Kovacs CE, Butler JP *et al.* (1995) The avian lung: is there an aerodynamic expiratory valve? *Journal of Experimental Biology* **198**, 2349–2357

Burgmann PM (1994) Pulmonary fibrosarcoma with hepatic metastases in a cockatiel (*Nymphicus hollandicus*). *Journal of American Medicine and Surgery* **8**, 81–84

Buyukmihci NC, Murphy CJ, Paul-Murphy J *et al.* (1990) Eyelid malformation in four cockatiels. *Journal of the American Veterinary Medicine Association* **196**, 1490–1492

Campbell VL, Drobatz KJ and Perkowski SZ (2003) Postoperative hypoxemia and hypercarbia in healthy dogs undergoing routine ovariohysterectomy or castration and receiving butorphanol or hydromorphone for analgesia. *Journal of the American Veterinary Medicine Association* **222**, 330–336

Carpenter MB (1978) *Core Text of Neuroanatomy, 2nd edition*. Williams and Wilkins, Baltimore, Maryland

Chitty JR (2002a) A novel disinfectant in psittacine respiratory disease *Proceedings of the Annual Conference and Expo of the Association of Avian Veterinarians*, pp. 25–27

Chitty JR (2002b) Cytological sampling in avian skin disease. *Proceedings of the 23rd Annual Conference and Exposition of the Association of Avian Veterinarians, Monterey, August 26–30*, pp. 355–358

Ciembor P, Murray MJ, Gregory CR *et al.* (1999) Sex determination in Psittaciformes. *Proceedings of the 20th Annual Conference Association of Avian Veterinarians*, pp. 37–39

Clark P (2000) The optimal environment. Part IV: The social climate. *Pet Bird Report* **9** (6), 26–31

Clippinger TL, Bennett RA and Platt SR (1996) The avian neurological examination and ancillary neurodiagnostic techniques. *Journal of Avian Medicine and Surgery* **10**, 221–247

Clubb KJ, Skidmore D, Schubot RM and Clubb SL (1992) Growth rates of handfed psittacine chicks. In: *Psittacine Aviculture: Perspectives, Techniques, and Research*, ed. RM Schubot, SL Clubb and KJ Clubb, pp. 14.1–14.19. Avicultural Breeding and Research Center, Loxahatchee, Florida

Clubb KJ and Swigert T (1992) Common sense incubation. In: *Psittacine Aviculture: Perspectives, Techniques, and Research*, ed. RM Schubot, SL Clubb and KJ Clubb, pp. 9.1–9.15. Avicultural Breeding and Research Center, Loxahatchee, Florida

Clubb SL, Clubb KJ, Skidmore D, Wolf S and Phillips A (1992) Psittacine neonatal care and hand-feeding. In: *Psittacine Aviculture: Perspectives, Techniques, and Research*, ed. RM Schubot, SL Clubb and KJ Clubb, pp. 11.1–11.12. Avicultural Breeding and Research Center, Loxahatchee, Florida

Clubb SL and Karpinski L (1993) Aging in macaws. *Journal of the Association of Avian Veterinarians* **7**, 31–33

Clubb SL and Phillips A (1992) Psittacine embryonic mortality. In: *Psittacine Aviculture: Perspectives, Techniques, and Research*, ed. RM Schubot, SL Clubb and KJ Clubb, pp. 10.1–10.9. Avicultural Breeding and Research Center, Loxahatchee, Florida

Clyde VL and Patton S (2000) Parasitism of caged birds. In: *Manual of Avian Medicine*, ed. GH Olsen and SE Orosz, pp. 424-448. Mosby, St Louis, Missouri

Coles B (1996) Wing problems. In: *BSAVA Manual of Psittacine Birds*, ed. PE Beynon, NA Forbes and MPC Lawton, pp. 134–146. BSAVA, Cheltenham

Collar NJ (1997) Psittacidae (Parrots). In: *Handbook of the Birds of the World, Volume 4: Sandgrouse to Cuckoos*, ed. J del Hoyo, A Elliot and J Sargatal, pp. 290–339. Lynx Edicions, Barcelona

Colombini S *et al.* (2000) Intradermal skin testing in Hispaniolan parrots. *Veterinary Dermatology* **11**, 271–276

Cooper JE and Harrison GJ (1994) Dermatology. In: *Avian Medicine: Principles and Application*, ed. BW Ritchie, GJ Harrison and LR Harrison, pp. 607–639. Wingers, Lake Worth, Florida

Cray C (1997) Plasma protein electrophoresis: an update. *Proceedings of the Annual Conference and Expo of the Association of Avian Veterinarians*, pp. 209–212

Cray C, Bossart G and Harris D (1995) Plasma protein electrophoresis: principles and diagnosis of infectious disease. *Proceedings of the Annual Conference and Expo of the Association of Avian Veterinarians*, pp. 55–59

Cray C and Tatum LM (1998) Applications of protein electrophoresis in avian diagnostics. *Journal of Avian Medicine and Surgery* **12**, 4–10

Cray C, Zielezienski-Roberts K and Roskos J (2003) Nicotine metabolites in birds exposed to second-hand smoke. *Proceedings of 24th Annual Conference of the Association of Avian Veterinarians*, pp. 13–14

Cribb PH (1984) Cloacal papilloma in an Amazon parrot. *Proceedings of the Annual Conference of the Association of Avian Veterinarians, Denver, USA*, pp. 35–37

Cruickshank AJ, Gautier JP and Chappuis C (1993) Vocal mimicry in wild African Grey Parrots *Psittacus erithacus*. *Ibis* **135**, 293–299

Curro TG, Brunson DB and Paul-Murphy J (1994) Determination of the ED50 of isoflurane and evaluation of the isoflurane-sparing effect of butorphanol in Cockatoos (*Cacatua* spp.). *Veterinary Surgery* **23**, 429–433

Dahlhausen E, Lindstrom JG and Radabaugh S (2000) The use of terbinafine hydrochloride in the treatment of avian fungal disease. *Proceedings of the Annual Conference and Expo of the Association of Avian Veterinarians*, pp. 35–39

Davis C (1997) Behavior. In: *Avian Medicine and Surgery*, ed. RB Altman, SL Clubb, GM Dorrestein and KJ Quesenberry, pp. 96–100. WB Saunders, Philadelphia

Dawson CO, Wheeldon BE and McNeil PE (1976) Air sac and renal mucormycosis in an African grey parrot (*Psittacus erithacus*). *Avian Diseases* **20**, 593–600

De Voe RS, Trogdon M and Flammer K (2003) Diet modification and L-carnitine supplementation in lipomatous Budgerigars. *Proceedings of the Annual Conference of the Association of Avian Veterinarians 2003*, pp. 161–163

De Wit M, Schoemaker NJ, Kik M and Westerhof I (2003) Hypercalcaemia in two Amazons with malignant lymphoma. *Proceedings of 7th European Association of Avian Veterinarians Conference, Tenerife*, pp. 9–10

Dennis PM, Bennett RA, Newell SM and Heard DJ (1999) Diagnosis and treatment of tracheal obstruction in a cockatiel (*Nymphicus hollandicus*). *Journal of Avian Medicine and Surgery* **13**, 275–278

Doneley RJT (2001) Acute pancreatitis in parrots. *Australian Veterinary Journal* **79**, 409–411

Doolen M (1994) Crop biopsy – a low risk diagnosis for neuropathic gastric dilation. *Proceedings of the Annual Conference of the Association of Avian Veterinarians, Denver, USA*, pp. 193–196

Dorrestein GM (1996) Cytology and haemocytology. In: *Manual of Psittacine Birds*, ed. PH Beynon, NA Forbes and MPC Lawton, pp. 38–48. BSAVA, Cheltenham

Dorrestein GM (1997) Diagnostic necropsy and pathology. In: *Avian Medicine and Surgery*, ed. RB Altman, SL Clubb, GM Dorrestein and K Quesenberry, pp. 158–169. WBSaunders, Philadelphia

Driggers JC and Comar CL (1949) The secretion of radioactive calcium in the hen's egg. *Poultry Science* **28**, 420–424

Dvorak L, Bennett A and Cranor K (1998) Cloacotomy for excision of cloacal papillomas in a Catalina Macaw. *Journal of Avian Medicine and Surgery* **12**, 11–15

Echols SM (1999) Collecting diagnostic samples in avian patients. *Veterinary Clinics of North America: Exotic Animal Practice* **2**, 621–649

Echols SM (2002) Surgery of the avian reproductive tract. *Seminars in Avian and Exotic Pet Medicine* **11**, 177–195

Echols SM (2003) Practical gross necropsy of exotic animal species: introduction. *Seminars in Avian and Exotic Pet Medicine* **12**, 57–58

Edling TM (2001) Gas anesthesia – how to successfully monitor and keep them alive. *Proceedings of the Annual Conference and Expo of the Association of Avian Veterinarians*, 289–301

Edling TM, Degernes L, Flammer K and Horne WB (2001) Capnographic monitoring of African Grey Parrots during positive pressure ventilation. *Journal of the American Veterinary Medical Association* **219**, 1714–1717

Eger EI (1993) New inhalational agents – desflurane and sevoflurane. *Canadian Journal of Anaesthesia* **40**(5), R3–R5

Evans HE (1969) Anatomy of the Budgerigar. In: *Diseases of Cage and Aviary Birds*, ed. ML Petrak, pp. 45–112. Lea and Febiger, Philadelphia

Fillipich LJ, Bucher A and Charles B (1999) The pharmackinetics of cisplatin in Sulfur-crested Cockatoos (*Cacatua galerita*). *Proceedings of 20th Annual Conference of the Association of Avian Veterinarians*, pp. 229–233

Flammer K (1994) Antimicrobial therapy. In: *Avian Medicine: Principles and Application*, ed. BW Ritchie, GJ Harrison and LR Harrison, pp. 434–456. Wingers, Lake Worth, Florida

Flammer K and Clubb S (1994) Neonatology. In: *Avian Medicine: Principles and Application*, ed. BW Ritchie, GJ Harrison and LR Harrison, pp. 805–838. Wingers, Lake Worth, Florida

Forbes NA (1992) Diagnosis of avian aspergillosis and treatment with itraconazole. *Veterinary Record* **130**, 519–520

Franchetti DR and Kilde AM (1978) Restraint and anaesthesia. In: *Zoo and Wild Animal Medicine*, ed. ME Fowler, pp. 359–364. WB Saunders, Philadelphia

Fraser M (2002) Avian allergic skin disease. *Proceedings of the British Veterinary Dermatology Study Group Spring Meeting, Birmingham, 3rd April*, pp. 31–34

Friedman SG and Brinker B (2000) Early socialization: a biological need and the key to companionability. *The Original Flying Machine* **2**, 7–8

Fudge AM (1997) Avian clinical pathology – haematology and chemistry. In: *Avian Medicine and Surgery*, ed. RB Altman, SL Clubb, G Dorrestein and K Quesenberry K, p. 151. WB Saunders, Philadelphia

Fudge AM (2000a) Laboratory reference ranges for selected avian, mammalian, and reptilian species. In: *Laboratory Medicine – Avian and Exotic Pets*, ed AM Fudge, pp. 376–400. WB Saunders, Philadelphia

Fudge AM (2000b) Liver and gastrointestinal testing. In: *Laboratory Medicine – Avian and Exotic Pets*, ed. AM Fudge, pp. 47–55. WB Saunders, Philadelphia

Garner M (2003) Air sac adenocarcinomas in birds: 7 cases. *Proceedings of 24th Annual Conference of the Association of Avian Veterinarians*, pp. 55–57

Gerlach H (1994) Chlamydia. In: *Avian Medicine: Principles and Application*, ed. BW Ritchie, GJ Harrison and LR Harrison, pp. 984–996. Wingers, Lake Worth, Florida

Gerlach H (1994) Bacteria. In: *Avian Medicine: Principles and Application*, ed. BW Ritchie, GJ Harrison and LR Harrison, pp. 949–983. Wingers Publishing, Lake Worth, Florida

Gfeller RW and Messonnier SP (2004) *Small Animal Toxicology and Poisonings. 2nd edition*. Mosby, St Louis

Gilardi JB (1996) Ecology of parrots in the Peruvian Amazon: habitat use, nutrition and geophagy. PhD Thesis, University of California, Davis, California

Gilardi JD, Duffrey SS, Munn CA and Tell LS (1999) Biochemical functions of geophagy in parrots: detoxification of dietary toxins and cytoprotective effects. *Journal of Chemical Ecology* **25**, 898–899

Gill JH (2001) Avian skin diseases. *Veterinary Clinics of North America: Exotic Animal Practice* **4**, 463–492

Gionfriddo JP and Best LB (1995) Grit use by house sparrows: effects of diet and grit size. *The Condor* **97**, 57–67

Girling SJ (2002) Plasma protein electrophoresis: variations in health and disease in the family Psittaciformes (a study into the variation in blood protein electrophoresis distribution in differing species and ages of healthy and *Aspergillus fumigatus* infected Psittaciformes). Dissertation for RCVS Diploma of Zoological Medicine (Avian). Royal College of Veterinary Surgeons Library

Girling SJ (2003) Diagnosis and management of viral diseases in psittacine birds. *In Practice* **25**, 402–405

Girling SJ (2003) Viral diseases of psittacine birds. *Journal of Veterinary Postgraduate Clinical Study – In Practice* **25**, 396–407

Goldstein DL and Skadhauge E (2000) Renal and extrarenal regulation of body fluid composition. In: *Sturkie's Avian Physiology, 5th edn*, ed. GC Whittow, pp. 265–297. Academic Press, Harcourt Science and Technology, California

Graham DL (1991) Internal papillomatous disease – a pathologist's view. *Proceedings of the Annual Conference of the Association of Avian Veterinarians*, pp. 141–143

Graham DL and Heyer GW (1992) Diseases of the exocrine pancreas in pet, exotic and wild birds: a pathologist's perspective. *Proceedings of the Annual Conference of the Association of Avian Veterinarians, Denver*, pp. 190–193

Greenacre CB (2004) Physiologic responses of Amazon Parrots (*Amazona* species) to manual restraint. *Journal of Avian Medicine and Surgery* **18**, 19–22

Greenacre CB and Behrend EN (1999) Evaluation of total T4 levels in selected psittacines using a new testing method. *Proceedings of the 20th Annual Conference and Expo of the Association of Avian Veterinarians, New Orleans, September 1–3*, pp. 25–28

Greenacre CB, Latimer KS and Ritchie BW (1992) Leg paresis in a black palm cockatoo (*Probosciger aturimus*) caused by aspergillosis. *Journal of Zoo and Wildlife Medicine* **23**, 122–126

Greenacre CB and Lusby AL (2004) Physiological responses of Amazon Parrots (*Amazona* species) to manual restraint. *Journal of Avian Medicine and Surgery* **18**, 19–22

Greenacre CB and Quandt JE (1997) Comparison of sevoflurane to isoflurane in psittaciformes. *Proceedings of the Annual Conference and Expo of the Association of Avian Veterinarians*, pp. 124

Greenacre CB, Watson E and Ritchie BW (1993) Choanal atresia in an African grey parrot (*Psittacus erithacus erithacus*) and an umbrella cockatoo (*Cacatua alba*). *Journal of the Association of Avian Veterinarians* **7**, 19–22

Harcourt-Brown NH (1996a) Torsion and displacement of the oviduct as a cause of egg-binding in four psittacine birds. *Journal of Avian Medicine and Surgery* **10**, 262–267

Harcourt-Brown NH (1996b) Leg problems. In: *BSAVA Manual of Psittacine Birds*, ed PE Beynon, NA Forbes and MPC Lawton, pp. 123–133. BSAVA, Cheltenham

Harcourt-Brown NH (2003) The incidence of juvenile osteodystrophy in hand-reared grey parrots (*Psittacus e. erithacus*). *Veterinary Record* **152**, 438–439

Harcourt-Brown NH (2004) Development of the skeleton and feathers of dusky parrots (*Pionus fuscus*) in relation to their behaviour. *Veterinary Record* **154**, 42–48

Hargis AM, Stauber E, Casteel S and Eitner D (1989) Avocado intoxication in caged birds. *Journal of the American Veterinary Medical Association* **194**, 64–66

Harris D (1999) Resolution of choanal atresia in African Grey Parrots. *Exotic DVM Veterinary Magazine* **1**, 13–17

Harris J (1997) The human–avian bond. In: *Avian Medicine and Surgery*, ed. RB Altman, SL Clubb, GM Dorrestein and K Quesenberry, pp. 993–1002. WB Saunders, Philadelphia

References and further reading

Harrison GJ (1989) Medroxyprogesterone acetate-impregnated silicone implants: preliminary results in pet birds. *Proceedings of the Annual Conference of the Association of Avian Veterinarians*, pp. 6–10

Harrison GJ (1994) Perspective on parrot behavior. In: *Avian Medicine: Principles and Application*, ed. BW Ritchie, GJ Harrison and LR Harrison, pp. 96–108. Wingers, Lake Worth, Florida

Hawkins MG and Machin KL (2004) Avian pain and analgesia. *Proceedings of the Association of Avian Veterinarians*, pp.165–174

Hellner CF, Barrie KL and Ball RL (2000) Bilateral phacoaspiration in two greater sulphur-crested cockatoos (*Cacatua galerita*). *Proceedings of the American Association of Zoo Veterinarians and International Association of Aquatic Animal Medicine Joint Conference, New Orleans*, p. 310

Hernandez-Divers SJ (2002) Endosurgical debridement and diode laser ablation of lung and air sac granulomas in psittacine birds. *Journal of Avian Medicine and Surgery* **16**,138–145

Hess L, Mauldin G and Rosenthal K (2002) Estimated nutrient content of diets commonly fed to pet birds. *Veterinary Record* **150**, 399–403

Hillyer EV (1997) Clinical manifestations of respiratory disorders. In: *Avian Medicine and Surgery,* ed. RB Altman, SL Clubb, GM Dorrestein and K Quesenberry, pp. 394–411. WB Saunders, Philadelphia

Hillyer EV, Quesenberry KE and Baer K (1989) Basic avian dermatology. *Proceedings of the Annual Conference of the Association of Avian Veterinarians*, pp. 101–121

Hochleithner M (1994) Biochemistries. In: *Avian Medicine: Principles and Application*, ed. BW Ritchie, GJ Harrison and LR Harrison, pp. 242–244. Wingers, Lake Worth Florida

Hoefer HL (1997) Diseases of the gastrointestinal tract. In: *Avian Medicine and Surgery*, ed. RB Altman, SL Clubb, GM Dorrestein and K Quesenberry, pp. 419–453. WB Saunders, Philadelphia

Holick MF (1981) The cutaneous photosynthesis of previtamin D3: a unique photoendocrine system. *Journal of Investigative Dermatology* **77**, 51

Hooijmeier J (2003) Organizing parrot walks/picnics as prevention, as therapy, to educate and for fun. *Proceedings of the 7th Conference of the European Association of Avian Veterinarians, Tenerife, April 22–26*, pp. 385–386

Horwitz D (1999) Playtime: how to have fun with your pet. *Proceedings of the North American Veterinary Conference*, p. 1

Ivey ES (2000) Serologic and plasma protein electrophoresis findings in 7 psittacine birds with aspergillosis. *Journal of Avian Medicine and Surgery* **14**, 103–106

Jenkins J (1991) Use of computed tomography (CT) in pet bird practice. *Proceedings of the 1991 Annual Conference of the Association of Avian Veterinarians*, pp. 276–279

Jenkins JR (1997) Avian critical care and emergency medicine. In: *Avian Medicine and Surgery*, ed. RB Altman, SL Clubb, GM Dorrestein and K Quesenberry, pp. 839–863. WB Saunders, Philadelphia

Johne R, Konrath A, Krautwald-Junghanns ME *et al.* (2002) Herpesviral, but no papovaviral sequences, are detected in cloacal papillomas of parrots. *Archives of Virology.* **147**,1869–1880

Johnson CA (1987) Chronic feather picking: a different approach to treatment. *Proceedings of the 1st International Conference of Zoological and Avian Medicine*, pp. 125–142

Johnson-Delaney CA (1992) Feather picking: diagnosis and treatment. *Journal of the Association of Avian Veterinarians* **6**, 82–83

Jones MP and Orosz SE (1996) Overview of avian neurology and neurological diseases. *Seminars of Avian Exotic Pet Medicine* **5**, 150–164

Jones MP, Orosz SE, Richman LK *et al.* (2001) Pulmonary carcinoma with metastases in a Moluccan cockatoo (*Cacatua moluccensis*). *Journal of Avian Medicine and Surgery* **15**,107–113

Joseph VJ (2000) Vomiting and regurgitation. In: *Manual of Avian Medicine*, ed. GH Olsen and SE Orosz, pp. 70–85. Mosby, St Louis

Joyner KL (1994) Theriogenology. In: *Avian Medicine: Principles and Application*, ed. BW Ritchie, GJ Harrison and LR Harrison, pp. 748–804. Wingers, Lake Worth, Florida

Kern JJ, Paul-Murphy J, Murphy CJ *et al.* (1996) Disorders of the third eyelid in birds: 17 cases. *Journal of Avian Medicine and Surgery* **10**, 12–18

King AS and McLelland J (1975) Respiratory system. In: *Outlines of Avian Anatomy*, ed. AS King and McLelland, pp. 43–64. Baillière Tindall, London

Klein DR, Novilla MN, Watkins KL *et al.* (1994) Nutritional encephalomalacia in turkeys: diagnosis and growth performance. *Avian Diseases* **38**, 653–659

Kollias GV (1984) Liver biopsy techniques in avian clinical practice. *Veterinary Clinics of North America Small Animal Practice* **14**, 287–298

Korbel R (1993) Tonometry in avian ophthalmology. *Proceedings of the Association of Avian Veterinarians, Nashville*, p. 44

Korbel R, Milovanovic A, Erhardt W *et al.* (1993) Aerosacular perfusion with isoflurane – an anesthetic procedure for head surgery in birds. *Proceedings of the 2nd Annual Conference of the European Association of Avian Veterinarians*, pp. 9–37

Koski MA (2002) Dermatologic diseases in psittacine birds: an investigational approach. *Seminars in Avian and Exotic Pet Medicine* **11**, 105–124

Koutsos EA, Matson KD and Klasing KC (2001b) Nutrition of birds in the order Psittaciformes. *Journal of Avian Medicine and Surgery* **15**, 257–275

Koutsos EA, Smith J, Woods L and Klasing KC. (2001a) Adult cockatiels (*Nymphicus hollandicus*) metabolically adapt to high protein diets. *Journal of Nutrition* **131**, 2014–2020

Krautwald-Junghans ME (1990) Befiederungsstoerungen bei Ziervoegeln (Plumage disorders in ornamental birds). *Der Praktische Tierarzt* **71**(10), 5

Krautwald-Junghans ME, Kaleta EF, Marshang RE and Pieper K (2000) Untersuchungen zur Diagnostik und Therapie der papillomatose des aviaren gastrointestinaltraktes. *Tierärztiliche Praxis.* **28**(K), 272–278

Krautwald-Junghans M, Riedal U and Neumann W (1991) Diagnostic use of ultrasonography in birds. *Proceedings of the 1991 Annual Conference of the Association of Avian Veterinarians*, pp.269–275

LaBonde J (2003) Anaesthesia and intraoperative support of the avian patient. *AAV Newsletter and Clinical Forum*, pp. 9–11

Latimer SL and Rakich PM (1994) Necropsy examination. In: *Avian Medicine: Principles and Application*, ed. BW Ritchie, GJ Harrison and LR Harrison, pp. 355–379. Wingers, Lake Worth, Florida

Lawton MPC (1991) Avian ophthalmology. *Proceedings of the Association of Avian Veterinarians, European Conference, Vienna*, pp. 154–158

Lawton MPC (1993) Avian anterior segment disease. *Proceedings of the Association of Avian Veterinarians, Nashville*, pp. 223–228

Leijnieks DV (2004) Treatment of a mandibular fracture using a steel plate in a lesser sulfur-crested cockatoo. *Exotic DVM* **6**(4), 15–17

Lennox AM and Van Der Heyden N (1993) Haloperidol for use in treatment of psittacine self mutilation and feather picking. *Proceedings of the Annual Conference of the Association of Avian Veterinarians*, pp. 119–120

Levine J (1955) Consensual light response in birds. *Science* **122**, 690

Lichtenberger M, Chavez W, Cray C *et al.* (2003) Mortality and response to fluid resuscitation after acute blood loss in mallard ducks. *Proceedings of the Annual Conference of the Association of Avian Veterinarians*, pp. 7–10

Lindenstruth and Forst (1993) Enrofloxacin (Baytril) – an alternative for official prophylaxis and treatment of psittacosis in imported psittacine birds. *Deutsche Tierärztliche Wochenschrift* **100**, 364–368

Ludders JW and Matthews N (1996) Birds. In: *Lumb and Jones Veterinary Anesthesia, 3rd edition*, ed. JC Thurmon, WJ Tranquilli and JG Benson, pp. 645–669. Williams and Wilkins, Baltimore, Maryland

Ludders JW, Mitchell GS and Rode J (1990) Minimal anaesthetic concentration and cardiopulmonary dose response of isoflurane in ducks. *Veterinary Surgery* **19**, 304–307

Ludders JW, Rode J and Mitchell GS (1989a) Isoflurane anaesthesia in sandhill cranes (*Grus canadensis*): minimal anaesthetic concentration and cardiopulmonary dose-response during spontaneous and controlled breathing. *Anesthesia and Analgesia* (Cleveland) **68**, 511–516

Ludders JW, Rode JA and Mitchell GS (1989b) Effects of ketamine, xylazine and a combination of ketamine and xylazine in Pekin ducks. *American Journal of Veterinary Research* **50**, 245–249

Luescher UA (2004) Avian husbandry and behaviour. *The NAVTA Journal*, Spring, 37–41

Lumeij JT (1987) The diagnostic value of plasma proteins and non-protein nitrogen substances in birds. *Veterinary Quarterly* **9**, 262–268

Lumeij JT (1994a) Gastroenterology. In: *Avian Medicine: Principles and Application*, ed. BW Ritchie, GJ Harrison and LR Harrison, pp. 482–521. Wingers, Lake Worth, Florida

Lumeij JT (1994b) Hepatology. In: *Avian Medicine: Principles and Application*, ed. BW Ritchie, GJ Harrison and LR Harrison, pp. 522–537. Wingers Publishing, Lake Worth, Florida

Lumeij JT (1994c) Nephrology. In: *Avian Medicine: Principles and Application*, ed. BW Ritchie, GJ Harrison and LR Harrison, pp. 538–555. Wingers Publishing, Lake Worth, Florida

Lumeij JT (2003) Pathophysiology and clinical features of avian cardiac disease, with an emphasis on electrocardiology. *Proceedings of 7th European Association of Avian Veterinarians Conference, Tenerife*, pp. 407–415

Lumeij JT and Overduin LM (1990) Plasma chemistry reference values in psittaciformes. *Avian Pathology* **19**, 234–244

MacCoy DM (1989) Excision arthroplasty for management of coxofemoral luxation in pet birds. *Journal of the American Veterinary Medical Association* **194**, 95–97

Machin KL and Caulkert NA (1996) The cardiopulmonary effects of propofol in mallard ducks. *Proceedings of the American Association of Zoo Veterinarians*, pp. 149–154

Macmillen RE (1990) Water economy of granivorous birds: a predictive model. *Condor* **92**, 379–392

MacWhirter P (1994) Malnutrition. In: *Avian Medicine: Principles and Application*, ed. BW Ritchie, GJ Harrison and LR Harrison, pp. 842–861. Wingers, Lake Worth, Florida

Malley AD (1996) Feather and skin problems. In: *BSAVA Manual of Psittacine Birds*, ed PH Beynon, NA Forbes and MPC Lawton, pp. 96–105. BSAVA Publications, Cheltenham

Mansour A, Khachaturian LME, Akil H and Watson SJ (1988) Anatomy of CNS opioid receptors. *Trends in Neuroscience* **11**, 301–314

Matthews K, Danova G, Newman A *et al.* (2003) Ratite cancellous xenograft: effects on avian fracture healing. *Journal of Veterinary Comparative Orthopaedics and Traumatology* **12**, 50–58

McCluggage D (1992) Proventriculotomy: a study of selected cases. In: *Proceedings of the Annual Conference of the Association of Avian Veterinarians, Denver, USA*, pp. 195–200

McDonald DL (2002a) Evaluation of the use of organic formulated bird foods for large psittacines. *Proceedings of the Joint Nutrition Symposium, Antwerp*, p. 110

McDonald DL (2002b) Dietary considerations for iron storage disease in birds and implications for high vitamin A contents of formulated bird foods. *Proceedings of the Joint Nutrition Symposium, Antwerp*, p. 162

McLelland J (1989) Anatomy of the lungs and air sacs. In: *Form and Function in Birds, Vol. 4*, ed. AS King and J McLelland, pp. 221–279. Academic Press, London

McNab BK and Salisbury CA (1995) Energetics of New Zealand's temperate parrots. *New Zealand Journal of Zoology* **22**, 339–349

Meehan CL, Millam JR and Mench JA (2003) Foraging opportunity and increased physical complexity both prevent and reduce psychogenic feather picking by young Amazon parrots. *Applied Animal Behavioural Science* **80**, 71–85.

Monks D (2002) Microchipping birds. *Veterinary Times* **32**(40), 14

Moore SJ (1998) Use of an artificial gizzard to investigate the effect of grit on the breakdown of grass. *Journal of Zoology London* **246**, 119–124

Morse, DH (1975) Ecological aspects of adaptive radiation in birds. *Biological Reviews* **50**, 167–214

Moulton JE (ed.) (1990) *Tumours in Domestic Animals, 3rd edition*. University of California Press, Berkley, California

Muir WW and Hubbell LA (2000a) Inhalation anesthesia. In: *Handbook of Veterinary Anesthesia*, ed. WW Muir and LA Hubbell, pp. 154–163. Mosby, St Louis, Missouri

Muir WW and Hubbell LA (2000b) Pharmacology of inhalation anesthetic drugs. In: *Handbook of Veterinary Anesthesia*, ed. WW Muir and LA Hubbell, pp. 164–181. Mosby, St Louis

Muir WW and Hubbell LA (2000c) Anesthetic machines and breathing systems. In: *Handbook of Veterinary Anesthesia*, ed. WW Muir and LA Hubbell, pp. 210–231. Mosby, St Louis

National Research Council (1994) *Nutrient Requirements of Poultry*. National Academy Press, Washington DC

Nett CS, Hodgin EC, Foil CS *et al.* (2003) A modified biopsy technique to improve histopathological evaluation of avian skin. *Veterinary Dermatology* **14**, 147–152

Nett CS and Tully TN (2003) Hypersensitivity and intradermal allergy testing in psittacines. *Compendium on Continuing Education for the Practicing Veterinarian* **25**, 348–357

Neville PF (1997) Preventing problems and producing better puppies. *Proceedings of the North American Veterinary Conference*, pp. 31–32

Oliver JE and Lorenz MD (1993) Neurological history and examination. In: *Handbook of Veterinary Neurology*, ed. JE Oliver and MD Lorenz, pp. 3–45. WB Saunders, Philadelphia

Olsen GH and Clubb S (1997) Embryology, incubation, and hatching. In: *Avian Medicine and Surgery*, ed. RB Altman, SL Clubb, GM Dorrestein and K Quesenberry, pp. 54–71. WB Saunders, Philadelphia

Oppenheimer J (1991) Feather picking: systematic approach. *Proceedings of the Annual Conference of the Association of Avian Veterinarians*, pp. 314–315.

Orosz SE (1996) Principles of avian clinical neuroanatomy. *Seminars in Avian and Exotic Pet Medicine* **5**, 127–139

Orosz SE (2000) Overview of aspergillosis pathogenesis and treatment options. *Seminars in Avian and Exotic Pet Medicine* **9**, 59–65

Orosz SE and Frazier DL (1995) Antifungal agents: a review of their pharmacology and therapeutic indications. *Journal of Avian Medicine and Surgery* **9**, 8–18

Orosz SE, Frazier DL, Schroeder EC *et al.* (1996) Pharmacokinetic properties of itraconazole in blue-fronted Amazon parrots (*Amazona aestiva aestiva*). *Journal of Avian Medicine and Surgery* **10**, 168–173

Orosz SE and Johnson-Delaney CA (2003) Self-injurious behavior (SIB) of primates as a model for feather damaging behavior (FDB) in companion psittacine birds. *Proceedings of the Annual Conference of the Association of Avian Veterinarians: Another Feather Picker: That Sinking Feeling: Avian Specialty Advanced Program*, pp. 39–50

Overall KL (1997) Appendix F Terminology: necessary and sufficient conditions for behavioural diagnoses. In: *Clinical Behavioral Medicine for Small Animals*, ed. KL Overall. Mosby, St Louis, Missouri

Paul-Murphy JR, Koblik PD, Stein G and Pennick DG (1990) Psittacine skull radiography, anatomy, radiographic technique and patient application. *Veterinary Radiology* **31**, 218–224

Pees M, Straub J and Krautwald-Junghans M-E (2004) Echocardiographic examinations of 60 African grey parrots and 30 other psittacine birds. *Veterinary Record* **155**, 73–76

Pessacq-Asenjo TP (1984) The nerve endings of the glycogen body of embryonic and adult avian spinal cord: on the existence of two different varieties of nerve fibers. *Growth* **48**, 385–390

Phalen DN (2000) Avian renal disorders. In: *Laboratory Medicine – Avian and Exotic Pets*, ed. AM Fudge, pp. 61–68. WB Saunders, Philadelphia

Phalen DN, Lau MT and Filippich LJ (1997) Considerations for safely maintaining the avian patient under prolonged anaesthesia. *Proceedings of the Annual Conference and Expo of the Association of Avian Veterinarians*, pp. 111–116

Phillips A and Clubb SL (1992) Psittacine neonatal development. In: *Psittacine Aviculture: Perspectives, Techniques, and Research*, ed. RM Schubot, SL Clubb and KJ Clubb, pp. 12.1–12.26. Avicultural Breeding and Research Center, Loxahatchee, Florida

Poore SO, Ashcroft A, Sanchez-Haiman A and Goslow GE (1997) The contractile properties of the m. supracoracoideus in the pigeon and starling: a case for long axis rotation of the humerus. *Journal of Experimental Biology* **200**, 2987–3002

Poore SO, Sanchez-Haiman A and Goslow GE (1997) Wing upstroke and the evolution of flapping flight. *Nature* **387**, 799–802

Powell FL and Scheid P (1989) Physiology of gas exchange in the avian respiratory system. In: *Form and Function in Birds, Vol. 4*, ed. AS King AS and J McLelland, pp. 393–437. Academic Press, London

Proulx J (2002) Nutrition in critically ill animals. In: *The ICU Book*, pp. 202–217. Teton NewMedia, Jackson, Wyoming

Pye GW, Bennett RA, Newell SM *et al.* (2000) Magnetic resonance imaging in psittacine birds with chronic sinusitis. *Journal of Avian Medicine and Surgery* **14**, 243–256

Quesenberry K (1997) Treatment of neoplasia . In: *Avian Medicine and Surgery*, ed. RB Altman, SL Clubb, GM Dorrestein and K Quesenberry, pp. 600–603. WB Saunders, Philadelphia

Rae M (2000) Avian endocrine disorders. In: *Laboratory Medicine – Avian and Exotic Pets*, ed. AM Fudge, pp. 76–89. WB Saunders, Philadelphia

Rae MA (2003) Practical avian necropsy. *Seminars in Avian and Exotic Pet Medicine* **12**, 62–70

Raffe MR and Wingfield W (2002) Hemorrhage and hypovolemia. In: *The ICU Book*, pp. 453–477. Teton NewMedia, Jackson, Wyoming

Ramsay EC and Grindlinger H (1992) Treatment of feather picking with clomipramine. *Proceedings of the Annual Conference of the Association of Avian Veterinarians*, pp. 379–382

Raymond JT, Topham K, Shirota K *et al.* (2001) Tyzzer's disease in a neonatal Rainbow Lorikeet (*Trichoglossus haematodus*). *Veterinary Pathology* **38**, 326–327

Reavill D (2003) A review of psittacine squamous cell carcinomas submitted during 1998–2001. *Proceedings of 7th European Association of Avian Veterinarians Conference, Tenerife*, pp. 237–240

Redig PT (1983) Aspergillosis. In: *Kirk's Current Veterinary Therapy VII*, ed. RW Kirk, pp. 611–613. WB Saunders, Philadelphia

Redig PT (1993) Avian aspergillosis. In: *Zoo and Wild Animal Medicine: Current Therapy 3*, ed. ME Fowler, pp. 178–180. WB Saunders, Philadelphia

Redig PT (1996) Avian emergencies. In: *Manual of Raptors, Pigeons and Waterfowl*, ed. PH Beynon, NA Forbes and NH Harcourt-Brown, pp. 30–41. BSAVA, Cheltenham

Redig PT, Brown PA and Talbot B (1997) The ELISA as a management guide for aspergillosis in raptors. *Proceedings of the 4th Conference of the European Association of Avian Veterinarians*, pp. 223–226

Reidarson TH and McBain J (1995) Serum protein electrophoresis and aspergillus antibody titre as an aid to diagnosis of aspergillosis in penguins. *Proceedings of the Annual Conference and Expo of the Association of Avian Veterinarians*, pp. 61–64

Remple JD (1980) Avian malaria with comments on other hemosporidia in large falcons. In: *Recent Advances in the Study of Raptor Diseases. Proceedings of the International Symposium of Diseases of Birds of Prey*, ed. JE Cooper and AG Greenwood, pp. 15–19. London

Ritchie BW (1995) *Avian Viruses – Function and Control*. Wingers, Lake Worth, Florida

Ritchie BW (2003) Management of avian infectious diseases. In: *Proceedings of the 7th European Conference of the Association of Avian Veterinarians and 5th ECAMS Scientific Meeting, Tenerife, Spain*

Ritchie BW, Harrison GJ and Harrison LR (1994) *Avian Medicine: Principles and Application*. Wingers, Lake Worth,

Ritchie PA, Anderson IL and Lambert DM (2003) Evidence for specificity of psittacine beak and feather disease virus among avian hosts. *Virology* **306**, 109–115

References and further reading

Ritzman TK (2000) Pancreatic hypoplasia in Eclectus Parrot (*Eclectus roratus polychloros*). *Proceedings of the Annual Conference of the Association of Avian Veterinarians, Denver*, pp. 83–87

Rivera S, Reavill D and McClearen J (2002))Treatment of cutaneous lymphosarcoma in an Umbrella Cockatoo. *Proceedings of the Annual Conference of the Association of Avian Veterinarians*, pp. 99–100

Rodriguez-Quiros J, SanRoman F and Rodriguez-Bertos A (2001) Clinical and pathological changes induced by the use of corticocancellous autograft during healing process in experimental fractures of tibiotarsus in pigeons (*Columba livia*). *Proceedings of the 6th Conference of the European Association of Avian Veterinarians*, pp. 50–54

Romagnano A (1996) Avian obstetrics. *Seminars in Avian and Exotic Pet Medicine* 5, 180–188

Rosskopf WJ and Woerpel R(1996) *Diseases of Cage and Aviary Birds, 3rd edition*. Williams and Wilkins, Baltimore, Maryland

Rowley I (1997) Cacatuidae (Cockatoos) In: *Handbook of Birds of the World, Volume 4, Sandgrouse to Cuckoos*, ed. J del Hoyo, A Elliot and J Sargatal, pp. 246–279. Lynx Edicions, Barcelona

Roze M (1990) Comparative electroretinography in several species of raptors. *Transactions of the American College of Veterinary Ophthalmology* 21, 45–48

Scheid P and Piiper J (1989) Aerodynamic valving in the avian lung. *Acta Anaesthesia Scandinavica* 33, 28–31

Schlumberger HG (1954) Neoplasia in the parakeet. I. Spontaneous chromophobe pituitary tumours. *Cancer Research* 14, 237–245

Schmidt RE, Reavill DR and Phalen DN (2003) *Pathology of Pet and Aviary Birds*. Iowa State Press, Ames, Iowa

Schmitt PM, Gobel T and Trautvetter E (1998) Evaluation of pulse oximetry as a monitoring method in avian anesthesia. *Journal of Avian Medicine and Surgery* 12, 91–99

Schoemaker NJ, Dorrestein GM, Latimer KS *et al.* (2000) Severe leukopenia and liver necrosis in young African grey parrots (*Psittacus erithacus erithacus*) infected with psittacine circovirus. *Avian Diseases* 44, 470–478

Sibley CG and Ahlquist JE (1990) *Phylogeny and Classification of Birds. A Study in Molecular Evolution*. Yale University Press, New Haven, Connecticut

Simpson VR (1996) Post-mortem examination. In: *Manual of Psittacine Birds*, ed. PH Beynon, NA Forbes and MPC Lawton pp. 69–86. BSAVA Publications, Cheltenham

Sims MH (1996) Clinical electrodiagnostic evaluation in exotic animal medicine. *Seminars in Avian and Exotic Pet Medicine* 5, 140–149

Smith IL (1999) Basic behavioral principles for the avian veterinarian. *Proceedings of the Annual Conference of the Association of Avian Veterinarians*, pp. 47–55

Spearman R and Hardy J (1985) Integument. In: *Form and Function in Birds*, ed. AS King and J McLelland, pp. 1–56. Academic Press, London

Speer BL (1998) A clinical look at the avian pancreas in health and disease. In: *Proceedings of the Annual Conference of the Association of Avian Veterinarians, Denver, USA*, pp. 57–64

Speer B (2003a) Trans-sinus pinning technique for the correction of chronic mandibular prognathism in psittacines. *Proceedings of the 5th Scientific Meeting of the European College of Avian Medicine and Surgery*, p. 3

Speer B (2003b) Trans-sinus pinning technique to address scissor beak deformity in psittacine species. *Proceedings of the 7th Conference of the European Association of Avian Veterinarians*, pp. 347–352

Speer BL and Spadafori G (1999) *Birds for Dummies*, pp. 288. IDG Books Worldwide, Indianapolis

Stamp JT, McEwen AD, Watt JAA and Nisbet DJ (1950) Enzootic abortion in ewes. *Veterinary Record* 62, 251–254

Stanford M (2002) Effects of dietary change on faecal Gram stains in the Grey Parrot. *British Veterinary Zoological Society Proceedings November, Edinburgh Zoo*, p. 39

Stanford M (2003) The significance of serum ionized calcium and 25-hydroxy-cholecalciferol (vitamin D₃) assays in African grey parrots. *Proceedings of the International Conference on Exotics*, pp. 1–6

Stanford MD (2003a) Measurement of 25-hydroxycholecalciferol in captive grey parrots (*Psittacus e erithacus*). *Veterinary Record* 153, 58–59

Stanford MD (2003b) Measurement of ionized calcium in African grey parrots (*Psittacus e erithacus*): the effect of diet. *Proceedings, European Association of Avian Veterinarians, Tenerife*, pp. 269–275

Stanford MD (2003c) The effect of husbandry on calcium metabolism in the grey parrot (*Psittacus e erithacus*). *Proceedings of the European Association of Avian Veterinarians, Tenerife*

Stanford MD (2004a) The effect of UV-B supplementation on calcium metabolism in psittacine birds. *Proceedings of the International Conference of Exotics, Naples, Florida*, pp. 57–60

Stanford M (2004b) Interferon treatment of circovirus infection in grey parrots (*Psittacus e erithacus*). *Veterinary Record* 154, 435–436

Steffey EP and Howland D (1978) Isoflurane potency in the dog and cat. *American Journal of Veterinary Research* 39, 573–577

Steffey EP, Howland D, Giri S and Eger EI (1977) Enflurane, halothane, and isoflurane potency in horses. *American Journal of Veterinary Research* 38, 1037–1039

Stiles J and Greenacre C (2001) Infraorbital cyst in a white cockatoo (*Cacatua alba*). *Journal of Avian Medicine and Surgery* 15, 40–43

Sturkie PD (1986) Heart and circulation: anatomy, hemodynamics, blood pressure, blood flow. In: *Avian Physiology, 4th edition*, ed. PD Sturkie, pp. 130–166. Springer-Verlag, New York

Styles DK, Phalen DN and Tomaszewski EK (2002) Elucidating the etiology of avian mucosal papillomatosis in psittacine birds. *AAV Proceedings Monterey, California*, pp. 175–178

Sundberg JP, Junge RE, O'Banion MK *et al.* (1986) Cloacal papillomatosis in psittacines. *American Journal of Veterinary Research* 47, 928–932

Taylor EJ (1996) An evaluation of the importance of insoluble versus soluble grit in the diet of canaries. *Journal of Avian Medicine and Surgery* 10, 248–251

Taylor M and Murray M (1999) A diagnostic approach to the avian cloaca. *Proceedings of the Annual Conference of the Association of Avian Veterinarians, Denver*, pp. 301–304

Tomaszewski E, Wilson van G, Wigle WL and Phalen DN (2001) Detection and heterogeneity of herpesviruses causing Pacheco's disease in parrots. *Journal of Clinical Microbiology* 39, 533–538

Tudor DC and Yard C (1978) Retinal atrophy in a parakeet. *Veterinary Medicine/Small Animal Clinician* 73, 1456

Tully TN and Carter JD (1993) Bilateral supraorbital abscesses associated with sinusitis in an orange-winged Amazon parrot (*Amazona amazonica*). *Journal of the Association of Avian Veterinarians* 7, 157–158

Tully TN and Harrison GJ (1994) Pneumonology. In: *Avian Medicine: Principles and Application*, ed. BW Ritchie, GJ Harrison and LR Harrison, pp. 556–581. Wingers, Lake Worth, Florida

Turner R (1993) Trexan (Naltrexone hydrochloride) use in feather picking in avian species. *Proceedings of the Annual Conference of the Association of Avian Veterinarians*, pp. 116–118

Tyler JW (1990a) Hepatoencephalopathy. Part I. Clinical signs and diagnosis. *Compendium on Continuing Education for the Practicing Veterinarian* 12, 1069–1073

Tyler JW (1990b) Hepatoencephalopathy. Part II. Pathophysiology and treatment. *Compendium on Continuing Education for the Practicing Veterinarian* 12, 1260–1270

Van der Mast H, Dorrestein GM and Westerhof J (1990) A fatal treatment of sinusitis in an African grey. *Journal of the Association of Avian Veterinarians* 4, 189

Van Wettere A and Redig PT (2001) A review of methods used to induce molting in raptors. *Hawk Chalk* 30(2), 46–56

VanDerHeyden N (1988) Psittacine papillomas. *Proceedings of the Annual Conference of the Association of Avian Veterinarians, Lake Worth, Florida*, pp. 23–25

VanDerHeyden N (1993) Jejunostomy and jejuno-cloacal anastomosis in macaws. *Proceedings of the Annual Conference of the Association of Avian Veterinarians, Denver*, pp. 35–37

Verschueren CP and Lumeij JT (1991) Mydriatics in birds. *Journal of Veterinary Pharmacology and Therapeutics* 14, 206–208

Voith VL and Borchelt PL (1985) Fears and phobias in companion animals. *Compendium on Continuing Education for the Practicing Veterinarian* 7, 209–218

Wade LL, Simpson K, McDonough P *et al.* (2003) Identification of oral spiral bacteria in Cockatiels (*Nymphicus hollandicus*). *AAV Proceedings Pittsburgh, Pennsylvania*, pp. 23–25

Walsh M (1986) Radiology. In: *Clinical Avian Medicine and Surgery*, ed. G Harrison and L Harrison, pp. 201–233. WB Saunders, Philadelphia

Ward MP, Ramer JC, Proudfoot J *et al.* (2003) Outbreak of salmonellosis in a zoologic collection of lorikeets and lories (*Trichoglossus, Lorius* and *Eos* spp.). *Avian Diseases* 47, 493–498

Welle KR (1997) Avian obedience training. *Proceedings of the Annual Conference of the Association of Avian Veterinarians*, pp. 297–303

Welle KR (1998) Psittacine behavior. *Proceedings of the Annual Conference of the Association of Avian Veterinarians*, pp. 371–377

West GD, Garner M and Talcott P (2001) Haemochromatosis in several species of lories with high dietary iron. *Journal of Avian Medicine and Surgery* 15, 297–301

Williams D (1994) Ophthalmology. In: *Avian Medicine: Principles and Application*, ed. BW Ritchie, GJ Harrison and LR Harrison, pp. 673–694. Wingers, Lake Worth, Florida

Willis AM and Wilkie DA (1999a) Avian ophthalmology, part 1: anatomy, examination and diagnostic techniques. *Journal of Avian Medicine and Surgery* 13, 160–166

Willis AM and Wilkie DA (1999b) Avian ophthalmology, part 2: review of ophthalmic diseases. *Journal of Avian Medicine and Surgery* 13, 245–251

Wilson FE (1997) Photoperiodism in American tree sparrows; role of the thyroid gland. In: *Perspectives in Avian Endocrinology*, ed. S Harvey and R Etches, pp. 159–172. Society for Endocrinology, Bristol

Wilson H, Graham J, Roberts R *et al.* (2000) Integumentary neoplasms in psittacine birds. *Proceedings of the Annual Conference of the Association of Avian Veterinarians, Portland, Oregon*

Wilson L (1999) What to do with biters and screamers. *Proceedings of the Annual Conference of the Association of Avian Veterinarians*, pp. 71–76

Wilson L (2000) The one person bird – prevention and rehabilitation. *Proceedings of the Annual Conference of the Association of Avian Veterinarians*, pp. 69–73

Wingfield W (2002) Fluid and electrolyte therapy. In: *The ICU Book*, pp. 453–477. Teton NewMedia, Jackson, Wyoming

Wishnow KI, Johnson DE, Grignon DJ *et al.* (1989) Regeneration of the urinary bladder mucosa after complete surgical denudation. *De Voe Journal of Urology* **141**, 1476–1479

Woerpel RW and Rosskopf WJ (1997) Heavy metal intoxication in caged birds – parts I and II. In: *Practical Avian Medicine – The Compendium Collection*, pp. 99–111. Veterinary Learning Systems, Trenton, New Jersey

Wolf ED, Amass K and Olsen J (1983) Survey of the conjunctival flora in the eye of clinically normal, captive exotic birds. *Journal of the American Veterinary Medical Association* **183**, 1232–1233

Wolf S and Clubb SL (1992) Clinical management of beak malformations in handfed psittacine chicks. In: *Psittacine Aviculture: Perspectives, Techniques, and Research*, ed. RM Schubot, SL Clubb and KJ Clubb, pp. 17.1–17.12. Avicultural Breeding and Research Center, Loxahatchee, Florida

Woolf CJ and Chong MS (1993) Preemptive analgesia – treating postoperative pain by preventing the establishment of central sensitization. *Anesthesia and Analgesia* **77**, 362–369

Further reading

Anderson-Brown AF and Robbins GES (2002) *The New Incubation Book*. World Pheasant Association, Reading, UK

Athan MS (1993) *Guide to a Well-Behaved Parrot*. Barron's, Hong Kong

Athan MS (1997) *Guide to the Quaker Parrot*. Barron's, Hong Kong

Athan MS and Deter D (2000) *The African Grey Parrot Handbook*. Barron's, Hong Kong

Bauck L (1997) Avian dermatology. In: *Avian Medicine and Surgery*, ed. RB Altman, SL Clubb, GM Dorrestein and K Quesenberry, pp. 548–562. WB Saunders, Philadelphia

Baumel JJ (ed.) (1993) *Handbook of Avian Anatomy: Nomina Anatomica Avium, 2nd edition*. Nuttall Ornithological Club, Harvard University, Massachusetts

Bennett RA (1994) Neurology. In: *Avian Medicine: Principles and Application*, ed. BW Ritchie, GJ Harrison and LR Harrison, pp. 723–787. Wingers, Lake Worth, Florida

Brue RN (1994) Nutrition. In: *Avian Medicine: Principles and Application*, ed. BW Ritchie, GJ Harrison and LR Harrison, pp. 63–95. Wingers, Lake Worth, Florida

Campbell TW (1995) *Avian Hematology and Cytology, 2nd edition*. Iowa State University Press, Ames, Iowa

Clubb S (1986) Therapeutics. In: *Clinical Avian Medicine and Surgery*, ed. GJ Harrison and LR Harrison, pp. 327–355. WB Saunders, Philadelphia

Clubb S (1997) Psittacine pediatric husbandry and medicine. In: *Avian Medicine and Surgery*, ed. RB Altman, SL Clubb, GM Dorrestein and K Quesenberry, pp. 73–95. WB Saunders, Philadelphia

Coles B (1997) *Avian Medicine and Surgery, 2nd edition*. Blackwell Scientific, Oxford

Cooper ME (1987) *An Introduction to Animal Law*. Academic Press, London

Deeming DC (ed.) (2001) *Avian Incubation – Behaviour, Environment and Evolution*. Oxford University Press, Oxford

Deeming DC (2002) *Nests, Birds and Incubators*. Brinsea Products Ltd, Sandford, UK

Del Hoyo J, Elliott A and Sargatal J (1997) *Handbook of the Birds of the World: Volume 4: Sandgrouse to Cuckoos*. Lynx Edicions, Barcelona

Dickinson EC (ed.) (2003) *The Howard and Moore Complete Checklist of Birds of the World*. Christopher Helm, London

Forbes NA (1996) Fits, incoordination and coma. In: *BSAVA Manual of Psittacine Birds*, ed. PH Beynon, NA Forbes and MPC Lawton, pp. 190–197. BSAVA, Cheltenham

Forshaw JM and Cooper WT (1989) *Parrots of the World*. Landsdowne Editions, Melbourne

Gill FB (1995) *Ornithology, 2nd edition*. WH Freeman, New York

Higgins PJ (ed.) (1999) *Handbook of Australian, New Zealand and Antarctic Birds, Volume 4*. Oxford University Press,

Juniper T and Parr M (1998) *Parrots: A Guide to Parrots of the World*. Pica Press, London

King AS and McLelland J (1979–1989) *Form and Function in Birds, Volumes I –IV*. Academic Press, London

King AS and McLelland J (1984) *Birds: Their Structure and Function, 2nd edition*. Baillière Tindall, London

Klasing K (1998) *Comparative Avian Nutrition*. CAB International, Wallingford, UK

Lucas AM and Stettenheim PR (1972) *Avian Anatomy: Integument*. US Department of Agriculture Handbook 362, Washington DC

McLelland J (1990) *A Colour Atlas of Avian Anatomy*. Wolfe Publishing, Aylesbury, UK

Olsen GH and Orosz SE (2000) *Manual of Avian Medicine*. Mosby, St Louis, Missouri

Pepperberg IM (1999) *The Alex Studies: Cognitive and Communicative Abilities of Grey Parrots*. Harvard University Press, Cambridge, Massachusetts

Petrak ML (1969) *Diseases of Cage and Aviary Birds*. Lea and Febiger, Philadelphia

Proctor NS and Lynch PJ (1993) *Manual of Ornithology*. Yale University Press, New Haven, Connecticut

Rach JA (1998) *Why Does my Bird Do That: A Guide to Parrot Behavior*. Howell Book House, New York

Romagnano A and Heard D (2000) Avian dermatology. In: *Manual of Avian Medicine*, ed. G Olsen and S Orosz, pp. 95–123. Mosby, St Louis

Rubel G, Isenbugel E and Wolvekamp P (1991) *Atlas of Diagnostic Radiology of Exotic Pets*. Wolfe Publishing, London

Rupley AE (1997) *Manual of Avian Practice*. WB Saunders, Philadelphia

Samour J (2000) *Avian Medicine*. Mosby (Harcourt Publishers), London

Smith SA and Smith BJ (1992) *An Atlas of Radiographic Anatomy*. WB Saunders, Philadelphia

Snyder NFR, Wiley JW and Kepler CB (1987) *The Parrots of Luquillo: Natural History and Conservation of the Puerto Rican Parrot*. Western Foundation of Vertebrate Zoology, Los Angeles

Stark JM and Ricklefs RE (eds) (1998) *Avian Growth and Development*. Oxford University Press, Oxford

Surai PF (2002) *Natural Antioxidants in Avian Nutrition and Reproduction*. Nottingham University Press, Nottingham, UK

Voitkevic, AA (1966) *The Feathers and Plumage of Birds*. Sidgwick & Jackson, London

Welle KR (1999) *Psittacine Behavior Handbook*. Association of Avian Veterinarians Publication Office, Bedford, Texas

Welty JC (ed.) (1982) *The Life of Birds, 3rd edition*. Saunders College Publishing, Philadelphia

Whittow GC (ed.) (2000) *Sturkie's Avian Physiology, 5th edition*. Academic Press, Harcourt Science and Technology, California

Formularies

Bishop Y (2004) *The Veterinary Formulary, 6th Edition*. Pharmaceutical Press, London

Carpenter JW, Mashima TY and Rupiper DJ (2001) *Exotic Animal Formulary, 2nd edition*. WB Saunders, Philadelphia

Hawk CT and Leary SL (1999) *Formulary for Laboratory Animals, 2nd edition*. Iowa State University Press, Ames, Iowa

Marx KL and Roston MA (1996) *The Exotic Animal Drug Compendium; An International Formulary*. Veterinary Learning Systems, Trenton NJ

Tully TN (1997) Formulary. In: *Avian Medicine and Surgery*, ed. RB Altman, SL Clubb, GM Dorrestein and KE Quesenberry, pp. 671–687. WB Saunders, Philadelphia

Appendix 1
Clinical approaches for some clinical presentations

John Chitty

It is sometimes daunting to be faced with a sick bird and a long list of differential diagnoses. These flowcharts do not represent the only way to approach the following presentations but they are designed to give a structured approach to each case, biased towards giving the clinician the maximum chance of diagnosing the more commonly seen conditions. The numbers in circles refer to the chapter(s) in the Manual where diagnostic techniques are described or more information is given.

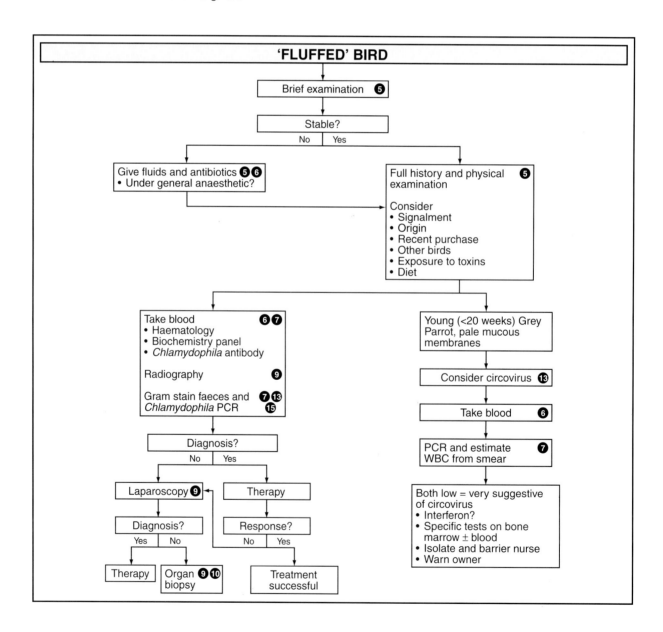

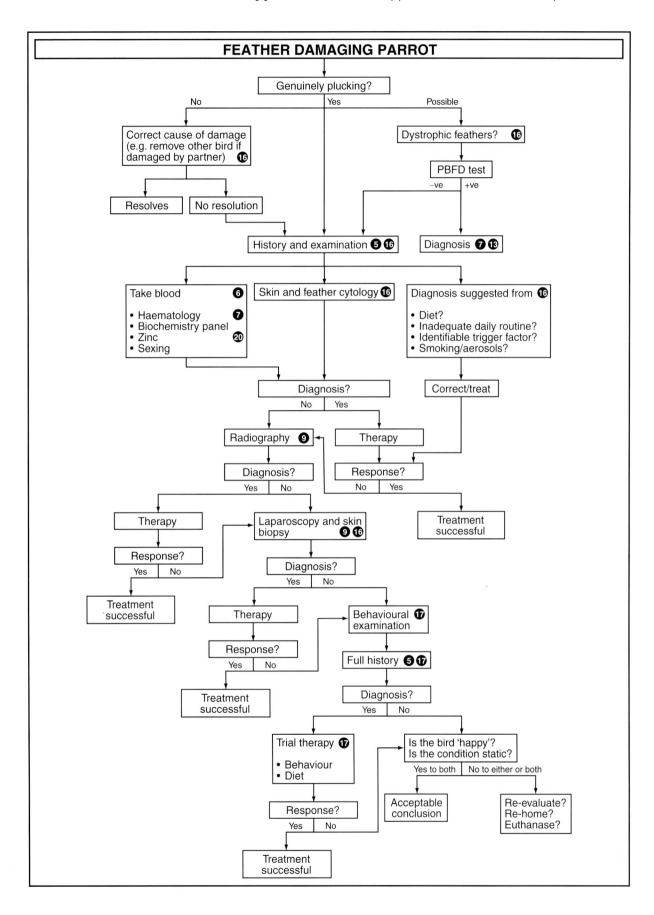

Appendix 1 Clinical approaches for some clinical presentations

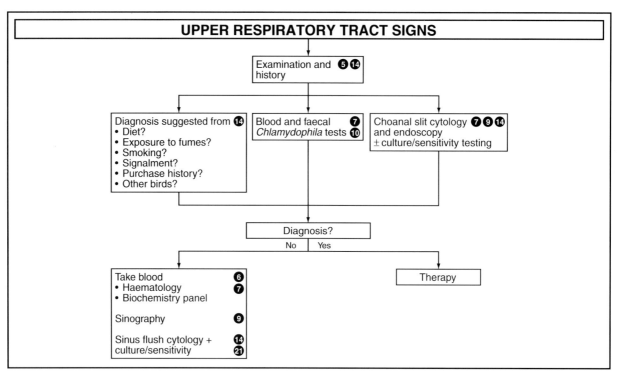

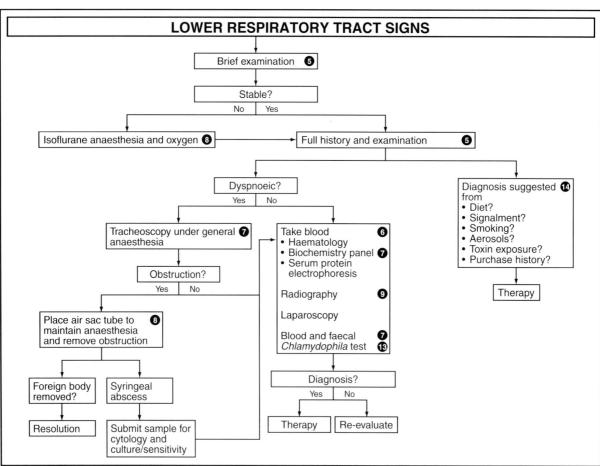

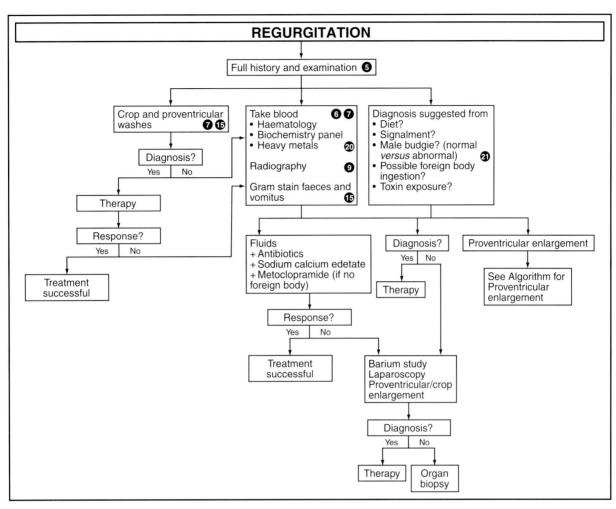

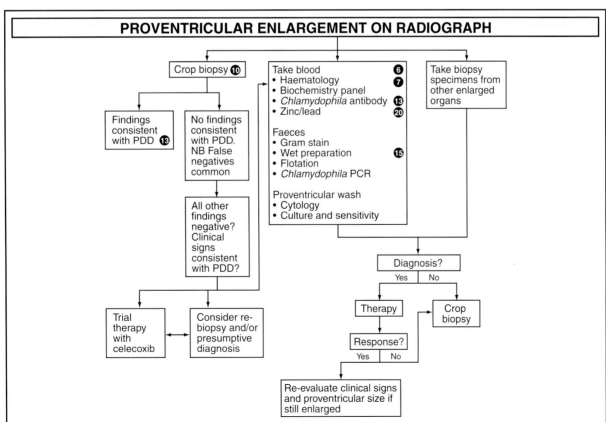

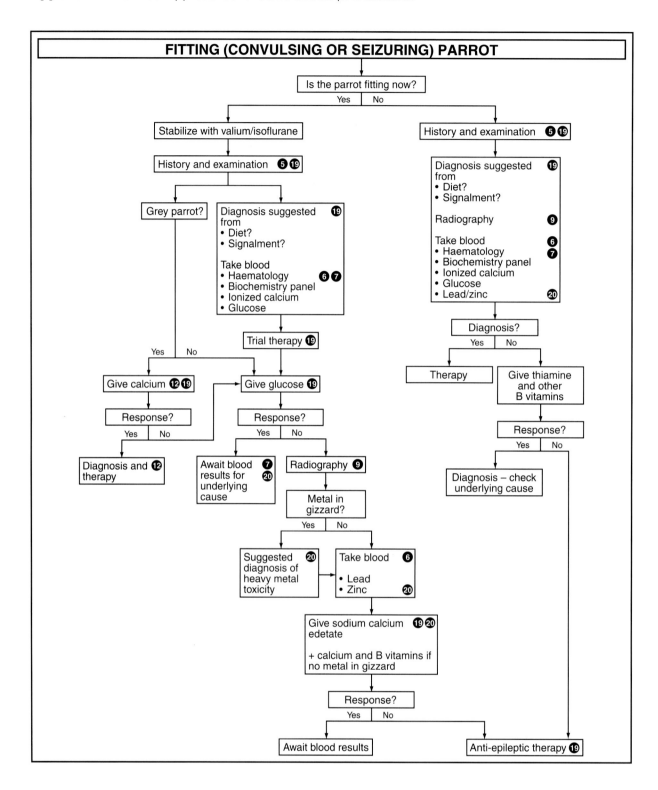

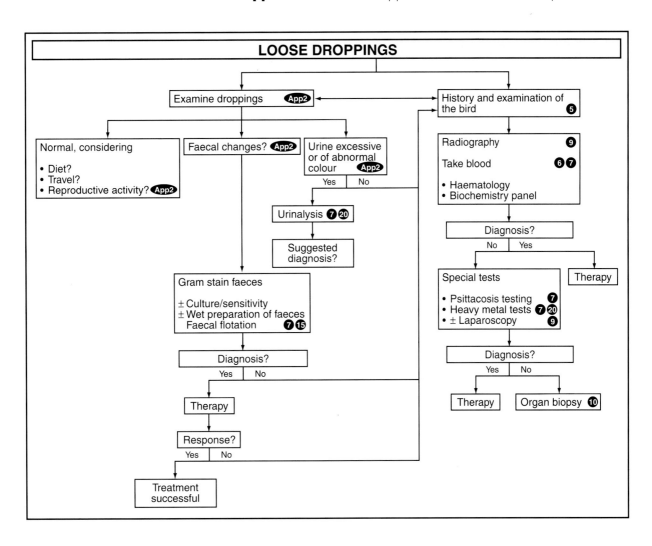

Appendix 2

The cage floor: in sickness and health

Nigel Harcourt-Brown

Introduction

In many cases where a parrot is thought to be unwell, examination of the floor of the cage is as useful as an examination of the parrot itself. Many birds have newspaper on the floor of their cages on to which droppings fall. Droppings are a mixture of excreted products that leave the body through the vent at the same time. In the majority of parrots the faeces are vermiform,

corresponding to the shape of the coprodeum (Chapter 2). Faecal size is also determined by the type and quantity of food the bird has eaten, as this affects the roughage and water content of the droppings. The urinary portion is formed from insoluble urates and whatever quantity of liquid urine has not been reabsorbed from the bowel. Birds may also vomit or regurgitate food or other crop contents and these can also be found in the cage, on perches or on the floor.

Droppings from healthy birds

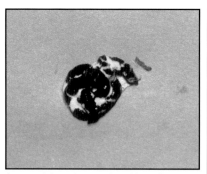

A normal dropping produced by a Pionus Parrot that had been fed on seed for the previous 5 days. This diet is low in fibre and is quite dry. Therefore the faecal component is small and vermiform. The urates are white. Any urine has been reabsorbed before the dropping is passed.

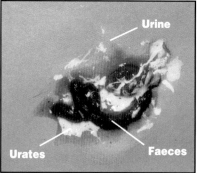

A normal dropping from the same Pionus parrot fed on a pulse based diet for 5 days. As this diet has more fibre and contains more water than seed, the faecal mass is larger and wetter; because of the increased water content there is urine as well as urates.

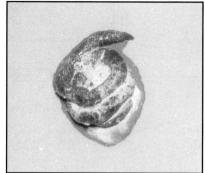

This parrot has been fed on a proprietary dry complete diet. Most complete diets are low in water and high in fibre. The faeces are brown (the colour of the diet) and voluminous. There is little urine and the urates are white.

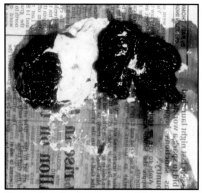

Single dropping from a normal Green-winged Macaw on a moist food diet.

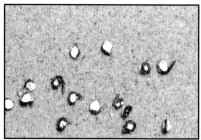

Normal small dry droppings, with comma-shaped faeces and urates and no urine, passed by a Budgerigar on a dry seed diet. Such droppings are typical of many small Australian parakeets, especially the xerophilic birds.

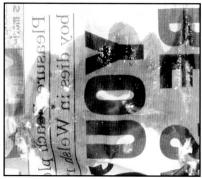

A single dropping from a normal lorikeet on a nectar diet. Note the abundant liquid urine, limited urates and small faecal moist mass.

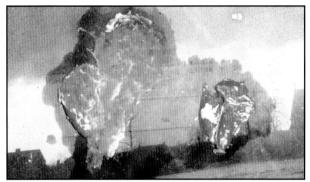

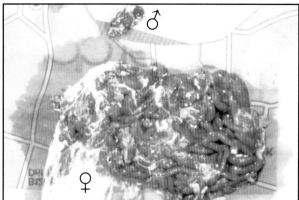

These two droppings are from the same healthy parrot. The dropping on the left was produced during transport to the surgery, whereas the dropping on the right was produced before the bird was moved. When birds are frightened they void the contents of the cloaca. Because the urine has not been in the intestine long enough to be reabsorbed (see Chapter 2) the faecal mass is very wet. This normal appearance could be confused with polyuria. The presence of normal droppings is a helpful guide.

Incubating parrots leave the nest box once or twice a day and void a voluminous dropping. The lower dropping was produced by a female Pionus Parrot incubating 5 eggs. A dropping from her mate is included for comparison. The birds were fed on a pulse based diet. A change in the size of droppings occurs in females a few days prior to laying the first egg.

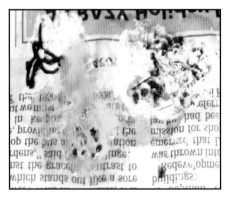

Many substances can influence the colour of the droppings of a normal bird. Foods such as elderberries or beetroot will lead to red or purple faeces but normal urine/urates. At other times the urine/urates can be discoloured either by abnormal levels of metabolites (see later) or by substances absorbed by the body. Occasionally dye from the newspaper can soak into a dropping.

This parrot had had a wound dressed with oil of proflavine and then bandaged. The yellow proflavine was absorbed and excreted in the urine; the faeces are still a normal colour. The two normal droppings were produced before treatment. This experience appeared to have no effect on the bird.

Droppings from ill birds

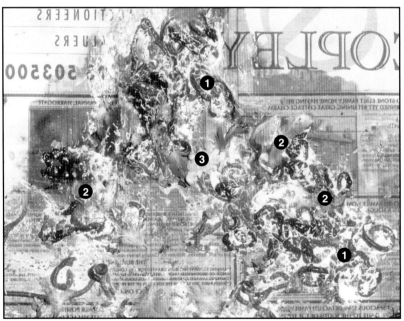

On many occasions the 'mess' beneath an ill bird is as useful as the clinical history. This bird appears to have been eating well (some normal droppings, ❶) but suddenly it has become ill. The bowel is inflamed and the faeces are watery, of low volume and contain mucus or protein (❷) — it has bowel disease. From the history and droppings this has happened over several days. The urates have continued to be white: there is no liver involvement so far. The bird has regurgitated its crop contents (❸), so it has eaten recently. The regurgitation was probably due to the illness but could also have been caused by motion sickness as the bird had recently been transported to the surgery. Smears from the normal faeces were stained and showed mainly Gram-positive cocci, but the diarrhoea showed mostly Gram-negative coccobaccili — *Escherichia coli* on culture. A wet preparation of the faeces and a McMaster slide technique failed to show any parasites. This parrot had a bacterial enteritis and responded to enrofloxacin.

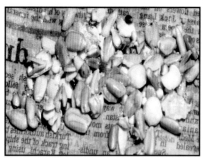

Many conditions cause birds to regurgitate their crop contents: proventricular dilatation disease; intestinal obstruction; motion sickness; irritant drugs administered orally or parenterally.

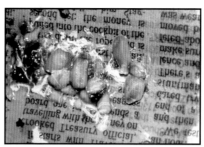

This cockatoo was losing weight and passing undigested seeds in its droppings. The seeds are bile-stained and surrounded by urates, proving their faecal origin. The cause was proventricular dilatation disease.

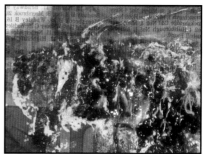

Diarrhoea, as seen here, is uncommon in parrots. The urates from this bird were normal but there was increased water. The faeces were not formed and were a variable brown/green colour.

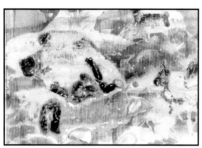

An unwell parrrot had small amounts of soft faeces that were formed normally but the urates were 'apple green' denoting a mild obstructive bacterial hepatitis.

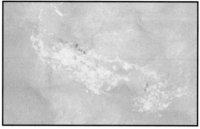

A very ill young Blue and Gold Macaw was producing polyuric droppings. The bird had no faeces, which means that it had not eaten for 24hrs+. The yellow/green urates are a sign of hepatitis; polyuria could be due to nephritis.

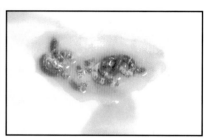

Acute *Chlamydophila* infection in an 8-week-old Amazon. Droppings like these are described as green diarrhoea – in reality the faeces are soft and pale but the urine and urates are heavily stained with biliverdin.

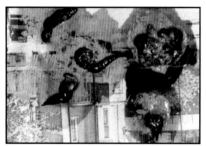

Droppings with bright green urates like this denote a serious hepatitis that is nearly always caused by *Chlamydophila* infection.

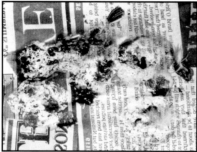

Drops of blood from cloacal papilloma. Urates and faeces are normal.

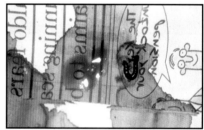

This parrot has passed a normal faecal mass with extra bile staining. The urine is full of haemoglobin but no erythrocytes. The bird was anaemic and its erythrocytes autoagglutinated.

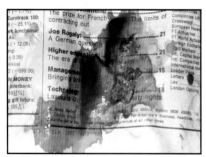

An Amazon passed deformed, enlarged faecal masses mixed with urates and surrounded by bloody fluid. The urodeum was filled by a soft cloacolith.

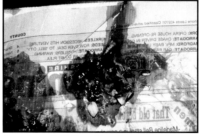

An extremely ill Grey Parrot was passing urates, faeces and blood. It then stopped passing faeces. Radiography showed intestinal gas. Surgery allowed the intussusception to be corrected.

Appendix 3

Formulary

This formulary is not intended to be a complete listing of drugs used in parrots; rather, it is a summary of drugs mentioned within this manual. More comprehensive drug listings are to be found in Marx and Roston (1996), Carpenter *et al.* (2001) and Bishop (2004). Generic names are generally used, as product formulations and trade names vary widely between countries.

Drugs	Dosages and routes	Notes
Antiviral agent		
Aciclovir	80 mg/kg orally, i.v., i.m. q8h 240 mg/kg in food in aviaries	For Pacheco's disease
Antibacterial agents		
Amoxicillin	150–175 mg/kg orally q12h 150 mg/kg i.m. q24h	Use long-acting preparations for injection
Amoxicillin/clavulanate	125 mg/kg orally q12h 125 mg/kg i.m. q24h	
Chlortetracycline	2500–5000 mg/kg in feed for 45 days	One of the statutory recommended therapies for psittacosis in Germany
Clindamycin	25 mg/kg orally q8h 50 mg/kg orally q12h 100 mg/kg orally q24h	
Doxycycline	15–50 mg/kg orally q24h 1000 mg/kg in dehulled seed or soft food Vibravenos: 75–100 mg/kg q7d	Ornicure (Genitrix): In the UK this is the only licensed product for psittacosis in cage birds. Licensed dose rate = 25 mg/kg orally q24h for 45 days. This may be given in water, in feed or directly by mouth. In-water is NOT recommended, as water intake of parrots may be unreliable. Genitrix produces a useful booklet describing therapeutics of Ornicure Vibravenos (Pfizer): This is recommended for psittacosis in larger parrots. Macaws may be more sensitive to side effects than other psittacids. Side-effects include vomiting/regurgitation. Injection may cause significant irritant reactions. If large injection volume required, divide dose between several sites. If given s.c. skin slough may result. In Germany Vibravenos is one of the statutory therapies recommended for psittacosis, when it should be given at 75 mg/kg i.m. q5d X6, then q4d X3. Many texts suggest 75–100 mg/kg q7d X6 is sufficient to achieve clearance of *Chlamydophila psittaci* from the body, although this is not totally reliable. In the UK Vibravenos is only available on a **Special Treatment Authorisation** from the Veterinary Medicines Directorate
Enrofloxacin	10–15 mg/kg orally, i.m. q12h 100–200 mg/l in drinking water Psittacosis: many texts recommend 15 mg/kg i.m. or orally q12h for 45 days Psittacosis in Germany: 10 mg/kg i.m. q24h for 21 days; in food at 1000 mg/kg corn (or nectar food for lories/lorikeets); sole diet for 21 days or at 500 ppm in drinking water for 21 days for Budgerigars	Preparations licensed for use in birds in the UK: licensed dose rate = 10 mg/kg q12h orally or i.m. (many authors recommend higher) Injection may cause irritant reactions, so advised to switch from systemic to oral as soon as possible. **Injectable preparations >2.5% concentration should NOT be used** Enrofloxacin may cause vomition Enrofloxacin is one of the statutory treatments for psittacosis is Germany

Drugs	Dosages and routes	Notes
Antibacterial agents (continued)		
Marbofloxacin	10 mg/kg orally, i.m. q24h	
Neomycin	80–100 mg/l q24h in drinking water	
Oxytetracycline	50 mg/kg i.m. q24h	Use long-acting preparation. Some preparations may cause irritant reactions
Polymyxin B	10–15 mg/kg i.m. q24h 50,000 IU/l in drinking water	Not absorbed from the gut
Trimethoprim/ Sulphonamide	8 mg/kg i.m. q12h 20–100 mg/kg orally q8h–q12h	If regurgitation occurs, reduce dose
Antifungal agents		
Amphotericin B	1.5 mg/kg i.v. q8h for 3 days 1 mg/kg intratracheally q8h–q12h Megabacteriosis: 100–300 mg/kg orally q12h–q24h	Nephrotoxic (unless oral). **Use with care.** Concurrent fluid therapy advised Useful adjunctive therapy to azoles in aspergillosis. Not absorbed from gut; therefore oral route not used for systemic infections
Clotrimazole	10 mg/kg applied directly via endoscope to fungal lesions in the air sacs; 10 mg/ml as nasal flush (volume of flush 20 ml/kg)	Dilute with propylene glycol to 2.5 mg/ml before application. Dose may be repeated if required, but take care not to overdose. **May be toxic, especially to Grey Parrots**
Fluconazole	5 mg/kg orally q24h	May be hepatotoxic. May cause vomition
Itraconazole	5–10 mg/kg orally q12h	Less hepatotoxic than ketoconazole, though many **Grey Parrots have an idiosyncratic reaction that may prove lethal.** Some will tolerate the lower dose
Ketoconazole	30 mg/kg orally q12h	May be hepatotoxic. May cause vomition
Nystatin	300,000 IU/kg orally q12h	NOT absorbed from the gut
Terbinafine	15 mg/kg orally q12h	Less toxic to Grey Parrots than itraconazole. May have faster onset of action than azoles
Antiparasitic agents		
Carnidazole	30–50 mg/kg orally, repeat after 14 days	For trichomoniasis
Chloroquine	25 mg/kg orally at 0 h, then 15 mg/kg orally at 12, 24 and 48 h	For *Plasmodium* infections
Fenbendazole	GI nematodes: 20–100 mg/kg orally once (may repeat after 14 days) Giardiasis: 50 mg/kg orally q24h for 3 days	
Fipronil	Apply spray to cotton wool and dab behind head, under wings and at base of tail	Ectoparasites. **Do not soak bird – may cause hypothermia.** Spot-on preparations not recommended
Ivermectin	200 µg/kg s.c., orally q2–4wk	In the UK a 0.1% form is available as a spot-on for smaller birds: place a drop on bare skin at back of head. Some practitioners have used a drop of undiluted cattle injectable product in the same way with no apparent side-effects. Active against mites, especially *Cnemidocoptes*, and gut nematodes. **Take care not to overdose birds when injecting;** oral or cutaneous routes may be safer
Levamisole	GI nematodes: 20 mg/kg orally once Capillariasis: 40 mg/kg orally once	May cause vomition
Metronidazole	30 mg/kg orally q12h	Active against *Giardia*
Permethrin/ Pyriproxyfen spray	Apply to environment	For tick or *Dermanyssus* control
Praziquantel	10 mg/kg i.m., orally, repeat after 10 days	For trematode and cestode infections
Pyrantel	7 mg/kg orally, repeat after 14 days	For GI nematodes

Drugs	Dosages and routes	Notes
Antiparasitic agents (continued)		
Pyrimethamine	0.5 mg/kg orally q12h for 14 days	For *Leucocytozoon* infections
Toltrazuril	7 mg/kg orally q24h for 3 days	For coccidiosis
Analgesics/Anti-inflammatories		
Acetylsalicylic acid	5 mg/kg orally q8h 325 mg/250 ml in drinking water	
Butorphanol	1 mg/kg i.m. once 0.02–0.04 mg/kg i.v. once	
Carprofen	5 mg/kg i.m., orally q24h	
Celecoxib	1–10 mg/kg orally q12h or q24h	Used in proventricular dilatation disease
Dexamethasone	Anti-inflammatory: 1 mg/kg i.m. once Shock: 2–4 mg/kg i.v. once	Especially useful for tick reactions; use short-acting preparations (e.g. Dexadreson, Intervet)
Flunixin meglumine	1 mg/kg i.m. q24h	**Take care with peri-anaesthetic use**
Glucocorticoids		**All glucocorticoids should be used with great care in birds as they may cause immunosuppression, hepatopathy and a diabetes mellitus-like syndrome. Topical agents should be totally avoided as these have been associated with the most side-effects**
Ibuprofen	5–10 mg/kg orally q8h–q12h	
Ketoprofen	2 mg/kg i.m., s.c. q8h–q24h	
Lidocaine	MAXIMUM 1–4 mg/kg as local nerve block	Must not contain epinephrine. Dilute at least 1:10 with saline
Meloxicam	200 µg/kg i.m. once 200 µg/kg orally q24h	Oral dose roughly equivalent to 1 drop daily of 1.5 mg/ml suspension for a Grey Parrot. Various authors describe the safe long-term use of this drug
Phenylbutazone	3.5–7 mg/kg orally q8h	
Piroxicam	0.5 mg/kg orally q12h	
Prednisolone	1 mg/kg orally q12h	For pruritus. **Reduce to minimum effective dose as quickly as possible. ESSENTIAL to rule out underlying infectious disease (e.g. aspergillosis, psittacosis) BEFORE use. Must be sure bird is pruritic and all other therapies have failed before using this drug**
Psychotropic drugs/Sedatives		
Atropine	Supraventricular tachycardia: 0.01–0.02 mg/kg i.v. once Premedicant: 0.02–0.08 mg/kg i.m. once	Causes mucous secretions to become thicker, therefore increasing the chances of endotracheal tube blockage
Clomipramine	0.5–1 mg/kg orally q6–8h	Antihistamine antipruritic as well as psychoactive effects
Diazepam	Convulsions/ seizures: 0.1–1.0 mg/kg i.v., i.m. once Premedicant: 0.2–0.5 mg/kg i.m.; 0.05–0.15 mg/kg i.v. Anxiolytic: 0.5 mg/kg orally q8h–q12h once	
Diphenhydramine	2–4 mg/kg orally q12h	Antihistamine antipruritic and sedative
Doxepin	0.5–1 mg/kg orally q12h Organophosphate toxicity: 0.2 mg/kg i.m. q4h	May cause arrhythmias
Fluoxetine	1 mg/kg orally q24h	
Glycopyrrolate	0.01 mg/kg i.m., i.v.	Premedicant. See Atropine
Haloperidol	0.15–0.2 mg/kg orally q12h; 1–2 mg/kg i.m. q21 days	May cause drowsiness, especially injectable form. Most useful in self–mutilation syndromes
Midazolam	0.1–0.5 mg/kg i.m. 0.05–0.15 mg/kg i.v.	Premedicant

Drugs	Dosages and routes	Notes
Psychotropic drugs/Sedatives (continued)		
Naltrexone	1.5 mg/kg orally q12h	
Phenobarbital	3.5–7 mg/kg orally q12h	Anticonvulsant. Used in epilepsy or where feather plucking associated with seizures
Miscellaneous		
Acetic acid	5 ml/600 ml in drinking water	Organic cider apple vinegar. Gut acidifier, especially for megabacteriosis
Allopurinol	10 mg/30 ml q24h in drinking water	For gout
Ascorbic acid	20–40 mg/kg i.m. q24h	
Calcium gluconate	50–100 mg/kg slow i.v. injection prn	For hypocalcaemia
Cisapride	0.5–1.5 mg/kg orally q8h	Prokinetic
Colchicine	0.04 mg/kg orally q12h	For gout, hepatic cirrhosis/fibrosis
Deferoxamine	20 mg/kg orally q4h	Toxin chelating agent
Dextrose	500 mg/kg slow i.v. injection prn	Hypoglycaemia
Digoxin	0.02 mg/kg q24h	For cardiovascular disease where a positive inotrope is required
Doxapram	5–10 mg/kg i.v., i.m. once	For respiratory arrest. **Oral drops do not appear to be as effective in birds as they are in mammals**
Edetate calcium disodium	35 mg/kg i.m. q12h	For heavy metal toxicosis. In chronic zinc toxicosis 100 mg/kg i.m. weekly has been described as effective
Enalapril	0.5 mg/kg q24h	ACE-inhibitor for use in cardiovascular disease
Epinephrine	0.1 mg/kg i.v., intra-osseous, intracardiac or intratracheal once	For cardiac arrest
F10	Nasal flush: dilute 1:250 and use at 20 ml/kg prn For skin infections: dilute 1:250, spray or bathe	Disinfectant. Contents: 0–<10% quaternary ammonium compounds, 0–<10% poly (hexamethylene biguanide) HCl, 10–<30% nonylphenol ethylene oxide condensate, 10–<30% tetrasodium EDTA
Heparin	300 IU/kg i.v. once	For PTFE toxicosis
Insulin	0.002–1.4 IU/kg i.m.	Repeat as required in 'true' diabetes mellitus
Interferon	1,000,000 IU q24h i.m. for 90 days	For acute circovirus infection. Use avian interferon; feline interferon unsuccessful at this dose though may be successful at higher dosage
Iohexol	1 ml of 300 mg iodine/ml i.v. for a 500 g parrot	For intravenous positive contrast imaging
Kaolin	2 ml/kg orally q8h	Gut protectant
Lactulose	0.3 ml/kg orally q8h	For hepatic encephalopathy
Leuprolide acetate	250–750 µg/kg i.m. q2–6wk	Use the 30-day depot product in cases of chronic egg laying. Expensive, but once reconstituted, aliquots may be frozen and remain active for up to 6 months
Lugol's iodine	Prepare 1 ml iodine: 15 ml water stock solution. Dose at 1 drop per 250 ml drinking water daily	For iodine deficiency goitres
Medroxyprogesterone acetate	5–25 mg/kg i.m. q4–6wk	Suppresses sexual activity. Side-effects include liver damage, obesity and diabetes mellitus
Metoclopramide	0.5 mg/kg i.m. q8h	Prokinetic drug
Milk thistle extract	5 mg/kg orally q8h	For liver disease. Active constituent silymarin
Penicillamine	55 mg/kg orally q12h	Chelating agent for use in heavy metal toxicosis. Low therapeutic index. Overdosage may result in vomition, hypoglycaemia and death. The dose should, therefore, be accurately titrated and the bird monitored for side-effects.
Pralidoxime	10–100 mg/kg i.v. q24h	For organophosphate or carbamate toxicity
Prostaglandin E2 gel	0.1 ml/100 g applied directly to oviduct sphincter	To relax sphincter and increase uterine tone in egg retention
Sucralfate	25 mg/kg orally q8h	Coating agent for GI ulcers

Drugs	Dosages and routes	Notes
Miscellaneous (continued)		
L-Thyroxine	0.02 mg/kg q24h or q12h	For hypothyroidism
D-Tubocurarine	0.01–0.03 ml of 3% sterile solution injected into anterior chamber of eye using 27–30 G needle	Use as mydriatic (for ocular examination) and for treatment of uveitis **Very dangerous compound; supplied as dry powder. Reconstitute in a fume cabinet and DO NOT inhale**
Vitamin A	2000 IU/kg orally or i.m.	For hypovitaminosis A and as adjunctive therapy in poxvirus infections. Systemic dosing associated with toxicity, so best given q12h. Where the injectable route is employed, the dose should not be repeated
Vitamin B1	3 mg/kg i.m. q7d	For thiamine deficiency
Vitamin B Complex	1–3 mg/kg i.m. once	For multi-vitamin B deficiencies
Vitamin D3	6600 IU/kg i.m. once	For hypocalcaemia
Vitamin K1	2.5 mg/kg i.m. q24h	For coumarol anticoagulant toxicity
Topical preparations		
Aloe vera	Apply q24h to skin lesions	For skin infections and polyfolliculosis. May add heparin at 1000 IU heparin/150 mg aloe vera
Chlorhexidine	1:50 dilution used as spray for skin infections q24h	
Echinacea cream	Apply q24h to chronic infections	Immunomodulator? Use herbal form
F10 ointment	Apply q24h to infected areas	Barrier cream *(see F10 re ingredients)*
Flurbiprofen	1 drop q12h	NSAID. Excellent for uveitis or ocular pain, especially in corneal damage
Fusidic acid	Skin: apply q24h Ophthalmic preparations: apply q12–24h	Various formulations exist; **avoid those containing corticosteroids**
Ofloxacin	1 drop q12h	Fluoroquinolone antibiotic
Silver sulfadiazine cream	Apply to infected areas q24h	Barrier cream
Vecuronium	1 drop of 0.8 mg/ml solution in 0.9% saline. Repeat after 2 min	Mydriatic: enables examination of posterior segment of the eye **Ensure solution does NOT contain surface-acting penetrating agent**

Appendix 4

List of bird names

Latin names are the zoologist's standard and there is usually only one Latin name for a species. Common names vary with the language of the country and then, often, within the language. There have been many attempts to produce 'standard' lists of common names in English, in both the UK and USA. *The Handbook of Birds of the World* (Del Hoyo *et al.*, 1997) has an excellent set of names in English, Spanish, German and French; these names are given for every species of psittacid (as well as other birds).

- The English names used in this Manual are those used most commonly by bird keepers and breeders.
- The Latin names and taxonomy used in this Manual are taken from *The Howard and Moore Complete Checklist of Birds of the World* (Dickinson, 2003).

English name	Latin name	English name	Latin name
Blue-crowned Hanging Parrot	*Loriculus galgulus*	***Lovebirds***	*Agapornis* spp.
		Madagascar Lovebird	*Agapornis cana*
Pygmy parrots	*Micropsitta* spp.	Abyssinian Lovebird	*Agapornis taranta*
		Fischer's Lovebird	*Agapornis fischeri*
Cockatoos		Peach-faced Lovebird	*Agapornis roseicollis*
Palm Cockatoo	*Probosciger aterrimus*		
Galah	*Elophus roseicapilla*	Vasa Parrot (Greater)	*Coracopsis vasa*
Slender-billed Cockatoo	*Cacatua tenuirostris*	Vasa Parrot (Lesser)	*Coracopsis nigra*
Greater Sulphur-crested Cockatoo	*Cacatua galerita*		
Triton Cockatoo	*Cactua galerita triton*	Grey Parrot	*Psittacus erithacus*
Lesser Sulphur-crested Cockatoo	*Cacatua sulphurea*	Timneh Parrot	*Psittacus erithacus timneh*
Citron-crested Cockatoo	*Cacatua sulphurea citronocristata*		
Umbrella Cockatoo	*Cacatua alba*	Cape Parrot	*Poicephalus robustus*
Moluccan or Salmon-crested Cockatoo	*Cacatua moluccensis*	Myer's Parrot	*Poicephalus myeri*
		Senegal Parrot	*Poicephalus senegalus*
Cockatiel	*Nymphicus hollandicus*	***Macaws***	
		Hyacinth Macaw	*Anodorhynchus hyacinthus*
Lories and lorikeets		Blue and Gold Macaw	*Ara ararauna*
Red Lory	*Eos rubra*	Scarlet Macaw	*Ara macao*
Rainbow Lorikeet	*Trichoglossus haematodus*	Green-winged Macaw	*Ara chloropterus*
		Severe Macaw	*Ara severa*
Parakeets		Red-bellied Macaw	*Orthopsittaca manilata*
Red-fronted Kakariki	*Cyanoramphus novaezelandiae*	Yellow-collared Macaw	*Propyrrhura auricollis*
Yellow-fronted Kakariki	*Cyanoramphus auriceps*	Noble (Red-shouldered) Macaw	*Diopsittaca nobilis*
		Hahn's Macaw	*Diopsittaca nobilis cumanensis*
Rosella	*Platycercus* spp.		
		Sun Conure	*Aratinga solstitialis*
Grass parakeets		Jenday (or Janday) Conure	*Aratinga jendaya*
Bourke's Parakeet	*Neosephotus bourkii*	Brown-throated Conure	*Aratinga pertinax*
Turquoisine Parakeet	*Neophema pulchella*	Patagonian Conure	*Cyanoliseus patagonus*
Splendid Parakeet	*Neophema splendida*	Blue-throated Conure	*Pyrrhura cruentata*
Budgerigar	*Melopsittacus undulatus*	Quaker (Monk) Parakeet	*Myiopsitta monachus*
Eclectus Parrot	*Eclectus roratus*	Black-headed Caique	*Pionites melanocephalus*
		White-bellied Caique	*Pionites leucogaster*
Alexandrine Parakeet	*Psittacula eupatria*		
Ringneck Parakeet	*Psittacula krameri*	Yellow-faced Parrotlet	*Forpus xanthops*
Blossom-headed Parakeet	*Psittacula roseata*	Blue-winged Parrotlet	*Forpus xanthopterigius*
		Celestial Parrotlet	*Forpus coelestis*
		Grey-cheeked parakeet	*Brotgeris pyrrhoptera*

English name	Latin name	English name	Latin name
Pionus parrots		Red-lored Amazon	*Amazona autumnalis*
Blue-headed Pionus Parrot	*Pionus menstruus*	Blue-fronted Amazon	*Amazona aestiva*
Coral-billed Pionus Parrot	*Pionus sordidus*	Yellow-headed Amazon	*Amazona oratrix*
Maximilian's Pionus Parrot	*Pionus maximilani*	Yellow-crowned (or Yellow-fronted) Amazon	*Amazona ochrocephala*
White-capped Pionus Parrot	*Pionus senilis*		
Bronze-winged Pionus Parrot	*Pionus chalcopterus*	Orange-winged Amazon	*Amazona amazonica*
Dusky Pionus Parrot	*Pionus fuscus*	Mealy Amazon	*Amazona farinosa*
		Festive Amazon	*Amazon festiva*
Amazons		Hawk-headed Parrot	*Deroptyus accipitrinus*
Hispaniolan Amazon	*Amazona ventralis*		
White-fronted Amazon	*Amazona albifrons*	Fig parrots	*Cyclopsitta* spp.

CITES Listed birds: common names

The names below do not conform entirely with those common names used by DEFRA; to be safe the Latin should be used

English name	Latin name	English name	Latin name
Appendix I		Illiger's Macaw	*Propyrrhura maracana*
Goffin's Cockatoo	*Cacatua goffini*	Thick-billed Parrot	*Rhynchpsitta pachyryncha*
Red-vented Cockatoo	*Cacatua haematuropygia*	Maroon-fronted Parrot	*Rhynchpsitta terrisi*
Moluccan Cockatoo	*Cacatua mouluccensis*	Yellow-eared Conure	*Ognorhynchus icterotis*
Palm Cockatoo	*Probsciger aterrimus*	Queen of Bavaria's Conure	*Guarouba guarouba*
Red and Blue Lory	*Eos histrio*	Blue-throated Conure	*Pyrrhura cruentata*
Ultramarine Lorikeet	*Vini ultramarina*	Pileated Parrot	*Pionpsitta pileata*
Kakapo	*Strigops habroptilus*	There is also a Pileated Parakeet (*Purpureicephalus spurius*), which is very different but is often confusingly called a Pileated Parrot as well	
Southern or Blue-browed Fig-parrot	*Cyclopsitta diopthalmia coxeni*		
Horned Parakeet	*Eunymphicus coornutus*		
Red-fronted Kakariki (or Parakeet)	*Cyanorhamphus novaezelandiae*	Red-necked Amazon	*Amazona arausiaca*
Chatam Kakariki (or Parakeet)	*Cyanorhamphus forbesi*	Yellow-shouldered Amazon	*Amazona barbadensis*
Hooded Parakeet	*Psephotus dissimilis*	Red-tailed Amazon	*Amazona brasiliensis*
Golden-shouldered Parakeet	*Psephotus chrysopterygius*	St Vincent Amazon	*Amazona guildingii*
Paradise Parakeet (? extinct)	*Psephotus pulcherrimus*	Imperial Amazon	*Amazona imperialis*
Orange-bellied Grass-parakeet	*Neophema chrysogaster*	Cuban Amazon	*Amazona leucocephala*
Ground Parrot	*Pezoprus wallicus*	Yellow-naped Amazon	*Amazona ochrocephala auropalliata*
Night Parrot	*Geopsittacus occidentalis*	Belize Yellow-crowned Amazon	*Amazona o. belizensis*
Mauritius Parakeet	*Psittacula echo*	No common name	*Amazona o. caribaea*
Spix's Macaw	*Cyanopsitta spixii*	Parvipes Amazon	*Amazona o. parvipes*
Blue macaws:	*Anodorhynchus* spp.	Tresmarias' Amazon	*Amazona o. tresmariae*
Hyacinth Macaw	*Anodorhynchus hyacinthus*	Pretre's or Red-spectacled Amazon	*Amazona pretrei*
Lears Macaw	*Anodorhynchus leari*	Red-topped Amazon	*Amazona rhodocorytha*
Glaucous Macaw	*Anodorhynchus glaucus*	Tucuman Amazon	*Amazona tucumana*
Buffon's Macaw	*Ara ambigua*	St Lucia Amazon	*Amazona versicolor*
Military Macaw	*Ara militaris*	Vinaceous Amazon	*Amazona vinacea*
Caninde Macaw (Blue-throated Macaw)	*Ara glaucogularis*	Green-cheeked Amazon	*Amazona viridigenalis*
		Puerto Rican Amazon	*Amazona vittata*
Red-fronted Macaw	*Ara rubrogenys*		
Scarlet Macaw	*Ara macao*	***Appendix III***	
Blue-headed Macaw	*Propyrrhura couloni*	Ringneck Parakeet	*Psittacula krameri*

309

Appendix 5

Conversion tables

Biochemistry

	SI unit	Conversion	Conventional unit
Alanine transferase	IU / l	x 1	IU / l
Albumin	g / l	x 0.1	g / dl
Alkaline phosphatase	IU / l	x 1	IU / l
Aspartate transaminase	IU / l	x 1	IU / l
Bilirubin	µmol / l	x 0.0584	mg / dl
BUN	mmol / l	x 2.8	mg / dl
Calcium	mmol / l	x 4	mg / dl
Carbon dioxide (total)	mmol / l	x 1	mEq / l
Cholesterol	mmol / l	x 38.61	mg / dl
Chloride	mmol / l	x 1	mEq / l
Cortisol	nmol / l	x 0.362	ng / ml
Creatine kinase	IU / l	x 1	IU / l
Creatinine	µmol / l	x 0.0113	mg / dl
Glucose	mmol / l	x 18.02	mg / dl
Insulin	pmol / l	x 0.1394	µIU / ml
Iron	µmol / l	x 5.587	µg / dl
Magnesium	mmol / l	x 2	mEq / l
Phosphate	mmol / l	x 3.1	mg / dl
Potassium	mmol / l	x 1	mEq / l
Sodium	mmol / l	x 1	mEq / l
Total protein	g / l	x 0.1	g / dl
Thyroxine (T4) (free)	pmol / l	x 0.0775	ng / dl
Thyroxine (T4) (total)	nmol / l	x 0.0775	µg / dl
Tri-iodothyronine (T3)	nmol / l	x 65.1	ng / dl
Triglycerides	mmol / l	x 88.5	mg / dl

Temperature

	Celsius	Conversion	Fahrenheit
	°C	(x 9/5) + 32	°F

Haematology

	SI unit	Conversion	Conventional unit
Red blood cell count	10^{12} / l	x 1	10^6 / µl
Haemoglobin	g / l	x 0.1	g / dl
MCH	pg / cell	x 1	pg / cell
MCHC	g / l	x 0.1	g / dl
MCV	fl	x 1	$µm^3$
Platelet count	10^9 / l	x 1	10^3 / µl
White blood cell count	10^9 / l	x 1	10^3 / µl

Hypodermic needles

	Metric	Non-metric
External diameter	0.8 mm	21 G
	0.6 mm	23 G
	0.5 mm	25 G
	0.4 mm	27 G
Needle length	12 mm	$^1/_2$ inch
	16 mm	$^5/_8$ inch
	25 mm	1 inch
	30 mm	$1^1/_4$ inch
	40 mm	$1^1/_2$ inch

Suture material sizes

Metric	USP
0.1	11/0
0.2	10/0
0.3	9/0
0.4	8/0
0.5	7/0
0.7	6/0
1	5/0
1.5	4/0
2	3/0
3	2/0
3.5	0
4	1
5	2
6	3

Index

Page numbers in **bold** indicate main sections; page numbers in *italics* indicate illustrations.

Index

Index

Index

Index

Index

Index

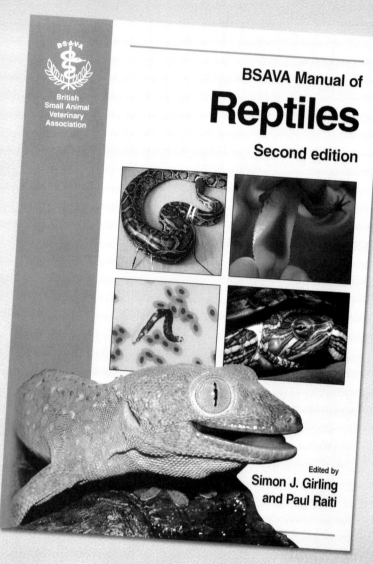
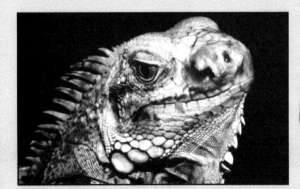
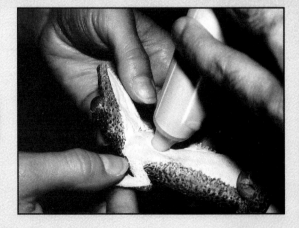

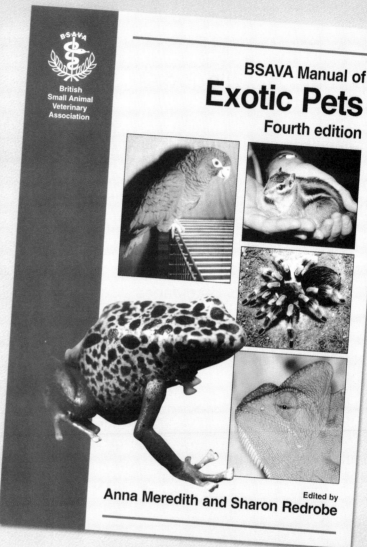
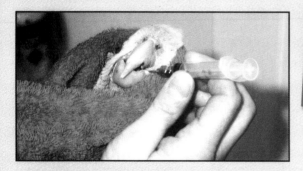
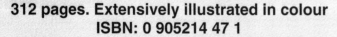
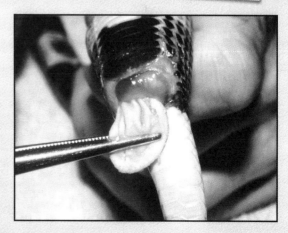

BSAVA Manual of
Ornamental Fish
Second Edition

Edited by
William H. Wildgoose
BVMS CertFHP MRCVS

Completely revised and expanded NEW edition

29 international contributors

Detailed overview of husbandry and filter systems

Aquatic trade, farming, hobby and public aquaria

Diseases by system and cause

Practical approach to diagnosis and treatment

Details of anaesthetic systems and surgery

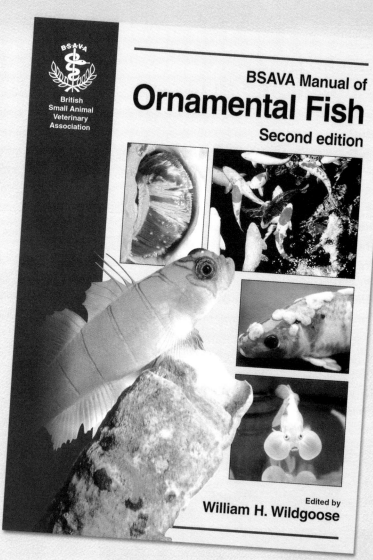

BSAVA Manual of
Ornamental Fish
Second edition

Edited by
William H. Wildgoose

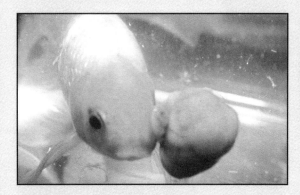

312 pages. Extensively illustrated in colour
ISBN: 0 905214 57 9

Price to members of BSAVA, BVNA and FECAVA £52.00
Price to non-members £80.00
BSAVA reserves the right to alter prices at any time.
Prices include postage & packaging charges on orders for UK and EIRE

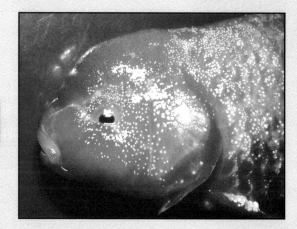

For information and to order please contact us at:
British Small Animal Veterinary Association • Woodrow House
1 Telford Way • Waterwells Business Park • Quedgeley • Gloucester • GL2 2AB
Tel: 01452 726709 • e-mail: publications@bsava.com • www.bsava.com